Fast Food Chains & Restaurants

The Ultimate
Calorie Counter
&
DIET JOURNAL

Lose weight by knowing and recording how many CALORIES, FATS & CARBS you eat from AMERICA'S MOST POPULAR RESTAURANTS

BY ALEX A. LLUCH
HEALTH & FITNESS EXPERT AND
AUTHOR OF OVER 3 MILLION BOOKS SOLD

WS Publishing Group
San Diego, California 92119

THE ULTIMATE CALORIE COUNTER & DIET JOURNAL

BY ALEX A. LLUCH

Published by WS Publishing Group
San Diego, California 92119
Copyright © 2009 by WS Publishing Group

Nutritional and fitness guidelines based on information provided by the United States Food and Drug Administration, Food and Nutrition Information Center, National Agricultural Library, Agricultural Research Service, and the U.S. Department of Agriculture.

Designed by: David Defenbaugh, WS Publishing Group

Photo credits:
Front cover image: © iStockphoto/NiDerLander
Food llustration, pg.153 : © iStockphoto/Viviyan

For inquiries:
Log on to www.WSPublishingGroup.com
E-mail info@WSPublishingGroup.com

ISBN-13: 978-1-934386-53-8

Printed in China

CONTENTS

CONTENTS

RESTAURANTS & FAST-FOOD CHAINS (CONT.)

INTRODUCTION

By purchasing this book, you have taken the first and most important step to lose weight, stay in shape, feel better, and have more energy than you ever thought possible. Research has shown, again and again, that the best way to accomplish your health and weight-loss goals is to track the calories, fat, and carbs in the foods you eat on a daily basis.

THE BENEFITS OF LOSING WEIGHT

Losing weight has major benefits that can improve your way of life. Weight loss can lower the risk of numerous diseases, including heart disease, stroke, cancer, and diabetes.

However, it is difficult in today's society to make the right choices regarding your health and diet. Our jobs promote sedentary lifestyles, our days are busier than ever, and fast-food, while usually unhealthy, is convenient and inexpensive. Many food companies use larger portions as a selling point, making the claim that bigger is better. It then becomes the consumer's responsibility to monitor what and how much he or she eats.

We know how difficult it can be to choose wisely when you are eating out, dining with friends, and planning meals. It is extremely hard to locate a healthy option on many restaurant menus. Additionally, it has been scientifically proven that most people will consume hundreds of extra calories when dining in a group or social setting.

Think back to the last dinner you attended with a group of friends: Did you order an extra cocktail, partake in a fatty appetizer, or share a large dessert? The answer is probably yes. But have you ever thought about how many extra calories you are consuming during these get-togethers?

The wonderful thing about *The Ultimate Calorie Counter & Diet Journal* is that it takes the guesswork out of ordering a healthy meal when you dine out. The book's portable size makes it easy to put in your purse or car so you can quickly and conveniently look up the nutritional values for any menu item.

INTRODUCTION

The Ultimate Calorie Counter & Diet Journal is the most comprehensive book on the market, providing nutritional information and serving sizes for over 200 restaurants and fast-food chains. Better still, this book highlights the most healthy and least healthy food choices in every category.

USING THIS BOOK WHEN DINING OUT OR PLANNING MEALS AT HOME

Refer to this book when planning to eat out, and you will be able to determine the restaurant that best suits your needs. For instance, if you are in the mood for a hamburger, you can browse this book and choose a restaurant that has the healthiest burger choices.

If you have decided where to go, you can use the information provided in this book to choose the best options from the restaurant's menu. For example, you may find that the steak and potato entrée has fewer calories than a chicken salad made with high-fat mayonnaise-based dressing. Wouldn't it be nice to enjoy the steak dish you crave, knowing that you're making the healthy choice?

You should also use this book when planning to cook meals at home. You will be able to plan healthy, hearty meals and buy only items that contribute to eating smart, losing weight, and feeling better.

By using The Ultimate Calorie Counter & Diet Journal you can stop relying on fad diets or depriving yourself of the things you love to eat. With this handy book, you can easily compare and contrast foods to make the best selections, even while dining out or on-the-go.

You will find that by monitoring what you eat on a daily basis, you will lose weight and feel great, almost effortlessly. When you write down everything you eat, you hold yourself accountable for your food consumption, so not even the tiniest bite of a cookie should slip by!

INTRODUCTION

FILLING OUT THE DIET JOURNAL PAGES

With this nutritional information and diet journal as your companion, you can make better, more informed choices that will help you lose weight, look better, and improve your health. Here is how to use the journal pages to record what you eat and drink every day.

Weight: Document your daily weight on each journal page. Invest in a scale so you can accurately measure your progress. Weigh yourself unclothed when you wake up in the morning, before breakfast, so you can get a fresh reading for the day. Write this number in the space provided. Gradually, as you make your progress, you will see this number move closer to your goal.

Daily Nutritional Intake: Write down all the foods you eat on a daily basis, including all meals, snacks, sauces, dressings, condiments, and beverages. This book provides the values for more than 200 restaurants and fast-food chains. Look up each item you eat and drink, and record the total amount of calories, fat, and carbs in the diet journal pages. Once you have made all of your documentation for the day, use the Daily Totals section to calculate the total number of calories, fat, and carbs you have consumed.

Water Intake: Strive for a total of eight 8-ounce glasses of water per day. Check off a box for each 8-ounce glass you drink each day. Many times, people believe that they are hungry when they are actually thirsty!

Vitamins & Supplements: If you choose to incorporate vitamins and supplements into your diet program, be sure to keep track on a daily basis. You can assess the effectiveness of your supplements over time by comparing your energy levels to the vitamins that you have taken. When in doubt about specific vitamin recommendations, consult with a health care professional.

Energy Level: Determine the relationship that your body has with food. Document your daily overall energy by checking one of the three boxes in this section. See how your energy correlates to the types of foods you have eaten that day. As you discover these relationships, make adjustments as needed to help you feel your best.

INTRODUCTION

Calories Burned: This section will encourage you to participate in physical activities on a daily basis. All physical activity burns calories, so be sure to write down the approximate number of calories utilized by your body. This information can help you recognize behaviors or habits that may lead to a successful weight-loss journey.

Weight loss is determined by the amount of calories consumed versus the amount burned. If you happen to have a "bad eating" day, you can try to make up for the excess calories by adding an additional exercise routine the following day. Since you will be recording this number on a daily basis, motivate yourself by incorporating the activities that you enjoy the most.

Notes/Reminders: This section will help you observe obstacles and solutions throughout your diet journey. Record your thoughts and feelings as you gradually achieve your weight-loss goals. Stay motivated by recording positive results and reflecting on your progress. If for any reason you did not meet your daily goal, reflect on the factors that kept you from your goal and write them down in this section. You can then decide on any changes to your diet plan that will help you stay on track. Incorporate these improvements into the following day.

End-of-the-Week Wrap-Up: At the end of each week, use the End-of-the-Week Wrap-Up pages to record your start and end weight, energy level for the week, and total calories burned for the week. Also record how many days you successfully tracked your diet (although you should aim to do it every day). There is also space to write down how you felt for the week and goals for the following week. Assessing your mood, progress, achievements, and also setbacks will help you prepare for the upcoming week. Don't get bogged down in minor setbacks or obstacles; instead, reward yourself for each small step of success along the way. The End-of-the-Week Wrap-Up pages will give you an accurate picture of how you did and how you felt for each week.

Congratulations on taking an important step toward increased energy, better health, and weight loss! Happy eating!

A&W Restaurant	Cal	Fat	Cbs
Dipping Sauces			
• BBQ, 28 g	40	0	10
Honey Mustard, 28 g	100	6	12
• Ranch, 28 g	160	17	2
Sweet & Sour, 28 g	45	0	12
Hot Dogs			
Cheese Dog, 126 g	320	20	25
• Coney (Chili) Cheese Dog, 154 g	350	21	27
Coney (Chili) Dog, 126 g	310	18	24
• Dog (plain), 90 g	280	17	22
Root Beer			
A&W Diet Root Beer, 20 fl.oz.	0	0	0
A&W Regular Root Beer, 20 fl.oz.	290	0	76
Root Beer Floats			
A&W Root Beer Float, 468 g	350	5	77
A&W Diet Root Beer Float, 468 g	170	5	30
Sandwiches & Strips			
Chicken Strips (3 pieces), 159 g	500	29	32
Crispy Chicken Sandwich, 219 g	590	29	54
Grilled Chicken Sandwich, 213 g	440	19	34
Kids Cheeseburger, 175 g	460	24	39
• Kids Hamburger, 161 g	420	22	35
Original Bacon Cheeseburger, 223 g	570	33	41
• Original Bacon Double Chzburger, 303 g	800	48	47
Original Double Cheeseburger, 288 g	720	42	46
Papa Burger, 288 g	720	42	46
Sides			
• Cheese Curds, 142 g	570	40	27
Cheese Fries, 170 g	380	19	50
• Chili Bowl, 225 g	190	6	22
Chili Cheese Fries, 198 g	400	19	51
Chili Fries, 170 g	370	16	49
Kids Fries, 113 g	310	13	45
Large Fries, 156 g	430	18	61
Onion Rings, 113 g	350	16	45
Sweets & Treats - Medium			
A&W Root Beer Freeze, 510 g	480	10	89
Caramel Sundae, 189 g	340	9	57
Chocolate Milkshake, 475 g	700	29	100
Chocolate Sundae, 189 g	320	8	53
Hot Fudge Sundae, 189 g	350	11	54
M&M Polar Swirl, 340 g	710	25	107
Oreo Polar Swirl, 340 g	690	24	107
• Reese's Polar Swirl, 340 g	740	31	97
Strawberry Milkshake, 475 g	670	29	90
Strawberry Sundae, 189 g	300	8	47
• Vanilla Cone, 157 g	260	7	41
Vanilla Milkshake, 475 g	720	31	97
Vanilla Sundae, 189 g	310	8	52

Amazon Café	Cal	Fat	Cbs
Smoothie			
Amazon Power Boost, 16 oz.	229	1	68
Bananarama, 16 oz.	239	1	65
Chocolate Nirvana, 16 oz.	225	1	76
Citrus Sunrise, 16 oz.	254	2	88
Coffee Utopia, 16 oz.	251	0	43
Coldblaster, 16 oz.	247	1	65
Orange Outrage, 16 oz.	215	1	65
Orange Sensation, 16 oz.	242	2	63
Paradise Lust, 16 oz.	265	3	60
• Piña Colada, 16 oz.	320	4	63
Raspberry Rage, 16 oz.	234	1	69
Raspberry Razzle, 16 oz.	207	1	62
• Skinny Delight, 16 oz.	186	1	44

Amazon Café (cont.)	Cal	Fat	Cbs
Smoothie (cont.)			
Soy Smoothie, 16 oz.	191	0	50
Strawberry Supreme, 16 oz.	221	0	55
Tropical Passion, 16 oz.	236	1	71
Soup			
Broccoli & Cheese, 8 oz.	110	6	10
Chicken & Sausage Gumbo, 8 oz.	100	3	12
Chicken & Wild Rice, 8 oz.	120	3	17
• Chili Con Carne, 8 oz.	250	7	29
Chipotle Black Bean, 8 oz.	130	1	21
Classic Chicken Noodle, 8 oz.	80	2	9
Corn Chowder, 8 oz.	110	4	19
Cream of Broccoli, 8 oz.	110	5	14
Cream of Potato with Bacon, 8 oz.	120	4	18
Hearty Vegetable, 8 oz.	70	1	15
Italian Wedding, 8 oz.	130	4	16
Mushroom Barley, 8 oz.	80	2	14
New England Clam Chowder, 8 oz.	90	2	15
Rosemary Chicken Dumpling, 8 oz.	80	1	12
Rustic Beef & Mushroom, 8 oz.	70	2	6
Split Pea with Ham, 8 oz.	160	5	22
Sweet Pepper & Beef, 8 oz.	90	2	14
Three Bean Chili, 8 oz.	130	0	47
• Tomato & Three Cheese, 8 oz.	60	2	7

Applebee's	Cal	Fat	Cbs
Angus Burgers or Chicken Sandwiches			
Bruschetta	780	N/A	N/A
• Chicken Bruschetta	600	N/A	N/A
Chicken Cowboy	950	N/A	N/A
Chicken Quesadilla	1240	N/A	N/A
Cowboy	1140	N/A	N/A
• Quesadilla	1420	N/A	N/A
Appetizers			
• Appetizer Sampler	2540	N/A	N/A
Boneless Buffalo Wings	1460	N/A	N/A
Buffalo Chicken Wings	1130	N/A	N/A
Chicken Quesadilla Grande	1320	N/A	N/A
Crunchy Onion Rings	1230	N/A	N/A
Mini Bacon Cheeseburgers	1470	N/A	N/A
• Mozzarella Sticks	930	N/A	N/A
Nachos Nuevos	2070	N/A	N/A
Veggie Patch Pizza	940	N/A	N/A
Burgers, Sandwiches & Rollups			
• Blacken Tilapia Sandwiches	710	N/A	N/A
• Brewtus Steak Burger	1390	N/A	N/A
Chicken Fajita Rollup	1080	N/A	N/A
Oriental Chicken Rollup	1170	N/A	N/A
Roasted Turkey and Bacon Ciabatta	1370	N/A	N/A
Zesty Ranch Chicken Sandwich	1170	N/A	N/A
Chicken			
Chicken Fingers Basket	1050	N/A	N/A
Chicken Fingers Platter	1300	N/A	N/A
Chicken Fried Chicken	1280	N/A	N/A
Chicken Parmesan	1430	N/A	N/A
Fiesta Lime Chicken	1290	N/A	N/A
Riblet and Chicken Fingers Basket	1360	N/A	N/A
• Riblet and Chicken Fingers Platter	1950	N/A	N/A
• Roasted Garlic & Asiago Chicken	770	N/A	N/A
Fresh-Made Sides			
• Baked Potato	380	N/A	N/A
Caesar Salad	220	N/A	N/A
Garden Salad	310	N/A	N/A
Garlic Mashed Potatoes	110	N/A	N/A
• Seasonal Vegetables	50	N/A	N/A

Applebee's (cont.)

	Cal	Fat	Cbs
Pasta			
• Cheddar-Jack Mac & Cheese with Chicken	1110	N/A	N/A
Chicken Broccoli Pasta Alfredo Bowl	1220	N/A	N/A
• Crispy Orange Chicken Bowl	1910	N/A	N/A
Grilled Shrimp Pesto Alfredo Fettuccine	1790	N/A	N/A
Three-Cheese Chicken Penne	1210	N/A	N/A
Ribs & Fajitas			
• Applebee's Riblets	1740	N/A	N/A
• Applebee's Riblets Basket	1120	N/A	N/A
Honey BBQ Baby Backs	1430	N/A	N/A
Sizzling Fajitas	1440	N/A	N/A
Salads			
Blue Cheese Dressing, Full	460	N/A	N/A
Blue Cheese Dressing, Half	230	N/A	N/A
Buffalo Chicken Salad, Full	830	N/A	N/A
Buffalo Chicken Salad, Half	590	N/A	N/A
California Shrimp Salad, Full	370	N/A	N/A
California Shrimp Salad, Half	310	N/A	N/A
Creamy Avocado Dressing, Full	350	N/A	N/A
Creamy Avocado Dressing, Half	180	N/A	N/A
Garlic Caesar Dressing, Full	420	N/A	N/A
Garlic Caesar Dressing, Half	190	N/A	N/A
Grilled Chicken Caesar Salad, Full	380	N/A	N/A
• Grilled Chicken Caesar Salad, Half	210	N/A	N/A
Grilled Shrimp 'N Spinach Salad, Full	850	N/A	N/A
Grilled Shrimp 'N Spinach Salad, Half	580	N/A	N/A
Hot Bacon Vinaigrette Dressing, Full	310	N/A	N/A
Hot Bacon Vinaigrette Dressing, Half	150	N/A	N/A
Mexi-Ranch Dressing, Full	380	N/A	N/A
Mexi-Ranch Dressing, Half	190	N/A	N/A
Oriental Chicken Salad, Full	840	N/A	N/A
Oriental Chicken Salad, Half	450	N/A	N/A
Oriental Grilled Chicken Salad, Full	630	N/A	N/A
Oriental Grilled Chicken Salad, Half	350	N/A	N/A
Oriental Vinaigrette Dressing, Full	590	N/A	N/A
Oriental Vinaigrette Dressing, Half	290	N/A	N/A
• Santa Fe Chicken Salad, Full	900	N/A	N/A
Santa Fe Chicken Salad, Half	800	N/A	N/A
Seafood			
• Double Crunch Shrimp	1330	N/A	N/A
• Garlic Herb Salmon	700	N/A	N/A
Parmesan Tilapia	880	N/A	N/A
Steak Toppings			
• Grilled Onions	90	N/A	N/A
Sauteed Garlic & Mushrooms	130	N/A	N/A
• Shrimp 'N Parmesan	350	N/A	N/A
Steaks			
Bourbon Street, 10 oz.	1570	N/A	N/A
• Chop Steak, 10 oz.	1820	N/A	N/A
• House Sirloin, 9 oz.	410	N/A	N/A
New York Strip, 12 oz.	590	N/A	N/A
Ribeye, 12 oz.	590	N/A	N/A
Shrimp 'N Parmesan Sirloin, 9 oz.	1420	N/A	N/A
Steak & Friend Shrimp, 7 oz.	1390	N/A	N/A
Steak & Grilled Shrimp, 7 oz.	530	N/A	N/A
Steak & Honey BBQ Chicken, 7 oz.	1280	N/A	N/A
Steak & Riblets, 7 oz.	1710	N/A	N/A
Ultimate Trios			
• Boneless Buffalo Wings	840	N/A	N/A
Dynamite Shrimp	730	N/A	N/A
Mini Bacon Cheese Burgers	750	N/A	N/A
Mini Chicken Ranchers	770	N/A	N/A
• Mozzarella Sticks	420	N/A	N/A
Spinach & Artichoke Dip	580	N/A	N/A
Steak Quesadilla Towers	690	N/A	N/A

Applebee's (cont.)

	Cal	Fat	Cbs
Ultimate Trios (cont.)			
Traditional Buffalo Wings	680	N/A	N/A

Arby's

	Cal	Fat	Cbs
Arby's Chicken Naturals®			
BBQ Dipping Sauce, 28 g	44	0	11
Buffalo Dipping Sauce, 28 g	10	1	2
Chicken Bacon & Swiss - Crispy, 214 g	624	29	52
Chicken Bacon & Swiss - Grilled, 209 g	462	17	38
Chicken Fillet Sandwich - Crispy, 249 g	577	30	50
Chicken Fillet Sandwich - Grilled, 244 g	414	17	36
Chicken Tenders - 3 piece, 131 g	379	18	28
Chicken Tenders - 5 piece, 218 g	630	31	47
• Chkn Cordon Bleu Sand - Crispy, 250 g	657	32	49
Chkn Cordon Bleu Sand - Grilled, 245 g	495	19	35
Honey Mustard Dipping, 28 g	129	12	6
Popcorn Chicken - Large, 184 g	531	26	39
• Popcorn Chicken - Regular, 126 g	365	18	27
Popcorn Chicken Shakers™, 240 g	585	27	51
Arby's® Roast Beef Sandwiches & Melts			
Arby's Melt, 146 g	302	12	36
Arby's Sauce, 14 g	15	0	4
Bacon Beef 'n Cheddar Sandwich, 212 g	521	27	45
BBQ Bacon 'n Jack 2 for, 169 g	360	16	42
Beef 'n Cheddar Sandwich, 195 g	445	21	44
French Dip & Swiss Sandwich, 224 g	473	18	38
• Ham & Swiss Melt Sandwich, 131 g	268	5	35
Kids Meal - Jr. Roast Beef Sand, 125 g	272	10	34
• Large Roast Beef Sandwich, 281 g	547	28	41
Medium Roast Beef Sandwich, 210 g	415	21	34
Regular Roast Beef, 154 g	320	14	34
Sourdough Ham Melt, 165 g	380	13	39
Sourdough Roast Beef Melt, 166 g	355	14	40
Super Roast Beef, 198 g	398	19	40
Swiss Melt, 146 g	303	12	37
Arby's® Toasted Subs			
Chicken Parmesan Toasted Sub, 317 g	843	38	80
Classic Italian Toasted Sub, 379 g	828	46	69
French Dip & Swiss Toasted Sub, 337 g	622	20	68
• Meatball Toasted Sub, 325 g	1000	62	71
Philly Beef Toasted Sub, 281 g	739	37	64
• Turkey Bacon Club Toasted Sub, 341 g	619	18	65
Breakfast			
Bacon & Egg Croissant, 120 g	337	22	23
Bacon Biscuit, 95 g	340	21	29
Bacon, Egg & Cheese Biscuit, 158 g	461	28	30
Bacon, Egg & Cheese Croissant, 133 g	378	22	23
Bacon, Egg & Cheese Sourdough, 173 g	437	16	40
Bacon, Egg & Cheese Wrap, 193 g	515	29	50
Biscuit - Plain, 82 g	273	15	28
Blueberry Muffin, 85 g	320	12	49
Breakfast Syrup, 28 g	78	0	20
Chicken Biscuit, 132 g	417	23	39
Croissant, 57 g	190	10	21
Egg & Cheese Sourdough, 164 g	392	12	40
French Toastix, 124 g	312	13	44
Ham & Cheese Croissant, 113 g	274	12	22
Ham Biscuit, 132 g	323	17	29
Ham, Egg & Cheese Biscuit, 195 g	444	24	31
Ham, Egg & Cheese Croissant, 220 g	441	24	25
Ham, Egg & Cheese Sourdough, 214 g	442	14	41
Ham, Egg, & Cheese Wrap, 249 g	575	31	51
Sausage & Egg Croissant, 147 g	433	32	23
Sausage Biscuit, 122 g	436	31	28
• Sausage Gravy Biscuit, 238 g	961	68	107
• Sausage Patty, 51 g	210	20	0

Arby's (cont.)

Breakfast (cont.)	Cal	Fat	Cbs
Sausage, Egg & Cheese Biscuit, 185 g	557	38	30
Sausage, Egg & Cheese Croissant, 160 g	475	32	23
Sausage, Egg & Cheese Sourdough, 204 g	556	28	40
Sausage, Egg & Cheese Wrap, 239 g	689	45	50
Kids Menu			
Fruit Cup, 57 g	35	0	9
Junior Roast Beef Sandwich, 125 g	272	10	34
Market Fresh™ Mini Tkey & Chz Sandwich, 119 g	244	5	28
• Market Fresh™Mini Ham & Chz Sandwich, 119 g	235	5	28
• Popcorn Chicken, 95 g	274	13	20
Market Fresh™ Salads			
Buttermilk Ranch Dressing, 64 g	325	34	4
• Chicken Club Salad, 345 g	426	23	26
Garlic & Cheese Croutons, 14 g	77	5	7
Light Buttermilk Ranch Dressing, 64 g	112	6	13
Martha's Vineyard Salad™, 330 g	277	8	24
Raspberry Vinaigrette, 64 g	194	14	18
Santa Fe Ranch Dressing, 64 g	296	31	4
Santa Fe Salad™ w/ Grilled Chkn, 350 g	283	9	21
Santa Fe Salad™, 344 g	416	18	37
• Seasoned Tortilla Strips, 14 g	71	3	9
Sliced Almonds, 14 g	81	8	2
Market Fresh™ Sandwiches & Wraps			
Corned Beef Reuben Sandwich, 295 g	590	32	55
Corned Beef Reuben Wrap, 266 g	560	29	42
• Fish Sandwich, 210 g	535	25	59
Pecan Chicken Salad Sandwich, 322 g	769	39	79
Pecan Chicken Salad Wrap, 277 g	638	38	48
Roast Beef & Swiss Sandwich, 339 g	777	41	73
Roast Ham & Swiss Sandwich, 345 g	691	31	75
• Roast Tkey Ranch & Bacon Sand, 367 g	818	38	75
Roast Turkey & Swiss Sandwich, 345 g	708	30	74
Roast Turkey Ranch & Bacon Wrap, 302 g	683	37	44
Roast Turkey Reuben Sandwich, 295 g	594	30	56
Roast Turkey Reuben Wrap, 266 g	564	27	43
Southwest Chicken Wrap, 254 g	567	29	42
Spicy Cajun Fish Sandwich, 217 g	595	32	59
Ultimate BLT Sandwich, 294 g	779	45	75
Ultimate BLT Wrap, 249 g	648	44	45
Shakes & Desserts			
Apple Turnover, 128 g	377	16	65
Cheesecake Poppers, 69 g	270	15	30
Cherry Turnover, 128 g	377	15	65
• Chocolate Chip Cookie, 45 g	202	10	26
Chocolate Shake - Regular, 397 g	507	13	83
Jamocha Shake - Regular, 397 g	498	13	81
Raspberry Dipping Sauce, 28 g	60	0	14
Strawberry Banana Swirl Shake, 482 g	567	16	87
Strawberry Shake - Regular, 397 g	498	13	81
Vanilla Shake - Regular, 369 g	437	13	66
Sides & Sidekickers®			
Bronco Berry Dipping Sauce®, 57 g	122	0	30
Cheddar Cheese Sauce - side, 21 g	30	2	2
• Cheddar Fries - Medium, 170 g	465	28	51
Chile Lime Ranch Dipping Sauce, 43 g	190	19	2
Cool Ranch Sour Crm Dipping Sauce, 43 g	158	16	2
Curly Fries - Medium, 125 g	397	24	46
Homestyle Fries - Medium, 142 g	377	25	55
• Jalapeño Bites® - Regular (5), 110 g	305	21	29
Ketchup Packet, 14 g	13	0	3
Loaded Potato Bites® Regular (5), 112 g	353	22	27
Marinara Sauce, 43 g	30	2	4
Mozzarella Sticks - Regular (4), 137 g	426	28	38
Onion Petals - Regular, 113 g	331	23	35

Arby's (cont.)

Sides & Sidekickers® (cont.)	Cal	Fat	Cbs
Potato Cakes (2), 100 g	246	18	26
SW Egg rolls - Small (4 pieces), 90 g	225	7	29
Tangy Southwest Sauce®, 57 g	333	35	5
T.J. Cinnamons®			
• Chocolate Twist, 71 g	250	12	34
Cinnamon Twist, 71 g	260	14	33
Original Gourmet Cinnamon Roll®, 149 g	507	10	73
Pecan Sticky Bun 4 Pack, 738 g	2751	90	363
• Pecan Sticky Bun, 184 g	688	22	91
T.J. Cinnamons Mocha Chill®, 354 g	306	7	48
T.J. Icing, 28 g	117	5	18

Atlanta Bread Company

Baked Goods: Bagels	Cal	Fat	Cbs
Apple Spice, 4 oz.	360	3	73
• Asiago Cheese, 4 oz.	380	10	53
Blueberry, 4 oz.	270	1	55
Cinnamon Crisp, 4 oz.	330	3	68
Cinnamon Raisin, 4 oz.	270	1	56
Everything, 9 oz.	320	4	60
• Lower Carb Cranberry Walnut, 2 oz.	110	4	16
Onion, 4 oz.	290	1	59
Plain, 3 oz.	270	1	55
Poppy Seed, 4 oz.	320	5	57
Sesame, 4 oz.	360	9	57
Wheat, 4 oz.	270	2	54
Baked Goods: Breads			
ABC Roll, 4 oz.	260	1	54
Asiago Loaf, 2 oz.	160	2	29
Asiago Strip, 2 oz.	160	2	28
Challah, 2 oz.	160	3	29
Cinnamon Raisin Loaf, 2 oz.	150	2	28
Cracked Wheat, 2 oz.	160	2	30
Foccacia Round, Asiago, 2 oz.	180	5	26
Foccacia Round, Basil Pesto, 2 oz.	190	8	26
Foccacia Round, Tomato Onion, 2 oz.	150	3	27
Foccacia, Rosemary Tomato, 3 oz.	350	12	50
French Baguette, 2 oz.	140	1	30
French Loaf, 2 oz.	140	1	28
French Roll, 2 oz.	160	1	33
Honey Wheat, 2 oz.	150	2	28
Lower Carb Multigrain Bread, 2 oz.	100	2	16
Nine Grain, 2 oz.	160	3	28
Pumpernickel, 2 oz.	140	2	26
Rye, 2 oz.	150	2	28
• Sourdough Baguette, 2 oz.	140	0	29
• Sourdough Bread Bowl, 7 oz.	550	2	113
Sourdough Loaf, 2 oz.	140	0	29
Sourdough Roll, 2 oz.	160	0	34
Baked Goods: Cream Cheese Spreads			
Garden Vegetable Cream Cheese, 2 oz.	170	17	4
Onion & Chive Cream Cheese, 2 oz.	190	17	4
• Plain Cream Cheese, 2 oz.	190	19	1
• Plain Cream Cheese, Light, 2 oz.	120	10	6
Strawberry Cream Cheese, 2 oz.	190	15	12
Beverages: Cold			
• Caramel Latte Caffechillo, 19 oz.	250	10	32
• Frozen Spiced Chai Tea, 16 oz.	260	6	43
Kona Mocha Caffechillo, 19 oz.	250	10	32
Vanilla Caffechillo, 19 oz.	250	10	32
Beverages: Hot			
Café Latte, tall, 16 oz.	170	6	18
Café Mocha, tall, 16 oz.	340	8	57
• Cappuccino, tall, 16 oz.	130	5	14
Caramel Macchiato, tall, 16 oz.	390	8	69

Atlanta Bread Company (cont.)	Cal	Fat	Cbs
Beverages: Hot (cont.)			
Espresso, single shot, 2 oz.	5	0	1
• Hot Chocolate, tall, 16 oz.	450	10	78
Hot Spiced Chai Tea, 15 oz.	260	6	43
House Latte, tall, 16 oz.	380	10	65
Beverages: Smoothies			
• Pineapple Mango Banana, 16 oz.	290	0	72
Strawberry Banana, 16 oz.	290	0	71
• Strawberry Blueberry Banana, 16 oz.	280	0	69
Breakfast: Gourmet Breakfast			
Belgian Waffle w/ syrup, 7 oz.	480	13	82
Belgian Waffle w/o syrup, 5 oz.	320	13	41
• French Toast w/ syrup, 9 oz.	560	9	103
French Toast w/o syrup, 7 oz.	400	9	61
• Scrambled eggs, 5 oz.	220	16	2
Breakfast: Hot Sandwiches			
Bacon, Egg & Cheese on Croissant, 5 oz.	530	34	39
• Egg & Cheese on Croissant, 5 oz.	480	30	39
Ham, Egg & Cheese on Croissant, 7 oz.	540	31	41
• Sausage, Egg & Cheese on Croissant, 7 oz.	690	48	39
Breakfast: Omelets			
Florentine, 8 oz.	350	24	6
• Greek, 8 oz.	290	20	5
• Ham and Swiss, 8 oz.	390	26	4
Spanish, 8 oz.	350	24	6
Tomato Bacon, 8 oz.	370	27	4
Breakfast: Side Orders			
Bacon (3 slices), 1 oz.	80	7	0
Breakfast Potatoes, 4 oz.	170	9	20
• Ham, 2 oz.	60	2	2
Sausage (2 patties), 3 oz.	310	27	1
Pastas			
Asiago Cream, 14 oz.	860	51	63
• Basil Pesto, 14 oz.	940	53	69
Chicken Parmesan, 15 oz.	780	27	75
• Kid's Pasta, 9 oz.	410	12	56
Pasta Puttanesca, 14 oz.	590	21	63
Penne Pomodoro Pasta, 18 oz.	920	44	66
Pastries & Sweets: Cheesecakes			
• Carrot Cake Cheesecake, 1 slice	680	49	53
Chocolate Truffle Cheesecake, 1 slice	640	40	63
Oreo Cheesecake, 1 slice	630	39	60
Pecan Turtle Cheesecake, 1 slice	640	42	56
Plain Cheesecake, 1 slice	570	36	42
• Pumpkin Praline Cheesecake, 1 slice	510	31	50
Snickers Cheesecake, 1 slice	620	40	54
Pastries & Sweets: Cookies			
Chocolate Chunk, 3 oz.	400	19	51
• Chocolate Dipped Peanut, 4 oz.	530	30	52
Chocolate Dipped Shortbread, 4 oz.	440	23	55
• Oatmeal Raisin, 3 oz.	360	15	50
Peanut Butter, 3 oz.	430	24	42
Shortbread, 3 oz.	370	18	47
Toffee Chocolate Chunk, 3 oz.	400	21	49
White Macadamia, 3 oz.	410	22	49
Pastries & Sweets: Croissants			
• Almond Croissant, 6 oz.	660	38	67
Apple Croissant, 5 oz.	430	17	65
Cheese Croissant, 6 oz.	510	29	56
Chocolate Croissant, 4 oz.	520	27	61
• Plain Croissant, 3 oz.	360	20	39
Raspberry Cheese Croissant, 5 oz.	440	19	63
Pastries & Sweets: Danish			
Apple, 4 oz.	450	18	66
Cheese, 4 oz.	480	22	65

Atlanta Bread Company (cont.)	Cal	Fat	Cbs
Pastries & Sweets: Danish (cont.)			
• Gooey Butter, 4 oz.	550	25	73
• Raspberry, 4 oz.	430	18	62
Pastries & Sweets: Muffins and Tops			
Banana Nut Muffin Top, 3 oz.	420	26	39
Banana Nut Muffin, 5 oz.	560	33	57
• Blueberry Muffin Top, 2 oz.	250	12	31
Blueberry Muffin, 4 oz.	430	21	54
Bran Raisin Muffin, 4 oz.	410	18	55
Chocolate Chip Muffin Top, 3 oz.	400	19	52
Chocolate Chip Muffin, 5 oz.	560	27	73
Cranberry Apple Muffin, 5 oz.	490	23	64
• Cranberry Orange Muffin, 5 oz.	560	34	55
Low Fat Apple Muffin, 4 oz.	340	5	66
Low Fat Pumpkin Muffin, 4 oz.	320	5	65
Mocha Muffin Top, 3 oz.	410	20	53
Mocha Muffin, 5 oz.	560	27	73
Pumpkin Muffin Top, 3 oz.	350	13	54
Pumpkin Muffin, 5 oz.	470	18	73
Pastries & Sweets: Scones			
Cinnamon Scone, 4 oz.	350	11	57
Raspberry Scone, 4 oz.	360	13	56
Pastries & Sweets: Other			
Austrian Pretzel, 4 oz.	550	34	55
Banana Nut Bread, 2 oz.	230	14	24
Bear Claw, 4 oz.	540	24	73
• Boston Cream Pound Cake, 2 oz.	200	12	21
Cinnamon Roll, 5 oz.	630	26	91
Cranberry Orange Bread, 2 oz.	240	14	24
Key Lime Pie, 3 oz.	450	13	52
Lower Carb Chocolate Cake, 2 oz.	200	15	17
Marble Pound Cake, 2 oz.	230	15	22
• Pecan Roll, 6 oz.	860	60	72
Pumpkin Bread, 2 oz.	210	8	33
Sticky Bun, 5 oz.	560	30	66
Walnut Brownies, 4 oz.	490	24	63
Pizzas			
BBQ Chicken, 1/2 pizza	320	5	53
• Cheese (Kid's), 1/2 pizza	300	7	44
• Four Cheese, 1/2 pizza	530	23	46
Pepperoni, 1/2 pizza	340	10	44
White Pizza, 1/2 pizza	460	22	47
Salad Dressings			
• Balsamic Vinaigrette Dressing, 2 tbsp.	150	16	1
Bleu Cheese Dressing, 2 tbsp.	120	12	1
Caesar Dressing, 2 tbsp.	150	15	3
• Fat-Free Raspberry Vinaigrette, 2 tbsp.	35	0	8
Greek Dressing, 2 tbsp.	100	10	1
Honey Mustard Dressing, 2 tbsp.	130	12	6
Ranch Dressing, 2 tbsp.	130	13	2
Sesame Ginger Dressing, 2 tbsp.	130	11	8
Thousand Island Dressing, 2 tbsp.	120	11	5
Salads (w/o dressing)			
Add Grilled Chicken, 3 oz.	70	2	2
Balsamic Bleu Salad, 10 oz.	330	18	35
Caesar Salad, 8 oz.	190	10	11
Chicken Salad on Lettuce, 4 oz.	280	21	2
Chopstix Chicken Salad, 13 oz.	280	13	24
Extra Croutons, 1 oz.	50	2	6
Fruit Salad, 10 oz.	130	0	34
Greek Salad, 12 oz.	200	13	13
• House, 10 oz.	50	0	11
• Tuna Salad on Lettuce, 4 oz.	360	32	4
Sandwiches			
• Chicken Salad (Scoop), 4 oz.	280	21	2

Atlanta Bread Company (cont.)

Sandwiches (cont.)	Cal	Fat	Cbs
Chicken Salad on Sourdough, 10 oz.	540	19	62
Grilled Cheese on French Bread, 5 oz.	390	11	57
Honey Maple Ham on Honey Wheat, 10 oz.	410	5	63
w/ Cheese and Mayo, 11 oz.	620	26	64
w/ Mayo, 10 oz.	520	17	64
w/ Cheddar Cheese, 11 oz.	520	15	63
Peanut Butter & Jelly on Fren Bread, 7 oz.	600	14	99
Roasted Turkey Breast on 9 Grain, 10 oz.	430	7	61
• w/ Cheese and Mayo, 11 oz.	630	26	62
w/ Cheese, 11 oz.	530	15	61
w/ Mayo, 10 oz.	530	18	62
Tuna Salad (Scoop), 4 oz.	360	32	4
Tuna Salad on French Bread, 10 oz.	610	29	62
Veggie Sandwich on Nine Grain, 9 oz.	340	5	63
w/ Cheese and Dill Sauce, 11 oz.	500	19	63
w/ Dill Sauce, 10 oz.	401	11	63

Sandwiches: Paninis (Full)			
• Chicken Pesto, 12 oz.	800	35	83
Cordon Bleu, 10 oz.	660	18	82
Cuban Pork Loin, 10 oz.	660	19	81
• Italian Vegetarian, 12 oz.	640	16	93
Turkey Club, 12 oz.	750	27	83

Soups			
Black Bean and Ham, 10 oz.	250	9	40
Chicken Tortilla, 10 oz.	190	9	20
Chunky Baked Potato, 10 oz.	290	16	30
Classic Chicken Noodle, 10 oz.	140	3	21
Cream of Broccoli, 10 oz.	200	11	19
Creamy Tomato, 10 oz.	130	9	10
French Onion with Toppings, 10 oz.	200	10	16
• French Onion, 10 oz.	80	3	10
Garden Vegetable, 10 oz.	100	2	19
• Homestyle Chicken and Dumpling, 10 oz.	290	18	25
New England Clam Chowder, 10 oz.	280	16	24
Pasta Fagioli, 10 oz.	170	6	24
Spicy Chicken Gumbo, 10 oz.	120	3	16
Wisconsin Cheese, 10 oz.	240	14	21

Soups: Chili			
Frontier Chicken Chili, 10 oz.	270	10	26
Hearty Beef Chili, 10 oz.	350	15	33

Specialty Sandwiches			
ABC Special on French Roll, 12 oz.	420	5	61
w/ Cheese and Mayo, 14 oz.	680	28	62
w/ Cheese, 14 oz.	570	16	61
w/ Mayo, 13 oz.	530	16	62
Bella Basil on Tom & Rosemary Focaccia, 10 oz.	660	35	58
w/ Cheese, 11 oz.	760	44	58
California Avocado on Tom Onion Focaccia, 12 oz.	690	40	71
w/ Cheese, 14 oz.	790	48	71
Hot Pastrami, 8 oz.	460	10	59
w/ Swiss Cheese, 9 oz.	570	18	59
• Tangy Roast Beef, 10 oz.	390	4	56
w/ Horseradish Cheddar & Mayo, 12 oz.	790	39	60
w/ Horseradish Cheddar, 12 oz.	690	28	59

Au Bon Pain

Bakery: Bagels	Cal	Fat	Cbs
Asiago Cheese Bagel, 4 oz.	340	6	55
• Cinnamon Crisp Bagel, 4 oz.	410	7	76
Cinnamon Raisin Bagel, 4 oz.	310	1	66
Everything Bagel, 4 oz.	340	5	62
Honey 9 Grain Bagel, 5 oz.	360	4	71
Jalapeño Double Cheddar Bagel, 5 oz.	340	10	52
Onion Dill Bagel, 4 oz.	290	1	58
• Plain Bagel, 4 oz.	280	1	57

Au Bon Pain (cont.)

Bakery: Bagels (cont.)	Cal	Fat	Cbs
Poppy Bagel, 4 oz.	320	4	58
Sesame Seed Bagel, 4 oz.	320	4	58

Bakery: Cookies & Desserts			
Banana Nut Pound Cake, 5 oz.	520	28	60
Blondie, 4 oz.	330	19	61
Blueberry Tulip, 3 oz.	370	20	44
Cappuccino Poundcake, 5 oz.	530	26	68
Chocolate Bundt Cake, 4 oz.	440	21	61
Chocolate Cheesecake Brownie, 4 oz.	370	14	58
Chocolate Chip Brownie, 4 oz.	380	17	62
Chocolate Chip Cookie, 2 oz.	260	12	37
Choco Dipped Cranberry Almond Macaroon, 3 oz.	320	16	42
Chocolate Dipped Shortbread, 3 oz.	350	20	38
Chocolate Pound Cake, 134 g	500	29	58
Chocolate Raspberry Tulip, 4 oz.	430	21	55
Confetti Cookie With M&M's, 2 oz.	310	14	42
Crème De Fleur, 5 oz.	490	25	57
Crumb Cake, 4 oz.	470	25	56
English Toffee Cookie, 2 oz.	210	11	26
Gingerbread Cookie, 3 oz.	300	9	50
• Hazelnut Creme Pastry, 5 oz.	540	34	50
Hazelnut Dream Cookie, 3 oz.	390	24	41
Hazelnut Fudge Cookie, 2 oz.	290	16	34
Hazelnut Mocha Brownie, 4 oz.	430	21	58
Hazelnut Monkey Bread, 4 oz.	510	28	57
Holiday Tree Cookie, 2 oz.	170	5	31
Iced Cinnamon Roll, 4 oz.	400	15	60
Key Lime Sugar Cookie, 2 oz.	250	9	39
Key Lime Tulip, 4 oz.	440	22	55
Lemon Pound Cake, 139 g	520	27	64
Marble Pound Cake, 134 g	490	27	59
Mini Chocolate Chip Cookie, 1 oz.	70	3	9
• Mini Oatmeal Raisin Cookie, 1 oz.	60	2	9
• Mint Chocolate Pound Cake, 5 oz.	530	28	65
Oatmeal Raisin Cookie, 2 oz.	230	8	36
Palmier, 4 oz.	440	23	53
Pecan Roll, 6 oz.	630	32	80
Rocky Road Brownie, 4 oz.	410	17	62
Shortbread Cookie, 2 oz.	310	18	34
Wh Choc Chunk Macadamia Nut Cookie, 2 oz.	280	15	34

Bakery: Croissants			
• Almond Croissant, 5 oz.	600	38	55
• Apple Croissant, 4 oz.	270	11	44
Chocolate Croissant, 4 oz.	430	22	58
Ham And Cheese Croissant, 4 oz.	400	20	38
Plain Croissant, 3 oz.	300	17	31
Raspberry Cheese Croissant, 4 oz.	320	15	41
Spinach And Cheese Croissant, 4 oz.	290	16	28
Sweet Cheese Croissant, 4 oz.	380	19	48

Bakery: Danish			
Cherry Danish, 4 oz.	420	20	54
Lemon Danish, 4 oz.	440	20	57

Bakery: Kids			
All Natural Grilled Chicken Sandwich, 7 oz.	490	14	59
• Chicken Nuggets, 3 oz.	180	7	14
• Grilled Cheese, 7 oz.	670	41	55
Kid's Buttered Penne Pasta, 4 oz.	260	12	31
Macaroni And Cheese, 6 oz.	220	14	15
Smoked Turkey Sandwich, 7 oz.	450	13	56

Bakery: Muffins			
Blueberry Muffin, 6 oz.	510	19	76
Carrot Walnut Muffin, 6 oz.	520	25	66
Corn Muffin, 6 oz.	460	16	69
Cranberry Walnut Muffin, 6 oz.	500	24	61

Au Bon Pain (cont.)	Cal	Fat	Cbs
Bakery: Muffins (cont.)			
• Double Chocolate Chunk Muffin, 5 oz.	590	20	83
• Low-fat Triple Berry Muffin, 4 oz.	290	2	61
Mushroom, Gorgonzola & Rd Pepper Muffin, 5 oz.	490	28	50
Pumpkin Muffin, 6 oz.	490	17	75
Raisin Bran Muffin, 6 oz.	410	9	74
Southwest Jalapeño Muffin, 5 oz.	560	30	64
Bakery: Scones			
Cinnamon Scone, 4 oz.	530	27	60
Orange Scone, 4 oz.	470	23	57
Bakery: Strudel			
Apple Strudel, 4 oz.	430	24	48
Cherry Strudel, 5 oz.	460	26	49
Beverages: Blasts & Smoothies			
Banana Wildberry Smoothie Lg., 24 fl.oz.	530	8	119
Banana Wildberry Smoothie Medium, 16 fl.oz.	340	7	72
Caramel Blast Large, 24 fl.oz.	760	21	151
Caramel Blast Medium, 16 fl.oz.	540	17	104
Coffee Blast Large, 24 fl.oz.	690	29	119
Coffee Blast Medium, 16 fl.oz.	440	21	71
Mocha Blast Large, 24 fl.oz.	690	22	137
Mocha Blast Medium, 16 fl.oz.	440	17	80
Peach Smoothie Large, 24 fl.oz.	470	1	104
Peach Smoothie Medium, 16 fl.oz.	310	1	69
Strawberry Smoothie Large, 24 fl.oz.	470	1	100
Strawberry Smoothie Medium, 16 fl.oz.	310	1	66
• Vanilla Blast Large, 24 fl.oz.	760	21	152
Vanilla Blast Medium, 16 fl.oz.	540	17	104
Wildberry Smoothie Large, 24 fl.oz.	530	8	104
Wildberry Smoothie Medium, 16 fl.oz.	380	7	71
Beverages: Coffee & Espresso			
• Caffe Americano Medium, 16 fl.oz.	10	0	2
Caffe Latte Medium, 16 fl.oz.	260	14	21
Cappuccino Medium, 16 fl.oz.	150	8	13
• Caramel Macchiato Medium, 16 fl.oz.	430	12	68
Chai Latte Medium, 16 fl.oz.	380	14	51
Iced Caffe Latte Medium, 16 fl.oz.	150	8	13
Iced Caramel Macchiato Med, 16 fl.oz.	390	10	65
Iced Chai Latte Medium, 16 fl.oz.	260	7	42
Iced Decaf French Roast Coffee Med, 22 fl.oz.	10	0	2
Iced French Roast Coffee Med, 22 fl.oz.	10	0	2
Iced French Vanilla Coffee Med, 22 fl.oz.	10	0	2
Iced Mocha Latte Medium, 16 fl.oz.	300	15	40
Iced Vanilla Latte Medium, 16 fl.oz.	330	7	59
Iced White Chocolate Latte Medium, 16 fl.oz.	330	13	51
Mocha Latte Medium, 16 fl.oz.	390	20	48
Vanilla Latte Medium, 16 fl.oz.	410	12	66
White Chocolate Latte Medium, 16 fl.oz.	410	17	58
Breads			
Artisan Baguette Salad Size, 3 oz.	240	2	47
Artisan Baguette Sandwich Size, 4 oz.	310	2	62
Artisan Hny Multigrain Baguette Salad Size, 4 oz.	250	3	49
Artisan Hny Multigrain Baguette Sand Size, 5 oz.	340	4	66
Artisan Multigrain Bread, 4 oz.	280	3	53
Artisan Sundried Tomato Bread, 4 oz.	270	1	55
Asiago Breadstick, 2 oz.	180	4	28
Bacon And Cheese Mini Loaf, 5 oz.	570	33	52
Basil Pesto Cheese Toasts, 55 g	140	2	26
• Bread Bowl, 9 oz.	620	3	121
• Cheddar Jalapeño Breadstick, 2 oz.	130	2	25
Cheese Bread, 5 oz.	300	8	57
Ciabatta Small, 3 oz.	180	1	37
Cinnamon Raisin Breadstick, 2 oz.	180	0	40
Country White Bread, 4 oz.	270	1	56
Everything Breadstick, 2 oz.	170	3	31

Au Bon Pain (cont.)	Cal	Fat	Cbs
Breads (cont.)			
Farm House Rolls, 5 oz.	320	6	57
Focaccia, 5 oz.	350	7	61
Lahvash, 4 oz.	280	4	56
Rosemary Garlic Bread Stick, 2 oz.	180	5	30
Sesame Breadstick, 2 oz.	180	4	30
Soft Roll, 5 oz.	410	11	65
Breakfast Sandwiches			
• Bacon And Bagel, 4 oz.	340	6	57
Bacon And Egg Melt On Ciabatta, 8 oz.	500	26	40
Breakfast Quesadilla Sandwich, 8 oz.	550	24	56
Egg On A Bagel With Bacon And Cheese, 8 oz.	500	15	59
Egg On A Bagel With Bacon, 7 oz.	420	8	60
Egg On A Bagel With Cheese, 8 oz.	430	10	58
Egg On A Bagel, 7 oz.	360	4	59
Mediterranean Spinach Breakfast Sandwich, 8 oz.	520	15	19
Portobello, Egg And Cheddar, 8 oz.	490	26	41
Prosciutto & Egg On Asiago Bagel, 9 oz.	530	17	59
• Sausage, Egg & Cheddar On Asiago Bagel, 10 oz.	810	47	58
Smoked Salmon & Wasabi On Onion Dill Bgl, 7 oz.	430	11	64
Breakfast: Café Sandwiches			
Arizona Chicken Sandwich, 12 oz.	750	29	61
Baja Turkey Sandwich, 13 oz.	640	24	63
Caprese Sandwich, 12 oz.	700	35	65
Chicken Pesto Sandwich, 13 oz.	720	26	62
Chicken Tarragon Sandwich, 11 oz.	740	31	61
• Chilean Chicken Sandwich, 14 oz.	790	29	64
Ham & Cheddar Sandwich (On Ciabatta), 12 oz.	650	20	80
Mozzarella Chicken Sandwich, 14 oz.	750	25	67
Portobello And Goat Cheese Sandwich, 10 oz.	560	26	61
Prosciutto Mozzarella Sandwich, 12 oz.	770	41	64
Roast Beef Caesar Sandwich, 10 oz.	680	27	65
Smoked Turkey Club Sandwich, 12 oz.	780	43	56
• Spicy Tuna Sandwich, 10 oz.	500	18	59
The Montana, 13 oz.	560	23	62
Turkey And Cranberry Chutney Sandwich, 11 oz.	530	10	77
Turkey And Swiss Sandwich (On Baguette), 12 oz.	650	24	66
Breakfast: Hot Sandwiches and Melts			
• BBQ Chicken On Farmhouse Roll, 14 oz.	860	31	78
Cajun Shrimp Hot Wrap, 15 oz.	660	20	95
Eggplant & Mozzarella Sandwich, 12 oz.	670	31	70
• Mayan Chicken Hot Wrap, 14 oz.	590	15	92
Steak Teriyaki Hot Wrap, 14 oz.	620	15	96
Steakhouse On Ciabatta, 13 oz.	720	31	71
Tuna Melt, 13 oz.	670	30	62
Turkey Melt, 12 oz.	780	34	73
Breakfast: Wraps			
Cajun Shrimp Hot Wrap, 15 oz.	660	20	95
Chicken Caesar Asiago Wrap, 11 oz.	660	28	62
Chopped Turkey Cobb Wrap, 12 oz.	620	31	63
Fields And Feta Wrap, 13 oz.	500	21	67
Mayan Chicken Hot Wrap, 14 oz.	590	15	92
• Mediterranean Wrap, 13 oz.	360	31	73
• Southwest Tuna Wrap, 14 oz.	760	42	65
Steak Teriyaki Hot Wrap, 14 oz.	620	15	96
Thai Peanut Chicken Wrap, 13 oz.	620	22	76
Turkey Spinach Sonoma Wrap, 12 oz.	530	13	83
Dressings			
Balsamic Vinaigrette Dressing, 2 oz.	190	16	11
Blue Cheese Dressing, 2 oz.	230	24	2
Caesar Dressing, 2 oz.	280	28	4
• Fat Free Raspberry Vinaigrette (Low Fat), 2 oz.	70	0	17
• Hazelnut Vinaigrette Dressing, 2 oz.	330	31	10
Light Olive Oil Vinaigrette, 2 oz.	130	10	9
Light Ranch Dressing, 2 oz.	150	15	3

Au Bon Pain (cont.)

Dressings (cont.)	Cal	Fat	Cbs
Lite Honey Mustard Dressing, 2 oz.	180	11	21
Sesame Ginger Dressing, 2 oz.	280	25	13
Thai Peanut Dressing, 2 oz.	230	13	24
Harvest Rice Bowls			
Cajun Shrimp, 20 oz.	520	17	69
Cajun Shrimp w/ Brwn Rice, 20 oz.	560	20	73
• Mayan Chicken, 19 oz.	490	14	67
Mayan Chicken w/ Brown Rice, 19 oz.	540	16	71
Steak Teriyaki, 19 oz.	540	15	76
• Steak Teriyaki w/ Brown Rice, 19 oz.	590	18	80
Hot Entrées			
Beef Stroganoff, 1 oz.	35	3	2
Brown Rice, 1 oz.	35	1	6
Cheese Tortellini Primavera, 13 oz.	580	30	54
Chicken In Burgundy Wine Sauce, 1 oz.	30	1	2
Chicken Marsala, 1 oz.	30	2	2
• Chicken Penne Broccoli Alfredo, 17 oz.	700	31	47
Meat Lasagna, 11 oz.	480	28	29
Mediterranean Spinach & Chickpea Ragout, 1 oz.	20	0	4
Penne Marinara w/ Chicken And Vegetables, 1 oz.	30	1	3
Penne Marinara With Vegetables, 13 oz.	350	11	52
Penne w/ Chkn & Fire-Rsted Pepper Sauce, 17 oz.	620	19	58
Quinoa, 1 oz.	25	0	4
Roasted Carrots, 1 oz.	15	0	3
Roasted Green Beans With Almonds, 1 oz.	20	1	2
• Roasted Vegetable Provencal, 1 oz.	15	1	2
Salmon Provencal, 1 oz.	20	1	2
Spinach And Artichoke Lasagna, 12 oz.	410	16	43
White Bean Cacciatore, 1 oz.	20	1	3
Oatmeal			
• Oatmeal Large, 16 oz.	270	5	50
Oatmeal Medium, 12 oz.	210	4	38
• Oatmeal Small, 9 oz.	150	3	28
Pizzettas			
Spinach And Artichoke Pizzetta, 7 oz.	520	27	56
• Three Cheese Pizzetta, 9 oz.	700	41	55
Tomato, Mozzarella, Basil Pizzetta, 8 oz.	650	41	53
Portions			
Apples, Blue Cheese & Cranberries, 5 oz.	200	10	27
• Asparagus And Almonds, 3 oz.	70	6	5
BBQ Chicken, 5 oz.	170	2	13
Brie, Fruit And Crackers, 4 oz.	190	10	17
Cheddar, Fruit And Crackers, 4 oz.	190	11	17
Chickpea And Tomato Salad, 6 oz.	100	1	19
Herb Cheese, Fruit And Crackers, 4 oz.	180	11	19
Honey Mustard Chicken, 4 oz.	170	2	12
Hummus And Cucumber, 4 oz.	130	8	10
Mediterranean Tuna Salad, 4 oz.	120	8	4
• Mozzarella And Tomato, 5 oz.	200	15	5
Mozzarella, Olives, Roasted Peppers & Tom, 4 oz.	180	14	4
Smkd Tkey, Asprgs, Cran Chutney & Grgnzla, 5 oz.	140	5	10
Thai Peanut Chicken And Snow Peas, 5 oz.	200	7	7
Salads			
Caesar Asiago Salad (Side), 3 oz.	120	6	11
Caesar Asiago Salad, 6 oz.	210	12	18
Chef's Salad, 9 oz.	250	15	8
Chickpea & Tom Cucumber Salad, 11 oz.	230	12	23
Garden Salad, 7 oz.	70	2	12
Green Bean And Beet Salad, 12 oz.	210	8	27
Grilled Chicken Caesar Asiago, 9 oz.	340	13	19
• Mandarin Sesame Chicken Salad, 10 oz.	350	18	30
Mediterranean Chicken Salad, 10 oz.	330	16	12
Riviera Salad, 10 oz.	260	7	46
• Side Garden Salad, 4 oz.	50	2	8

Au Bon Pain (cont.)

Salads (cont.)	Cal	Fat	Cbs
Thai Peanut Chicken Salad, 11 oz.	240	8	19
Tuna Garden Salad, 11 oz.	250	13	14
Turkey Medallion Cobb Salad, 11 oz.	340	19	15
Turkey Spinach Sonoma Salad, 9 oz.	230	11	16
Snacks			
Assorted Nuts, 4 oz.	730	64	24
Chocolate Covered Almonds, 2 oz.	220	14	24
Chocolate Covered Pretzels, 30 g	140	6	20
• Chocolate Covered Strawberry, 1 oz.	30	2	4
Chocolate Nonpareils, 1 oz.	190	12	25
Dark Chocolate Cranberries, 1 oz.	170	9	27
Fruit Cup Small, 6 oz.	70	0	16
Fruit Sours, 4 oz.	400	0	105
Kookaburra Red Licorice, 1 oz.	140	1	30
Majuka Fruit Trail Mix, 1 oz.	140	7	17
Maple Roasted Cashews, 4 oz.	650	49	45
Muesli, 8 oz.	390	8	76
New Trail Mix, 1 oz.	120	5	20
Peach Gummies, 1 oz.	150	0	36
Summit Blend, 4 oz.	500	27	63
Tamari Almonds, 1 oz.	180	14	5
• Tamari Roast, 4 oz.	770	61	41
The 19th Hole Snack Mix, 1 oz.	160	9	15
Turkish Apricots, 1 oz.	120	0	29
Walnuts, 4 oz.	740	74	16
Soups - Medium			
• Baked Stuffed Potato, 12 oz.	350	21	30
Broccoli Cheddar Soup, 12 oz.	310	21	20
Carrot Ginger Soup, 12 oz.	130	5	21
Chicken And Dumpling Soup, 12 oz.	210	7	28
Chicken Florentine Soup, 12 oz.	240	13	25
Chicken Gumbo Soup, 12 fl.oz.	200	9	24
Chicken Noodle Soup (Low Fat), 12 oz.	130	3	20
Clam Chowder, 12 oz.	320	18	27
Corn And Green Chili Bisque, 12 oz.	250	14	29
Corn Chowder Medium, 12 oz.	350	18	40
Cream Of Chicken & Wild Rice Soup, 12 oz.	260	15	24
Curried Rice & Lentil Soup (Low Fat), 12 oz.	150	2	30
French Moroccan Tomato Lentil Soup, 12 oz.	180	2	32
French Onion Soup, 12 oz.	130	5	19
• Garden Vegetable Soup (Low Fat), 12 oz.	80	2	14
Gazpacho, 12 oz.	90	5	14
Harvest Pumpkin Soup, 12 oz.	190	10	26
Hearty Cabbage Soup, 12 oz.	110	5	14
Italian Wedding Soup, 12 oz.	170	7	19
Jamaican Black Bean Soup, 12 oz.	180	1	45
Mediterranean Pepper Soup, 12 oz.	100	3	18
Old Fashioned Tomato Rice, 12 oz.	120	1	24
Pasta E Fagioli Soup, 12 oz.	240	8	36
Portuguese Kale Soup, 12 oz.	120	5	15
Potato Cheese Soup, 12 oz.	250	14	25
Potato Leek Soup, 12 oz.	300	20	28
Rd Beans, Italian Sausage & Rice Soup, 12 oz.	200	5	38
Southern Black-eyed Pea Soup (Low Fat), 12 oz.	180	2	31
Southwest Tortilla Soup, 12 oz.	200	11	24
Southwest Vegetable Soup, 12 oz.	100	3	17
Split Pea With Ham Soup (Low Fat), 12 oz.	210	2	42
Thai Coconut Curry Soup, 12 oz.	150	7	20
Tomato Basil Bisque (Reduced Sodium), 12 oz.	210	8	29
Tomato Cheddar Soup, 12 oz.	240	15	17
Tomato Florentine Soup (Low Fat), 12 oz.	120	3	19
Tuscan Vegetable Soup, 12 oz.	170	5	24
Vegetable Beef Barley Soup (Low Fat), 12 oz.	140	3	21
Vegetarian Chili (Low Fat, Gluten Free), 12 oz.	230	3	40

Au Bon Pain (cont.)

	Cal	Fat	Cbs
Soups - Medium (cont.)			
Vegetarian Lentil Soup, 12 oz.	140	2	32
Vegetarian Minestrone Soup (Low Fat), 12 oz.	120	2	21
Wild Mushroom Bisque, 12 oz.	190	9	23
Stews			
Beef Stew Medium, 12 oz.	300	16	25
• Chicken Vegetable Stew Medium, 12 oz.	290	17	26
• Macaroni And Cheese Medium, 12 oz.	440	26	31
Toppings			
All Natural Chicken Breast, 4 oz.	150	2	2
Bacon, 1 oz.	80	7	0
Bagged Croutons, 2 oz.	180	5	29
Brie Cheese, 2 oz.	150	14	0
Cheddar Cheese, 2 oz.	160	13	1
Goat Cheese, 1 oz.	110	9	1
Gorgonzola Cheese, 2 oz.	210	18	1
Granola Topping, 2 oz.	220	6	37
Guacomole, 30 g	60	6	2
Ham, 4 oz.	100	4	0
Mozzarella Cheese, 2 oz.	160	9	3
Prosciutto, 2 oz.	105	6	2
Provolone Cheese, 2 oz.	140	10	1
Roast Beef, 4 oz.	150	6	0
Roasted Red Pepper Hummus, 2 oz.	80	5	6
• Roasted Red Peppers, 2 oz.	45	4	4
Sausage Patty, 2 oz.	210	20	0
Swiss Cheese, 2 oz.	150	12	1
• Tarragon Mayonnaise Sauce, 2 oz.	420	45	2
Tuna Salad Mix, 4 oz.	180	12	2
Turkey Breast, 4 oz.	120	2	4
Toppings: Dressings			
Balsamic Vinaigrette Dressing, 2 oz.	190	16	11
Blue Cheese Dressing, 2 oz.	230	24	2
Caesar Dressing, 2 oz.	280	28	4
• Fat Free Raspberry Vinaigrette, 2 oz.	70	0	17
• Hazelnut Vinaigrette Dressing, 2 oz.	330	31	10
Light Ranch Dressing, 2 oz.	150	15	3
Lite Honey Mustard Dressing, 2 oz.	180	11	21
Sesame Ginger Dressing, 2 oz.	280	25	13
Thai Peanut Dressing, 2 oz.	230	11	24
Toppings: Spreads			
Artichoke Aioli, 1 oz.	70	7	2
Basil Pesto, 1 oz.	140	15	1
Chili Dijon, 1 oz.	120	12	3
Herb Bagel Spread, 56 oz.	130	11	5
• Herb Mayonnaise, 1 oz.	210	23	1
Honey Mustard, 3 oz.	210	13	23
Honey Pecan Cream Cheese, 2 oz.	120	10	5
Jalapeño Mayonnaise, 1 oz.	60	6	1
Lite Cream Cheese Spread, 2 oz.	120	9	5
Mayonnaise, 1 oz.	90	8	1
• Mustard, 6 g	0	0	0
Plain Cream Cheese, 2 oz.	170	16	4
Strawberry Cream Cheese, 2 oz.	180	15	9
Sundried Tomato Cream Cheese, 2 oz.	120	10	5
Sun-dried Tomato Spread, 1 oz.	70	6	4
Vegetable Cream Cheese, 2 oz.	170	16	3
Yogurt - Small			
• Blueberry Yogurt w/ Granola & Fruit, 9 oz.	310	6	56
Blueberry Yogurt With Fruit (Low Fat), 8 oz.	220	2	44
Strawberry Yogurt w/ Granola & Blueberries, 9 oz.	310	6	56
Strawberry Yogurt w/ Blueberries (Low Fat), 8 oz.	220	2	44
Vanilla Yogurt w/ Granola & Blueberries, 9 oz.	310	6	56
• Vanilla Yogurt w/ Blueberries (Low Fat), 8 oz.	190	2	3

Auntie Anne's

	Cal	Fat	Cbs
Beverages			
Auntie Anne's Lemonade, 22 fl.oz.	180	0	43
Auntie Anne's Strawberry Lemonade, 22 fl.oz.	190	0	48
• Blue raspberry Dutch Ice®, 14 fl.oz.	165	0	38
Blue raspberry Dutch Smoothie, 14 fl.oz.	230	8	34
Caramel Dutch latté™, 14 fl.oz.	350	15	49
Chocolate Dutch Shake, 14 fl.oz.	580	27	75
Coffee Dutch latté™, 14 fl.oz.	290	14	38
Coffee Dutch Shake, 14 fl.oz.	590	27	77
Grape Dutch Ice®, 14 fl.oz.	180	0	43
Grape Dutch Smoothie, 14 fl.oz.	230	8	36
Kiwi-Banana Dutch Ice®, 14 fl.oz.	190	0	44
Kiwi-Banana Dutch Smoothie, 14 fl.oz.	240	8	38
Lemonade Dutch Ice®, 14 fl.oz.	315	0	77
Lemonade Dutch Smoothie, 14 fl.oz.	300	8	53
Mocha Dutch Ice®, 14 fl.oz.	400	10	74
Mocha Dutch latté™, 14 fl.oz.	360	17	47
Mocha Dutch Smoothie, 14 fl.oz.	330	13	50
Orange Creme Dutch Ice®, 14 fl.oz.	280	0	64
Orange Creme Dutch Smoothie, 14 fl.oz.	280	8	46
Piña Colada Dutch Ice®, 14 fl.oz.	220	0	53
Piña Colada Dutch Smoothie, 14 fl.oz.	260	8	44
Strawberry Dutch Ice®, 14 fl.oz.	220	0	50
• Strawberry Dutch Shake, 14 fl.oz.	610	27	78
Strawberry Dutch Smoothie, 14 fl.oz.	250	8	40
Strawberry Lemonade Dutch Ice, 14 fl.oz.	330	0	81
Vanilla Dutch Shake, 14 fl.oz.	510	27	58
Watermelon Dutch Ice®, 14 fl.oz.	200	0	50
Wild Cherry Dutch Ice®, 14 fl.oz.	210	0	48
Wild Cherry Dutch Smoothie, 14 fl.oz.	250	8	41
Dip Flavors			
• Caramel Dip, 2 oz.	135	3	27
Cheese Sauce Dip, 1 oz.	100	8	4
Hot Salsa Cheese Dip, 1 oz.	100	8	4
Light Cream Cheese Dip, 1 oz.	70	6	1
• Marinara Sauce Dip, 1 oz.	10	0	4
Sweet Mustard Dip, 1 oz.	60	2	8
Sweet Pretzel Dip, 1 oz.	40	0	10
Pretzels & More			
Almond Pretzel, 1 oz.	400	8	72
Almond Pretzel, no Butter, 1 oz.	350	2	72
Cinnamon Sugar Pretzel, 1 oz.	450	9	83
Cinnamon Sugar Pretzel, no Butter, 1 oz.	350	2	74
Garlic Pretzel, 1 oz.	350	5	68
Garlic Pretzel, no Butter, 1 oz.	320	1	66
• Glazin' Raisin®	510	4	107
Glazin' Raisin®, no Butter	470	1	104
Jalapeño	310	5	59
• Jalapeño, no Butter	270	1	58
Original	370	4	72
Original, no Butter	340	1	72
Pretzel Dog	290	16	25
Sesame	410	12	64
Sesame, no Butter	350	6	63
Sour Cream & Onion	340	5	66
Sour Cream & Onion, no butter	310	1	66
Stix, 6 sticks	370	4	72
Stix, no Butter, 6 sticks	340	1	72
Whole Wheat	370	5	72
Whole Wheat, no Butter	350	2	72

Baja Fresh

	Cal	Fat	Cbs
Americano Soft Taco			
Breaded Fish, 129 g	240	11	23
Carnitas, 142 g	250	12	21
• Chicken, 142 g	230	10	20

Baja Fresh (cont.)

	Cal	Fat	Cbs
Americano Soft Taco (cont.)			
Mahi Mahi, 150 g	240	10	20
Shrimp, 150 g	230	10	21
• Steak, 142 g	260	13	21
Baja Burrito			
Breaded Fish, 426 g	850	44	78
Carnitas, 440 g	830	45	67
Chicken, 440 g	790	38	65
Mahi Mahi, 451 g	780	38	66
• Shrimp, 454 g	760	37	66
• Steak, 437 g	850	46	67
Baja Ensalada®			
Charbroiled Chicken, 473 g	310	7	18
• Charbroiled Shrimp, 445 g	230	6	18
• Charbroiled Steak, 473 g	450	18	18
Savory Pork Carnitas, 473 g	370	18	20
Baja Fish Taco - Fried			
• Breaded Fish, 134 g	250	13	27
Complimentary Chips, 43 g	210	9	29
• Mahi Mahi Taco - Grilled, 177 g	230	9	26
Bean and Cheese Burritos			
Breaded Fish, 477 g	1030	41	108
Carnitas, 491 g	1010	42	98
Chicken, 491 g	970	35	96
Mahi Mahi, 502 g	960	35	96
• No Meat, 392 g	840	33	96
Shrimp, 505 g	950	34	96
• Steak, 488 g	1030	43	97
Burrito Mexicano			
Breaded Fish, 499 g	850	19	129
Carnitas, 514 g	830	20	119
Chicken, 514 g	790	13	117
Mahi Mahi, 525 g	791	13	117
• Shrimp, 528 g	770	13	117
• Steak, 511 g	860	21	118
Burrito Ultimo			
Breaded Fish, 465 g	940	42	96
Carnitas, 480 g	920	44	86
Chicken, 481 g	880	36	84
Mahi Mahi, 491 g	880	36	84
• Shrimp, 494 g	860	36	85
• Steak, 477 g	950	44	85
Chicken Tortilla Soup			
With Charbroiled Chicken, 388 g	320	14	29
Without Charbroiled Chicken, 354 g	270	14	29
"Enchilado" Style			
To Burrito add, 420 g	630	40	45
To "Burrito Dos Manos"® add, 839 g	1260	80	91
Fajitas			
Breaded Fish w/ Corn Tortillas, 817 g	1060	37	130
• Breaded Fish w/ Flour Tortillas, 876 g	1340	46	172
Breaded Fish w/ Mix Tortillas, 869 g	1260	43	162
Carnitas w/ Corn Tortillas, 788 g	920	34	108
Carnitas w/ Flour Tortillas, 847 g	1190	43	150
Carnitas w/ Mix Tortillas, 840 g	1120	40	140
Chicken w/ Corn Tortillas, 788 g	860	24	105
Chicken w/ Flour Tortillas, 847 g	1140	33	147
Chicken w/ Mix Tortillas, 840 g	1070	30	137
• Mahi Mahi w/ Corn Tortillas, 794 g	840	23	105
Mahi Mahi w/ Flour Tortillas, 853 g	1120	32	147
Mahi Mahi w/ Mix Tortillas, 846 g	1050	29	138
Shrimp w/ Corn Tortillas, 817 g	840	23	106
Shrimp w/ Flour Tortillas, 876 g	1120	32	148
Shrimp w/ Mix Tortillas, 869 g	1040	29	138
Steak w/ Corn Tortillas, 788 g	960	36	107

Baja Fresh (cont.)

	Cal	Fat	Cbs
Fajitas (cont.)			
Steak w/ Flour Tortillas, 847 g	1240	45	149
Steak w/ Mix Tortillas, 840 g	1170	42	139
Grilled Veggie			
Grilled Veggie, 506 g	800	33	94
Kids' Faves			
Chicken Taquitos, 304 g	630	33	60
Mini Bean & Cheese Burrito w/ Chicken, 382 g	590	15	84
• Mini Bean & Cheese Burrito, 348 g	540	14	84
• Mini Cheese Quesadilla w/ Chicken, 317 g	650	27	72
Mini Cheese Quesadilla, 283 g	610	26	72
Nachos			
Breaded Fish, 867 g	2090	116	176
Charbroiled Chicken, 882 g	2020	110	164
Charbroiled Mahi Mahi, 893 g	2020	110	164
Charbroiled Shrimp, 893 g	2000	110	164
• Charbroiled Steak, 879 g	2120	118	163
• Cheese, 782 g	1890	108	163
Savory Pork Carnitas, 882 g	2060	117	166
Original Baja Taco			
Carnitas, 116 g	220	7	29
Chicken, 116 g	210	5	28
• Shrimp, 125 g	200	5	28
• Steak, 113 g	230	8	28
Quesadilla			
Breaded Fish, 539 g	1400	86	96
Charbroiled Chicken, 553 g	1330	80	84
Charbroiled Mahi Mahi, 565 g	1330	79	84
Charbroiled Shrimp, 567 g	1310	79	84
• Charbroiled Steak, 550 g	1430	87	84
• Cheese, 454 g	1200	78	84
Savory Pork Carnitas, 553 g	1370	87	86
Veggie, 565 g	1260	78	96
Salad Dressing			
• Fat Free Salsa Verde, 71 g	15	0	3
• Olive Oil Vinaigrette, 71 g	290	31	2
Ranch Dressing, 71 g	260	26	4
Sides			
Black Beans, 327 g	360	3	61
Corn Tortilla Chips, 43 g	210	9	29
Pinto Beans, 300 g	320	1	56
• Pronto Guacamole, 170 g	560	34	60
Rice and Beans Plate, 325 g	420	5	72
Rice, 181 g	280	4	55
• Side Salad, 186 g	130	6	16
Tostada Salad			
Breaded Fish, 744 g	1200	61	111
Charbroiled Chicken, 758 g	1140	55	98
Charbroiled Mahi Mahi, 769 g	1130	55	99
Charbroiled Shrimp, 772 g	1120	55	99
• Charbroiled Steak, 755 g	1230	63	98
• No Meat, 659 g	1010	53	98
Savory Pork Carnitas, 758 g	1180	62	100

Baker's Drive-Thru

	Cal	Fat	Cbs
American Menu: Chicken Specialties			
• Caribbean Chicken Sandwich	398	18	41
• Grilled Chicken Sandwich w/o Dressing	273	8	31
Grilled Chicken Sandwich	380	18	35
Teriyaki Chicken Sandwich	386	18	36
American Menu: French Fries			
1/2 Pound Fries	759	40	96
• Budget Meal French Fries	223	12	28
• Chili Cheese Fries	988	59	102
Regular French Fries	357	19	45

Baker's Drive-Thru (cont.)

American Menu: Hamburgers	Cal	Fat	Cbs
Boca Burger w/Cheese & Dressing	391	19	39
• Boca Burger w/o Cheese & Dressing	211	2	35
Budget Meal Hamburger	294	12	28
Chicken Sandwich w/o Dressing	273	8	31
• Double Baker	696	43	34
Grilled Boca Burger w/o Cheese or Dressing	211	2	35
Grilled Boca Burger	391	19	39
Grilled Cheese Sandwich	363	22	28
Grilled Cheese	363	22	28
Old Fashioned Cheeseburger	462	26	33
Old Fashioned Hamburger	382	20	33
American Menu: Platters			
Chicken Burrito Platter	1013	47	108
Chicken Mexican Salad	678	38	50
Chicken Soft Taco Platter	726	34	71
• Combination Burrito Platter	1089	47	123
Ground Beef Mexican Salad	762	47	49
Ground Beef Taco Platter	753	38	69
Shredded Beef Burrito Platter	1035	44	107
Shredded Beef Mexican Salad	695	38	50
Shredded Beef Soft Taco Platter	672	26	72
• Vegetarian Mexican Salad - (all beans)	642	33	64
Breakfast			
Add Potato to any Breakfast Burrito	247	13	32
Chili & Egg Burrito	534	23	55
Chorizo & Egg Burrito	657	34	55
• Egg Burrito w/Beans & Meat	744	31	75
Egg Burrito	535	24	56
Egg Sandwich	467	31	33
• Egg Taco	177	11	11
Hash Browns	433	23	56
Machaca Burrito	623	26	57
Sausage & Egg Burrito	639	32	56
Sausage & Egg Sandwich	579	40	34
Mexican: Burritos			
• All Chicken Burrito w/o Cheese	438	14	56
All Chicken Burrito	524	21	57
Bean & Cheese Burrito	442	10	70
Cheese Burrito	650	35	54
Combination Burrito	601	22	72
Green Burrito	621	17	90
Ground Beef Burrito	675	32	55
Make it Big!	73	6	4
Mexican Rice & Bean Burrito	442	13	74
Red Burrito	621	17	90
Shredded Beef Burrito	546	18	57
• Veggie Wrap	736	27	108
Mexican: Extras			
Bean Cup w/o cheese	229	3	37
Bean Cup	315	10	37
Cheese Quesadilla	588	39	45
• Chili & Bean Cup	222	9	26
Guacamole & Chips	426	28	44
Mexican Rice Cup	284	6	52
• Nachos	1407	81	120
Taco Burger	270	10	30
Tostada	285	10	38
Mexican: Tacos			
Bean Taco	150	6	18
Chicken Soft Taco	169	9	12
• Soft Taco w/Shredded Beef	141	5	12
• Taco	182	11	11
Milkshake			
Butterfinger® Milkshake	715	36	88

Baker's Drive-Thru (cont.)

Milkshake (cont.)	Cal	Fat	Cbs
• Chocolate Milkshake	624	29	84
Oreo® Milkshake	718	35	90
• Snickers® Milkshake	722	38	85
Strawberry Milkshake	637	28	88
Vanilla Milkshake	634	28	86
Vegetarian			
• Boca Burger w/o Cheese or Dressing	211	2	35
Cheese Burrito	650	35	54
Green Burrito	621	17	90
Grilled Boca Burger	391	19	39
Grilled Cheese Sandwich	363	22	28
Red Burrito	621	17	90
Tostada Salad - Vegetarian Style	700	36	61
Vegetarian Combination w/o cheese	478	8	76
Vegetarian Combination	563	15	77
Vegetarian Sandwich	240	5	35
Vegetarian Soft Taco	145	3	19
Vegetarian Taco	170	6	19
• Veggie Wrap	736	27	108

Baker's Square

Breakfast	Cal	Fat	Cbs
Rise & Shine Breakfast	510	19	66
Sunrise Omelette	650	25	70
Entrees			
Chicken and Vegetable Stir-Fry	465	14	61
• Grilled Catch of the Day	390	19	32
Lemon Chicken	440	20	33
• Small Sirloin Steak	500	25	32
Pitas & Wraps			
Fajita Pita	610	22	65
Stir-Fry Pita	660	23	74
Salads			
Chicken Caesar Salad	315	15	14
Stir-Fry Salad	555	22	53

Baskin Robbins

Cappuccino Blasts®	Cal	Fat	Cbs
Caramel Medium, 24 fl.oz.	720	24	121
• Low Fat Small, 16 fl.oz.	220	2	45
Mocha Medium, 24 fl.oz.	240	18	87
Mocha w/ Whipped Cream Medium, 24 fl.oz.	620	21	100
Nonfat Medium, 24 fl.oz.	340	0	78
• Oreo® N' Cookies Medium, 24 fl.oz.	800	31	118
Original Medium, 24 fl.oz.	460	19	66
Turtle - Medium, 24 fl.oz.	710	23	121
Whipped Cream Medium, 24 fl.oz.	480	21	67
Fruit Blast - Medium			
• Berry Pomegranate Fruit Blast, 24 fl.oz.	210	0	128
• Strawberry Citrus Fruit Blast, 24 fl.oz.	480	1	122
Wild Mango Fruit Blast, 24 fl.oz.	470	2	116
Fruit Blast Smoothie - Medium			
Berry Pomegranate Banana, 24 fl.oz.	710	1	172
• Mango Fruit Blast Smoothie, 24 fl.oz.	620	2	148
• Strawberry Banana, 24 fl.oz.	730	2	178
Holiday & Special Occasion Ice Cream Cakes			
• Choco Chip Ice Cream/Devil's Food Heart, 125 g	330	18	40
• Vanilla Ice Crm/Devil's Food Heart, 125 g	340	19	39
Ice Cream: Classic Flavors			
Cherries Jubilee, 4 oz.	240	12	30
Choco Chip Cookie Dough Ice Crm, 4 oz.	290	15	36
Chocolate Chip Ice Cream, 4 oz.	270	16	28
Chocolate Fudge Ice Cream, 4 oz.	270	15	35
Chocolate Ice Cream, 4 oz.	260	14	33
French Vanilla Ice Cream, 4 oz.	280	18	26

Baskin Robbins (cont.)

	Cal	Fat	Cbs
Ice Cream: Classic Flavors (cont.)			
Gold Medal Ribbon® Ice Cream, 4 oz.	260	13	34
Heath® Bar Crunch Ice Cream, 4 oz.	300	15	38
Jamoca® Almond Fudge Ice Cream, 4 oz.	270	15	31
Jamoca® Ice Cream, 4 oz.	240	13	26
Mint Chocolate Chip Ice Cream, 4 oz.	270	16	28
Nutty Coconut Ice Cream, 4 oz.	300	20	28
Old Fashioned Butter Pecan Ice Crm, 4 oz.	280	18	24
Oreo® Cookies 'n Cream Ice Crm, 4 oz.	280	15	32
• Peanut Butter 'n Chocolate Ice Crm, 4 oz.	320	20	31
Pistachio Almond Ice Cream, 4 oz.	290	19	25
Pralines 'n Cream Ice Cream, 4 oz.	270	14	34
Reese's® PB Cup Ice Cream, 4 oz.	300	18	31
Rocky Road Ice Cream, 4 oz.	290	15	36
Strawberry Cheesecake Ice Cream, 4 oz.	270	14	32
Vanilla Ice Cream, 4 oz.	260	16	26
• Very Berry Strawberry Ice Cream, 4 oz.	220	11	28
World Class® Chocolate Ice Cream, 4 oz.	280	16	31
Ice Cream: Seasonal Flavors			
Baseball Nut™ Ice Cream, 4 oz.	270	14	32
Black Walnut Ice Cream, 4 oz.	280	19	25
Chocolate Almond Ice Cream, 4 oz.	300	18	30
• Choco Mousse Royale® Ice Cream, 4 oz.	310	18	35
Chocolate Oreo® Ice Cream, 4 oz.	300	16	38
Creole Cream Cheese Ice Cream, 4 oz.	190	7	28
Egg Nog Ice Cream, 4 oz.	200	7	30
German Chocolate Cake Ice Cream, 4 oz.	300	16	37
Icing on the Cake Ice Cream, 4 oz.	290	15	35
Jamoca® Oreo® Ice Cream, 4 oz.	270	12	36
Lemon Custard Ice Cream, 4 oz.	260	13	30
Mississippi Mud Ice Cream, 4 oz.	270	13	38
New York Cheesecake Ice Cream, 4 oz.	230	10	30
Peppermint Ice Cream, 4 oz.	270	14	32
Pink Bubblegum Ice Cream, 4 oz.	260	12	36
• Pumpkin Pie Ice Cream, 4 oz.	180	6	29
Quarterback Crunch Ice Cream, 4 oz.	250	12	33
Rum Raisin Ice Cream, 4 oz.	250	11	34
Winter White Chocolate Ice Cream, 4 oz.	220	9	30
Lighter Side: Ice			
Lime Daiquiri Ice, 4 oz.	130	0	33
Lighter Side: Low Fat Ice Cream - No Sugar Added			
• Berries 'n Banana, 4 oz.	110	2	25
• Chocolate Chocolate Chip, 4 oz.	150	5	31
Pineapple Coconut, 4 oz.	120	2	27
Lighter Side: Low Fat Yogurt			
Raspberry Cheese Louise Frozen Yogurt, 4 oz.	190	4	35
Lighter Side: Nonfat Soft Serve Yogurt - No Sugar Added			
• Truly Free® Cafe Mocha, 88 g	90	0	18
• Truly Free® Chocolate, 1/2 cup, 88 g	80	0	15
Truly Free® Vanilla, 1/2 cup, 88 g	90	0	17
Lighter Side: Nonfat Yogurt			
Vanilla Nonfat Yogurt, 4 oz.	150	0	32
Lighter Side: Sherbet			
Orange Sherbet, 4 oz.	160	2	34
Rainbow Sherbet, 4 oz.	160	2	34
• Rock 'n Pop Swirl Sherbet, 4 oz.	190	4	37
• Wild 'N Reckless Sherbet, 4 oz.	160	2	33
Roll Ice Cream Cakes			
Chocolate Chip Ice Cream/Chocolate, 117 g	290	15	41
Mint Chocolate Chip Ice Cream/Chocolate, 117 g	290	14	36
• Vanilla Ice Cream/Chocolate, 117 g	270	14	39
Round Ice Cream Cakes			
• Choco Chp Cookie Dgh Ice Crm/Dvl's Fd 6, 161 g	460	23	59
Choco Chip Ice Cream/Devil's Food 9, 161 g	410	23	51
Oreo® Cookies 'n Crm Ice Crm/Dvl's Fd 6, 161 g	440	23	56

Baskin Robbins (cont.)

	Cal	Fat	Cbs
Round Ice Cream Cakes (cont.)			
Oreo® Cookies 'n Crm Ice Crm/Dvl's Food 9, 161 g	430	23	55
Pralines 'n Cream Ice Crm/White Sponge 9, 161 g	430	20	65
• Vanilla & Choco Ice Cream/Fudge Crunch 9, 123 g	340	18	41
Shakes - Medium			
• Choco Oreo® Shake, 633 g	1350	69	172
Choco Shake with Choco Ice Cream, 24 fl.oz.	990	40	149
Choco Shake with Vanilla Ice Cream, 24 fl.oz.	1000	45	133
Heath® Bar Crunch Shake, 24 fl.oz.	1340	66	167
Jamoca® Oreo® Shake, 625 g	1170	44	177
Mint Chocolate Chip Shake, 24 fl.oz.	970	47	116
Peppermint Shake, 612 g	930	32	145
Reese's® Peanut Butter Cup Shake, 24 fl.oz.	1340	92	105
• Strawberry w/ Very Brry Strwbrry Ice Crm, 24 fl.oz.	650	19	104
Vanilla Shake, 24 fl. oz.	980	45	125
Sheet Ice Cream Cakes			
Chocolate Chip Ice Cream/Devil's Food, 126 g	330	18	41
Mint Chocolate Chip Ice Cream/Devil's Food, 126 g	330	18	41
Oreo® Cookies 'n Crm Ice Crm/Wh Spnge, 126 g	350	16	47
• Pralines 'n Cream Ice Cream/White Sponge, 126 g	360	16	49
Vanilla & Choco Ice Cream/Fudge Crunch, 126 g	330	18	40
Vanilla Ice Cream/Devil's Food, 126 g	340	19	39
• Very Brry Strawberry Ice Crm/White Spnge, 126 g	310	13	44
Sundaes			
• 2 Scoop Hot Fudge Sundae, 203 g	530	29	62
3 Scoop Hot Fudge Sundae, 288 g	750	41	86
Banana Royale Sundae, 316 g	630	27	91
Banana Split Sundae, 570 g	1030	39	168
Brownie Sundae, 303 g	890	42	123
Candy Rush Sundae, 258 g	850	40	115
Heath® Bar Crunch Sundae, 370 g	1210	59	160
Oreo® Sundae, 347 g	1030	47	147
• Peppermint Brownie Sundae, 512 g	1580	75	221
Reese's® Peanut Butter Cup Sundae, 372 g	1400	90	124

BD's Mongolian Barbecue

	Cal	Fat	Cbs
Meats			
Chicken, 3 oz.	102	3	0
Lamb, 3 oz.	126	7	0
• NY Strip, 3 oz.	79	1	1
Pork, 3 oz.	123	5	0
Ribeye, 3 oz.	123	4	0
• Sausage, 3 oz.	273	26	2
Turkey, 3 oz.	102	3	0
Noodles			
• Lo Mein, 2 oz.	161	1	33
• Pasta, 2 oz.	210	1	42
Rice			
Rice, 3/4 cup	160	0	35
Salad Dressings			
Balsamic Vinaigrette, 1 oz.	60	5	4
• Blue Cheese, 1 oz.	160	17	2
Caesar, 1 oz.	150	16	29
• FAT FREE French, 1 oz.	30	0	8
Greek Feta, 1 oz.	70	5	1
Honey Mustard, 1 oz.	160	16	5
Raspberry Vinaigrette, 1 oz.	35	0	8
Sauces			
Barbecue, 1 oz.	41	0	9
Black Bean, 1 oz.	34	1	3
Chili Garlic, 1 oz.	40	3	3
Fajita, 1 oz.	27	2	2
Kung Pao, 1 oz.	34	1	7
Lemon, 1 oz.	23	0	6
• Lite Soy, 1 oz.	10	0	1
Mongo Marinara, 1 oz.	17	0	3

BD's Mongolian Barbecue (cont.)

	Cal	Fat	Cbs
Sauces (cont.)			
Mongolian Ginger, 1 oz.	42	1	7
• Peanut, 1 oz.	96	8	4
Sesame Oil, 0.5 oz.	60	7	0
Shiitake Mushroom, 1 oz.	27	0	5
Spicy Buffalo, 1 oz.	40	5	0
Sweet & Sour, 1 oz.	35	0	8
Teriyaki, 1 oz.	27	0	7
Seafood			
Calamari, 3 oz.	78	1	3
Cod, 3 oz.	69	1	0
Crawfish, 3 oz.	80	2	0
Krab (Surimi), 3 oz.	85	1	9
• Salmon, 3 oz.	156	10	0
Scallops, 3 oz.	84	1	3
• Shrimp, 3 oz.	65	0	0
Tuna, 3 oz.	112	4	0
Soups			
• Chicken Noodle, 8 oz.	70	2	10
Clam Chowder, 8 oz.	200	9	18
Country Potato, 8 oz.	220	10	21
Hearty Vegetable, 8 oz.	60	5	12
Hot and Sour, 8 oz.	90	4	10
Mangia Mangia Mushroom, 8 oz.	220	15	18
Mushroom Bisque, 8 oz.	180	9	16
• Tomato Bisque, 8 oz.	310	26	17
Vegetarian Chili, 8 oz.	140	2	26
Tortillas			
Tortillas, 1 oz.	100	3	15
Vegetables			
Artichoke, 1 oz.	8	0	2
Bean Sprouts, 1 oz.	29	0	2
Beets, 1 oz.	10	0	2
Black Olives, 1 oz.	53	5	2
Bok Choy, 1 oz.	2	1	0
Broccoli, 1 oz.	8	1	2
Cabbage (Green), 1 oz.	7	1	2
Cabbage (Red), 1 oz.	6	1	1
Carrots, 1 oz.	12	1	3
Celery, 1 oz.	5	0	1
• Cheddar Cheese, 1 oz.	120	10	1
• Cilantro, 1 tsp	0	0	0
Corn (Baby), 1 oz.	6	0	1
Crouton, 7 pieces	35	2	4
Cucumbers, 1 oz.	4	1	1
Head Lettuce, 1 leaf	1	0	0
Lemons, 1 wedge	2	0	1
Limes, 1 lime	20	1	7
Mushrooms, 1 oz.	7	1	1
Onions (Yellow), 1 oz.	11	1	2
Pea Pods, 1 oz.	11	1	3
Peppers (Green), 1 oz.	8	0	2
Peppers (Red), 1 oz.	9	1	2
Pineapple, 1 oz.	14	0	3
Romaine Lettuce, 1 oz.	1	0	0
Water Chestnuts, 1 oz.	9	0	2

Ben & Jerry's

	Cal	Fat	Cbs
Scoop Shop			
Banana Split, 85 g	210	12	22
Bananas On The Run, 90 g	210	10	27
• Berry Berry Extraordinary Sorbet, 92 g	100	0	27
Black Raspberry Frozen Yogurt, 93 g	140	2	28
Butter Pecan, 86 g	260	25	17
Cake Batter, 92 g	243	15	25
Cherry Garcia, 87 g	200	11	23

Ben & Jerry's (cont.)

	Cal	Fat	Cbs
Scoop Shop (cont.)			
Chocolate Chip Cookie Dough, 87 g	220	12	26
Chocolate Fudge Brownie Frozen Yogurt, 94 g	160	3	32
Chocolate Fudge Brownie, 87 g	220	11	27
Chocolate Peanut Butter Swirl, 89 g	250	17	22
Chocolate Therapy, 86 g	210	12	25
Chocolate, 88 g	200	12	21
Chunky Monkey, 87 g	240	14	24
Cinnamon Buns, 88 g	240	12	30
Coconut Almond Fudge Chip, 88 g	230	17	21
• Coconut Seven Layer Bar, 92 g	277	18	26
Coffee, 88 g	190	11	18
Coffee, Coffee BuzzBuzzBuzz!, 88 g	230	14	23
Half Baked Frozen Yogurt, 85 g	160	3	31
Imagine Whirled Peace, 1/2 cup	252	15	27
Jamaican Me Crazy Sorbet, 144 g	140	0	37
Lemonade Sorbet, 88 g	100	0	26
Mango Mango Sorbet, 91 g	100	0	27
Mint Chocolate Chunk, 88 g	230	14	23
New York Super Fudge Chunk, 1/2 cup	250	17	24
One Cheesecake Brownie, 92 g	235	14	24
Phish Food, 88 g	230	11	33
Pumpkin Cheesecake, 88 g	230	12	26
Strawberry Cheesecake, 87 g	210	11	24
Strawberry Kiwi Sorbet, 92 g	100	0	27
Strawberry, 87 g	170	9	20
Sweet Cream & Cookies, 88 g	220	13	24
Triple Cream Chunk, 88 g	230	12	28
Vanilla Frozen Yogurt, 94 g	130	2	25
Vanilla Fudge Chip, 80 g	180	13	20
Vanilla Heath Bar Crunch, 82 g	240	14	24
Vanilla, 88 g	190	12	18

Big Apple Bagels

	Cal	Fat	Cbs
BAB's Choice Bagels			
Blueberry Cobbler, 70 g	196	4	35
• Cheddar Nacho, 70 g	176	3	30
Cinnamon Apple Pie, 70 g	193	4	34
• Cinnamon Bun, 70 g	200	4	35
Cinnamon Danish, 70 g	198	4	36
French Toast, 70 g	186	2	37
Quiche Lorraine, 70 g	177	4	27
Strawberry White Chocolate, 70 g	182	2	36
Swiss Melt, 70 g	184	4	29
White Chocolate Swirl, 70 g	198	4	35
Big Apple Bagels® Regular Bagels			
Apple Cinnamon, 70 g	166	1	35
Banana Nut, 70 g	170	1	34
Blueberry, 70 g	165	1	34
Cheddar Herb, 70 g	176	3	30
Chocolate Chip, 70 g	174	1	34
Cinnamon Raisin, 70 g	168	1	35
Cinnamon Sugar, 70 g	175	1	37
Cranberry Walnut, 70 g	176	1	36
Egg, 70 g	164	1	33
Everything, 70 g	168	1	34
Garlic, 70 g	165	1	34
Honey Oat, 70 g	160	1	34
Jalapeño, 70 g	175	3	30
Onion, 70 g	168	1	35
Plain, 70 g	167	1	34
Poppy, 70 g	172	1	34
Pumpernickel, 70 g	166	1	34
Salt, 70 g	162	1	33
• Sesame, 70 g	179	2	33

Big Apple Bagels (cont.)	Cal	Fat	Cbs
Big Apple Bagels® Regular Bagels (cont.)			
Spinach, 70 g	178	1	36
Strawberry, 70 g	171	1	36
Tomato Basil, 70 g	161	1	33
• Vegetable, 70 g	159	1	33
Wheat, 70 g	165	1	34
Breakfast Sandwiches			
• Breakfast B.L.T., 9 oz.	704	31	83
Lox & Cream Cheese, 11 oz.	602	21	78
• Morning Classic, 8 oz.	486	11	73
Northern Omelette, 10 oz.	699	31	73
So. Tradition (w/bacon), 8 oz.	566	18	73
So. Tradition (w/ham), 9 oz.	547	15	73
So. Tradition (w/sausage), 10 oz.	696	31	73
Build Your Own Sandwiches			
Ham, 10 oz.	490	9	77
Roast Beef, 10 oz.	480	6	77
• Tuna, 10 oz.	547	14	77
• Turkey, 10 oz.	465	3	77
Classic Recipe Cream Cheese			
Cheddar Jalapeño, 30 g	90	8	2
• Garden Vegetable, 30 g	90	9	2
Onion Chive, 30 g	80	8	2
• Plain Lite, 30 g	60	5	3
Plain, 30 g	90	9	2
Strawberry, 30 g	90	7	5
Gourmet Salads			
Calypso Chicken Salad, 14 oz.	637	49	34
Chicken Caesar Salad, 12 oz.	524	41	15
Classic Caesar Cafe Salad, 4 oz.	225	19	9
Classic Caesar Salad, 8 oz.	414	36	12
• Garden Mix Cafe Salad (w/o egg), 7 oz.	63	2	9
Garden Mix Cafe Salad, 7 oz.	100	5	9
Garden Mix Salad (w/o egg), 12 oz.	123	4	18
Garden Mix Salad, 12 oz.	197	9	18
Grilled Chicken Club Salad, 18 oz.	820	69	16
• Mediterranean Bread Salad, 19 oz.	973	73	52
Gourmet Sandwiches			
Classic Turkey, 10 oz.	552	14	74
• Holey Guacamole, 11 oz.	476	5	76
• Kick-N Roast Beef, 11 oz.	579	15	79
Mediterranean Veg-Out, 11 oz.	506	9	90
Icepresso Drinks			
Caramel Decadence Icepresso, 16 oz.	300	12	42
• Classic Icepresso, 16 oz.	300	5	52
• Java Chip Icepresso, 16 oz.	360	18	48
Latte Icepresso, 16 oz.	300	12	42
Mocha Icepresso, 16 oz.	301	12	42
Strawberry Icepresso, 16 oz.	340	12	56
Low Carb Entrees			
Chicken Caesar Salad, 11 oz.	482	39	9
Deli Meat & Cheese Plate, 8 oz.	533	37	3
Garden Mix Salad, 15 oz.	564	51	12
Ham & Cheese Omelette, 13 oz.	679	49	6
Kick-n Chicken Plate, 9 oz.	382	22	10
• Three Cheese Omelette, 13 oz.	860	61	8
Tuna Salad Plate, 9 oz.	356	25	3
Muffins			
• Fat Free Blueberry, 55 g	108	0	26
Fat Free Cherry Pie, 55 g	109	0	24
Fat Free Chocolate Marble, 55 g	125	0	29
• Fat Free Cinnamon Bun, 55 g	168	0	42
Fat Free Raspberry Amaretto, 55 g	127	0	31
My Favorite Muffin® Bagels			
• Blueberry, 113 g	320	2	66

Big Apple Bagels (cont.)	Cal	Fat	Cbs
My Favorite Muffin® Bagels (cont.)			
Cinnamon Raisin, 113 g	310	1	66
Honey Grain, 113 g	310	3	61
Plain, 113 g	310	1	64
Russian Black Bread, 113 g	320	1	67
• Sour Dough, 113 g	310	1	64
Whole Wheat, 113 g	310	2	66
Other Specialty Drinks			
• Americano, 16 oz.	12	0	2
Black Forest Coffee, 16 oz.	198	5	37
• Cafe Caramello, 16 oz.	212	8	31
Overstuffed Sandwiches			
Classic Reuben, 14 oz.	962	43	57
Corned Beef, 11 oz.	661	19	77
Ham and Cheese, 14 oz.	889	36	79
• Manhattan Club, 16 oz.	1122	40	120
• Pastrami, 11 oz.	661	19	77
TD California Club, 16 oz.	759	12	113
TD Classic Club, 19 oz.	1119	43	122
TD The Clubhouse, 15 oz.	1079	37	117
Pizzaah! Sandwiches (per piece)			
• Bruschetta Pizzaah, 13 oz.	162	12	7
Cheese Pizzaah, 11 oz.	189	7	23
Grilled Chicken Bruschetta Pizzaah, 14 oz.	343	21	24
• Pepperoni Pizzaah, 14 oz.	398	26	23
Sausage Pizzaah, 14 oz.	211	17	6
Veggie Pizzaah, 12 oz.	238	10	32
Regular Muffins			
Pumpkin Spice, 55 g	181	8	26
Lemon Poppyseed, 55 g	201	10	25
Golden Corn Bread, 55 g	197	9	26
Double Chocolate, 55 g	201	9	28
Deep Dish Apple Pie, 55 g	177	8	25
• Cinnamon Swirl Cheesecake, 55 g	214	11	28
Cinnamon Crumb Cake, 55 g	212	13	21
Chocolate Chip, 55 g	211	11	27
Chocolate Cheesecake, 55 g	202	12	22
Cherry Cheesecake, 55 g	170	10	19
Boston Cream Pie, 55 g	176	7	26
• Blueberry, 55 g	168	8	22
Blueberry Cheesecake, 55 g	199	12	20
Banana Nut, 55 g	195	11	21
Salads: Prepared with Lite Italian Dressing			
Calypso Chicken Salad, 14 oz.	317	17	22
Chicken Caesar Salad, 12 oz.	268	12	17
• Classic Caesar Salad, 8 oz.	158	8	14
Grilled Chicken Club Salad, 18 oz.	500	31	18
• Mediterranean Bread Salad, 19 oz.	626	32	55
Snacks			
• Enchilada Bagellata, 8 oz.	522	11	84
• Pizza Bagel, 8 oz.	481	6	85
Soups			
Beef Barley Mushroom, 8 oz.	100	3	12
Beef Pot Roast, 8 oz.	110	4	12
Boston Clam Chowder, 8 oz.	210	13	20
California Medley, 8 oz.	170	9	16
• Cheese & Bacon, 8 oz.	310	21	18
Chicken & Dumplings, 8 oz.	250	14	20
Chicken & Wild Rice, 8 oz.	190	9	22
Chicken Gumbo, 8 oz.	130	3	19
Chicken Noodle, 8 oz.	110	4	12
Country Bean, 8 oz.	140	2	24
Cream of Broccoli (w/Cheese), 8 oz.	170	11	15
Cream of Broccoli (w/o Cheese), 8 oz.	230	17	17
Cream of Potato, 8 oz.	240	14	24

RESTAURANTS & FAST-FOOD CHAINS

Big Apple Bagels (cont.)

	Cal	Fat	Cbs
Soups (cont.)			
• French Onion, 8 oz.	60	2	9
Garden Vegetable, 8 oz.	110	1	22
Hearty Vegetable Beef, 8 oz.	100	1	16
Minestrone, 8 oz.	150	3	26
Navy Bean w/Ham, 8 oz.	110	2	23
New England Clam Chowder, 8 oz.	220	13	21
Potato Chowder, 8 oz.	210	13	20
Sirloin Beef w/Pasta, 8 oz.	190	7	22
Split Pea w/Ham, 8 oz.	90	2	15
Turkey & Sausage Gumbo, 8 oz.	190	10	14
Vegetable Beef, 8 oz.	110	3	16
Wisconsin Cheese, 8 oz.	210	11	20
Specialty Drinks (prepared with 2% milk)			
Cappuccino, 16 oz.	195	7	20
Cinnamon Toast Latte, 16 oz.	299	7	45
Creme Caramel Latte, 16 oz.	303	7	47
Italiano, 16 oz.	131	5	13
Jittery Monkey, 16 oz.	482	11	82
Latte, 16 oz.	212	7	22
Mocha w/whipped cream, 16 oz.	454	12	71
Oregon Chai® Tea Latte, 16 oz.	274	5	48
Raspberry Cheesecake Latte, 16 oz.	319	7	51
• Turtle Mocha, 16 oz.	577	17	91
Vanilla Creme Latte, 16 oz.	275	7	39
Specialty Drinks (prepared with fat free milk)			
Cappuccino, 16 oz.	133	1	18
Cinnamon Toast Latte, 16 oz.	240	1	44
Creme Caramel Latte, 16 oz.	244	1	45
• Italiano, 16 oz.	89	1	12
Jittery Monkey, 16 oz.	429	6	80
Latte, 16 oz.	145	1	20
Mocha w/whipped cream, 16 oz.	392	6	70
Oregon Chai® Tea Latte, 16 oz.	231	1	47
Raspberry Cheesecake Latte, 16 oz.	259	1	50
Turtle Mocha, 16 oz.	522	12	90
Vanilla Creme Latte, 16 oz.	132	1	18
Specialty Sandwiches			
All-American Duo, 13 oz.	752	28	78
• Big Apple Club, 11 oz.	797	37	75
Chicken Caesar, 11 oz.	611	19	78
• Grilled Chicken, 10 oz.	571	17	77
Roma Italian, 13 oz.	764	34	76
Turkey Club, 11 oz.	782	34	75
Toasted Sandwiches			
• Cafe Chicken Melt, 14 oz.	815	32	80
Deli-Style Turkey, 12 oz.	732	25	76
• Roast Beef Parmesan Grinder, 11 oz.	583	15	76
Spicy Italian Sub, 14 oz.	770	34	77
Tuna Melt, 10 oz.	641	23	75
Whipped Cream Cheese			
Brown Sugar Cinnamon, 20 g	70	5	5
• Classic Plain, 20 g	70	7	1
• Reduced Fat Spring Veggie, 20 g	60	5	2

Big Boy

	Cal	Fat	Cbs
Beverages			
Chocolate Float w/Pepsi	195	5	38
Chocolate Malt	290	16	31
Chocolate Milk Shake, Plain	276	15	30
w/ Chocolate Syrup	382	16	57
w/ Fudge Topping	377	18	48
French Vanilla Malt	300	17	29
French Vanilla Milk Float w/Pepsi	200	6	37
French Vanilla Milk Shake, Plain	286	16	28
Strawberry Waffle Topping Add	386	16	53

Big Boy (cont.)

	Cal	Fat	Cbs
Beverages (cont.)			
w/ Caramel Topping	387	19	46
• w/ Chocolate Syrup	392	17	55
w/ Fudge Topping	387	19	46
French Vanilla Root Beer Float	202	6	36
• Frozen Yogurt Shake	158	0	33
Fruit Works Large, 16 fl.oz.	168	0	43
Sierra Mist Float	200	6	36
Strawberry Float w/Pepsi	190	5	37
Strawberry Malt	280	16	31
Strawberry Milk Shake, Plain	266	15	29
w/ Strawberry Topping	366	15	54
Breakfast			
Belgian Waffle w/Powdered Sugar, 1 waffle	526	25	65
w/ Apple Topping, 1 waffle	746	26	122
w/ Strawberry Topping, 1 waffle	836	26	145
Big Boy Fave No Meat No Grain Product , 2 eggs	440	32	25
Biscuits Buttered, 2 Biscuits	460	24	54
Biscuits Plain, 2 Biscuits	424	20	54
Canadian Bacon, 2 sl.	146	7	2
Cinnamon French Toast, 2 sl.	472	8	88
Cinnamon Roll, 2 oz.	218	8	34
Country Biscuits& Sausage Gravy	924	54	93
Country Gravy w/ Sausage, 2 oz.	96	8	4
Danish, Pieces, 1 oz.	100	4	15
Deli Rye Bread Toasted Buttered, 2 sl.	284	7	45
Deli Rye Bread Toasted Plain, 2 sl.	248	3	45
Egg (Texas Toast) Bread Plain, 2 sl.	284	4	52
Egg (Texas Toast) Buttered, 2 sl.	320	8	52
Eggs Benedict	947	61	60
English Muffin Plain, 1 muffin	140	2	27
English Muffin w/ Butter, 1 muffin	176	6	27
French Toast, 2 sl.	365	7	363
H.S Egg Beaters Chz Omelet w/2 Sl. Dry Toast	322	8	39
H.S Egg Beaters Plain Omelet w/2 Sl. Dry Toast	283	6	38
H.S Egg Beaters Scrambled Eggs w/2 Sl. Dry Toast	283	6	38
H.S Egg Beaters Veggie Omelet w/2 Sl. Dry Toast	317	6	45
Hash Brown Potatoes, 4 oz.	254	18	23
Hot Cakes w/ Apple Top, no syrup, 3 hot cakes	1330	26	243
Hot Cakes w/ Blueberries, no syrup, 3 hot cakes	1115	26	187
• Hot Cakes w/ Strwbrry Top, no syrup, 3 hot cakes	1420	26	266
Hot Cakes, No Syrup, 3 hot cakes	1110	25	186
Multi-Grain Hot cakes Plain, 1 order	698	25	105
Omelet Cheese w/ Toast	866	53	61
w/ 2-2 oz. Hotcakes, No Syrup	1002	54	87
w/ Biscuits	1092	70	79
Omelet Farmer's w/ Toast	899	51	69
w/ 2-2 oz. Hotcakes, No Syrup	1035	53	95
w/ Biscuits	1125	68	87
Omelet Ham &Cheese w/ Toast	902	53	61
w/ 2-2 oz. Hotcakes, No Syrup	1038	54	87
w/ Biscuits	1128	70	79
Omelet Mexican Fiesta w/ Toast	896	52	67
w/ 2-2 oz. Hotcakes, No Syrup	1032	53	93
w/ Biscuits	1112	69	85
Omelet Plain w/ Toast	749	44	59
w/ 2 Hotcakes, No Syrup	885	45	85
w/ Biscuits	975	61	77
Omelet Southern Country w/ Toast	1102	70	72
w/ 2-2 oz. Hotcakes, No Syrup	1234	71	98
w/ Biscuits	1328	87	90
Omelet Vegetarian w/ Toast	782	44	66
w/ 2-2 oz. Hotcakes, No Syrup	918	46	92
w/ Biscuits	1008	61	84
Pecan Roll Plain, 1 Roll	419	30	35

RESTAURANTS & FAST-FOOD CHAINS

Big Boy (cont.)

Breakfast (cont.)	Cal	Fat	Cbs
Pork Sausage Links, 2 links	133	11	1
Pork Sausage Patties, 1 patty	134	11	3
Potato Pancakes Plain, 1 order	404	14	68
Seasoned Brawny Lad Patty, 1 patty	246	17	0
• Sliced Bacon, 2 sl.	75	1	0
Sliced Breakfast Ham, 1/2 sl.	311	21	1
White Bread Toasted Buttered, 2 sl.	234	7	36
White Bread Toasted Plain, 2 sl.	198	3	36
Whole Wheat Bread Toasted Buttered, 2 sl.	228	7	36
Whole Wheat Bread Toasted Plain, 2 sl.	192	3	36
Desserts			
Apple and Ice Cream Puff	579	30	73
Banana Cream Pie, 1 slice	368	22	39
• Banana Split	709	26	114
Butter Pecan Ice Cream, 2 scoops	200	12	20
Butter Pecan Super Sunday	221	13	23
w/ Caramel Topping	433	19	62
w/ Chocolate Syrup	433	14	76
w/ Fudge Topping	422	19	59
Chocolate Ice Cream, 2 scoops	190	10	22
Chocolate Super Sundae, Plain	211	11	25
w/ Caramel Topping	421	17	64
w/ Chocolate Syrup	423	12	78
w/ Fudge Topping	412	17	61
Coconut Cream Pie, 1 slice	402	29	34
Crumb Cherry Pie, 1 slice	466	10	60
French Silk Cream Pie, 1 slice	524	35	48
French Vanilla Ice Cream	200	11	20
French Vanilla Sundae, Plain	121	7	13
French Vanilla Super Sundae, Plain	221	12	23
w/ Caramel Topping	431	18	62
w/ Chocolate Syrup	433	13	76
w/ Fudge Topping	422	18	59
w/ Strawberry Topping	421	12	73
• Frozen Yogurt, 2 scoops	118	0	27
Hot Fudge Cake, 1 slice	662	27	100
No Sugar Added (NSA) Apple Pie, 1 slice	329	14	47
Oreo Mud Pie, 1 slice	495	24	66
Peanut Butter Ice cream Pie, 1 slice	607	42	47
Plain Cheese Cake, 1 slice	360	26	27
Pumpkin Pie Plain, 1 slice	366	16	48
Strawberry Cheese Cake, 1 slice	475	26	55
Strawberry Ice Cream, 2 scoops	180	10	21
Strawberry Pie, 1 slice	404	12	70
Strawberry Super Sundae, Plain	201	11	24
w/ Strawberry Topping	401	11	74
Dinner			
Baked Spaghetti Dinner	1056	47	108
Broiled Chicken Crumb Cod No Potato	671	51	14
Broiled Lemn Cod w/ Plain Bkd Potato	446	4	66
Cajun Chicken w/ Plain Baked Potato	396	5	57
Chicken & Veggie Stir Fry w/ Plain Baked Potato	717	8	128
Chicken Breast Mozz w/ Plain Baked Potato	436	8	58
Chicken Breast Tenders Only, 2 tenders	280	11	24
Chicken Parmesan Dinner	904	44	95
Chicken Pasta Primavera Dinner	919	28	117
Chicken Wisconsin Dinner No Potato	307	17	3
Country Fried Steak Dinner	990	66	68
• Fish & Chips	1252	84	87
Fried Lake Perch No Potato	504	55	15
Meatloaf (no Vegetable)	479	22	32
N.Y. Strip Steak No Potato	845	45	37
• Pot Roast Dinner, No Veg, No Potato	251	7	8
Sauteed Lake Perch No Potato	645	49	25

Big Boy (cont.)

Dinner (cont.)	Cal	Fat	Cbs
Shrimp (7 Pieces) No Potato	512	20	55
Spaghetti Dinner	612	13	105
Spaghetti Marinara Dinner	364	4	71
Turkey Dinner	642	18	83
Veal Parmesan	833	31	92
Vegetable Stir Fry w/ Plain Baked Potato	567	3	128
Kiddie Menu			
Cinnamon French Toast, 1 slice	236	4	44
Combination Plate	685	31	69
Fish& Chips	796	60	44
• French Toast, 1 slice	183	4	32
Hot Cakes w/ App Waffle Top, No Syrup, 2 ht cks	894	18	162
Hot Cakes w/ Blueberries, No Syrup, 2 hot cakes	743	17	125
• Hot Cakes w/ Strawberry Top, No Syrup, 2 ht cks	957	17	177
Hot Cakes, No Syrup, 2 hot cakes	740	17	124
Macaroni & Cheese	330	12	45
Salads			
3 -Cheese Grilled Chicken Montreal Salad	749	58	10
Blackened Chicken & Melon Salad	599	8	102
Buffalo Chicken Tenders Salad	1196	93	55
Caesar Salad, Side	66	4	7
Chicken Breast Caesar Salad	278	12	13
Chicken Fajita Salad w/Salsa Ranch Dressing	800	55	29
Chipotle Krab Salad	1106	100	39
Cole Slaw	120	10	9
• Dinner Salad, No Dressing	44	0	6
• Grilled Chicken Chipotle Salad	1697	152	32
Grilled Ham Steak w/ Grilled Melons & Pineapple	702	29	66
Lo Carb Cheddar Burger Salad	1081	87	10
Trop Garden Chicken w/ Roll & Promise Margarine	577	16	74
Turkey Club Super Salad	421	24	7
Sandwiches			
Bacon Lettuce & Tomato Sandwich	535	33	39
BBQ Pot Roast Sandwich Only	895	26	122
Big Cheese& Bacon Chicken w/ am Cheese (only)	847	50	40
w/ Mozz. Cheese (only)	849	50	40
w/ Swiss Cheese (only)	876	52	40
Big Ringer Burger (only)	958	59	50
Big Ringer Chicken (only)	615	30	50
Big Shrooms & Onion's (only)	801	44	45
Brawny Lad (only)	471	25	36
Breast of Chicken Fillet (only)	621	41	54
Chkn Brst & Mozz. Pita (only) w/ Greek Pita Bread	463	13	48
Chkn Brst & Mozz. Pita (only) w/ Med Pita Bread	494	11	57
Chkn Club Ciabatta Wrap	1103	66	76
Chkn Santa Fe Ciabatta Wrap	926	40	90
Club Sandwich Only	778	39	58
• Corned Beef Reuben Sandwich Only	1132	78	57
Grilled Cheese Sandwich Only	531	22	58
Hot Meat Loaf	677	25	68
Hot Turkey w/ Gravy	477	11	59
• Kiddie Grilled Cheese Only	312	13	37
Patty Melt	900	54	36
Philly Steak & Cheese Sandwich Only	620	28	38
Plain Big Topping Burger (only)	694	38	38
Plain Chicken Burger Sandwich (only)	351	9	39
Roast Beef Ciabatta Wrap	1052	59	80
Sandwich Only	635	40	35
Slim Jim (only)	548	27	51
Super Big Boy (only)	853	55	35
Super Slim Jim Sandwich	858	44	77
Swiss Miss (only)	604	37	33
Tuna Melt Sandwich Only	791	48	51
Tuna salad Pita (only) w/ Greek Pita Bread	546	29	47

Big Boy (cont.)	Cal	Fat	Cbs
Sandwiches (cont.)			
Tuna Salad Pita (only) w/ Med Pita Bread	577	27	56
Tuna Salad Sandwich Only	524	29	40
Turkey & Swiss Ciabatta Wrap	1040	58	78
Turkey Pita (only) w/ Greek Pita Bread	394	6	48
Turkey Pita (only) w/ Med Pita Bread	425	5	57
Sides			
6 Mozzarella Cheese Sticks- Plain	480	21	87
Beef Gravy, 2 oz.	31	1	3
Big Boy Sauce, 2 oz.	250	25	8
Big Boy Special Chili, 7 oz.	212	7	18
Broccoli Plain, 4 oz.	32	0	6
• Buffalo Style Chkn Tenders w/ Hot Sauce	658	30	52
Caesar Salad, Dressing, 2 oz.	338	32	12
Café Crackers, 1 pkg	25	1	3
• Cauliflower Plain, 4 oz.	21	0	4
Chicken Gravy, 2 oz.	57	3	7
Corn Plain, 4 oz.	104	1	25
Dinner Roll Plain, 1 Roll	123	3	20
Flavoured Sauce - Chipotle, 2 fl.oz.	424	44	4
Flavoured Sauce - Horseradish, 2 fl.oz.	324	33	6
French Fries (Combo & Side), 5 oz.	490	26	57
French Fries, (Kiddie Portion), 2 1/2 oz.	245	13	29
Garlic & Oil Dressing, 2 oz.	250	27	2
Green Beans Plain, 4 oz.	32	0	8
Grilled Grecian Roll (Garlic), 1 Roll	203	7	32
Grilled Texas Toast (Garlic), 1 slice	178	6	26
Mashed Potatoes Plain, 1 #8 Scoop	112	5	18
Ohio Big Boy Sauce, 2 oz.	354	38	2
Onion Rings, 8 Rings	304	16	36
Oyster Crackers, 1 pkg	60	3	9
Peas Plain, 4 oz.	91	7	16
Plain Bagel Plain, 1 Bagel	363	2	71
Plain Baked Potato, 8 oz.	246	0	57
Salsa Ranch Dressing, 2 fl.oz.	123	11	6
Shrimp Sauce, 2 oz.	54	0	15
Sour Cream, 1 oz.	60	6	2
Stir Fry Sauce, 2 oz.	222	1	55
Stir Fry Vegetables Plain, 6 oz.	53	0	11
Sweet Baby Rays Barbecue Sauce, 2 oz.	160	0	40
Tarter Sauce, 2 oz.	340	36	0
Tomato & Spice Dressing, 2 oz.	290	30	7
Turkey Gravy, 2 oz.	32	1	3
Vegetable Rice Pilaf, 5 oz.	206	4	38
Soups & Chili			
Bean w/ Bacon Soup, 6 oz.	170	13	8
• Cabbage Soup, 6 oz.	42	0	8
• Canadian Cheese Soup, 6 oz.	270	17	18
Chicken Noodle Soup, 6 oz.	110	2	11
Chicken w/ Rice Soup, 6 oz.	60	2	6
Chili Original, 6 oz.	230	11	20
Clam Chowder Soup, 6 oz.	109	6	10
Cream of Broccoli w/ Ham Soup, 6 oz.	110	9	8
Cream of Potato Soup, 6 oz.	180	10	17
Minestrone Soup, 6 oz.	70	2	12
Split Pea w/ Ham Soup, 6 oz.	80	3	9
Vegetable Beef Barley Soup, 6 oz.	80	3	10
Vegetarian Vegetable Soup, 6 oz.	45	1	9

Blackjack Pizza	Cal	Fat	Cbs
Pizza			
Blackjack Pizza 14" Lg Cheese Pepperoni, 108 g	250	9	28
Blackjack Pizza 14" Lg Cheese Sausage, 109 g	240	8	28
Blackjack Pizza 14 Large Cheese, 98 g	200	5	28
• Cheesebread, 163 g	410	15	52
• Cinnabread, 2 oz.	190	5	31

Blackjack Pizza (cont.)	Cal	Fat	Cbs
Pizza (cont.)			
Mediterranean Chicken, 78 g	190	11	15
Santa Fe, 98 g	210	11	17

Blimpie	Cal	Fat	Cbs
Breads/Wraps			
Cheddar Jalapeño, 6", 3 oz.	213	4	36
Ciabatta, 4 oz.	230	3	43
Honey Oat 6", 4 oz.	259	8	41
Marble Rye 6", 4 oz.	242	2	46
• Wheat, 6", 3 oz.	190	4	34
White, 6", 3 oz.	213	3	40
Wrap, Spinach Herb 12", 4 oz.	310	8	52
• Wrap, Traditional 12", 4 oz.	310	8	52
Zesty Parmesan, 6", 3 oz.	236	4	39
Breakfast Items			
Biscuit, Bacon Egg & Cheese, 5 oz.	387	21	33
Biscuit, Egg & Cheese, 4 oz.	339	18	33
Biscuit, Golden Buttermilk, 2 oz.	224	9	31
Biscuit, Ham Egg & Cheese, 5 oz.	375	19	34
Biscuit, Sausage Egg & Cheese, 6 oz.	489	32	33
Bluffin, Bacon Egg & Cheese, 5 oz.	293	14	27
Bluffin, Egg & Cheese, 4 oz.	245	10	27
Bluffin, Ham Egg & Cheese, 5 oz.	280	11	29
• Bluffin, Plain, 2 oz.	129	1	25
Bluffin, Sausage Egg & Cheese, 6 oz.	395	24	27
Burrito, Bacon Egg & Cheese, 10 oz.	553	24	56
Burrito, Egg & Cheese, 10 oz.	506	20	56
Burrito, Ham Egg & Cheese, 12 oz.	559	21	58
Burrito, Sausage Egg & Cheese, 12 oz.	656	34	56
Croissant, Bacon Egg & Cheese, 5 oz.	393	24	29
Croissant, Egg & Cheese, 4 oz.	345	21	29
Croissant, Ham Egg & Cheese, 5 oz.	381	21	30
Croissant, Plain, 2 oz.	232	12	27
Croissant, Sausage Egg & Cheese, 6 oz.	495	35	29
Donut, Long John Cream Filled, 4 oz.	370	15	51
Donut, Yeast, 4 oz.	404	25	52
Gourmet Cinnamon Roll, 6 oz.	566	233	9
Muffin, Banana Walnut, 4 oz.	420	19	56
Muffin, Blueberry, 4 oz.	440	23	54
Panini Breakfast, 4", 8 oz.	494	14	67
• Panini Breakfast, 6", 13 oz.	773	24	96
Cheese			
American Y&W, 1 oz.	104	9	1
• Cheddar, serving, 1 oz.	75	6	1
Four Blend, serving, 0.5 oz.	52	4	1
• Mild Cheddar Shredded, serving, 1 oz.	114	9	0
Pepper Jack, serving, 1 oz.	77	7	0
Provolone, serving, 1 oz.	76	6	0
Swiss, serving, 1 oz.	79	6	0
Desserts			
• Brownie, Chocolate Chip, 4 oz.	430	18	63
Cookie, Chocolate Chunk, 2 oz.	191	9	25
• Cookie, Oatmeal Raisin Walnut, 2 oz.	191	8	28
Cookie, Peanut Butter, 2 oz.	220	12	23
Cookie, Sugar, 3 oz.	327	17	41
Cookie, White Chocolate Macadamia Nut, 2 oz.	206	10	26
Strudel Stick, Apple, 3 oz.	264	16	27
Strudel Stick, Cherry, 3 oz.	289	16	33
Strudel Stick, Raspberry, 3 oz.	290	18	29
Strudel Stick, Strawberry Cream Cheese, 3 oz.	289	182	27
Turnover, Apple, 4 oz.	357	23	35
Turnover, Cherry, 4 oz.	358	23	35
Dressings/Sauces			
• Dressing, Blue Cheese, 2 oz.	230	24	2
• Dressing, Buttermilk Ranch, 2 oz.	230	24	2

Blimpie (cont.)	Cal	Fat	Cbs
Dressings/Sauces (cont.)			
Dressing, Creamy Caesar, 2 oz.	210	21	2
Dressing, Creamy Italian, 2 oz.	180	18	4
Dressing, Dijon Honey Mustard, 2 oz.	180	17	8
Dressing, Fat-Free Italian, 2 oz.	25	0	5
Dressing, Honey French, 2 oz.	210	18	14
Dressing, Light Buttermilk Ranch, 2 oz.	70	4	8
Dressing, Light Italian, 2 oz.	20	1	2
Dressing, Special, 1 oz.	70	7	0
Dressing, Thousand Island, 2 oz.	210	20	6
Mayonnaise, 1 oz.	202	22	0
Mayonnaise, Chipotle, 1 oz.	100	10	0
Mayonnaise, Horseradish, 1 oz.	100	10	4
Mustard, Deli Style, 0.5 oz.	5	0	0
Mustard, Honey, 1 oz.	43	1	7
• Mustard, Spicy Brown, 0.5 oz.	5	0	0
Oil, Blend, 0.5 oz.	130	14	0
Red Hot Original Sauce, 1 oz.	10	0	2
Red Wine Vinegar, 0.5 oz.	5	0	1
Kids Meals			
3" Ham & American Cheese, 6 oz.	262	9	32
• 3" Tuna, 6 oz.	277	11	30
• 3" Turkey, 5 oz.	187	2	31
Meats/Protein			
Bacon, 1 oz.	105	8	0
Cappacola, 1 oz.	18	1	0
Chicken Strips, 3 oz.	93	3	0
Corned Beef, 3 oz.	106	2	2
Egg, 2 oz.	45	3	2
Ham, 1 oz.	35	1	2
Meatballs, 5 oz.	220	15	10
Pastrami, 3 oz.	114	6	1
Pepperoni, 0.5 oz.	66	6	1
• Prosciuttini, 0.5 oz.	13	0	1
Roast Beef, 2 oz.	46	1	0
Salami, serving, 0.5 oz.	36	3	0
Seafood Salad, 4 oz.	92	4	10
Steak & Onion, 4 oz.	210	15	5
• Tuna, 3 oz.	241	18	0
Turkey, 1 oz.	30	0	1
Salads			
Chef Regular, 9 oz.	176	7	10
Chef Stacked, 10 oz.	209	8	12
Chicken Caesar Regular, 9 oz.	124	3	7
Chicken Caesar Stacked, 10 oz.	170	5	7
Chicken, 4 oz.	260	20	9
Cole Slaw, 4 oz.	160	9	20
• Garden Vegetable, 7 oz.	55	2	8
Macaroni, 5 oz.	330	22	28
Northwest Potato, 5 oz.	260	17	22
Potato, 5 oz.	230	12	28
Seafood, Regular, 9 oz.	122	4	17
Seafood, Stacked, 10 oz.	168	6	22
Sicilian Regular, 10 oz.	351	25	11
• Sicilian Stacked, 12 oz.	404	28	13
Tuna, Regular, 9 oz.	272	18	7
Tuna, Stacked, 10 oz.	393	28	7
Sandwiches/Wraps			
Blimpie Best, 6" Regular, 10 oz.	420	14	49
Blimpie Best, 6" Stacked, 12 oz.	478	16	51
BLT, 6" Regular, 8 oz.	346	11	46
BLT, 6" Stacked, 8 oz.	399	15	46
Buffalo Chicken, 6" Regular, 11 oz.	521	23	46
Buffalo Chicken, 6" Stacked, 13 oz.	591	25	47
Chicken Teriyaki (LTO), 8 oz.	428	9	50

Blimpie (cont.)	Cal	Fat	Cbs
Sandwiches/Wraps (cont.)			
Ciabatta, Buffalo Chicken (LTO), 12 oz.	583	27	50
Ciabatta, Grilled Chicken Caesar, 11 oz.	617	24	63
Ciabatta, The Mediterranean, 10 oz.	447	8	65
Ciabatta, The Sicilian, 11 oz.	637	25	68
Ciabatta, The Tuscan, 10 oz.	600	23	65
Ciabatta, Turkey Italiano, 10 oz.	502	11	64
Club, 6" Regular, 10 oz.	386	10	49
Club, 6" Stacked, 11 oz.	419	10	51
Cuban, 6" Regular, 8 oz.	413	11	43
Cuban, 6" Stacked, 20 oz.	515	12	55
Garden Burger, White 6", 10 oz.	382	8	64
Grilled Chicken, 6" Regular, 10 oz.	334	6	46
Grilled Chicken, 6" Stacked, 11 oz.	380	7	46
Ham & Swiss, 6" Regular, 10 oz.	391	10	50
Ham & Swiss, 6" Stacked, 11 oz.	427	11	51
Ham, Salami & Cheese, 6" Regular, 10 oz.	443	16	49
Ham, Salami & Cheese, 6" Stacked, 11 oz.	498	20	50
Meatball 6" Regular, 9 oz.	509	24	50
Meatball 6" Stacked, 14 oz.	706	40	54
Pastrami Special, 6" Regular, 11 oz.	463	14	47
Pastrami Special, 6" Stacked, 12 oz.	524	16	47
Pastrami, 6" Regular, 11 oz.	454	17	48
Pastrami, 6" Stacked, 13 oz.	522	20	49
Reuben, 6" Regular, 10 oz.	571	24	54
Reuben, 6" Stacked, 11 oz.	624	25	54
Roast Beef & Cheese, 6" Regular, 11 oz.	408	11	47
Roast Beef & Cheese, 6" Stacked, 13 oz.	454	12	47
Roast Beef, Turkey & Cheese, 6" Regular, 11 oz.	571	30	47
Roast Beef, Turkey & Cheese, 6" Stacked, 12 oz.	609	31	48
• Seafood, 6" Regular, 10 oz.	333	7	56
Seafood, 6" Stacked, 12 oz.	379	9	61
Steak & Onion, 6" Regular, 7 oz.	499	24	45
Steak & Onion, 6" Stacked, 11 oz.	709	39	50
Tuna, 6" Regular, 10 oz.	483	21	46
Tuna, 6" Stacked, 12 oz.	603	30	46
Turkey & Cheese, 6" Regular, 11 oz.	393	10	49
Turkey & Cheese, 6" Stacked, 13 oz.	431	10	51
Turkey Italian 6" Regular, 11 oz.	459	17	47
Ultimate Club, 6" Regular, 6 oz.	395	13	43
Ultimate Club, 6" Stacked, 8 oz.	443	14	44
Veggie Supreme, 6", 10 oz.	553	28	48
Wrap, Chicken Caesar, Regular, 10 oz.	607	29	56
Wrap, Chicken Caesar, Stacked, 11 oz.	653	30	56
Wrap, Roast Beef & Cheddar, Regular, 12 oz.	684	36	59
Wrap, Roast Beef & Cheddar, Stacked, 14 oz.	729	37	59
Wrap, Southwestern Regular, 10 oz.	530	22	61
Wrap, Southwestern Stacked, 11 oz.	575	23	63
Wrap, Steak & Onion, Regular, 11 oz.	774	47	62
• Wrap, Steak & Onion, Stacked, 15 oz.	984	62	67
Wrap, Ultimate BLT, Regular, 12 oz.	703	39	60
Wrap, Ultimate BLT, Stacked, 13 oz.	755	42	61
Wrap, Zesty, Regular, 10 oz.	569	26	59
Wrap, Zesty, Stacked, 11 oz.	655	31	61
Soups			
Bean w/ Ham, 9 oz.	140	1	23
Beef Steak & Noodle, 9 oz.	120	3	14
Beef Stew, 9 oz.	170	4	18
Captain's Corn Chowder, 9 oz.	210	7	29
Cheddar Cauliflower, 9 oz.	130	6	15
Chicken & Dumpling, 9 oz.	170	5	19
Chicken Gumbo, 9 oz.	90	2	13
Chicken Noodle, 9 oz.	130	4	18
• Chicken w/ White & Wild Rice, 9 oz.	250	10	15
Cream of Broccoli w/ Cheese, 9 oz.	190	8	15

Blimpie (cont.)

	Cal	Fat	Cbs
Soups (cont.)			
Cream of Potato, 9 oz.	190	9	24
French Onion, 9 oz.	80	4	11
Grande Chili w/ Bean & Beef, 9 oz.	250	9	30
Harvest Vegetable, 9 oz.	100	1	19
Italian Style Wedding, 9 oz.	130	4	17
Minestrone, 9 oz.	90	3	14
New England Clam Chowder, 9 oz.	170	3	28
Pasta Fagioli w/ Sausage, 9 oz.	150	5	22
Pilgrim Turkey Vegetables w/ Rice, 9 oz.	110	2	19
Seafood Gumbo, 9 oz.	100	2	16
Split Pea w/ Ham, 9 oz.	130	2	21
Tomato Basil w/ Raviolini, 9 oz.	110	1	22
• Yankee Pot Roast, 9 oz.	80	2	12
Toppings			
• Guacamole, 1 oz.	45	4	2
Lettuce, serving, 2 oz.	6	0	1
Olives, serving, 0.5 oz.	16	2	1
Onion, serving, 3 oz.	11	0	3
• Peppers, Hot Ring, 12 pcs., 1 oz.	0	0	1
Peppers, Jalapeño, 18 pcs., 1 oz.	10	0	1
Peppers, Red Roasted, serving, 2 oz.	11	0	2
Peppers, Sweet Strips, 6 pcs., 1 oz.	20	0	5
Tomato, serving, 2 oz.	7	0	2

Bob Evans Restaurants

	Cal	Fat	Cbs
Breakfast			
Bacon & Cheese Omelet, 10 oz.	825	66	6
Bacon & Cheese Omelet, egg beaters, 10 oz.	615	47	7
Blueberry Hotcake, 6 oz.	328	9	55
• Bob Evans Sausage Country Benedict, 14 oz.	936	66	40
Border Scramble Burrito, 21 oz.	110	64	80
Border Scramble Omelet, 15 oz.	756	58	15
Border Scramble Omelet, egg beaters, 15 oz.	517	37	16
Buttermilk Hotcake, 6 oz.	318	9	53
Cinnamon Hotcake, 6 oz.	417	15	66
Country Biscuit Breakfast, 10 oz.	659	45	40
Egg Beaters, 3 eggs, 7 oz.	173	12	3
Egg Beaters, omelet shell, 7 oz.	173	12	3
Farmer's Market Omelet, 15 oz.	778	60	13
Farmer's Market Omelet, egg beaters, 15 oz.	569	41	14
French toast, 2 oz.	131	2	13
Fruit & Yogurt Plate, 21 oz.	403	2	93
Garden Harvest Omelet, 14 oz.	654	50	13
Garden Harvest Omelet, egg beaters, 14 oz.	444	31	14
Grits, 7 oz.	178	7	28
Ham & Cheddar Omelet, 11 oz.	634	48	3
Ham & Cheddar Omelet, egg beaters, 11 oz.	426	29	5
Ham & Cheese Benedict, 15 oz.	826	52	44
• Hard Cooked Eggs, 2 oz.	60	4	1
Multigrain Hotcake, 6 oz.	322	10	52
Mush, 2 oz.	79	3	11
Oatmeal, 11 oz.	172	3	32
Omelet Shell, 7 oz.	383	31	2
Over Easy Egg, 2 oz.	101	8	1
Plain Crepe, 5 oz.	459	36	27
Pot Roast Hash, 13 oz.	652	39	34
Raspberry Crepes, 13 oz.	102	72	81
Roasted Apple Crepes, 13 oz.	102	73	76
Sausage & Cheddar Omelet, 10 oz.	741	61	3
Sausage & Cheddar Omelet, egg beaters, 10 oz.	502	40	4
Sausage & Egg Sandwich, breakfast, 7 oz.	577	37	32
Sausage Gravy, bowl, 10 oz.	268	17	21
Sausage Gravy, cup, 5 oz.	134	9	10
Sausage Link, 1 oz.	125	11	0
Sausage Patty, 2 oz.	141	11	0

Bob Evans Restaurants (cont.)

	Cal	Fat	Cbs
Breakfast (cont.)			
Scrambled Eggs, 6 oz.	255	17	2
Smoked Ham, 4 oz.	87	2	2
Spinach, Bacon & Tom Country Benedict, 12 oz.	729	48	42
Stacked & Stuffed Crml Apple Crm Htcks, 24 oz.	128	50	192
Stacked & Stuffed Crml Banaca Pcn Htcks, 23 oz.	154	77	198
Stacked & Stuffed Cinnamon Crm Htcks, 16 oz.	103	49	136
Strawberry Yogurt, 5 oz.	145	1	28
Stuffed French Toast, plain, 10 oz.	599	20	53
Sunshine Skillet, 17 oz.	842	60	36
Sweet Cream Waffles, 10 oz.	598	12	100
Three Cheese Omelet, 9 oz.	645	52	4
Three Cheese Omelet, egg beaters, 9 oz.	435	34	5
Turkey Florentine Omelet, 14 oz.	736	54	6
Turkey Florentine Omelet, egg beaters, 14 oz.	496	33	7
Turkey Sausage (1 link), 11 oz.	329	13	35
Turkey Sausage, (1 link), 2 oz.	72	4	1
Western Omelet, 13 oz.	654	48	8
Western Omelet, egg beaters, 14 oz.	447	30	10
Breakfast Condiments			
Apple Butter, 1 oz.	33	0	8
Apple Jelly, 1 oz.	35	0	9
Butter Cups (1), 0.5 oz.	37	4	0
Captain Wafers Crackers, 1 oz.	65	2	8
• Diet Blackberry Jam, 0.5 oz.	5	0	2
Grape Jelly, 1 oz.	36	0	9
Half and Half Cups, 1 oz.	40	3	1
Honey, 1 oz.	43	0	12
• Margarine Buttery Taste Sprd Cp, 0.5 oz.	102	3	0
Condiments			
Mayonnaise, 1 oz.	90	10	0
• Non-Dairy Creamer Cups, 1 oz.	19	1	1
Non-Dairy Creamer, 2 oz.	44	3	4
Orange Marmalade, 1 oz.	35	0	9
Saltine Crackers, 1 oz.	52	2	8
Sour Cream, 1 oz.	57	5	2
Desserts			
Apple Dumpling Pie a la mode, 13 oz.	769	37	105
Apple Dumpling Pie, 9 oz.	589	28	83
Coconut Cream Pie, 7 oz.	534	27	65
French Silk Pie, 6 oz.	693	47	62
NSA Apple Pie, 11 oz.	650	38	74
NSA Apple Pie, 7 oz.	491	30	55
• Pecan Pie, 8 oz.	909	46	127
Pumpkin Pie, 8 oz.	575	30	71
• Vanilla Ice Cream, 3 oz.	116	6	14
Dinner			
Bacon, 1 oz.	36	4	0
Chicken Parmesan, 23 oz.	611	29	45
Chicken Salad Plate, 21 oz.	763	46	72
Chicken Stir-Fry, 27 oz.	636	20	77
Chicken-N-Noodles Deep-Dish, 21 oz.	845	43	67
Country Fried Steak with Gravy, 8 oz.	553	38	37
Country Fried Steak, no gravy, 5 oz.	496	33	31
Fried Chicken Breast (1), 5 oz.	285	13	13
Fried Chicken Strips (1), 2 oz.	137	8	10
Fried Haddock, 7 oz.	363	18	27
Fruit Dish, 5 oz.	71	0	18
Garden Vegetable Alfredo, 27 oz.	713	45	59
Garden Vegetable Alfredo, chicken, 27 oz.	764	44	45
Garden Vegetable Alfredo, salmon, 30 oz.	888	52	46
Garden Vegetable Alfredo, shrimp, 28 oz.	814	52	45
Green Pepper and Onion Pasta, 22 oz.	372	19	43
Grilled Chkn Breast, garlic butter, 5 oz.	271	16	3
Grilled Chkn Breast, plain, 4 oz.	232	13	0

Bob Evans Restaurants (cont.)

	Cal	Fat	Cbs
Dinner (cont.)			
Grilled Chkn Breast, Wildfire Sauce, 6 oz.	325	13	22
• Grilled Chkn Tenders (1), 2 oz.	93	6	0
Italian Sausage and Pepper Pasta, 22 oz.	636	40	37
Meatloaf, 5 oz.	282	19	9
Open-Faced Roast Beef Dinner, 10 oz.	510	25	24
Pot Roast Beef Stew Deep-Dish, 20 oz.	763	39	65
Potato-Crusted Flounder, 5 oz.	254	17	8
Salmon Stir-Fry, 29 oz.	750	27	77
Salmon, garlic butter, 9 oz.	326	16	2
Salmon, plain, 8 oz.	287	13	0
Salmon, Wildfire Sauce, 9 oz.	380	13	22
Sausage Sandwich Patty, 3 oz.	222	17	0
Shrimp Stir-Fry, 29 oz.	686	28	77
Sirloin Steak, 5 oz.	403	27	3
Slow-Roasted Chicken-N-Noodles, 11 oz.	296	16	23
Slow-Roasted Pork Loin, 2 pieces, 12 oz.	519	30	30
Slow-Roasted Pork Loin, 7 oz.	324	20	18
• Slow-Roasted Pot Pie, 19 oz.	908	60	64
Slow-Roasted Turkey, 3 oz.	114	4	1
Steak Tips and Noodles, 28 oz.	822	43	44
Steak Tips Stir-Fry, 30 oz.	102	47	84
Steak Tips, 4 oz.	279	16	3
Turkey and Dressing Dinner, 14 oz.	551	28	33
Vegetable Stir-Fry, 27 oz.	505	15	86
Kids Menu			
Fruit & Yogurt Dippers, 13 oz.	275	2	61
Fudge Blast Sundae, 4 oz.	244	11	33
Grilled Cheese Sandwich, 3 oz.	290	16	26
Hotcakes, 9 oz.	501	17	79
Macaroni and Cheese, kids, 7 oz.	320	11	45
• Pasta, 8 oz.	113	5	15
Reese I'm Smiling Sundae, 5 oz.	330	17	41
• Smiley Face Potatoes, 6 oz.	524	31	57
Salads			
Avocado Ranch Dressing, dinner, 3 oz.	411	43	3
Bleu Cheese Dressing, dinner, 3 oz.	440	47	6
Buttermilk Ranch Dressing, dinner, 3 oz.	312	31	3
Chili and Cheese Taco Salad, 17 oz.	715	46	62
• Chili and Cheese Taco Salad, 24 oz.	928	62	73
Cobb Salad, 13 oz.	469	30	10
Cobb Salad, 20 oz.	698	46	14
Colonial Dressing, dinner, 3 oz.	464	41	23
Colonial Dressing, side, 2 oz.	232	21	12
Cranberry Pecan Chicken Salad, 14 oz.	801	47	49
• Cranberry Pecan Chicken Salad, 22 oz.	114	64	63
French Dressing, dinner, 3 oz.	439	41	19
French Dressing, side, 2 oz.	219	21	10
Garden Salad, 5 oz.	137	4	22
Heritage Chef Salad, 11 oz.	259	15	9
Heritage Chef Salad, 17 oz.	456	26	14
Honey Mustard Dressing, dinner, 3 oz.	384	36	16
Honey Mustard Dressing, side, 2 oz.	192	18	8
Hot Bacon Dressing, dinner, 3 oz.	213	6	35
Hot Bacon Dressing, side, 2 oz.	106	3	18
Lite Ranch Dressing, dinner, 3 oz.	206	20	5
Lite Ranch Dressing, side, 2 oz.	103	10	2
Specialty Side Salad, 6 oz.	171	9	14
Spinach Salad, 10 oz.	504	35	11
Spinach Salad, 13 oz.	608	40	13
Sweet Italian Dressing, dinner, 3 oz.	346	21	16
Sweet Italian Dressing, side, 2 oz.	173	10	8
Swiss Bacon Dressing, dinner, 3 oz.	454	51	3
Swiss Bacon Dressing, side, 2 oz.	227	26	1
Thousand Island Dressing, dinner, 3 oz.	425	40	14

Bob Evans Restaurants (cont.)

	Cal	Fat	Cbs
Salads (cont.)			
Thousand Island Dressing, side, 2 oz.	213	20	7
Vinegar & Oil Dressing, dinner, 3 oz.	54	6	0
Vinegar & Oil Dressing, side, 2 oz.	27	3	0
Wildfire Chicken Salad, fried, 14 oz.	631	30	68
Wildfire Chicken Salad, fried, 19 oz.	789	38	81
Wildfire Chicken Salad, grilled, 14 oz.	541	26	49
Wildfire Chicken Salad, grilled, 20 oz.	654	32	53
Wildfire Ranch Dressing, dinner, 3 oz.	241	19	18
Wildfire Ranch Dressing, side, 2 oz.	121	9	9
Sandwiches			
Bacon Cheeseburger, 8 oz.	716	48	32
Bob's BLT & E, 9 oz.	645	38	27
Cheeseburger, 8 oz.	645	41	32
Chicken Salad Sandwich, 7 oz.	649	38	53
Chicken Salad Sandwich, half, 5 oz.	331	19	28
Double Sausage Sandwich, 9 oz.	716	46	31
Fried Chicken Club Sandwich, 9 oz.	660	35	44
Fried Chicken Sandwich, plain, 7 oz.	503	21	43
Fried Haddock Sandwich, 11 oz.	786	34	78
Grilled Cheese Sandwich, 5 oz.	396	16	25
Grilled Chicken Club Sandwich, 9 oz.	606	35	31
Grilled Chicken Sandwich, plain, 6 oz.	399	15	30
Hamburger Patty, 5 oz.	321	24	1
Hamburger, plain, 7 oz.	539	32	31
Homemade Meat Loaf Knife & Fork Sand, 16 oz.	716	38	41
Knife & Fork Meatloaf Sandwich, 16 oz.	716	38	41
Knife & Fork Pork Loin Sandwich, 17 oz.	844	48	58
Knife & Fork Turkey Sandwich, 15 oz.	696	36	46
Mini Cheeseburgers, 3 oz.	306	19	21
Pot Roast Sandwich, 9 oz.	610	28	58
Pot Roast Sandwich, half, 6 oz.	390	19	31
• Ranch Steak Burger, 11 oz.	937	68	35
Sausage Sandwich Patty, 6 oz.	494	29	31
Slow Roasted Pork Loin Knife & Fork Sand, 17 oz.	844	48	58
Turkey Bacon Melt, 9 oz.	617	29	53
• Turkey Bacon Melt, half, 4 oz.	306	14	26
Sauces & Toppings			
American Cheese, 1 oz.	53	4	1
Apple Butter, 1 oz.	33	0	8
Apple Jelly, 1 oz.	35	0	9
Beef Gravy, 2 oz.	22	1	3
Bleu Cheese, 1 oz.	97	8	0
Brown Sugar, 1 oz.	79	0	20
Butter Cups, 0.5 oz.	37	4	0
Chicken-Roasted Gravy, 2 oz.	53	4	3
Citrus Stir-Fry Sauce, 2 oz.	51	0	12
Country Gravy, 3 oz.	56	4	6
Cranberries, 1 oz.	68	0	17
Diet Blackberry Jam, 0.5 oz.	5	0	2
Garlic Butter, 1 oz.	40	3	2
Grape Jelly, 1 oz.	36	0	9
Hollandaise, 2 oz.	50	3	5
Honey Roasted Pecans, 1 oz.	142	14	6
Honey, 1 oz.	43	0	12
• Lettuce & Tomato, 1 oz.	4	0	1
Lettuce, Tomato and Pickle, 1 oz.	6	0	1
Margarine Buttery Taste Sprd Cup, 0.5 oz.	102	3	0
Marinara, 3 oz.	35	1	5
Mayonnaise, 1 oz.	90	10	0
Milk, 2 oz.	28	1	3
Monterey Jack Cheese, 1 oz.	76	6	0
Non-Dairy Creamer Cups (1), 1 oz.	19	1	1
Non-Dairy Creamer, 2 oz.	44	3	4
Orange Marmalade, 1 oz.	35	0	9

RESTAURANTS & FAST-FOOD CHAINS

Bob Evans Restaurants (cont.)

	Cal	Fat	Cbs
Sauces & Toppings (cont.)			
• Pancake Syrup, 3 oz.	213	0	55
Pork-Roasted Gravy, 2 oz.	63	5	3
Raisins, 1 oz.	70	0	17
Ranchero Picante, 1 oz.	38	0	0
Raspberry, 3 oz.	108	0	27
Roasted-Apple Topping, 3 oz.	102	1	24
Saltine Crackers, 1 oz.	52	2	8
Sour Cream, 1 oz.	57	5	2
Strawberry Jam, 1 oz.	36	0	9
Sugar Free Pancake Syrup, 3 oz.	39	0	10
Tarter Sauce, 1 oz.	166	18	1
Whipped Topping, 1 oz.	92	7	7
Wildfire Sauce, 2 oz.	94	0	22
Seniors			
Chicken Parmesan, 17 oz.	522	26	33
Chicken Stir-Fry, 16 oz.	368	13	44
Garden Vegetable Alfredo, 14 oz.	363	23	29
Garden Vegetable Alfredo, chicken, 16 oz.	452	26	29
Garden Vegetable Alfredo, shrimp, 17 oz.	537	37	29
Green Pepper and Onion Pasta, 14 oz.	259	14	28
Italian Sausage and Pepper Pasta, 14 oz.	523	36	21
Shrimp Stir-Fry, 17 oz.	456	24	44
• Steak Tip Stir-Fry, 18 oz.	560	26	48
Steak Tips and Noodles, 15 oz.	422	22	23
Turkey and Dressing Dinner, 11 oz.	438	23	33
• Vegetable Stir-Fry, 14 oz.	281	10	44
Sides			
Applesauce, 4 oz.	83	0	21
Baked Potato, 11 oz.	207	0	54
Bread and Celery Dressing, 6 oz.	272	15	29
Broccoli Florets, 4 oz.	32	0	6
Caramelized Onions, 2 oz.	38	2	6
Coleslaw, 4 oz.	209	14	19
Corn, 5 oz.	169	8	25
Cottage Cheese, 4 oz.	115	5	4
Cranberry Relish, 1 oz.	57	0	13
• Dill Pickle Slices, 1 oz.	1	0	0
French Fries, 5 oz.	354	15	51
Fruit Cup, 8 oz.	150	1	38
Garden Vegetables, 6 oz.	121	7	14
Glazed Carrots, 4 oz.	83	3	14
Green Beans, 6 oz.	79	3	9
Grilled Mushrooms, 8 oz.	152	12	10
Home Fries, 5 oz.	186	7	27
• Loaded Baked Potato, 12 oz.	373	13	56
Mashed Potatoes, 6 oz.	205	7	17
Rice Pilaf, 6 oz.	129	4	20
Tomato Slice, 1 oz.	4	0	1
Soups			
Bean Soup, bowl, 10 oz.	205	5	27
Bean Soup, cup, 7 oz.	144	3	19
Cheddar Baked Potato Soup, bowl, 14 oz.	371	25	24
Cheddar Baked Potato Soup, cup, 11 oz.	294	20	19
• Sausage Chili, bowl, 11 oz.	376	24	26
Sausage Chili, cup, 8 oz.	268	17	18
Vegetable Beef Soup, bowl, 10 oz.	193	7	25
• Vegetable Beef Soup, cup, 7 oz.	135	5	17

Bojangles

	Cal	Fat	Cbs
Biscuit Sandwiches			
Bacon	290	17	26
Bacon, Egg & Cheese	550	42	27
• Biscuit (plain)	243	12	29
Cajun Filet	454	21	46
Country Ham	270	15	26

Bojangles (cont.)

	Cal	Fat	Cbs
Biscuit Sandwichesz (cont.)			
Egg	400	30	26
Sausage	350	23	26
Smoked Sausage	380	26	27
• Steak	649	49	37
Cajun Spiced Chicken			
Breast	278	17	12
• Leg	264	16	11
Thigh	310	23	11
• Wing	355	25	11
Individual Fixin'			
Botato Rounds	235	11	31
Cajun Pintos	110	0	18
Corn on the Cob	140	2	34
Dirty Rice	166	6	24
• Green Beans	25	0	5
Macaroni & Cheese	198	14	12
Marinated Cole Slaw	136	3	26
Potatoes w/o gravy	80	1	16
• Seasoned Fries	344	19	39
Sandwiches			
Cajun Filet	337	11	41
• Cajun Filet w/mayo	437	22	41
• Grilled Filet	235	5	25
Grilled Filet w/mayo	335	16	25
Snacks			
Buffalo Bites	180	5	5
Chicken Supremes	337	16	26
Southern Style Chicken			
Breast	261	16	12
• Leg	254	15	11
Thigh	308	21	14
• Wing	337	21	19
Sweet Biscuits			
Bo Berry™	220	10	29
Cinnamon	320	18	37

Boston Market

	Cal	Fat	Cbs
Desserts			
Apple Pie (slice), 6 oz.	420	20	56
• Chocolate Cake, 5 oz.	600	32	75
Chocolate Chip Fudge Brownie, 5 oz.	580	23	81
• Cornbread, 2 oz.	180	5	31
Nestle Toll House Chocolate Chip Cookie, 3 oz.	370	19	49
Family Meals			
Award Winning Sirloin, 5 oz.	290	15	0
• Boneless Holiday Turkey Breast, 5 oz.	180	3	0
• Meatloaf, 8 oz.	480	33	23
Roasted Turkey, 5 oz.	180	3	0
Rotisserie Chicken, 6 oz.	290	14	4
Spiral Sliced Holiday Ham, 8 oz.	450	26	13
Whole Holiday Turkey, 8 oz.	310	18	0
Individual Meals			
1 Thigh & 1 Drumstick, 6 oz.	300	17	6
1/4 White Rotisserie Chicken, 6 oz.	290	11	4
1/4 White Rotisserie Chicken, No Skin, 6 oz.	210	2	6
3 Piece Dark (2 thighs & 1 drumstick), 9 oz.	510	30	8
3 Piece Dark Individual Meal, 7 oz.	380	19	7
3 Piece Dark Skinless (2 thighs & drumstick), 7 oz.	310	13	6
3 Piece Dark Skinless (thigh & 2 drumsticks), 6 oz.	240	8	7
Award Winning Roasted Sirloin, 5 oz.	290	15	0
Half Rotisserie Chicken, 348 g	590	27	10
Meatloaf, 8 oz.	480	33	23
• Pastry Top Chicken Pot Pie, 15 oz.	780	47	60
• Roasted Turkey, 5 oz.	180	3	0

Boston Market (cont.)

	Cal	Fat	Cbs
Salads			
• Caesar Salad Entree, 7 oz.	500	45	12
Dressing, 3 oz.	360	38	4
Lite Ranch Dressing, 2 oz.	70	4	8
Roasted Sirloin, 3 oz.	160	6	0
Roasted Turkey, 3 oz.	140	6	1
Rotisserie Chicken, 5 oz.	160	1	3
w/o dressing, 7 oz.	140	8	8
• Market Chopped Salad, 18 oz.	580	48	30
Dressing, 3 oz.	360	39	2
Lite Ranch Dressing, 2 oz.	70	4	8
Roasted Sirloin, 3 oz.	160	6	0
Roasted Turkey, 3 oz.	140	6	1
Rotisserie Chicken, 5 oz.	160	1	3
w/o dressing, 17 oz.	210	9	28
Sandwiches			
Beef Au jus, 4 oz.	20	0	4
Boston Chicken Carver, 11 oz.	700	29	68
Boston Meatloaf Carver, 15 oz.	940	45	96
• Boston Sirloin Dip Carver, 13 oz.	1000	51	70
Boston Turkey Carver, 14 oz.	770	27	68
Boston Turkey Dip Carver, 16 oz.	770	27	67
• Half Boston Chicken Carver, 7 oz.	340	15	29
Half Boston Sirloin Dip Carver, 7 oz.	500	25	35
Half Boston Turkey Carver, 7 oz.	390	14	34
Half Turkey Dip Carver, 7 oz.	380	14	33
Poultry Au Jus, 4 oz.	15	1	4
Soups & Sides			
Beef Gravy, 3 oz.	35	2	4
Broccoli with Garlic Butter, 4 oz.	80	6	6
Butternut Squash R, 5 oz.	140	5	25
Caesar Salad Dressing, 3 oz.	360	38	4
• Caesar Side Salad w/o Dressing, 3 oz.	40	2	3
Caesar Side Salad, 5 oz.	400	40	7
Chicken Noodle Soup, 6 oz.	170	5	17
Chicken Tortilla Soup with toppings, 6 oz.	340	22	24
Chicken Tortilla Soup w/o toppings, 6 oz.	90	5	7
Cinnamon Apples, 5 oz.	210	3	47
Cranberry Walnut Relish LF, 3 oz.	140	2	30
Creamed Spinach, 7 oz.	280	23	12
Fresh Steamed Vegetables LF, 5 oz.	60	2	8
Fresh Vegetable Stuffing, 5 oz.	190	8	25
Garden Fresh Coleslaw, 4 oz.	170	9	21
Garlic Dill New Potatoes LF, 5 oz.	140	3	24
Green Bean Casserole, 6 oz.	60	2	9
Green Beans, 6 oz.	60	4	7
Macaroni and Cheese, 8 oz.	330	12	39
Market Chopped Salad Dressing, 3 oz.	360	39	2
Market Chopped Side Salad w/o Dressing, 5 oz.	80	4	10
Market Chopped Side Salad, 7 oz.	440	43	12
Mashed Potatoes, 8 oz.	270	11	36
Poultry Gravy, 4 oz.	15	1	4
Seasonal Fresh Fruit Salad LF, 5 oz.	60	0	15
Spinach Artichoke Dip, 2 oz.	100	8	3
Spinach with Garlic Butter Sauce, 6 oz.	130	9	9
Squash Casserole, 8 oz.	320	24	21
Sweet Corn, 6 oz.	170	4	37
• Sweet Potato Casserole, 7 oz.	460	17	77

Brown's Chicken & Pasta

	Cal	Fat	Cbs
Main Chicken Items			
• Chicken breast	284	15	12
Chicken legs	287	16	9
Chicken thigh	355	24	13
• Chicken wing	385	25	17

Brown's Chicken & Pasta (cont.)

	Cal	Fat	Cbs
Miscellaneous Items			
• Chicken Gizzards	387	N/A	26
Chicken Livers	341	N/A	20
• Mushrooms	289	N/A	30
Pasta Items			
• Mostaccioli (in Marinara)	792	10	146
• Spaghetti (in Marinara)	792	10	146
Premium Side Items			
• Cheezy Potatoes, 12 oz.	188	11	16
• Mostaccioli (in Marinara)	792	10	146
Spaghetti (in Marinara)	792	10	146
Regular Side Items			
Cole slaw	131	10	9
• Corn fritters	415	25	42
• Potato salad	95	4	13

Bruegger's

	Cal	Fat	Cbs
Alternative Breads			
• Bruegger's Bagel Bowl, Per Container	720	9	133
• Single Ciabatta, 113 g	250	3	48
Wheat Wrap, 4 oz.	310	8	53
Bagels			
Asiago Parmesan, 123 g	330	4	62
Baked Apple Bagel, 113 g	310	2	65
Blueberry, 120 g	330	2	67
Chocolate Chip, 121 g	350	5	64
Cinnamon Raisin, 123 g	330	2	69
Cinnamon Sugar, 129 g	350	2	73
Cranberry Orange, 121 g	330	2	68
Everything, 123 g	320	2	64
Fortified, 130 g	350	4	68
Garlic, 122 g	320	2	65
Honey Grain, 124 g	330	3	65
Jalapeño, 121 g	320	2	64
Onion, 122 g	320	2	64
Plain, 121 g	320	2	64
Poppy, 122 g	320	3	64
Pretzel Bagel, 123 g	320	2	64
Pumpernickel, 124 g	330	3	67
• Pumpkin Bagel, 120 g	310	2	63
Rosemary Olive Oil, 123 g	350	7	64
Salt, 123 g	320	2	64
Sesame, 130 g	360	3	68
Sourdough, 134 g	340	2	68
Sun Dried Tomato, 121 g	320	2	64
• Whole Wheat, 136 g	390	6	73
Breakfast Sandwich			
Classic Wrap with Bacon, 269 g	520	45	52
Classic Wrap with Ham, 312 g	510	41	54
Classic Wrap with Sausage, 312 g	660	60	52
Denver, 272 g	460	18	74
• Egg & cheese, 208 g	420	18	71
Egg, cheese & bacon, 210 g	460	23	65
Egg, cheese & ham, 244 g	460	18	73
Egg, cheese & sausage, 265 g	640	38	72
Rio Grande Wrap with Bacon, 284 g	560	49	55
Rio Grande Wrap with Ham, 298 g	630	34	55
Rio Grande Wrap with Sausage, 284 g	510	47	53
• Western Wheat Softwich, 308 g	820	58	76
Bruegger's Salmon			
Smoked Salmon, 2 oz.	90	3	1
Cream Cheese			
Bacon Scallion, 43 g	140	12	5
Cucumber Dill, 43 g	140	13	3
Garden Veggie Light, 43 g	90	6	3
Garden Veggie, 43 g	130	11	5

Bruegger's (cont.)

	Cal	Fat	Cbs
Cream Cheese (cont.)			
Herb & Garlic Light, 43 g	100	6	4
• Honey Walnut, 43 g	150	12	8
Jalapeño, 43 g	140	13	4
Olive Pimento, 43 g	140	13	3
Onion and Chive, 43 g	140	13	3
Plain Light, 43 g	100	6	4
Plain, 43 g	130	11	6
Pumpkin, 43 g	120	11	4
• Smoked Salmon, 2 oz.	90	3	1
Strawberry, 43 g	140	13	4
Wildberry, 43 g	140	12	5
Deli Sandwiches			
BLT with Mayo, 213 g	570	23	72
Chicken Breast, 318 g	660	11	87
Chicken Salad, 268 g	630	26	73
Ham, 275 g	460	7	76
• Hummus, 54 g	110	6	10
• Roast Beef w/ Mayo, Lettuce & Tomato, 289 g	730	39	71
Tuna Salad, 247 g	620	27	73
Turkey, 261 g	510	14	70
Deli Softwiches			
BLT with Mayo, 218 g	600	25	73
Chicken Breast, 325 g	630	11	81
Chicken Salad, 316 g	670	27	76
• Ham, 302 g	510	6	85
Hummus, 288 g	540	13	85
• Roast Beef w/ Mayo, Lettuce & Tomato, 325 g	750	40	72
Roasted Tkey w/ Chz, Let, Tom & Mayo, 302 g	550	15	74
Tuna Salad, 288 g	720	34	76
Desserts			
Chocolate Chunk Brownies, 73 g	330	18	40
Chocolate Chunk Cookie, 113 g	500	22	71
Lemon Pound Cake, 94 g	320	13	48
Luscious Lemon Bars, 78 g	300	16	36
• Marshmallow Chew, 69 g	250	6	55
Oatmeal Raisin Cookie, 113 g	460	19	71
Oreo® Dream Bar, 107 g	470	28	49
Peanut Butter Cookie, 113 g	480	23	63
Pecan Chocolate Chunks, 34 g	310	19	32
Raspberry Sammies, 73 g	340	16	44
• Seven Layer Bar, 133 g	650	43	58
Toffee Almond Bars, 89 g	400	19	53
Triple Chocolate Chunk Cookie, 121 g	560	28	71
White Choco Macadamia Cookie, 121 g	580	31	70
Iced Coffee			
Raspberries and Cream, 20 fl.oz.	210	10	27
Muffins			
• Blueberry Muffin, 43 g	450	19	64
• Chocolate Muffin, 128 g	460	24	57
Salad Wraps			
• Tossed Chicken Caesar, 354 g	660	28	73
Tossed Mandarin Medley, 328 g	630	25	87
• Tossed Sesame Chicken, 338 g	77	36	80
Softwiches (Square Bagels)			
Asiago, 130 g	360	5	66
BLT, 218 g	600	25	73
Chicken Breast, 325 g	630	11	81
• Everything, 123 g	320	2	64
Garden Veggie, 285 g	380	3	76
Ham, 285 g	380	3	76
Hummus, 285 g	380	3	76
Plain, 5 oz.	350	2	70
Roast Beef, 285 g	380	3	76
Sesame, 5 oz.	360	3	68

Bruegger's (cont.)

	Cal	Fat	Cbs
Softwiches (Square Bagels) (cont.)			
• Tuna Salad, 288 g	720	34	76
Whole Wheat, 130 g	350	4	70
Soups			
Beef Chili, 8 oz.	190	8	18
Butternut Squash, 285 g	380	3	76
Chicken Spaetzle Soup, 8 oz.	200	12	15
Chicken Tortilla Soup, 8 oz.	140	8	11
Chicken Wild Rice Soup, 285 g	380	3	76
Fire Roasted Tomato Soup, 285 g	380	3	76
• Four Cheese & Broccoli Soup, 285 g	380	3	76
New England Clam Chowder, 8 oz.	230	14	16
• Steak and Onion Soup, 8 oz.	90	4	11
Speciality Bagel Sandwiches			
Chicken Fajita, 311 g	530	11	81
Cranberry Gobbler, 274 g	620	21	78
Cuban Chicken, 319 g	680	25	74
• Garden Veggie, 285 g	380	3	76
Herby Turkey, 259 g	560	14	78
Leonardo Da Veggie, 244 g	480	12	74
Radishy Roast Beef, 269 g	560	18	73
• Roadhouse Chicken, 315 g	710	19	84
Santa Fe Turkey, 294 g	490	9	75
Smoked Salmon, 253 g	490	10	74
Supreme Club, 250 g	470	9	72
Specialty Softwiches			
Chicken Fajita, 311 g	570	10	81
Cranberry Gobbler, 312 g	730	28	80
• Cuban Chicken, 376 g	810	32	77
Garden Veggie, 285 g	380	3	76
Herby Turkey, 276 g	580	14	80
Leonardo Da Veggie, 329 g	550	15	79
Mediterranean Softwich, 303 g	790	33	90
Radishy Roast Beef, 310 g	670	26	75
Roadhouse Chicken, 296 g	670	19	74
Santa Fe Turkey, 328 g	520	10	78
Smoked Salmon, 282 g	520	11	76
• Supreme Club, 219 g	270	8	21
Thai Peanut Chicken Softwich, 332 g	590	12	82
Tossed Salads			
• Caesar, 234 g	270	17	22
Chicken Caesar, 319 g	370	20	23
Mandarin Medley, 286 g	340	17	36
• Sesame Chicken, 298 g	480	28	30

Buca di Beppo

	Cal	Fat	Cbs
Entrees			
• Chicken Marsala, 1/6 of large serving	380	24	11
• Fresh Salmon, 1/2 of small serving	465	26	26
• Green Beans, 1/6 of large serving	70	5	7
Pasta			
Linguini Frutti Di Mare, 1/4 of sm serving	360	22	18
• Penne Campofiore, 1/4 of sm serving	380	19	41
• Spaghetti with Marinara Sauce, 1/4 of sm serving	260	2	50
Pizza			
Pizza Margherita, Small 2 slices	325	12	26
Salad			
Apple Gorgonzola Salad, 1/4 of sm serving	210	14	17
Warm Tomato and Spinach Salad, 1/4 of sm serving	90	6	7

Buck's Pizza

	Cal	Fat	Cbs
14 Canadian Bacon Pizza, 1 sl.	313	9	47
• 14 Cheese Pizza, 1 sl.	296	8	47
14 Pepperoni Pizza, 1 sl.	361	14	47
14 Sausage Pizza, 1 sl.	362	14	47
16 Cheese Pizza, 1 sl.	309	8	48

Buck's Pizza (cont.)

Buck's Pizza (cont.)	Cal	Fat	Cbs
16 Pepperoni Pizza, 1 sl.	374	14	48
• 16 Sausage Pizza, 1 sl.	377	15	49

Burger King

Burger King	Cal	Fat	Cbs
Breakfast			
Bacon, Egg & Cheese Biscuit, 146 g	410	25	31
Breakfast Syrup, 28 g	80	0	21
Cini-minis, 108 g	390	18	51
Croissan'wich® Bcn, Egg & Chz, 122 g	340	20	26
Egg & Cheese, 115 g	300	17	26
Ham, Egg & Cheese, 149 g	340	18	26
Sausage & Cheese, 106 g	370	25	23
Sausage, Egg & Cheese, 159 g	470	32	26
Double Croissan'wich™ w/Bcn, Egg, & Chz, 142 g	430	27	27
w/ Ham, Bcn, Egg, & Chz, 169 g	420	24	27
w/ Ham, Egg, & Cheese, 196 g	420	23	27
w/ Ham, Sausage, Egg, & Chz, 206 g	550	37	27
w/ Sausage, Bacon, Egg, & Chz, 179 g	550	39	27
w/ Sausage, Egg, & Cheese, 215 g	680	51	26
• Enormous Omelet Sandwich, 266 g	730	45	44
French Toast Kid's Meal (With Syrup), 494 g	680	24	100
• French Toast Sticks (3 Piece), 65 g	240	13	26
French Toast Sticks (5 Piece), 109 g	390	22	43
Grape Jam, 12 g	30	0	7
Ham Omelet Sandwich, 139 g	330	14	35
Ham, Egg, & Cheese Biscuit, 156 g	390	22	31
Hash Browns - Large, 202 g	620	40	60
Hash Browns - Medium, 140 g	430	28	42
Hash Browns - Small, 84 g	260	17	25
Sausage Biscuit, 118 g	390	26	28
Sausage, Egg, & Cheese Biscuit, 183 g	530	37	31
Strawberry Jam, 12 g	30	0	7
Vanilla Icing (For Cini-minis), 28 g	110	3	21
Desserts			
• Dutch Apple Pie, 108 g	300	13	45
• Hershey's® Sundae Pie, 79 g	310	19	32
Fire-grilled Burgers			
Bk™ Double Stacker, 190 g	610	39	32
• Bk™ Quad Stacker, 311 g	1000	68	34
Bk™ Triple Stacker, 250 g	800	54	33
Cheeseburger, 133 g	330	16	31
Double Cheeseburger, 189 g	500	29	31
Double Hamburger, 164 g	410	21	30
• Hamburger, 121 g	290	12	30
The Angus Steak Burger, 273 g	640	33	55
Salad Dressings & Toppings & Condiments			
Garlic Parmesan Croutons, 14 g	60	2	9
Ken's® Creamy Caesar Dressing, 2 oz.	210	21	4
Ken's® Fat Free Ranch Dressing, 2 oz.	60	0	15
• Ken's® Honey Mustard Dressing, 2 oz.	270	23	15
Ken's® Light Italian Dressing, 2 oz.	120	11	5
Ken's® Ranch Dressing, 2 oz.	190	20	2
• Ketchup (Packet), 10 g	10	0	3
Mayonnaise (Packet), 12 g	80	9	1
Salads			
Garden Salad (No Chicken), 184 g	90	5	7
• Side Garden Salad, 98 g	15	0	3
• Tendercrisp™ Chkn Garden Salad, 306 g	410	22	26
Tendergrill™ Chkn Garden Salad, 292 g	240	9	8
Shakes, Milk, & Iced Coffee			
• Chocolate Milk Shake - Medium, 447 g	690	20	114
• Mocha Bk Joe® Iced Coffee, 452 g	380	10	66
Oreo® Sundae Shake - Chocolate - Med, 369 g	680	24	105
Oreo® Sundae Shake - Strawberry - Med, 367 g	660	23	103
Oreo® Sundae Shake - Vanilla - Med, 351 g	610	24	87
Strawberry Milk Shake - Med, 444 g	660	19	111

Burger King (cont.)

Burger King (cont.)	Cal	Fat	Cbs
Shakes, Milk, & Iced Coffee (cont.)			
Vanilla Milk Shake - Medium, 412 g	560	21	79
Sides			
Cheesy Tots™ Potatoes - Medium (9 pcs.), 115 g	320	18	30
French Fries - Medium (Salt Not Added), 116 g	360	20	41
• French Fries - Medium (Salted), 116 g	360	20	41
• Mott's® Strawberry Flavored Apple Sauce, 113 g	90	0	23
Onion Rings - Medium, 91 g	310	15	37
Zesty Onion Ring Dipping Sauce (1 oz), 28 g	150	15	3
Whopper® Sandwiches			
Bacon (1 Strip), 3 g	15	1	0
Barbecue Dipping Sauce, 1 oz.	40	0	11
Bk Big Fish® Sandwich w/o Tartar Sauce, 220 g	470	13	65
Bk Big Fish® Sandwich, 249 g	640	32	67
Bk Veggie® Burger w/ Cheese, 228 g	470	20	47
Bk Veggie® Burger w/o Mayo, 205 g	340	8	46
Bk Veggie® Burger, 215 g	420	16	46
Bk™ Chicken Fries 12 pcs., 170 g	520	31	35
Bk™ Chicken Fries 6 pcs., 85 g	260	15	18
Bk™ Chicken Fries 9 pcs., 128 g	390	23	26
Buffalo Dipping Sauce (1 oz), 28 g	80	8	2
Chicken Tenders® 5 pcs., 77 g	210	12	13
Chicken Tenders® 8 pcs., 123 g	340	20	21
Chicken Tenders® Big Kid's Meal 6 pcs, 92 g	250	15	16
• Chicken Tenders® Kid's Meal 4 pcs., 62 g	170	10	11
Double Whopper® Sandwich, 373 g	900	57	51
w/o Mayo, 352 g	740	39	51
with Cheese w/o Mayo, 376 g	830	47	52
with Cheese, 398 g	990	64	52
Honey Mustard Dipping Sauce, 1 oz.	90	6	8
Original Chicken Sandwich w/o Mayo, 190 g	450	17	52
Original Chicken Sandwich, 219 g	660	40	52
Ranch Dipping Sauce, 1 oz.	140	15	1
Spicy Chick'n Crisp™ Sandwich w/o Mayo, 122 g	320	13	36
Spicy Chick'n Crisp™ Sandwich, 144 g	480	31	36
Sweet and Sour Dipping Sauce, 1 oz.	45	0	11
Tendercrisp® Chicken Sandwich, 284 g	790	44	68
w/ Mayo, 258 g	510	19	49
w/o Mayo, 244 g	400	7	49
Triple Whopper® Sandwich, 456 g	1130	74	51
w/o Mayo, 434 g	980	57	51
with Cheese w/o Mayo, 459 g	1070	65	52
with Cheese, 480 g	1230	82	52
Whopper Jr.® Sandwich, 158 g	370	21	31
w/o Mayo, 147 g	290	12	31
with Cheese w/o Mayo, 149 g	330	16	31
with Cheese, 170 g	410	24	32
Whopper® Sandwich, 290 g	670	39	51
w/o Mayo, 269 g	510	22	51
with Cheese w/o Mayo, 294 g	600	30	52
with Cheese, 315 g	760	47	52

Burgerville, USA

Burgerville, USA	Cal	Fat	Cbs
Breakfast			
2 Eggs, Any Style	200	14	2
American Cheese, 2 slices	90	7	0
Bagel, Bacon, Egg	450	11	64
Bagel, Ham, Egg	450	8	65
• Bagel, Sausage, Egg	600	26	64
Biscuit, Bacon, Egg	400	23	32
Biscuit, Ham, Egg	400	20	33
Biscuit, Sausage, Egg	470	29	32
Cheese Bagel	290	6	53
• Ham, 2 oz.	55	2	1
Hash Browns	220	13	23
Plain Bagel	310	1	63

Burgerville, USA (cont.)

	Cal	Fat	Cbs
Breakfast (cont.)			
Sausage Patty, 2 oz.	210	20	0
Tillamook Cheese, 1 slices	120	10	1
Condiments/Dressings			
BBQ Sauce Dip	60	1	13
Blue Cheese Dressing	240	24	3
Honey Mustard Dressing	210	20	6
Italian Dressing	140	15	1
Ranch Dressing	250	27	1
• Raspberry Vinaigrette	45	2	6
• Spread Cups, 2 oz.	280	30	4
Tartar Cups, 2 oz.	260	28	2
Cones			
Ice Cream Cone	250	11	32
Yogurt Cone	190	0	39
Cookies			
Chocolate Chunk	320	14	48
• Heath Toffee	340	14	46
• Oatmeal Raisin	290	8	50
White Chocolate Macadamia	340	16	46
Entrees			
Cheeseburger	350	19	29
Chicken Strips, 5 pcs.	550	30	36
Colossal	520	30	30
Crispy Chicken	450	18	55
Deluxe Crispy Chicken	610	30	56
Double Beef Cheeseburger	430	25	29
Gardenburger	460	19	53
Grilled Chicken	350	3	45
• Half Pound Colossal	730	45	31
Halibut Fillet Sandwich	480	27	42
Halibut Fish, 3 pcs.	330	16	25
Halibut Fish, 4 pcs.	410	20	32
• Hamburger	300	15	29
Pepper Bacon Cheeseburger	680	45	28
Protein Platter	530	40	6
Spicy Black Bean Gardenburger	550	32	45
Tillamook Cheeseburger	630	40	32
Turkey Burger	540	29	33
Turkey Club Sandwich	540	32	38
French Fries			
• Kid's	220	12	24
• Large	510	29	57
Regular	390	22	44
Kids Meal			
• Apple Slices	29	0	9
• Cheeseburger	370	20	29
Chicken Strips, 3 pcs.	200	8	15
Hamburger	320	16	29
Kid's French Fries	220	12	24
Kids Caramel Sundae	210	7	35
Kids Chocolate Sundae	180	6	31
Kids Hot Fudge Sundae	210	10	30
Milkshakes			
Black Forest	820	32	130
• Chocolate Hazelnut	900	44	117
Fresh Strawberry	770	31	116
Mocha Perk	830	39	112
NW Blackberry	870	36	129
NW Huckleberry	790	36	105
NW Raspberry	870	36	126
Pumpkin Spice	770	35	105
Regular Chocolate	520	23	73
• Regular Strawberry	500	20	74
Regular Vanilla	500	20	74

Burgerville, USA (cont.)

	Cal	Fat	Cbs
Salads			
• Chicken Strip Salad	750	51	39
Grilled Chicken Salad	520	35	18
NW Smoked Salmon Salad	540	34	20
NW Smoked Turkey Salad	500	36	25
• Side Salad	70	4	5
Seasonal			
Blackberry Shortcake	340	7	70
• Onion Rings, 5 pcs.	810	48	83
• Raspberry Shortcake	330	7	63
Strawberry Shortcake	290	5	62
Sweet Potato Fries	530	29	60
Walla Walla Onion Cheeseburger	679	44	39
Smoothies			
• Chocolate Hazelnut	460	4	93
Chocolate Monkey	450	3	100
Fresh Strawberry	410	0	90
NW Blackberry	420	0	92
NW Huckleberry	390	0	82
NW Raspberry	420	0	91
Pumpkin Spice	390	2	79
• Strawberry Splash	310	1	68
Triple Berry Blast	350	0	75
Sundaes			
Caramel	380	15	56
Chocolate	360	15	52
• Hot Fudge	380	18	51
• Raspberry	360	14	53

Captain D's Seafood

	Cal	Fat	Cbs
Appetizers			
Cheese Sticks w/o sauce, 133 g	440	24	32
• Cheese Sticks with sauce, 154 g	560	36	35
Fried Pickles w/ Ranch Dressing, 143 g	360	30	17
• Gumbo Soup with Rice, 227 g	210	8	26
Jalapeño Cheese Bites, 136 g	350	19	36
D's Classics			
2 Piece Fish & Chicken Dinner, 502 g	1460	93	121
2 Piece Fish Dinner, 443 g	1290	83	110
3 Piece Fish Dinner, 508 g	1450	93	120
Batter Dipped Fish, 65 g	160	10	10
Bite Size Shrimp Platter, 432 g	1140	62	121
• Butterfly Shrimp, 15 g	45	3	3
Catfish Dinner, 404 g	1040	63	87
• Catfish Feast, 737 g	1990	141	128
Chicken Dinner, 438 g	1200	72	102
Chicken Strip, 58 g	170	10	11
Clam Platter, 490 g	1440	87	134
Country Style Fish Dinner, 440 g	1180	69	99
Crab & Fish Dinner, 492 g	1320	83	118
Crab & Shrimp Dinner, 450 g	1080	63	104
Crab Dinner, 490 g	1050	60	106
Deluxe Seafood Platter, 630 g	1700	106	144
Fish & Fries, 330 g	1120	71	97
Fish & Shrimp Dinner, 516 g	1510	96	126
Fish, Shrimp & Chicken Platter, 568 g	1700	107	138
Flounder Dinner, 584 g	1530	94	116
Jumbo Fish Platter, 573 g	1610	102	130
Oyster Dinner, 416 g	1000	58	100
Shrimp Dinner, 409 g	1110	67	102
Stuffed Crab, 57 g	100	5	9
Super Shrimp Platter, 496 g	1380	83	122
Desserts			
Carrot Cake, 99 g	390	19	50
• Cheesecake w/ Strawberry Topping, 142 g	430	26	45
• Chocolate Cake, 85 g	300	11	49

Captain D's Seafood (cont.)

	Cal	Fat	Cbs
Desserts (cont.)			
Pecan Pie, 113 g	470	26	56
Pineapple Cream Cheese Pie, 106 g	320	14	43
Dressing Packets			
Blue Cheese Dressing, 2 oz.	230	24	2
• Fat Free Italian Dressing, 2 oz.	15	0	3
Fat Free Raspberry Vinaigrette, 2 oz.	50	0	13
• Honey Mustard Dressing, 2 oz.	250	25	8
Ranch Dressing, 2 oz.	180	18	2
Thousand Island Dressing, 2 oz.	180	17	8
Family Packs			
• 10 Piece Chicken Only, 146 g	440	26	27
10 Piece Chicken Pack, 406 g	1110	66	96
10 Piece Fish Only, 213 g	690	47	45
• 10 Piece Fish Value Pack, 473 g	1360	87	114
Seafood Feast, 456 g	1350	85	115
Slaw, Fries, Hush Puppies, 260 g	670	40	69
Kids Meal			
• Kid's Chicken, 535 g	680	32	85
• Kid's Fish, 593 g	960	55	105
• Kid's Shrimp, 562 g	740	33	100
Kitchen Selections			
Chicken Breast Combo, 288 g	470	15	54
• Coastal Flounder Dinner, 302 g	360	10	31
Mahi-Mahi, 315 g	490	15	52
Parmesan Chicken Scampi, 352 g	610	27	59
Premium Shrimp Dinner, 186 g	470	15	18
• Seafood Lover's Mixed Grill, 605 g	910	25	80
Seafood Scampi Platter, 409 g	530	20	36
Shrimp Skewers Combo, 315 g	510	10	53
Tilapia Combo, 316 g	490	14	52
Wild Alaskan Salmon, 330 g	590	22	56
Pasta			
Chicken Broccoli Alfredo, 540 g	900	37	98
• Chicken Broccoli Alfredo, 554 g	970	44	98
Classic Chicken Parmesan, 519 g	850	30	105
Savory Shrimp Scampi, 473 g	800	33	92
Shrimp Broccoli Alfredo, 517 g	870	36	97
• Shrimp Marinara, 502 g	670	15	94
Salads			
Blackened Chicken Salad, 325 g	250	9	10
Breadstick, 43 g	150	5	21
Crispy Chicken Caesar Salad, 440 g	920	70	52
Fried Chicken Salad, 335 g	500	29	31
Fried Shrimp Salad, 388 g	610	29	60
• Garden Salad, 218 g	150	8	9
• Grilled Chicken Caesar Salad, 510 g	910	68	44
Grilled Seasoned Shrimp, 400 g	420	12	41
Grilled Wild Alaskan Salmon, 466 g	570	25	44
Southern Style Fried Chicken Salad, 354 g	460	20	51
Sandwiches			
Deluxe Classic Fish Sandwich, 306 g	890	59	62
• Double Bacon Ranch Crispy Chkn Sand, 331 g	1000	67	67
Double Bacon Ranch Grilled Chkn Sand, 310 g	870	60	45
Grilled Alaskan Salmon Sandwich, 328 g	790	49	46
• Seasoned Tilapia Sandwich, 314 g	690	42	42
Sauces			
• Cocktail Sauce, 3/4 oz.	25	0	6
Ginger Teriyaki Sauce, 2 fl.oz.	60	0	13
• Honey Mustard Sauce, 3/4 oz.	120	12	3
Scampi Sauce, 2 fl.oz.	120	10	5
Sweet & Sour Sauce, 3/4 oz.	45	0	10
Sweet Chili Sauce, 2 fl.oz.	100	0	25
Tartar Sauce, 3/4 oz.	100	10	1

Captain D's Seafood (cont.)

	Cal	Fat	Cbs
Sides			
Baked Potato plain, 255 g	240	0	54
Breadstick, 85 g	300	11	42
Broccoli, 100 g	40	1	5
Cole Slaw, 109 g	170	12	13
Corn on the Cob, 163 g	190	3	37
French Fries, 3 oz.	310	15	38
Fried Okra, 113 g	230	14	23
Fried Pickles w/ Ranch Dressing, 143 g	360	30	17
Garlic Mashed Potatoes, 113 g	100	3	16
Green Beans, 113 g	60	2	10
• Hush Puppies, 99 g	400	26	36
Lemon Herb Rice, 113 g	150	1	31
Macaroni & Cheese, 113 g	160	7	17
Roasted Red Potatoes, 124 g	170	7	25
• Sliced Tomatoes, 60 g	10	0	2
Vegetable Medley, 144 g	140	11	9

Caribou Coffee

	Cal	Fat	Cbs
Amy's Blend Pink Ribbon Bagel, 113 g	310	4	61
Blackberry & White Choco Scone, 128 g	490	22	70
Blueberry Muffin, 135 g	410	18	55
Caprese Salad, 287 g	378	32	8
Caribou Coffee Snack Bars, 35 g	140	4	26
Cheddar Cheese Bagel, 113 g	290	4	53
Chocolate Chocolate Chip Muffin, 135 g	480	24	62
Chocolate Chunk Cookie, 94 g	441	22	58
Cinnamon Chip Scone, 120 g	500	22	68
Cinnamon Hoof Mints, 1 g	0	0	1
Cinnamon Raisin Bagel, 113 g	300	2	63
Cinnamon Roll Popover, 159 g	580	30	70
Cinnamon Streusel Muff w/ Wh Choco Chp, 135 g	530	25	71
Dark Chocolate Graham, 28 g	140	8	18
Double Chocolate Biscotti, 57 g	250	10	36
• Fruit Salad, 250 g	105	0	27
Italian Beef Sandwich, 272 g	626	30	56
Lemon Poppy Seed Loaf Cake, 128 g	470	26	56
Milk Chocolate Graham, 28 g	140	8	18
Multi Grain Bagel, 113 g	360	7	63
Orange Walnut White Chocolate Biscotti, 57 g	250	11	34
Original Almond Biscotti, 57 g	230	8	34
Peanut Butter Cookie, 94 g	450	23	55
Peppermint Hoof Mints, 1 g	0	0	1
Pumpkin Bread, 124 g	430	22	54
Reduced Fat Banana Bread, 129 g	380	11	72
Reduced Fat Cranberry Orange Scone, 128 g	450	14	78
Reduced Fat Mountain Brry Muffin, 135 g	300	6	54
Roasted Chicken Sandwich, 238 g	540	19	53
Roasted Vegetable Sandwich, 296 g	622	36	61
Rosemary Romano Chicken Salad Sandwich, 258 g	637	65	49
Smoked Turkey Sandwich, 245 g	590	29	53
Tomato Gorgonzola Pasta Salad, 258 g	397	19	45
• Tortellini Salad, 278 g	820	48	72
Turkey and Pesto Sandwich, 239 g	431	16	42
Turkey Cherry Pasta Salad, 247 g	571	33	44
White Chocolate Macadamia Nut Cookie, 94 g	420	20	55
White Chocolate Pretzel, 24 g	110	5	17
Wintergreen Hoof Mints, 1 g	0	0	1
Beverages			
Small Açaí Smoothie, 16 fl.oz.	290	3	65
• Small Americano, 12 fl.oz.	5	0	1
Small Blended Chai w/ 2% Milk, 16 fl.oz.	180	4	31
Small Blended Chai w/ Skim Milk, 16 fl.oz.	150	0	31
Small Breve, 12 fl.oz.	310	26	11
• Small Campfire Mocha, 12 fl.oz.	460	16	71
• Small Cappuccino, 12 fl.oz.	140	5	14

Caribou Coffee (cont.)

	Cal	Fat	Cbs
Beverages (cont.)			
Small Caramel Cooler, 16 fl.oz.	340	12	56

Carl's Jr.

	Cal	Fat	Cbs
Breakfast			
Bacon & Egg Burrito, 208 g	570	33	37
• Breakfast Burger™, 309 g	830	47	65
• French Toast Dips® - No Syrup (5 pieces), 129 g	430	18	58
Hash Brown Nuggets, 108 g	330	21	32
Loaded Breakfast Burrito, 328 g	820	51	52
Sourdough Breakfast Sandwich, 193 g	460	21	39
Steak & Egg Burrito, 322 g	660	36	44
Sunrise Croissant™ Sandwich, 172 g	560	41	27
Charbroiled Burgers			
Big Hamburger, 209 g	470	17	54
Double Western Bacon Cheeseburger™, 323 g	970	52	71
Famous Star™ with Cheese, 278 g	660	39	53
Jalapeño Burger™, 286 g	720	45	50
• Kid's Hamburger, 195 g	460	17	53
Philly Cheesesteak Burger, 297 g	830	55	52
Super Star® with Cheese, 385 g	930	59	54
The Bacon Cheese Six Dollar Burger™, 409 g	1070	76	50
• The Double Six Dollar Burger™, 602 g	1520	111	60
The Guacamole Bacon Six Dollar Burger™, 447 g	1140	85	54
The Low Carb Six Dollar Burger™, 267 g	490	37	6
The Original Six Dollar Burger™, 430 g	1010	68	60
The Western Bacon Six Dollar Burger®, 382 g	1130	66	83
Western Bacon Cheeseburger®, 241 g	710	33	70
Chicken & Other Choices			
• Bacon Swiss Crispy Chicken™ Sandwich, 318 g	720	35	64
Carl's Catch™ Fish Sandwich, 291 g	660	31	75
• Charbroiled BBQ Chicken™ Sandwich, 239 g	360	5	48
Charbroiled Chicken Club™ Sandwich, 264 g	550	25	43
Charbroiled Santa Fe Chicken™ Sandwich, 264 g	610	32	43
Chicken Breast Strips (3 pieces), 129 g	420	25	28
Chicken Breast Strips (5 pieces), 215 g	710	41	46
Spicy Chicken Sandwich, 213 g	560	30	59
Desserts			
Chocolate Cake, 85 g	300	12	48
• Chocolate Chip Cookie, 71 g	350	18	46
• Strawberry Swirl Cheesecake, 99 g	290	17	30
Hand-Scooped Ice Cream Shakes & Malts™			
Chocolate Malt, 414 g	780	35	98
Chocolate Shake, 397 g	710	33	85
OREO® Cookie Malt, 414 g	790	39	91
OREO® Cookie Shake, 397 g	720	37	79
Strawberry Malt, 414 g	770	35	97
• Strawberry Shake, 397 g	700	33	84
• Vanilla Malt, 414 g	780	35	99
Vanilla Shake, 397 g	710	33	86
Salad Dressings			
• Blue Cheese Dressing, 2 oz.	320	34	1
House Dressing, 2 oz.	220	22	2
• Low Fat Balsamic Dressing, 2 oz.	35	2	5
Thousand Island Dressing, 2 oz.	250	2	7
Salads - Without Dressings			
Charbroiled Chicken Salad, 417 g	260	7	16
Side Salad, 139 g	50	3	5
Sides			
• Chicken Stars™ (6 pieces), 85 g	260	16	14
CrissCut® Fries, 139 g	410	24	43
• Fish & Chips, 258 g	630	28	68
French Fries (Medium), 147 g	460	22	59
Fried Zucchini, 139 g	320	19	31
Onion Rings, 128 g	430	21	53

Carvel Ice Cream

	Cal	Fat	Cbs
Classic Sundaes (Regular)			
• Bittersweet Fudge	690	38	77
Caramel	670	34	81
Hot Fudge	670	38	73
No Fat Classic Sundae (Fudge)	380	0	81
• No Fat Classic Sundae (Strawberry)	320	0	69
Strawberry	580	33	63
Cones - Regular			
• Cake Cone with Chocolate	440	21	51
Cake Cone with Vanilla	470	26	50
Sugar Cone with Chocolate	460	21	59
Sugar Cone with Vanilla	500	26	58
Waffle Cone with Chocolate	500	22	66
• Waffle Cone with Vanilla	530	26	65
Fountain Regular			
Brown Bonnet®, 16 fl.oz.	370	21	40
Chipsters, 16 fl.oz.	330	16	44
Deluxe Flying Saucer™, 16 fl.oz.	330	15	47
Flying Saucer™ (Chocolate), 16 fl.oz.	230	10	33
Flying Saucer™ (Vanilla), 16 fl.oz.	240	11	33
• Mini Sundae (Chocolate Syrup), 16 fl.oz.	200	9	27
No Fat Carvelanche® (Strwbrry), 16 fl.oz.	430	0	91
No Fat Chocolate Shake, 16 fl.oz.	440	0	104
No Fat Mocha Shake, 16 fl.oz.	440	0	97
No Fat Vanilla Shake, 16 fl.oz.	300	0	62
Olde Fashion Sundae, 16 fl.oz.	340	15	47
• Sinful Love Bar, 16 fl.oz.	460	29	47
Sprinkle Cup, 16 fl.oz.	230	15	28
Ice Cream Regular Cup			
Chocolate, 7 oz.	410	21	48
No Fat Chocolate, 7 oz.	270	0	62
• No Fat Vanilla, 7 oz.	270	0	55
No Sugar Added Vanilla, 7 oz.	300	7	57
Sherbet, 7 oz.	300	3	66
• Vanilla, 7 oz.	450	26	47
Novelties			
• 98% Fat Free Flying Saucer™ (chocolate)	180	3	34
98% Fat Free Flying Saucer™ (vanilla)	180	3	35
No Fat Miniature Sundae	190	0	45
No Fat Olde Fashioned Sundae	300	0	67
No Fat Parfait	190	0	42
No Sugar Added Miniature Sundae	200	3	42
• No Sugar Added Olde Fashioned Sundae	360	5	76
No Sugar Added Parfait	200	3	42

Charley's Grilled Subs

	Cal	Fat	Cbs
Chicken Tenders			
5 piece	334	20	17
Kid's	200	12	10
Fries			
Cheddar & Bacon	1089	87	55
Cheddar Cheese	1054	84	55
• Cheddar, Ranch & Bacon	1249	103	57
Ranch & Bacon	1149	95	51
• Regular	611	46	42
Grilled Salads			
Buffalo Chicken	296	13	17
Chicken Teriyaki	292	13	16
• Fresh Garden	141	8	13
Grilled Chicken	281	13	14
Grilled Steak	291	16	14
Lemonade			
Kiwi or Strawberry, 16 oz.	202	0	50
Original, 16 oz.	162	0	40
Sandwiches			
• Bacon 3 cheese Steak	645	30	55

Charley's Grilled Subs (cont.)	Cal	Fat	Cbs
Sandwiches (cont.)			
Bacon 3 cheese Steak Low Fat	490	18	53
BBQ Cheddar Steak	586	20	70
BBQ Cheddar Steak Low Fat	476	11	69
Chicken Bacon Club	580	23	54
Chicken Bacon Club Low Fat	480	15	53
Chicken Buffalo	531	16	61
Chicken Buffalo Low Fat	431	8	60
Chicken Cordon Bleu	595	22	58
Chicken Cordon Bleu Low Fat	495	14	57
Chicken Teriyaki	527	16	60
Chicken Teriyaki Low Fat	427	8	59
Italian Deli	427	12	55
Italian Deli Low Fat	327	4	54
Philly Cheesesteak	526	19	58
Philly Cheesesteak Low Fat	426	11	57
Philly Chicken	519	16	59
Philly Chicken Low Fat	419	8	58
Philly Ham & Swiss	439	13	59
Philly Ham & Swiss Low Fat	339	5	58
Philly Steak Deluxe	529	19	59
Philly Steak Deluxe Low Fat	429	11	58
Philly Veggie	452	15	63
• Philly Veggie Low Fat	297	3	61
Steak Sicilian	570	24	54
Steak Sicilian Low Fat	520	20	54
Turkey Cheddar Melt	444	12	55
Turkey Cheddar Melt Low Fat	334	3	54
Ultimate Club	517	20	55
Ultimate Club Low Fat	407	11	54

Chevy's Fresh Mex	Cal	Fat	Cbs
Grande Salads			
Santa Fe Chopped Salad	682	41	25
No cheese	480	25	25
• No cheese, bacon or avocado	258	6	21
No cheese or bacon	338	13	25
• Tostada Salad with Chicken	1228	77	63
No tortilla strips	1088	71	44
No tortilla strips, cheese or sour cream	542	23	40
No tortilla strips, cheese, sour cream, or guac	463	16	35
No tortilla strips or cheese	663	35	42
Grilled Tacos			
Grilled Chicken Tacos	911	41	86
No tamalito	827	37	73
No tamalito or rice	651	32	44
No tamalito, rice, cheese or Chipotle Aioli	504	17	43
No tamalito, rice or cheese	595	27	44
• Grilled Fish Tacos (Salmon)	1092	64	70
No tamalito	1008	60	57
No tamalito or rice	832	55	28
No tamalito, rice or sour cream	711	43	26
No tamalito, rice, sour cream or guacamole	632	36	21
Grilled Fish Tacos (Sea Bass)	845	39	88
No tamalito	761	35	75
No tamalito or rice	585	30	46
No tamalito, rice or cheese	529	25	46
• No tamalito, rice, cheese or Chipotle Aioli	438	15	45
Grilled Steak Tacos	972	51	87
No tamalito	888	47	74
No tamalito or rice	712	42	45
No tamalito, rice or cheese	656	37	45
Homemade Beans			
Beans a la Charra	230	5	33
No cheese	202	3	33
No cheese or pico de gallo	198	3	32

Chevy's Fresh Mex (cont.)	Cal	Fat	Cbs
Homemade Beans (cont.)			
Black Beans	207	3	33
No cheese	179	1	33
• No cheese or pico de gallo	175	1	32
• Refried Beans	298	15	29
No cheese	270	13	29
No cheese or pico de gallo	266	13	28
Sizzling Fajitas			
• Juicy Shrimp Fajitas, no tortillas	1212	85	70
No tortillas or tamalito	1128	81	57
No tortillas, tamalito or rice	952	76	28
No tortillas, tamalito, rice or sour cream	831	64	26
No tortillas, tamalito, rice, sour crm or guac	752	57	21
Mix & Match (Chicken & Steak) Fajitas, no tortillas	959	52	67
No tortillas or tamalito	875	48	54
No tortillas, tamalito or rice	699	43	25
No tortillas, tamalito, rice or sour cream	578	31	23
No tortillas, tamalito, rice, sour cream or guac	499	24	18
Original Famous Chicken Fajitas, no tortillas	913	45	67
No tortillas or tamalito	829	41	54
No tortillas, tamalito or rice	653	36	25
No tortillas, tamalito, rice or sour cream	532	24	23
No tortillas, tamalito, rice, sour cream or guac	453	17	18
Portobello Mushroom & Asprgs Fajitas, no tortillas	878	57	86
No tortillas or tamalito	794	53	73
No tortillas, tamalito or rice	618	48	44
No tortillas, tamalito, rice or sour cream	497	36	42
• No tortillas, tamalito, rice, sour cream or guac	418	29	37
Sizzling Steak Fajitas, no tortillas	1066	59	67
No tortillas or tamalito	922	55	54
No tortillas, tamalito or rice	746	50	25
No tortillas, tamalito, rice or sour cream	625	38	23
No tortillas, tamalito, rice, sour cream or guac	546	31	18

Chick-Fil-A	Cal	Fat	Cbs
Breakfast			
Bacon Egg & Cheese Biscuit, 6 oz.	470	26	39
Biscuit with Gravy, 7 oz.	330	15	43
Chicken, Egg & Chz on Sunflower Mltgrn Bagel, 8 oz.	500	20	49
Chick-Fil-A Chicken Burrito, 7 oz.	410	16	42
Chick-Fil-A Chicken, 5 oz.	420	19	44
Chick-Fil-A Chick-N-Minis (3 Count), 3 oz.	280	11	29
Chick-Fil-A Chick-N-Minis (4 Count), 4 oz.	370	15	38
Chick-Fil-A Sausage Burrito, 7 oz.	450	23	39
Cinnamon Cluster, 4 oz.	400	15	61
• Fruit Cup (medium), 4 oz.	70	0	16
Hashbrowns, 3 oz.	260	17	25
Hot Buttered Biscuit, 3 oz.	270	12	38
• Sausage & Egg Biscuit, 7 oz.	570	37	39
Sunflower Multigrain Bagel, 3 oz.	220	3	41
Chick-Fil-A Coolwrap			
Chargrilled Chicken Coolwrap, 9 oz.	410	12	46
• Chicken Caesar Coolwrap, 8 oz.	480	16	44
• Spicy Chicken Coolwrap, 8 oz.	410	12	44
Croutons/Kernels			
• Garlic & Butter Croutons, 0.5 oz.	70	3	9
• Honey Roasted sunflower Kernels, 0.5 oz.	80	7	3
Tortilla Strips, 0.5 oz.	70	4	9
Desserts			
Cheesecake (1 slice), 3 oz.	340	21	30
Fudge Nut Brownie (1 Brownie), 3 oz.	330	15	45
Hand-Spun Milk Shake (Chocolate), 20 oz.	760	28	113
• Hand-Spun Milk Shake (Cookies & Cream), 20 oz.	790	33	111
Hand-Spun Milk Shake (Strawberry), 20 oz.	730	28	109
Hand-Spun Milk Shake (Vanilla), 20 oz.	660	27	90
• Icedream (Small Cone), 5 oz.	160	4	28

RESTAURANTS & FAST-FOOD CHAINS

Chick-Fil-A (cont.)

	Cal	Fat	Cbs
Desserts (cont.)			
Icedream (Small Cup), 8 oz.	240	6	41
Lemon Pie (1 slice), 4 oz.	350	11	59
Dipping Sauces			
Barbecue Sauce, 1 oz.	45	0	11
• Buttermilk Ranch Sauce, 1 oz.	110	12	1
• Chick-Fil-A Buffalo Sauce, 1 oz.	15	2	1
Honey Mustard Sauce, 1 oz.	45	0	10
Honey Roasted BBQ Sauce, 0.5 oz.	60	6	2
Polynesian Sauce, 1 oz.	110	6	13
Dressings			
Blue Cheese, 29 g	150	16	1
Buttermilk Ranch, 30 g	160	16	1
• Caesar, 29 g	160	17	1
Fat Free Honey Mustard, 35 g	60	0	14
• Light Italian, 32 g	15	5	2
Reduced Fat Raspberry Vinaigrette, 37 g	80	2	15
Spicy, 29 g	140	14	2
Thousand Salad, 30 g	150	14	5
Salads			
• Chick-Fil-A Chargrilled Chicken Green Salad, 10 oz.	180	6	9
• Chick-Fil-A Chick-N-Strips Salad, 11 oz.	400	20	21
Chick-Fil-A Southwest Chargrilled Salad, 11 oz.	240	8	17
Sandwiches: Classics			
Chargrilled Chicken Club Sandwich, 8 oz.	221	11	33
Chick-Fil-A Chargrilled Chicken Sandwich, 7 oz.	270	4	33
Chick-Fil-A Chicken Salad Sandwich, 5 oz.	350	15	32
• Chick-Fil-A Chicken Sandwich, 6 oz.	410	16	38
Chick-Fil-A Chick-N-Strips, 5 oz.	310	15	15
Chick-Fil-A Nuggets, 4 oz.	260	13	10
Sides			
Carrot & Basin Salad (small), 4 oz.	170	6	28
• Chick-Fil-A Waffle Potato Fries (sm), 3 oz.	270	13	34
Cole Slaw, 5 oz.	260	21	17
Fruit Cup (small), 4 oz.	70	0	17
Hearty Breast of Chicken Soup, 9 oz.	140	4	18
• Side Salad, 4 oz.	60	3	4

Chili's Restaurant

	Cal	Fat	Cbs
Baby Back Ribs			
• Blazin' Habanero Ribs w/ Habanero BBQ Sauce	1220	66	94
Brown Sugar Chile Ribs w/ Sauce	1000	70	37
Honey BBQ Ribs w/ Honey BBQ Sauce	1060	65	82
Honey Chipotle Ribs w/ Sauce	1160	65	82
Memphis Dry Rub Ribs w/ Dijon BBQ Sauce	1000	70	37
• Original BBQ Ribs w/ Classic BBQ Sauce	970	66	33
Big Mouth Burgers®			
Bacon Burger	1080	71	54
• BBQ Ranch Burger	1110	71	60
Big Mouth Bun only (with butter)	460	20	55
• Burger Patty only (without bun or toppings)	360	25	0
Chipotle Bleu Cheese Bacon Burger	1090	71	57
Ground Peppercorn Burger	1050	68	61
Mushroom-Swiss Burger	1100	71	60
Oldtimer Burger®	800	44	54
Oldtimer Burger® w/ Cheese	880	51	54
Chicken			
Cajun Chicken Pasta w/ Garlic Toast	1500	78	123
Chicken Club Tacos	1140	45	126
Chicken Crispers®	1880	103	133
Chicken Tacos	1200	41	137
Country Fried Chicken Crispers (no dressing)	1660	101	141
• Crispy Honey Chipotle Crispers (no dressing)	1890	99	203
• Margarita Grilled Chicken	690	18	81
Monterey Chicken®	1130	67	67

Chili's Restaurant (cont.)

	Cal	Fat	Cbs
Create Your Own Combo			
Sizzle & Spice Classic Sirloin	540	42	1
Sizzle & Spice Firecracker Tilapia	270	7	16
• Sizzle & Spice Garlic & Lime Grilled Shrimp	260	13	6
Sizzle & Spice Half Rack Baby Back Ribs	490	33	16
• Sizzle & Spice Honey BBQ Sirloin	730	57	17
Sizzle & Spice Margarita Grilled Chicken	320	13	13
Sizzle & Spice Monterey Chicken®	460	27	14
Desserts			
Cheesecake	720	44	68
• Chocolate Chip Paradise Pie® w/ Vanilla Ice Cream	1600	78	215
Frosty Chocolate Shake w/ Chocolate Sprinkles	850	36	123
Molten Chocolate Cake w/ Vanilla Ice Cream	1270	62	172
Sweet Shot – Dutch Apple Caramel	230	6	41
Sweet Shot – Seven Layers of Chocolate	310	16	40
• Sweet Shot – Strawberry Vanilla Cheesecake	220	11	26
Dressings & Sauces			
Asian Sesame Ginger Dressing, 2 fl.oz.	260	26	6
Avocado Ranch Dressing, 2 fl.oz.	150	15	3
• Awesome Blossom Sauce, 2 fl.oz.	350	36	5
Balsamic Ranch Dressing, 2 fl.oz.	270	27	4
Balsamic Vinaigrette Dressing, 2 fl.oz.	270	27	4
Balsamic Vinaigrette Dressing, low fat, 2 fl.oz.	50	0	9
BBQ Sauce, 2 fl.oz.	80	0	18
Bleu Cheese Dressing, 2 fl.oz.	320	35	1
Caesar Dressing, 2 fl.oz.	350	37	3
Carolina BBQ Sauce, 2 fl.oz.	130	0	31
Chimichurri Sauce, 2 fl.oz.	250	29	3
Chipotle Ranch Dressing, 2 fl.oz.	170	18	2
Citrus Balsamic Vinaigrette Dressing, 2 fl.oz.	340	33	7
Creamy Cilantro Dressing, 2 fl.oz.	300	32	2
Dijon BBQ Sauce, 2 fl.oz.	145	0	35
Habanero BBQ Sauce, 2 fl.oz.	170	0	39
Honey Chipotle Sauce, 2 fl.oz.	200	0	49
Honey Lime Dressing, 2 fl.oz.	270	22	17
Honey Mustard Dressing, 2 fl.oz.	260	28	2
Honey Mustard Dressing, no fat, 2 fl.oz.	90	1	14
Jalapeño Ranch Sauce, 2 fl.oz.	200	20	3
Mango Sauce, 2 fl.oz.	170	15	9
Peanut Dipping Sauce (Lettuce Wraps), 2 fl.oz.	190	13	15
Ranch Dressing, 2 fl.oz.	240	25	3
Ranch Dressing, low fat, 2 fl.oz.	110	6	12
• Salsa Picante Sauce, 2 fl.oz.	40	0	4
Sesame-Ginger Dipping Sauce (Lett Wrps), 2 fl.oz.	70	1	11
Thousand Island Dressing, 2 fl.oz.	270	26	9
Wasabi-Ranch Dressing, 2 fl.oz.	180	18	3
Fire-Grilled Steaks			
Cajun Ribeye	870	76	3
• Classic Sirloin	540	42	1
• Country-Fried Steak w/ Sides	1890	107	148
Flame-Grilled Ribeye	960	87	1
Honey BBQ Sirloin	800	56	19
NY Strip	790	64	1
Guiltless Grill®			
Big Mouth Bun, unbuttered	330	6	55
• Black Bean Brgr Patty only (w/o bun or toppings)	200	2	25
• Guiltless Black Bean Burger	650	12	96
Guiltless Chicken Platter	580	9	85
Guiltless Chicken Sandwich	490	8	63
Guiltless Salmon	480	14	31
Small Whole Wheat Bun, unbuttered	80	2	16
Pepper Pals®			
Cheese Pizza, 1 Pizza	570	24	67
Corn Dog	250	17	18
Country-Fried Chipotle Crispers, 3 each	610	41	26

Chili's Restaurant (cont.)

	Cal	Fat	Cbs
Pepper Pals® (cont.)			
• Crispy Honey Chipotle Crispers, 3 each	770	41	65
Grilled Cheese Sandwich	420	27	26
• Grilled Chicken Platter	140	3	3
Grilled Chicken Sandwich	170	3	16
Kraft® Macaroni & Cheese	510	18	69
Little Chicken Crispers	590	42	19
Little Mouth Burger	280	15	14
Little Mouth Cheeseburger	350	21	14
Pepper Pals® Pasta w/ Alfredo Sauce	410	17	47
Pepper Pals® Pasta w/ Marinara Sauce	290	5	52
Ribs Basket, 1 basket	370	24	16
Pepper Pals Sides & Desserts			
Black Beans	115	0	19
Cinnamon Apples	210	8	35
• Frosty Choc-A-Lot Shake w/ Chocolate Sprinkles	640	27	92
Homestyle Fries	260	16	27
Mashed Potatoes	190	11	19
Rice	160	1	33
• Steamed Broccoli	80	6	6
Sweet Corn on the Cob	230	7	55
Vanilla Ice Cream, 1 Scoop	400	22	44
Salads			
Boneless Buffalo Chicken Salad	910	58	51
• Caesar Salad w/ Chicken & Dressing	1010	76	39
Caesar Salad w/ Lime Grlld Shrimp & Dressing	980	77	39
Dinner Salad – Caesar w/ Dressing	520	43	27
• Dinner Salad – House	140	7	12
Grilled Caribbean Salad	440	10	51
Lettuce Wraps w/ Dipping Sauces	580	35	55
Mesquite Chicken Salad	800	43	53
Quesadilla Explosion Salad w/ Ranch Drizzle	980	48	81
Southwestern Cobb Salad	970	60	56
Sandwiches & Pitas			
Cajun Chicken Sandwich	820	43	66
• Chicken Ranch Sandwich	1150	70	82
Chili's Cheesesteak Sandwich	1010	55	72
Grilled Chicken Sandwich	840	47	57
• Pita – Chicken Caesar	650	41	31
• Pita – Chicken Fajita	450	17	35
Pita – Steak Fajita	580	33	32
Smoked Turkey Sandwich	930	57	65
Smoked Turkey Sandwich w/ Bacon	1030	64	66
Seafood			
• Add On Garlic & Lime Grilled Shrimp, 4 each	160	10	3
Firecracker Tilapia	540	14	63
Grilled Salmon w/ Garlic & Herbs	700	33	53
• Grilled Shrimp Alfredo Pasta w/ Garlic Toast	1540	84	123
Southwest Cedar Plank Tilapia	680	34	53
Sides & Extras			
Black Beans w/ Pico de Gallo	115	0	19
Cinnamon Apples	210	8	35
Garlic Toast, 1 Piece	200	12	18
Homestyle Fries Basket	520	31	53
Homestyle Fries w/ Entrée	430	26	43
• Mashed Potatoes – Loaded	500	32	37
Mashed Potatoes w/ Black Pepper Gravy	450	28	44
Rice	210	2	45
Sautéed Mushrooms, Onions & Bell Peppers	120	10	6
Steamed Broccoli	80	6	6
Steamed Seasonal Veggies w/ Parmesan Cheese	80	5	8
• Steamed Seasonal Veggies w/ Parmesan Cheese	50	1	8
Sweet Corn on the Cob, unbuttered	180	2	55
Sizzling Fajitas & Quesadillas			
Add On Cadillac Style (rice & black beans only)	350	3	68

Chili's Restaurant (cont.)

	Cal	Fat	Cbs
Sizzling Fajitas & Quesadillas (cont.)			
Add On Guacamole	60	5	3
Buffalo Chicken Fajitas	1090	76	56
Citrus Fire Chicken & Shrimp Fajitas	720	42	34
• Classic Chicken Fajitas	330	11	23
Classic Combo Chicken & Steak Fajitas	560	30	21
Classic Steak Fajitas	790	49	20
Fajita Chicken Quesadillas	1830	95	151
Fajita Combo Chicken & Steak Quesadillas	1690	87	133
• Fajita Steak Quesadillas	1830	95	151
Fajita Trio - Garlic Lime Shrmp, Grlld Stk & Chkn	870	51	28
Flour Tortillas, 4 each	400	12	79
Guac, Sour Crm, Cheese & Pico de Gallo, 1 boat	240	19	8
Mushroom Jack Fajitas	750	45	31
Rice, Black Beans, Sour Cream & Pico de Gallo	480	10	79
Steak & Portobello Fajitas	1130	84	26
Soups			
Baked Potato Soup, 1 cup	220	16	12
Broccoli Cheese Soup, 1 cup	160	9	12
Chicken Enchilada Soup, 1 cup	220	14	11
• Chicken Noodle Soup, 1 cup	50	1	7
Chicken Tortilla Soup, 1 cup	140	7	10
Chili - Terlingua w/ Toppings, 1 cup	180	8	15
• New England Clam Chowder Soup, 1 cup	470	33	27
Southwestern Vegetable Soup, 1 cup	110	5	13
Starters			
• Awesome Blossom® w/ Seasoned Sauce	2710	203	194
Blazin' Boneless Bfflo Wng w/ Mango Sau, 9 ea.	1050	67	60
Boneless Bfflo Wings w/ Bleu Cheese, 9 ea.	1170	85	50
Boneless Shanghai Wngs w/ Wasabi-Ranch, 9 ea.	1140	62	91
Bottomless Tostada Chips w/ Ht Sauce, 1 basket	480	36	26
• Bottomless Tostada Chips, 1 basket	400	36	18
Classic Nachos w/ Fajita Beef	1740	127	55
Classic Nachos w/ Fajita Chicken	1630	112	55
Classic Nachos w/ Pico de Gallo & Sour Cream	1450	108	53
Fried Cheese w/ Marinara Sauce, 9 ea.	1210	89	82
Hot Spinach & Artichoke Dip	510	17	39
w/ Tostada Chips	905	36	74
Skillet Queso	670	53	12
w/ Tostada Chips	1071	89	30
SW Egg rolls w/ Avocado-Ranch Dressing, 3 each	810	51	59
Texas Cheese Fries w/ Jalapeño-Ranch, 1 skillet	2070	160	73
Triple Dipper - Blazin' BBQ Wngs w/Mngo Sau, 5	620	41	35
Boneless Bfflo Wings w/ Trtll Strips & Bleu Chz, 5	760	57	0
Chicken Crispers w/ Honey Mustard, 3	780	63	21
Country Fried Chicken Crispers, 3	610	41	26
Fried Cheese Option w/ Marinara, 5	680	50	34
Honey Fried Chicken Crispers w/ Honey-Chipotle, 3	960	41	115
Hot Spinach & Artichoke Dip w/ Tostada Chips	630	53	27
Shanghai Wings w/ Wasabi-Ranch, 5	780	45	63
SW Egg rolls w/ Avocado-Ranch Dressing, 2	550	35	39
Wings Over Buffalo® w/ Bleu Cheese, 5	740	67	3
Celery & Carrot Sticks Garnish	20	0	3
Wings Over Buffalo® w/ Bleu Cheese, 10	1340	117	4

Chipotle

	Cal	Fat	Cbs
Barbacoa, 4 oz.	170	7	2
Black Beans, 4 oz.	130	1	22
Burrito Size Flour Tortilla, 1 ea	290	9	44
Carnitas, 4 oz.	210	11	2
Cheese, 1 oz.	110	9	0
Chicken, 4 oz.	200	7	2
• Chips, 4 oz.	570	27	73
Corn Salsa, 4 oz.	100	1	22
Crispy Taco Shells, 3 ea	180	7	26
Fajita Vegetables, 3 oz.	100	8	6

Chipotle (cont.)

	Cal	Fat	Cbs
Green Tomatillo, 2 oz.	15	1	3
Guacamole, 4 oz.	140	10	10
• Lettuce, 1 oz.	5	0	0
Pinto Beans, 4 oz.	138	1	23
Red Tomatillo, 2 oz.	28	1	4
Rice, 4 oz.	160	4	30
Sour Cream, 2 oz.	120	10	2
Steak, 4 oz.	190	7	2
Taco Size Flour Tortilla, 3 ea	255	8	38
Tomato Salsa, 4 oz.	20	0	3
Vinaigrette, 2 oz.	330	31	12

Chuck E. Cheese

	Cal	Fat	Cbs
Appetizers			
• Buffalo Wings, 12 ea	660	45	3
Italian Bread Sticks, 1 stick	193	8	27
• Mozzarella Sticks, 1 stick	105	6	7
Birthday Cakes			
8" Chocolate/white, 1 slice	310	13	45
8" White/white, 1 slice	310	13	44
Desserts			
Apple Pie Pizza, 1 slice	194	2	40
Cinnamon Sticks, 1 stick	197	5	33
French Fries			
French fries, 5 oz.	241	9	37
French fries, ala carte, 10 oz.	482	17	74
Pizzas			
• Individual w/ cheese, 1 slice	155	5	22
Pepperoni, 1 slice	172	6	22
Large w/ cheese, 1 slice	262	8	36
• All Meat Combo, 1 slice	332	14	37
BBQ Chicken, 1 slice	296	8	47
Canadian Bacon & Pineapple, 1 slice	272	8	38
Pepperoni & Sausage, 1 slice	313	13	37
Pepperoni, 1 slice	289	10	36
Super Combo, 1 slice	305	12	39
Vegetarian, 1 slice	264	8	40
Medium w/ cheese, 1 slice	237	7	33
All Meat Combo, 1 slice	292	12	33
BBQ Chicken, 1 slice	269	8	43
Canadian Bacon & Pineapple, 1 slice	245	7	34
Pepperoni & Sausage, 1 slice	281	11	33
Pepperoni, 1 slice	263	10	33
Super Combo, 1 slice	270	10	35
Vegetarian, 1 slice	237	7	36
Small w/ cheese, 1 slice	192	6	27
All Meat Combo, 1 slice	227	9	27
BBQ Chicken, 1 slice	214	6	34
Canadian Bacon & Pineapple, 1 slice	199	6	28
Pepperoni & Sausage, 1 slice	230	9	27
Pepperoni, 1 slice	216	8	27
Super Combo, 1 slice	220	8	29
Vegetarian, 1 slice	194	6	30
Salad Dressings			
• Blue Cheese, 29 g	150	16	1
• French, 33 g	35	0	8
Lite Ranch, 30 g	80	8	1
Olive Oil & Vinegar, 31 g	100	11	1
Thousand Island, 30 g	150	15	5
Sandwiches			
Grilled Chicken Sub	652	31	70
Ham & Cheese	622	28	70
• Hot Dog	170	17	27
Hot Dog w/Cheese	335	30	28
• Italian Sub	729	40	69

Church's Chicken

	Cal	Fat	Cbs
Condiments			
BBQ Sauce, 21 g	30	0	7
Creamy Jalapeño Sauce, 21 g	100	11	1
Honey Mustard Sauce, 21 g	110	11	4
Honey, 9 g	27	0	7
• Hot Sauce, 7 g	18	0	0
Ketchup, 17 g	18	0	5
Purple Pepper Sauce, 21 g	45	0	12
• Ranch Sauce, 30 g	130	13	1
Sweet & Sour Sauce, 21 g	30	0	8
Desserts			
• Edward's Double Lemon Pie, 85 g	300	14	39
Edward's Strawberry Cream Cheese, 78 g	280	15	32
• Pie Apple Pie, 88 g	260	11	39
Main Course			
Bigger Better Chicken Sandwich w/ Cheese, 182 g	510	27	46
Chkn. Fried Steak w/ White Gravy, 164 g	470	28	36
• Chkn. Fried Steak, w/ White Gravy, 213 g	610	43	31
Chicken Fried Steak Sandwich, 142 g	490	32	38
Crunchy Tenders, 54 g	120	6	6
Original Breast, 1 piece	200	11	3
• Original Leg, 1 piece	110	6	3
Original Thigh, 1 piece	330	23	8
Original Wing, 1 piece	300	19	7
Spicy Breast, 1 piece	320	20	12
Spicy Crunchy Tenders, 54 g	135	7	7
Spicy Fish Fillet, 65 g	160	9	13
Spicy Fish Sandwich, 108 g	320	20	25
Spicy Leg, 1 piece	180	11	8
Spicy Thigh, 1 piece	480	35	20
Spicy Wing, 1 piece	430	27	17
Sides			
Cajun Rice, 88 g	130	7	16
Cole Slaw, 118 g	150	10	15
Collard Greens, 100 g	25	0	5
Corn on the Cob, 1 ear	140	3	24
French Fries, 100 g	290	14	38
Honey Butter Biscuits, 60 g	240	12	28
Jalapeño Bombers®, 113 g	240	10	29
Macaroni & Cheese, 150 g	210	11	23
Mashed Potatoes & Gravy, 104 g	70	2	12
Okra, 113 g	350	22	36
• Sweet Corn Nuggets, 210 g	600	29	72
• Whole Jalapeño Peppers, 36 g	10	0	2

Cici's Pizza

	Cal	Fat	Cbs
Extras & Desserts			
• Apple Pizza, 1 slice	149	4	26
Brownies, 1 slice	143	6	22
Cinnamon Rolls, 1 slice	139	6	20
• Garlic Bread, 1 slice	99	5	10
Pizza: 15" To-Go Pizzas			
Alfredo, 1 slice	216	2	27
Bacon Cheddar, 1 slice	257	8	36
BBQ, 1 slice	289	10	36
Beef, 1 slice	260	10	28
Cheese, 1 slice	223	8	28
Ham & Pineapple, 1 slice	225	8	27
• Ole, 1 slice	169	4	26
Pepperoni & Jalapeño, 1 slice	221	9	25
Pepperoni, 1 slice	240	10	27
• Sausage, 1 slice	290	10	28
Spinach Alfredo, 1 slice	243	8	32
Zesty Ham & Cheddar, 1 slice	229	11	24
Zesty Pepperoni, 1 slice	246	12	26
Zesty Tomato Alfredo, 1 slice	217	8	27

Cici's Pizza (cont.)	Cal	Fat	Cbs
Pizza: 15" To-Go Pizzas (cont.)			
Zesty Veggie, 1 slice	213	9	25
Pizza: Buffet Pizza			
12" Alfredo, 1 slice	139	5	18
12" Bacon Cheddar, 1 slice	145	5	18
12" BBQ, 1 slice	172	6	21
12" Beef, 1 slice	170	7	18
12" Cheese, 1 slice	152	5	20
12" Ham & Pineapple, 1 slice	141	4	19
• 12" Ole, 1 slice	108	4	13
12" Pepperoni & Jalapeño, 1 slice	163	6	20
12" Pepperoni, 1 slice	175	7	21
• 12" Sausage, 1 slice	197	7	19
12" Spinach Alfredo, 1 slice	151	5	20
12" Zesty Ham & Cheddar, 1 slice	153	6	18
12" Zesty Pepperoni, 1 slice	157	7	18
12" Zesty Tomato Alfredo, 1 slice	136	5	18
12" Zesty Veggie, 1 slice	124	4	17

Cinnabon	Cal	Fat	Cbs
Classic Cinnabon	813	32	117
• The Caramel Pecanbon	1100	56	141
• The Minibon	339	13	49

Cold Stone Creamery	Cal	Fat	Cbs
6" Cakes - per slice			
A Cheesecake Named Desire™, 145 g	420	19	56
Butterfinger® Bonanza, 140 g	450	21	59
• Cake Batter Confetti™, 130 g	350	17	46
Caramel Nut Nirvana™, 144 g	510	29	57
Chocolate Chipper™, 133 g	450	26	49
• Coffeehouse Crunch™, 146 g	530	31	59
Cookie Dough Delirium™, 136 g	420	21	49
Cookies & Creamery™, 129 g	390	20	49
Midnight Delight™, 151 g	510	28	60
MMMMMM Chip™, 127 g	380	19	46
Peanut Butter Playground™, 139 g	490	29	54
Raspberry Truffle Temptation™, 145 g	470	25	55
Strawberry Passion™, 141 g	390	19	50
Zebra Stripes Dark, 146 g	480	29	53
Zebra Stripes, 137 g	400	22	46
Grab and Go Ice Cream			
Chocolate Devotion™, 74 g	200	11	26
Coffee Lovers Only®, 74 g	210	13	22
Crème De La Berry™, 74 g	180	9	23
Founder's Favorite®, 74 g	210	12	24
Peanut Butter Cup Perfection™, 74 g	220	13	24
• Rocky Off Road™, 74 g	230	14	25
Shock-A-Cone™, 74 g	220	13	26
• Zenilla™, 74 g	170	11	17
Ice Cream (Love It)			
Amaretto Ice Cream, 227 g	530	31	53
Banana Ice Cream, 227 g	500	29	53
Black Cherry Ice Cream, 227 g	530	30	58
Bubble Gum Ice Cream, 227 g	520	27	64
Butter Pecan Ice Cream, 227 g	520	31	53
Cake Batter Ice Cream™, 227 g	550	30	66
Candy Cane Ice Cream, 227 g	560	32	64
Cheesecake Ice Cream, 227 g	520	29	59
Chocolate Ice Cream, 227 g	520	32	53
• Cinnamon Bun Ice Cream, 227 g	600	33	68
Cinnamon Ice Cream, 227 g	530	32	55
Coconut Ice Cream, 227 g	520	31	52
Coffee Ice Cream, 227 g	530	31	54
Cookie Batter Ice Cream, 227 g	600	32	71
Cotton Candy Ice Cream, 227 g	530	31	55

Cold Stone Creamery (cont.)	Cal	Fat	Cbs
Ice Cream (Love It) (cont.)			
Dark Chocolate Ice Cream, 227 g	540	32	51
Dark Chocolate Peppermint Ice Cream, 227 g	540	32	54
French Toast Ice Cream, 227 g	530	31	56
French Vanilla Ice Cream, 227 g	540	30	60
Irish Cream Ice Cream, 227 g	530	32	54
Macadamia Nut Ice Cream, 227 g	530	31	540
Mango Ice Cream, 227 g	490	29	53
Mint Ice Cream, 227 g	530	30	57
Mocha Ice Cream, 227 g	520	31	53
Oatmeal Cookie Batter Ice Cream, 227 g	540	31	58
Orange Dreamsicle Ice Cream, 227 g	510	30	55
Peach Ice Cream, 227 g	500	27	58
Peanut Butter Ice Cream, 227 g	590	39	53
Pecan Praline Ice Cream, 227 g	530	30	58
Pistachio Ice Cream, 227 g	520	31	54
Pumpkin Ice Cream, 227 g	460	24	53
Raspberry Ice Cream, 227 g	520	30	57
• Sinless Sans Fat™Sweet Cream, 227 g	220	0	55
Strawberry Ice Cream, 227 g	510	30	55
Sweet Cream Ice Cream, 227 g	530	32	53
Vanilla Bean Ice Cream, 227 g	530	31	52
White Chocolate Ice Cream, 227 g	520	31	53
Light Ice Cream (Love It)			
• Cake Batter Light Ice Cream, 227 g	390	10	68
Chocolate Light Ice Cream, 227 g	350	10	57
Coffee Light Ice Cream, 227 g	350	9	56
• Vanilla Light Ice Cream, 227 g	350	9	56
Mix-Ins: Candy			
Almond Joy® Candy, 35 g	170	9	21
Butterfinger® Candy, 30 g	140	6	22
Chocolate Chips, 1 oz.	130	7	16
Chocolate Shavings, 0.5 oz.	90	5	9
Gumballs, 1 oz.	90	0	23
Gummi Bears, 1 oz.	120	0	30
Heath® Candy Bar, 20 g	110	7	12
Kit Kat® Candy Bar, 20 g	110	5	13
• Kool-Aid® Infusions, 05 oz.	80	3	14
M&M's® Candy, 1 oz.	170	7	25
Nestle® Crunch Bar, 25 g	130	7	16
Peanut M&M's®, 1 oz.	150	8	18
• Reese's® Peanut Butter Cup, 35 g	190	11	19
Reese's® Pieces, 1 oz.	180	9	21
Snickers® Candy, 35 g	170	9	21
Twix® Candy, 30 g	150	7	20
White Chocolate Chips, 1 oz.	160	9	18
Whoppers® Candy, 1 oz.	120	4	19
York® Peppermint Patties, 1 oz.	120	2	24
Mix-Ins: Fruit			
Apple Pie Filling, 3/4 oz.	60	0	16
Bananas, 60 g	50	0	14
• Black Cherries, 3/4 oz.	80	0	18
Blackberries, 3/4 oz.	10	0	2
Blueberries, 3/4 oz.	10	0	2
Cherry Pie Filling, 3/4 oz.	50	0	13
• Maraschino Cherries, 1 g	5	0	1
Peach Pie Filling, 3/4 oz.	60	0	16
Pineapple Chunks, 3/4 oz.	15	0	4
Raisins, 1 oz.	70	0	20
Raspberries, 3/4 oz.	25	0	5
Strawberries, 3/4 oz.	20	0	7
Nuts			
Cashews, 1 oz.	170	14	9
Macadamia Nuts, 1 oz.	180	19	3
Peanuts, 1 oz.	210	18	5

Cold Stone Creamery (cont.)

	Cal	Fat	Cbs
Nuts (cont.)			
• Pecan Pralines, 1 oz.	210	21	5
Pecans, 1 oz.	140	15	3
Pistachio Nuts, 1 oz.	200	16	10
Roasted Almonds, 1 oz.	150	14	4
Sliced Almonds, 1 oz.	210	20	6
• Walnuts, 1 oz.	130	13	3
Other Mix-Ins			
Brownies, 40 g	170	4	32
Coconut, 0.5 oz.	80	5	7
• Cookie Dough, 40 g	180	8	26
Graham Cracker Pie Crust, 1 oz.	130	6	17
Granola, 1 oz.	120	2	23
Marshmallows, 1 oz.	100	0	24
• Nilla Wafers, 15 g	70	3	11
OREO® Cookies, 25 g	120	5	18
OREO® Pie Crust, 1 oz.	180	8	19
Peanut Butter, 3/4 oz.	150	13	5
Toasted Coconut, 0.5 oz.	90	7	7
Yellow Cake, 25 g	80	3	13
Shakes (Love It)			
Cake 'n Shake™, 629 g	1480	76	186
Cherry Cheeseshake™, 636 g	1290	66	157
Cream de Menthe™, 571 g	1280	74	138
Lotta Caramel Latte™, 660 g	1530	72	200
Milk and Cookies™, 598 g	1400	80	154
Oh Fudge!™, 773 g	1660	91	191
• PB&C™, 687 g	1690	111	149
• Savory Strawberry™, 636 g	1200	67	138
Very Vanilla™, 607 g	1390	69	173
Smoothies (Like It)			
2 to Mango™, 437 g	330	0	86
Berry Lemony™, 470 g	370	0	97
Berry Trinity™ (Soy), 437 g	270	3	57
• Berry Trinity™ (Yogurt), 417 g	260	0	60
Citrus Sunsation™, 549 g	420	0	107
• Dew Iced™, 390 g	570	0	151
Man-Go Bananas™ (Soy), 457 g	360	3	80
Man-Go Bananas™ (Yogurt), 437 g	360	0	83
On the YoGo™ (Soy), 445 g	370	3	82
On the YoGo™ (Yogurt), 425 g	360	0	85
Strawberry Bananza™, 516 g	350	0	91
Sorbet (Love It)			
Green Apple Gummy Bear, 227 g	250	0	65
• Lemon Sorbet™, 227 g	250	0	64
• Raspberry Sorbet™, 227 g	260	0	67
Watermelon Sorbet™, 227 g	260	0	66
Toppings			
Butterscotch Fat Free, 1 oz.	80	0	0
Caramel Fat Free, 1 oz.	80	0	0
Chocolate Sprinkles, 1 oz.	25	0	0
• Cinnamon, 1 oz.	0	0	0
Fudge Fat Free, 1 oz.	80	0	0
Honey, 1 oz.	90	0	0
Marshmallow Crème, 1 oz.	100	0	0
Rainbow Sprinkles, 1 oz.	25	0	0
Reddi Whip® Original, 20 g	45	3	0
Smuckers Caramel, 1 oz.	100	0	0
• Smuckers Fudge, 1 oz.	100	3	0
Waffle Products			
• Dipped Waffle, 68 g	310	15	46
• Sugar Cone, 13 g	50	0	11
Waffle Cone or Bowl, 38 g	160	4	29

Corner Bakery Café

	Cal	Fat	Cbs
Breakfast			
All American Scrambler no potatoes or bread	310	22	3
Anaheim Scrambler no potatoes or bread	490	36	10
Baked French Toast	570	15	86
Buckhead Cheese Grits	350	22	19
Crunchy Honey Banana Oatmeal	380	3	78
Farmer's Scrambler, no potatoes or bread	430	31	6
Fresh Berry Parfait	330	4	67
Ham & Cheddar Panini	720	34	57
Oatmeal	280	7	41
• Seasonal Fruit Medley	90	0	24
Smoked Bacon & Cheddar Panini	680	34	56
Swiss Oatmeal	330	1	79
• The Commuter Croissant	720	46	44
Entree Salads			
• Caesar Salad	520	44	19
with Roasted Chicken	640	49	19
with Roasted Chicken, no croutons	540	44	8
Chopped Salad, no bread	810	61	27
Harvest Salad	860	68	53
• with Roasted Chicken	980	72	53
Santa Fe Ranch	680	44	56
with Roasted Chicken	800	49	56
Panini			
• California Grille Panini	700	41	59
Chicken Pomodori Panini	890	45	74
Club Panini	900	48	72
• Corned Beef Reuben Panini	930	48	76
Grilled Ham & Swiss Panini	880	44	75
Pasta			
Chicken Carbonara	740	28	70
Half Moon Cheese Ravioli	550	21	63
• Penne with Marinara	550	11	92
• Pesto Cavatappi	930	40	93
Salad Dressings			
Balsamic Vinaigrette	300	31	4
• Caesar	310	32	2
House Dressing	280	27	8
• Ranch	160	16	2
Sandwiches			
Bavarian with Ham	720	25	78
Bavarian with Turkey	690	22	78
• Chicken Pesto	840	41	75
D.C. Chicken Salad	750	37	81
Southwest Roast Beef	840	37	78
Tomato Mozzarella	670	26	73
• Tuna Salad on Olive Bread	450	16	42
Turkey Derby	650	29	60
Turkey Harvest	560	7	91
Uptown Turkey	660	29	61
Side Salads			
Cucumber Tomato Salad, 6 oz.	140	9	13
D.C. Chicken Salad, 6 oz.	560	46	18
• Egg Salad, 6 oz.	570	53	2
Roasted Potato Bacon Salad, 6 oz.	370	23	29
• Seasonal Fruit Medley, 6 oz.	90	0	22
Tomato Mozzarella Pasta Salad, 6 oz.	205	8	24
Tuna Salad, 6 oz.	310	16	3
Soup			
Big Al's Chili with cheddar cheese, 10 oz.	380	17	29
• Butternut Bisque, 10 oz.	166	6	27
Cheddar Broccoli, 10 oz.	310	23	16
Chicken Wild Mushroom Brie Stew, 10 oz.	260	14	20
Chicken Wild Mushroom Brie Stew, bread bowl	420	30	21
Chkn. Wild Mushroom Brie Stew, Cup w/ Caesar	510	35	28

Corner Bakery Café (cont.)

	Cal	Fat	Cbs
Soup (cont.)			
Chkn. Wild Mushroom Brie Stew, Cup w/ Greens	480	31	35
Loaded Baked Potato, 10 oz.	420	29	29
Mom's Chicken Noodle lower fat, 10 oz.	170	4	23
Old Fashioned Beef Stew, 10 oz.	260	13	20
Old Fashioned Beef Stew, bread bowl	420	29	21
• Old Fashioned Beef Stew, Cup w/ Caesar Salad	510	34	28
Old Fashioned Beef Stew, Cup w/ Mixed Greens	480	29	34
Roasted Tomato Basil, 10 oz.	170	5	27
Zesty Chicken Tortilla w/ tortilla strips, 10 oz.	230	11	26

Cosi

	Cal	Fat	Cbs
Arctics			
Arctic Latte - Grande, 16 oz.	527	16	94
Arctic Mocha - Grande, 16 oz.	539	14	101
• Arctic Raspberry Chai - Grande, 16 oz.	404	11	75
• Double Oh! Arctic - Grande, 16 oz.	758	29	123
Smores Latte - Grande, 16 oz.	509	23	61
Bagels			
Asiago Cheese, 6 oz.	327	1	68
• Cinnamon Raisin, 6 oz.	438	1	90
Cranberry Orange, 6 oz.	372	1	80
Etruscan Whole Grain, 5 oz.	331	3	66
Everything, 6 oz.	353	3	71
• Plain, 6 oz.	326	1	68
Poppy Seed, 6 oz.	346	3	69
Sesame, 6 oz.	347	3	69
Baked Omelette Sandwiches			
• Bacon & Cheddar, 5 oz.	326	16	1
Ham & Swiss, 5 oz.	225	15	1
• Plain, 4 oz.	131	9	1
Spinach & Tomato, 5 oz.	142	9	3
Beverage Favorites			
Chai Tea Latte - Grande, 12 oz.	163	3	23
• Hot Chocolate - Grande, 16 oz.	502	31	49
Iced Tea - Grande, 12 oz.	22	0	6
Lemonade, 15 oz.	112	0	26
• Mint Hot Chocolate, 10 oz.	10	10	10
Mocha Latte - Grande, 13 oz.	358	18	40
Steamer, 10 oz.	10	10	10
Beverages: Coffee & Espresso			
• Café Americano, 10 oz.	10	10	10
Café Au Lait, 10 oz.	10	10	10
Cappuccino, 10 oz.	10	10	10
Caramel Mocha - Grande, 12 oz.	420	22	50
• Egg Nog Latte - Grande, 14 oz.	527	26	65
Espresso, 10 oz.	10	10	10
House Coffee, 10 oz.	10	10	10
Latté, 10 oz.	10	10	10
Mint Mocha, 10 oz.	10	10	10
Breakfast Favorites			
Apple Crumb Cake, 6 oz.	540	30	62
• Bagel Club Sandwich, 8 oz.	719	31	70
Biscotti Amaretto, 3 oz.	240	8	34
Biscotti Chocolate, 3 oz.	280	13	38
Cosi Break Bar, 1 oz.	463	24	54
Croissant - Almond, 3 oz.	340	16	42
Croissant - Butter, 3 oz.	330	17	38
Croissant - Chocolate, 3 oz.	370	18	45
Dried Fruits & Yogurt Parfait, 12 oz.	586	6	112
• Fruit Salad, 8 oz.	216	1	54
Granola Cereal, 9 oz.	564	12	107
Granola Peach Parfait, 12 oz.	389	6	74
Granola Strawberry Parfait, 12 oz.	426	6	84
Plain Crumb Cake, 6 oz.	600	36	61

Cosi (cont.)

	Cal	Fat	Cbs
Cream Cheese			
Fruit Trio, 2 oz.	159	14	7
Low Fat Plain, 2 oz.	121	12	2
• Low Fat Veggie, 2 oz.	113	9	2
• Plain, 2 oz.	182	18	2
Desserts			
Apple Tart, 6 oz.	396	6	83
Blondie Brownie, 4 oz.	570	36	57
Cheesecake Brownie, 4 oz.	470	26	55
Cheesecake, 6 oz.	567	33	62
Chocolate Chunk Cookie, 4 oz.	480	20	72
Cinnamon Apple Pie, 14 oz.	960	40	147
Creme Brulee Cheesecake, 3 oz.	307	21	25
• Double Scoop Ice Cream, 6 oz.	225	14	22
• Double Trouble Brownie Sundae, 18 oz.	1586	77	198
Extra chocolate Bar, 2 oz.	230	13	24
Large Sundae, 11 oz.	520	31	55
Medium Sundae, 8 oz.	408	24	43
Mississippi Mud Pie, 9 oz.	850	49	109
Oatmeal Raisin Cookie, 4 oz.	440	14	76
Plain Cheesecake, 3 oz.	307	21	25
Rocky Road Brownie, 6 oz.	550	33	49
S'mmm...Oreos ™ (For 4), 14 oz.	1535	45	271
S'mmm...Oreos ™ (For 2), 7 oz.	827	24	147
S'mores (For 4), 14 oz.	1382	39	244
S'mores (For 2), 7 oz.	751	21	133
Triple Scoop Ice Cream, 9 oz.	338	20	34
White Chocolate Mac Cookie, 4 oz.	520	24	72
Dinner Flatbread Pizza			
Margherita Pizza, 25 oz.	1656	71	228
• Meat Trio, 28 oz.	1986	97	227
Pan Asian Chicken, 33 oz.	1668	67	267
Pepperoni Pizza, 25 oz.	1829	86	226
• Traditional Cheese, 23 oz.	1539	62	225
Every Day Soups			
Pollo E Pasta (Reg/Cup), 10 oz.	122	3	12
Tomato Basil Aurora (Reg/Cup), 10 oz.	374	34	18
Fruit Smoothies			
Blueberry Pomegranate - Grande, 16 oz.	725	1	179
• Citrus Passion Fruit - Grande, 16 oz.	753	0	177
• Mango Mania - Grande, 16 oz.	715	0	177
Strawberry - Banana - Grande, 16 oz.	720	0	179
Hearth-Baked Dinners			
• Alpine Chicken, 13 oz.	973	63	28
Grilled Wild Alaskan Salmon, 11 oz.	623	13	35
• Turkey & Stuffing, 18 oz.	458	21	41
Individual Flatbread Pizza			
Margherita Pizza, 13 oz.	829	36	114
• Meat Trio, 14 oz.	994	49	113
Pan Asian Chicken, 16 oz.	833	33	133
Pepperoni Pizza, 13 oz.	911	43	112
• Traditional Cheese, 12 oz.	769	31	112
Kid's Pizza			
Cheese Pizza, 23 oz.	1257	34	187
Pepperoni Pizza, 28 oz.	1901	93	190
Kids Menu			
• Gooey Grilled Cheese, 4 oz.	357	21	26
Tuna Sandwich, 5 oz.	333	13	27
• Turkey Sandwich, 5 oz.	289	7	48
Melts			
Bacon Turkey Cheddar, 12 oz.	682	25	74
Chicken TBM Melt, 15 oz.	926	47	68
Grilled Chicken Parmesan, 12 oz.	701	27	64
Pesto Chicken, 12 oz.	809	39	64
• Tomato, Basil & Mozzarella Melt, 10 oz.	666	34	67

RESTAURANTS & FAST-FOOD CHAINS

Cosi (cont.)

Item	Cal	Fat	Cbs
Melts (cont.)			
• Tuna Melt, 13 oz.	1012	60	56
Muffins			
Banana Nut Muffin, 5 oz.	480	22	63
Blueberry Muffin, 5 oz.	440	19	60
Carrot Muffin, 5 oz.	470	22	62
• Chocolate Chocolate Chip Muffin, 5 oz.	506	27	67
Corn Muffin, 5 oz.	450	25	50
• Low Fat Bran Muffin, 5 oz.	351	6	70
Salads			
• Bombay Chicken, 13 oz.	176	3	13
Caesar Dressing, 2 oz.	301	32	2
Caesar w/ Grilled Chicken, 10 oz.	340	16	21
Caesar, 7 oz.	182	8	20
Cosi Cobb, 11 oz.	419	28	8
Cosi Vinaigrette, 2 oz.	357	39	2
Fat Free Balsamic Vinaigrette, 2 oz.	45	0	11
Greek Salad, 12 oz.	236	17	9
Italian Dressing, 2 oz.	279	30	2
Low Fat Ginger Soy Dressing, 2 oz.	74	2	13
Pepperanch Dressing, 2 oz.	262	28	2
Reduced Fat Roasted Shallot Sherry, 2 oz.	85	5	3
Roasted Shallot Sherry Vinaigrette, 2 oz.	308	31	8
• Salad Bruschetta, 18 oz.	474	13	67
Shanghai Chicken, 9 oz.	221	9	16
Signature Salad, 10 oz.	375	21	40
Wild Alaskan Salmon Salad, 15 oz.	339	15	20
Sandwiches			
Buffalo Blue, 10 oz.	649	30	57
Classic Turkey & Stuffing, 13 oz.	440	10	65
Cosi Club, 10 oz.	702	35	59
Green Market, 12 oz.	555	17	74
Grilled Chicken T.B.M., 10 oz.	791	43	60
• Hummus & Fresh Veggies, 12 oz.	432	8	77
Italiano, 10 oz.	834	47	58
Meatball Aurora, 11 oz.	796	40	63
Roasted Turkey & Brie, 11 oz.	772	36	71
Sesame Ginger Chicken, 11 oz.	508	11	70
Smoked Ham & Brie, 10 oz.	639	25	69
T.B.M., 11 oz.	729	42	61
Tandoori Chicken, 10 oz.	633	26	58
• Tuna Cheddar, 12 oz.	956	55	55
Turkey Light, 10 oz.	476	9	73
Turkey Rustica, 12 oz.	619	27	60
Tuscan Pesto Chicken, 10 oz.	571	22	58
Vegi Muffaletta, 12 oz.	824	51	24
Wasabi Roast Beef, 11 oz.	626	28	64
Scones			
Blueberry Scones, 4 oz.	410	17	60
Cranberry Scones, 4 oz.	400	15	61
Shareables			
• Brie & Fruit, 6 oz.	277	15	26
• Fresh Guacamole, 10 oz.	10	10	10
Hummus Dip, 4 oz.	121	4	18
Spinach Artichoke, 3 oz.	182	15	9
Weekly Soups			
• Autumn Vegetable & Mushroom, 10 oz.	93	3	14
Beef with Winter Garden Vegetable, 10 oz.	136	7	12
Moroccan Lentil, 10 oz.	199	3	32
• New England Clam Chowder, 10 oz.	440	29	24
Sausage, Chicken & Orzo, 10 oz.	238	10	10

Country Buffet

Item	Cal	Fat	Cbs
Bread and Other Items			
• Biscuits, 51 g	180	7	24
Breadsticks, 47 g	140	5	21

Country Buffet (cont.)

Item	Cal	Fat	Cbs
Bread and Other Items (cont.)			
Buns, Hot Dog, 43 g	120	2	22
• Cinnamon Bread, 50 g	45	1	10
Cinnamon Sugared Donut Holes, 11 g	50	3	5
Dinner Rolls, Wheat, 36 g	110	3	18
Dinner Rolls, White, 36 g	120	4	20
English Muffin, 26 g	60	1	13
Flour Tortilla, 38 g	120	3	20
French Toast, 74 g	170	8	24
Glazed Donuts, 34 g	130	7	16
Pancakes, 49 g	120	4	19
Taco Shells, 11 g	50	3	7
Waffles, 41 g	120	3	19
Condiments			
Bacon Bits, 7 g	25	2	0
Black Olives, sliced, 15 g	15	2	1
• Blueberry Syrup, 2 fl.oz.	250	0	63
Brown Sugar, 9 g	35	0	9
Butter, packet, 5 g	35	4	0
Cheese, Grated Parmesan, 7 g	30	2	0
Cheese, Shredded Cheddar, 10 g	40	4	0
Cherry Peppers, 11 g	4	0	1
Cocktail Sauce, 30 g	30	0	8
Coffee Creamers, packet, 11 g	15	1	0
Cranberry Sauce, 30 g	45	0	12
Crushed Red Pepper, 2 g	10	1	1
Diced Onions, 15 g	5	0	2
Hollandaise Sauce, 2 fl.oz.	130	13	3
Honey, packet, 14 g	45	0	11
Horseradish Sauce, 30 g	60	5	2
• Hot Sauce, 5 g	0	0	0
Jalapeño Peppers, 11 g	2	0	1
Jelly, packet, 14 g	35	0	9
Ketchup, 15 g	15	0	4
Lemons, 8 g	2	0	1
Lettuce, shredded, 14 g	0	0	0
Maple Syrup, 2 fl.oz.	180	0	47
Margarine, melted, 2 fl.oz.	410	45	1
Margarine, packet, 5 g	25	3	0
Mayonnaise, 14 g	100	11	0
Mustard, 15 g	10	1	1
Non-Dairy Creamers, packet, 11 g	10	1	1
Peanut Butter, 16 g	100	8	3
Pepperoncini Peppers, 11 g	2	0	1
Salsa, 30 g	10	0	2
Sautéed Green Peppers, 54 g	25	2	4
Sautéed Mushrooms, 51 g	30	3	2
Sautéed Onions, 51 g	30	1	5
Sliced Pickles, 11 g	2	0	1
Sliced/Diced Tomatoes, 15 g	2	0	1
Sour Cream, 12 g	25	3	1
Soy Sauce, 5 g	2	0	1
Sweet Pickle Relish, 15 g	25	0	6
Tabasco Sauce, 5 g	0	0	0
Desserts			
Apple Crisp, 94 g	150	4	31
Apple Pie, Reduced Sugar, 116 g	190	11	24
Bread Pudding, 96 g	190	8	27
Butterfinger Pieces, 15 g	70	3	11
Butterscotch Topping, 75 g	230	1	56
Cheesecake, Plain, 80 g	220	10	29
Chocolate Chips, 15 g	90	5	10
Chocolate Cream Pie-Reduced Sugar, 79 g	190	12	18
Chocolate Decadence Cake, 64 g	200	9	27
Chocolate Syrup, 37 g	80	0	21

Country Buffet (cont.)

Desserts (cont.)	Cal	Fat	Cbs
Cone, Ice Cream, 4 g	15	0	3
Cookie-Sugar Free Ranger, 20 g	100	5	11
FunE Chips, 15 g	80	3	12
Gummy Bears, 20 g	60	0	15
Honey Nut Topping, 28 g	150	12	7
Hot Fudge Sundae Cake, 86 g	160	4	32
Hot Fudge Topping, 41 g	120	3	23
Hydrox Cookies, Crushed, 8 g	35	2	6
Malted Milk Balls, Ground, 15 g	70	3	11
Nestle Crunch Pieces, 15 g	80	4	10
Pudding, Chocolate, 86 g	150	7	19
• Pudding, Chocolate, Reduced Sugar, 86 g	70	1	14
Pudding, Vanilla, 86 g	140	6	19
Pudding, Vanilla, Reduced Sugar, 86 g	70	1	14
• Pumpkin Pie, 119 g	270	9	31
Rainbow Sprinkles, 15 g	70	2	13
Reduced Sugar Pie-Cherry, 95 g	160	9	16
Reduced Sugar Pie-Lemon, 95 g	160	9	16
Reduced Sugar Pie-Lime, 95 g	160	9	16
Reduced Sugar Pie-Orange, 95 g	160	9	16
Reduced Sugar Pie-Raspberry, 95 g	160	9	16
Reduced Sugar Pie-Strawberry, 95 g	160	9	16
Soft Serve Froz Yog, Nonfat, Strawberry, 4 fl.oz.	100	0	23
Soft Serve Froz Yog, Nonfat, Vanilla, 4 fl.oz.	110	0	23
Soft Serve, Chocolate, 4 fl.oz.	140	5	24
Soft Serve, Vanilla, 4 fl.oz.	150	5	25
SS Froz Yog, Nonfat, Nutrasweet, Vanilla, 4 fl.oz.	80	0	17
Strawberry Topping, 47 g	100	0	23
Whipped Topping, Non-Dairy, 21 g	60	5	5
Dressings			
• Bleu Cheese, 30 g	170	18	1
Creamy Italian, 29 g	110	11	3
Fat Free French, 30 g	35	0	8
French, 33 g	150	12	12
Italian, 32 g	120	11	5
• Low Fat Italian, 30 g	25	2	2
Ranch, 30 g	110	11	1
Reduced Fat Ranch, 30 g	60	6	2
Entrees			
• BBQ Beef Ribs, 143 g	300	23	7
BBQ Smoked Sausage, 80 g	140	10	9
Beef Liver and Onion, 45 g	80	3	4
Carved Beef Brisket, 3 oz.	200	11	1
Carved Ham, 3 oz.	140	9	0
Carved Peppered Pork Loin, 3 oz.	160	8	0
Carved Roast Beef, 3 oz.	230	15	0
Carved Roast Turkey, 3 oz.	170	8	0
Carved Salmon Filet, 3 oz.	190	12	0
Chicken and Dumplings, 136 g	190	7	24
Chicken Cacciatore, 140 g	220	11	5
Chicken, Hand Breaded Fried-breast, 143 g	310	16	3
Chicken, Hand Breaded Fried-drumstick, 39 g	90	6	2
Chicken, Hand Breaded Fried-thigh, 89 g	210	14	4
Chicken, Traditional Baked-breast, 149 g	280	12	0
Chicken, Traditional Baked-drumstick, 40 g	90	6	0
Chicken, Traditional Baked-thigh, 91 g	160	11	0
Chinese Chicken Livers, 89 g	200	12	17
Country BBQ Chicken-breast, 143 g	300	12	5
Country BBQ Chicken-drumstick, 40 g	110	6	3
Country BBQ Chicken-thigh, 91 g	210	13	4
Country BBQ Chicken-wing, 37 g	70	3	2
Denver Scrambled Eggs, 77 g	140	11	2
Egg, Poached, 50 g	70	5	0
Eggs Benedict, 134 g	250	15	15

Country Buffet (cont.)

Entrees (cont.)	Cal	Fat	Cbs
Fish Patties, 73 g	160	9	13
Fish, Fried, 37 g	80	4	9
Hamburger Patties, 74 g	220	19	0
Hot Dogs, Turkey, 56 g	130	11	2
Hot Wings-Drummies, 15 g	35	2	0
• Hot Wings-Wing, 10 g	25	2	0
Mini Corn Dogs, 19 g	50	2	6
Mostaciolli, Baked, 102 g	120	5	13
Orange Chicken, 99 g	240	11	24
Quiche, Breakfast, 106 g	220	15	12
Sauerkraut , 28 g	5	0	1
Scrambled Eggs, 62 g	130	11	1
Shrimp, fried, 54 g	110	5	11
Smoked Sausage, 56 g	190	17	2
Spanish Rice, 86 g	140	9	9
Taco Meat, Beef, 2 fl.oz.	100	5	3
Teriyaki Chicken Wings-Drummie, 26 g	50	3	2
Teriyaki Chicken Wings-Wing, 13 g	50	3	2
Fruits			
Cantaloupe, 85 g	25	0	6
• Grapes, 80 g	60	0	15
Honeydew, 88 g	30	0	8
Pineapple, 78 g	35	0	10
Strawberries, 72 g	25	0	6
• Watermelon, 76 g	25	0	6
Gravies and Sauces			
• Au Jus, 2 fl.oz.	0	0	0
Gravy, Beef, 2 fl.oz.	30	2	2
Gravy, Chicken, 2 fl.oz.	30	1	5
• Gravy, Country, 2 fl.oz.	120	8	12
Gravy, Roasted Pork, 2 fl.oz.	50	4	3
Gravy, Turkey, 2 fl.oz.	10	0	2
Meat Sauce, 2 fl.oz.	70	3	4
Salad Toppers			
Bacon Bits, Imitation, 7 g	30	1	2
Black Olives, sliced, 15 g	15	2	1
Carrots, julienne, 8 g	5	5	1
Cherry Tomatoes, 17 g	5	0	1
Chow Mein Noodles, 7 g	35	2	4
Croutons, 7 g	35	2	5
Cucumbers, sliced, 15 g	2	0	1
Eggs, hard cooked, diced, 15 g	20	2	0
Feta Cheese, 40 g	35	3	1
• Mushrooms, sliced, 10 g	2	0	1
Parmesan Cheese, grated, 7 g	30	2	0
Peas, 15 g	10	0	2
Pepperoncini, 11 g	2	0	1
Raisins, 12 g	40	0	10
Red Onions, sliced, 6 g	2	0	1
Shredded Cheese, Imitation, 10 g	25	2	2
Spinach Leaves, 32 g	5	0	1
• Sunflower Seeds, 11 g	70	6	2
Salads			
Ambrosia, 89 g	140	5	23
BLT Salad, 70 g	150	14	3
Broccoli Apple Salad, 100 g	160	11	13
Caesar Salad, 65 g	80	6	5
California Coleslaw, 100 g	90	1	22
Carrot and Raisin Salad, 100 g	140	8	18
Chicken Pasta Salad, 100 g	230	18	11
Creamy Pea Salad, 100 g	160	11	11
Cucumber Tomato Salad, 100 g	30	1	6
Dilled Potato Salad, 83 g	110	8	9
Flavored Gelatin, 70 g	40	0	10

RESTAURANTS & FAST-FOOD CHAINS

Country Buffet (cont.)	Cal	Fat	Cbs
Salads (cont.)			
Gelatin Whip, 68 g	80	3	14
Greek Salad, 75 g	120	8	11
Macaroni Vegetable Salad, 100 g	230	15	20
Marinated Vegetables, 100 g	60	4	6
Oriental Pasta, 100 g	110	6	11
Pickled Beets, 100 g	100	0	25
Potato Salad, 75 g	110	5	14
Prunes, Stewed, 71 g	100	0	28
Raisin Fluff, 80 g	140	4	25
• Seafood Salad, 117 g	310	26	16
Seven Layer Salad, 75 g	180	17	4
Sicilian Pasta Salad, 100 g	150	9	15
• Spring Mix, 45 g	5	0	1
Strawberry Whip, 76 g	200	14	17
Strawberry-Banana Salad, 85 g	70	1	16
Strawberry-Peach-Banana, 79 g	80	1	20
Tarragon Potato Salad, 82 g	120	7	13
Three Bean Salad, 100 g	90	5	12
Tossed Green Salad, 45 g	5	0	1
Waldorf Salad, 60 g	110	7	12
Whipped Pineapple/Banana, 114 g	180	2	33
Sides			
Bacon, 6 g	30	3	0
Baked Beans, 110 g	120	1	29
Bread Dressing, 100 g	130	4	21
Cabbage, German Boiled, 85 g	40	4	3
Cabbage, Green, 85 g	40	3	3
Carrots, steamed, 85 g	40	0	9
Chesapeake Corn, 85 g	80	3	13
Corn on the Cob, 72 g	100	3	16
Corn, steamed, 85 g	100	1	21
Creamy Cheese Sauce, 2 fl.oz.	50	2	9
French Fries, 51 g	190	9	24
Fried Rice w/Ham, 100 g	170	6	23
Green Bean Casserole, 110 g	60	3	9
Green Beans El Greco, 85 g	20	0	5
• Green Beans, 85 g	15	0	3
Grits, 4 fl.oz.	70	0	16
Joe's Cracked Pepper Green Beans, 85 g	70	6	5
Montreal Vegetable Medley, 85 g	40	4	3
Oatmeal, 4 fl.oz.	70	1	13
Pinto Beans w/ Ham, 85 g	90	1	21
Potatoes, Baked Sweet, 192 g	160	0	47
Potatoes, Baked, 180 g	160	0	39
Potatoes, Hash Brown Patties, 57 g	120	8	11
Potatoes, Hash Browns, 80 g	110	6	13
Potatoes, Jo Jo, 84 g	210	15	18
Potatoes, O'Brien, 110 g	120	6	18
Potatoes, Red, 113 g	100	3	18
Red Beans w/ Ham, 85 g	90	1	18
Sausage Links, 25 g	100	10	0
Spaghetti, 85 g	90	1	19
• Spinach Marie, 110 g	210	17	8
Squash, winter, 85 g	150	9	18
Turnip or Collard Greens w/ Bacon, 110 g	40	3	2
Vegetable Stir Fry, 85 g	25	1	6
White Rice, 100 g	90	0	22
Wild Rice Vegetable Pilaf, 100 g	90	1	17
Yams, Candied, 118 g	140	2	30
Zucchini, Sautéed, 85 g	50	4	3
Soups			
Chicken Noodle Soup, 4 fl.oz.	70	2	7
Chicken Rice Soup, 4 fl.oz.	70	2	8
Chili Bean Soup, 4 fl.oz.	100	4	9

Country Buffet (cont.)	Cal	Fat	Cbs
Soups (cont.)			
Corn Chowder, 4 fl.oz.	140	8	15
Cream of Broccoli Soup, 4 fl.oz.	80	7	5
• Navy Bean Soup w/ Ham, 4 fl.oz.	50	1	10
• New England Clam Chowder, 4 fl.oz.	300	12	9
Potato Cheese Soup, 4 fl.oz.	130	9	11

Cousins Subs	Cal	Fat	Cbs
5" Mini Subs			
5" Mini BLT, 125 g	298	19	24
5" Mini Chicken Cheddar Deluxe, 169 g	329	19	26
5" Mini Club, 195 g	337	18	27
• 5" Mini Garden Veggie, 146 g	216	7	26
5" Mini Ham & Provolone, 174 g	316	18	26
5" Mini Hot Veggie, 144 g	254	10	28
• 5" Mini Italian Special, 178 g	403	25	25
5" Mini Meatball & Provolone, 140 g	361	19	27
5" Mini Pepperoni Melt, 169 g	348	21	26
5" Mini Pizza Sub, 157 g	336	18	28
5" Mini Seafood with Crab, 170 g	323	19	31
5" Mini Three Cheese, 156 g	363	23	25
5" Mini Tuna, 169 g	335	20	25
5" Mini Turkey Breast, 172 g	279	14	26
7 1/2" Subs			
7½" BLT, 225 g	591	38	47
7½" Cheese Steak, 290 g	503	19	49
7½" Chicken Breast, 314 g	569	27	50
7½" Chicken Cheddar Deluxe, 330 g	669	39	51
7½" Club, 361 g	657	35	51
7½" Double Cheese Steak, 393 g	747	36	49
• 7½" Garden Veggie, 253 g	390	12	51
7½" Gyro, 344 g	710	41	61
7½" Ham & Provolone, 308 g	612	34	50
7½" Hot Veggie, 277 g	472	17	55
• 7½" Italian Special, 343 g	817	51	50
7½" Meatball & Provolone, 280 g	723	38	54
7½" Pepperoni Melt, 331 g	730	45	50
7½" Philly Cheese Steak, 326 g	531	19	55
7½" Pizza Sub, 324 g	709	39	55
7½" Roast Beef, 301 g	607	30	50
7½" Seafood with Crab, 314 g	642	38	60
7½" Spicy Chicken Sedona, 308 g	530	18	54
7½" Three Cheese, 276 g	685	44	50
7½" Tuna, 312 g	666	40	49
7½" Turkey Breast, 301 g	537	28	50
Better Bunch Salads			
Chef Salad (Better Bunch), 295 g	131	3	10
Garden Salad (Better Bunch), 201 g	40	0	8
• Garden Salad w/Chicken Brst (Better Bunch), 315 g	154	1	10
• Side Salad (Better Bunch), 96 g	19	0	4
Better Bunch Subs			
5" Mini Club (Better Bunch), 169 g	193	3	26
• 5" Mini Garden Veggie (Better Bunch), 123 g	136	1	26
5" Mini Ham (Better Bunch), 149 g	178	2	26
5" Mini Hot Veggie (Better Bunch), 112 g	144	1	27
5" Mini Turkey Breast (Better Bunch), 157 g	177	2	26
7½" Chicken Breast (Better Bunch), 286 g	366	2	50
• 7½" Club (Better Bunch), 312 g	381	5	51
7½" Garden Veggie (Better Bunch), 218 g	266	2	50
7½" Ham (Better Bunch), 258 g	336	4	50
• 7½" Hot Veggie (Better Bunch), 223 g	287	2	55
• 7½" Roast Beef (Better Bunch), 272 g	405	6	50
7½" Turkey Breast (Better Bunch), 272 g	335	3	50
Limited Time Specials			
• 5" Mini Chicken Salad, 170 g	280	11	32
7½" Black Forest Bliss, 330 g	545	17	69

Cousins Subs (cont.)

	Cal	Fat	Cbs
Limited Time Specials (cont.)			
7½" Chicken Italiana, 371 g	520	12	57
• 7½" Chicken Salad, 314 g	556	23	62
Salads			
Chef Salad, 345 g	332	14	26
Chicken Sedona Salad, 365 g	232	5	16
Garden Salad, 251 g	241	11	24
w/ Chicken Breast, 365 g	355	12	26
Italian Salad, 329 g	409	24	25
Seafood Salad, 336 g	320	11	35
• Side Salad, 124 g	135	6	14
• Tuna Salad, 379 g	629	46	24
Sides & Other			
Chocolate Chip Cookie, 43 g	210	11	26
Chocolate Chip with M&Ms, 43 g	190	9	26
Coconut Toffee Chip Cookie, 43 g	200	9	23
Double Chocolate Chip Cookie, 43 g	190	9	25
• French Fries (Medium), 113 g	367	19	43
Oatmeal Cranberry Walnut Cookie, 43 g	170	7	26
• Oatmeal Raisin Cookie, 43 g	170	7	25
Peanut Butter w/ Reese's Pieces Cookie, 43 g	210	11	22
Snickerdoodle Cookie, 43 g	190	9	25
Sugar Cookie, 43 g	180	8	26
White Chunk Macadamia Nut Cookie, 43 g	200	11	24
Soups			
Beef Steak & Noodle (Regular), 198 g	105	3	12
Cheddar Cauliflower (Regular), 198 g	114	5	13
Cheddar Cheese (Regular), 198 g	201	11	18
Chicken & Dumplings (Regular), 198 g	149	4	17
Chicken Noodle (Regular), 198 g	114	4	16
Chicken with Wild Rice (Regular), 198 g	219	9	13
• Chili (Regular), 198 g	219	8	26
Cream of Broccoli w/ Cheese (Regular), 198 g	166	7	13
Cream of Mushroom (Regular), 198 g	193	11	13
Cream of Potato (Regular), 198 g	166	8	21
Eight Bean Soup with Ham (Regular), 198 g	105	1	18
Fiesta Tortilla Soup with Chicken (Regular), 198 g	114	5	11
New England Clam Chowder (Regular), 198 g	149	3	25
Tomato Basil w/ Raviolini (Regular), 198 g	96	1	19
• Vegetable Beef (Regular), 198 g	70	2	11

Culver's

	Cal	Fat	Cbs
ButterBurger Classics			
ButterBurger, Cheese, Double, 9 oz.	580	32	37
• ButterBurger, Cheese, Single, 6 oz.	398	20	36
ButterBurger, Cheese, Triple, 12 oz.	763	45	38
Bacon ButterBurger Deluxe, Double, 10 oz.	751	50	34
Bacon ButterBurger Deluxe, Single, 9 oz.	573	38	34
• Bacon ButterBurger Deluxe, Triple, 13 oz.	931	63	34
ButterBurger, Low Carb, 6 oz.	443	32	1
ButterBurger Original, Double, 8 oz.	480	23	36
ButterBurger Original, Single, 5 oz.	346	15	35
ButterBurger Original, Triple, 10 oz.	613	31	37
The Culver's ButterBurger Deluxe, Double, 10 oz.	671	43	34
The Culver's ButterBurger Deluxe, Single, 8 oz.	494	31	34
The Culver's ButterBurger Deluxe, Triple, 12 oz.	851	56	34
Classic Sundaes			
Banana Split, 2-Scoop, 18 oz.	1081	64	115
• Banana Split, 3-Scoop, 21 oz.	1345	75	152
• Bananas Foster Sundae, 1-Scoop, 8 oz.	420	20	53
Bananas Foster Sundae, 2-Scoop, 13 oz.	784	41	93
Bananas Foster Sundae, 3-Scoop, 18 oz.	1015	51	123
Caramel Cashew, 1- Scoop, 7 oz.	585	33	58
Caramel Cashew, 2-Scoop, 13 oz.	957	51	104
Caramel Cashew, 3-Scoop, 15 oz.	1133	62	121
Strawberry Shortcake Sundae, 1-Scoop, 9 oz.	577	28	73

Culver's (cont.)

	Cal	Fat	Cbs
Classic Sundaes (cont.)			
Strawberry Shortcake Sundae, 2-Scoop, 15 oz.	939	48	115
Strawberry Shortcake Sundae, 3-Scoop, 18 oz.	1115	58	132
Turtle Sundae, 1-Scoop, 7 oz.	605	41	53
Turtle Sundae, 2-Scoop, 13 oz.	977	60	97
Turtle Sundae, 3-Scoop, 15 oz.	1153	71	114
Concrete Mixers			
Chocolate Concrete Mixer, Medium, 16 oz.	992	49	122
• Turtle Concrete Mixer, Medium, 15 oz.	1153	71	114
• Vanilla Concrete Mixer, Medium, 13 oz.	832	49	82
Condiments			
BBQ Sauce, 1 oz.	48	0	12
Dill Pickles, Sliced, 0 oz.	1	0	0
Honey Mustard, 2 oz.	130	6	20
Horseradish Sauce, 1 oz.	150	14	6
Ketchup, 1 oz.	15	0	4
Mayonnaise, 0.5 oz.	100	11	0
Mustard, Mild, 0.5 oz.	0	0	0
• Mustard, Spicy Brown, 0.5 oz.	0	0	0
Picante Sauce, Mild and Medium, 1 oz.	10	0	2
Shrimp Cocktail Sauce, 2 oz.	50	0	12
Steak Sauce, 0.5 oz.	10	0	2
Sweet & Sour Dipping Sauce, 2 oz.	90	0	23
• Tartar Sauce, 1 oz.	188	18	1
Cones & Custard			
• Baby Scoop Chocolate Cake Cone, 3 oz.	193	8	25
Baby Scoop Vanilla Cake Cone, 3 oz.	200	10	22
Chocolate Cake Cone, 1-Scoop, 5 oz.	319	14	40
Chocolate Cake Cone, 2-Scoop, 10 oz.	592	27	73
Chocolate Cake Cone, 3-Scoop, 12 oz.	739	34	90
Chocolate Dipped Waffle Cone w/Sprinkles, 2 oz.	306	13	47
Chocolate Dipped Waffle Cone, 1-Scoop, 7 oz.	533	24	72
Chocolate Dipped Waffle Cone, 2 oz.	239	10	37
Chocolate, Dish, 1-Scoop, 5 oz.	294	14	35
Chocolate, Dish, 2-Scoop, 10 oz.	567	27	68
Chocolate, Dish, 3-Scoop, 12 oz.	714	34	85
Chocolate, Waffle Cone, 1-Scoop, 6 oz.	384	15	55
Chocolate, Waffle Cone, 2-Scoop, 10 oz.	657	28	88
Chocolate, Waffle Cone, 3-Scoop, 13 oz.	804	35	105
No Sugar Added Caramel Fudge Swirl, 3 oz.	205	11	30
Plain Cake Cone, 0.5 oz.	25	0	5
Plain Waffle Cone, 1 oz.	90	1	20
Vanilla Cake Cone, 1-Scoop, 5 oz.	332	18	35
Vanilla Cake Cone, 2-Scoop, 10 oz.	616	35	63
Vanilla Cake Cone, 3-Scoop, 12 oz.	770	44	78
Vanilla, Choc. Dipped Waffle Cone, 1-Scoop, 7 oz.	546	28	67
Vanilla, Dish, 1-Scoop, 5 oz.	307	18	30
Vanilla, Dish, 2-Scoop, 10 oz.	591	35	58
Vanilla, Dish, 3-Scoop, 12 oz.	745	44	73
Vanilla, Waffle Cone, 1-Scoop, 6 oz.	397	19	50
Vanilla, Waffle Cone, 2-Scoop, 10 oz.	681	36	78
• Vanilla, Waffle Cone, 3-Scoop, 13 oz.	835	45	93
Dinner Plates			
Beef Pot Roast Dinner, 21 oz.	635	24	74
Breaded Shrimp (about 8 pieces), 18 oz.	1250	61	148
Chicken, 2 pcs., 25 oz.	1755	94	140
• Chicken, 4 pcs., 32 oz.	2185	116	158
Chopped Steak Dinner, 22 oz.	683	29	67
Crispy Shrimp Basket, 8 pcs., 11 oz.	760	34	92
Fish n' Chips, 6 pcs., 16 oz.	1381	83	104
North Atlantic Cod Fillet, 2 pcs., 23 oz.	1831	116	135
North Atlantic Cod Fillet, 3 pcs., 28 oz.	2122	134	147
Favorites			
Angus Philly Steak Sandwich, 10 oz.	518	20	46
Beef Frank w/ Bun, 7 oz.	392	22	38

RESTAURANTS & FAST-FOOD CHAINS

Culver's (cont.)

	Cal	Fat	Cbs
Favorites (cont.)			
• Beef Pot Roast Sandwich, 6 oz.	363	16	33
Blackened Chicken Sandwich, 8 oz.	369	8	48
Cheese Dog w/ Bun, 6 oz.	461	31	27
Chicken Salad Wrap, 7 oz.	518	26	39
Chicken Tenders, Breaded, 4 pcs., 6 oz.	440	20	32
Chili Dog w/Bun, 6 oz.	379	24	28
Crispy Chicken Fillet Sandwich, 9 oz.	625	29	68
Grilled Chicken Breast, 8 oz.	374	8	47
Grilled Ham n' Swiss on Rye, 8 oz.	497	25	33
• North Atlantic Cod Fillet Sandwich, 10 oz.	740	42	58
Pork Tenderloin Sandwich, 9 oz.	593	29	62
Tuna Salad Wrap, 8 oz.	485	24	39
Turkey Sourdough BLT, 9 oz.	562	31	36
Turkey, Stacked, Sandwich, 8 oz.	450	19	47
Garden Fresh Salads			
Avocado Pecan Bleu w/ Blackened Chicken, 13 oz.	557	41	16
Chicken Cashew w /Grilled Chicken, 11 oz.	441	25	17
Classic Caesar w/ Grilled Chicken, 10 oz.	358	14	15
Cobb Salad, 13 oz.	531	31	19
• Crispy Chicken Salad, 11 oz.	616	42	34
Garden Fresco, 9 oz.	225	11	25
• Side Caesar, 3 oz.	82	4	5
Side Salad, 4 oz.	86	5	6
Kids Meals			
ButterBurger, 5 oz.	346	15	35
• ButterBurger, Cheese, 6 oz.	396	20	36
• Chicken Tenders, Breaded, 2 pcs., 3 oz.	220	10	16
Corn Dog, 3 oz.	260	14	26
French Fries, 4 oz.	275	12	38
Grilled Cheese on Sourdough, 4 oz.	290	14	33
Hot Dog w/Bun, 5 oz.	366	22	30
Malts & Shakes			
• Chocolate Malt, Medium, 16 oz.	968	45	122
Chocolate Shake, Medium, 16 oz.	912	44	114
• Old Fashioned Cherry Soda, 16 oz.	516	25	63
Vanilla Malt, Medium, 14 oz.	872	45	98
Vanilla Shake, Medium, 13 oz.	752	44	74
Salad Dressing			
• Bleu Cheese, Fancy, Chunky, 2 oz.	310	33	2
Caesar Dressing, 2 oz.	220	23	2
French, 2 oz.	190	13	19
French, Reduced Calorie, 2 oz.	140	9	16
Ranch, Buttermilk, Gourmet, 2 oz.	230	24	3
Ranch, Reduced Calorie, 2 oz.	130	12	5
• Raspberry Vinaigrette, 2 oz.	45	0	11
Sesame Ginger Dressing, 2 oz.	70	0	16
Thousand Island, Gourmet, 2 oz.	220	18	14
Sides			
Chili Cheddar Fries, 9 oz.	661	34	73
Cole Slaw, 5 oz.	350	21	37
Dinner Roll, 2 oz.	140	6	19
French Fries, Regular, 5 oz.	385	17	53
Green Beans, 7 oz.	203	18	12
Mashed Potatoes & Gravy, 7 oz.	140	2	26
• Mashed Potatoes, 6 oz.	120	1	24
Onion Rings, Breaded, 7 oz.	630	36	70
• Wisconsin Dairyland Cheese Curds, 7 oz.	670	38	54
Soups			
Baja Chicken Enchilada, 11 oz.	352	23	21
Bean with Ham, 11 oz.	190	3	33
Black Bean, 11 oz.	188	3	32
Boston Clam Chowder, 11 oz.	252	11	25
Bread Bowl, 9 oz.	665	3	135
Broccoli Cheese with Florets, 11 oz.	240	14	16

Culver's (cont.)

	Cal	Fat	Cbs
Soups (cont.)			
California Medley, 11 oz.	204	11	18
Cauliflower Cheese, 11 oz.	252	14	23
Cheesy Chicken Tortilla, 11 oz.	180	7	16
Chicken & Dumpling, 11 oz.	300	22	19
Chicken Gumbo, 11 oz.	120	6	13
Chicken Noodle, 11 oz.	112	2	14
Chicken Pot Pie, 11 oz.	260	16	22
Chicken Tortilla, 11 oz.	168	3	26
Corn Chowder, 11 oz.	276	13	35
Cream of Asparagus Spears, 11 oz.	250	11	26
Cream of Broccoli, 11 oz.	185	10	16
Cream of Potato, 11 oz.	288	13	26
Creamy Garden Vegetable, 11 oz.	188	11	19
Creamy Tomato Bisque, 11 oz.	180	9	20
Creamy Turkey Vegetable, 11 oz.	216	9	19
• Fire Roasted Vegetable, 11 oz.	72	2	12
French Onion, 11 oz.	155	8	12
• George's Chili Supreme, 11 oz.	456	30	27
George's Chili, 11 oz.	336	18	27
Harvest Grain w/ Portabello Mushrooms, 11 oz.	185	7	26
Italian Style Wedding, 11 oz.	275	6	44
Lumberjack Mixed Vegetable, 11 oz.	150	6	21
Minestrone, 11 oz.	100	1	19
Mushroom Medley, 11 oz.	252	16	20
Oven Roasted Turkey Noodle, 11 oz.	175	5	21
Pasta Fagioli, 11 oz.	172	3	28
Potato Au Gratin, 11 oz.	350	22	28
Potato with Bacon, 11 oz.	225	9	28
Seven Bean Medley, 11 oz.	150	2	25
Split Pea with Ham, 11 oz.	262	9	32
Stuffed Green Pepper with Beef, 11 oz.	150	3	25
Tomato Basil Ravioletti, 11 oz.	112	3	18
Tomato Florentine, 11 oz.	112	1	21
Vegetable Beef & Barley, 11 oz.	112	4	14
Wild and Brown Rice with Chicken, 11 oz.	452	22	27
Wisconsin Cheese, 11 oz.	375	24	29
Special Treats			
Cookies n' Cream Concrete Cake, 4 oz.	245	14	26
• Culver's Root Beer Float, 15 oz.	467	18	70
Lemon Ice Smoothie, 11 oz.	403	16	61
• Lemon Ice, 7 oz.	140	0	35
Turtle Concrete Cake, 4 oz.	280	17	30
Specialty Burgers & Sandwiches			
• Cheddar Burger with Bacon, 11 oz.	871	48	56
Cheddar Burger, Double, 8 oz.	641	37	31
Cheddar Burger, Single, 5 oz.	421	22	31
Cheddar Burger, Triple, 11 oz.	861	52	31
Grilled Reuben Melt, 11 oz.	588	31	41
Mushroom & Swiss Burger, Double, 9 oz.	633	35	35
Mushroom & Swiss Burger, Single, 6 oz.	417	21	33
Mushroom & Swiss Burger, Triple, 13 oz.	849	49	37
Sourdough Melt, Double, 9 oz.	636	35	33
Sourdough Melt, Single, 6 oz.	413	20	33
Sourdough Melt, Triple, 12 oz.	858	50	34
Wisconsin Swiss Melt, Double, 9 oz.	616	34	34
• Wisconsin Swiss Melt, Single, 6 oz.	403	20	33
Wisconsin Swiss Melt, Triple, 12 oz.	828	48	35
Toppings			
Almond, 0.5 oz.	84	8	3
Andes Creme De Menthe Thins, 1 oz.	151	10	16
Apple, 0.5 oz.	23	0	6
Black Cherry, 0.5 oz.	18	0	5
Blackberry, 0.5 oz.	14	0	4
Blueberry, 0.5 oz.	17	0	4

Culver's (cont.)

Toppings (cont.)	Cal	Fat	Cbs
• Brownie Pieces, 3 oz.	361	16	52
Butterfinger®, 1 oz.	110	5	18
Butterscotch, 0.5 oz.	43	0	10
Cashew, 0.5 oz.	90	7	4
Cherry, 0.5 oz.	20	0	5
Chocolate Chip Cookie Dough, 1 oz.	120	5	17
Crème De Menthe, 0.5 oz.	45	1	10
Culver's Chocolate Syrup, 1 oz.	64	0	16
Heath® Toffee Chunks, 1 oz.	155	9	17
Hershey's Take Five, 1 oz.	141	7	17
M&M Minis, 1 oz.	140	7	18
Marshmallow Creme, 0.5 oz.	39	0	10
Milk Chocolate Flakes, 1 oz.	142	9	17
Nestle Crunch, 1 oz.	140	7	19
Novelty Coating, 0.5 oz.	87	7	6
Oreo® Cookie Crumbs, 0.5 oz.	62	2	9
Peach, 0.5 oz.	15	0	4
Peanut Butter, 1 oz.	179	15	6
Pecan Halves, 0.5 oz.	100	11	2
Pineapple, 0.5 oz.	20	0	5
Raspberry, 0.5 oz.	18	0	4
Reese's Pieces® Minis, 1 oz.	142	7	16
Reese's® Peanut Butter Cups, 1 oz.	150	9	16
Snickers® Candy Bar Pieces, 0.5 oz.	67	4	8
Spanish Peanuts, 1 oz.	160	14	5
Sprinkles, Blue and White, 1 oz.	140	7	21
Sprinkles, King Decorette, 1 oz.	134	6	20
• Strawberry, 0.5 oz.	13	0	3

D'Angelo

D'Lite Sandwiches	Cal	Fat	Cbs
ChixSFry D'Lite, 354 g	426	6	57
Classic Veggie, 345 g	362	7	63
Fresh Veggie, 267 g	348	7	62
Grilled Chicken Breast, 261 g	388	7	52
Roast Beef, 234 g	338	5	51
• Turkey Cranberry, 291 g	444	4	75
• Turkey, 234 g	347	4	51
D'Lite Wraps			
• Chicken Caesar Salad, 373 g	374	7	43
• Tuna, 288 g	725	59	20
Turkey & Bacon, 263 g	491	30	19
Wrap LC Steak & Provolone, 227 g	469	27	15
Dressing			
Bleu Cheese, 30 g	152	15	3
• Caesar, 85 g	397	43	6
Creamy Italian, 85 g	340	37	9
• Fat Free Caesar, 85 g	57	0	9
Greek w/ Feta Cheese, 85 g	227	26	6
Honey Mustard, 30 g	150	14	7
Lite Ranch, 85 g	240	19	6
Olive Oil Vinaigrette, 85 g	170	17	9
Kidz Meals			
Cheeseburger Sub, 123 g	294	13	28
• Cookie Chocolate Chip, 43 g	171	6	26
Ham & Cheese Sub, 103 g	227	5	32
• Kidz Tuna Sub, 128 g	438	29	30
Meatball Sub, 153 g	330	15	37
Turkey D'Lite, 113 g	217	3	30
Pokket® Sandwiches			
Big Papi, 340 g	469	11	53
BLT & Cheese, 255 g	397	17	38
Caesar Salad, 312 g	616	39	54
Capicola & Cheese, 230 g	362	13	35
Cheese, 230 g	519	27	41

D'Angelo (cont.)

Pokket® Sandwiches (cont.)	Cal	Fat	Cbs
Cheeseburger, 231 g	459	25	31
Chicken Caesar Salad, 390 g	674	39	47
Chicken Club, 296 g	526	28	36
Chicken Honey Dijon, 323 g	508	20	40
Chicken Salad, 238 g	623	42	34
Chicken Stir Fry, 277 g	380	9	39
Classic Vegetable Pokket, 341 g	368	13	46
Classic Vegetable, 341 g	368	13	46
Classic Veggie No Cheese, 312 g	212	1	44
• Greek, 450 g	790	61	49
Grilled Chicken, 261 g	303	5	35
Ham & Salami, 202 g	386	17	34
Ham & Cheese, 222 g	326	10	38
Ham, 177 g	229	3	35
Hamburger, 212 g	399	20	29
Italian, 232 g	525	30	36
Lobster, 255 g	530	31	34
Meatball, 346 g	574	31	52
Mortadella & Cheese, 205 g	410	21	35
Number 9, 258 g	407	18	31
Pastrami, 184 g	438	25	33
Pepperoni, 184 g	407	20	35
Roast Beef, 202 g	247	3	33
• Salad, 298 g	196	1	40
Salami & Cheese, 216 g	509	30	33
Seafood Salad, 234 g	449	22	50
Steak & Cheese, 186 g	377	17	26
Steak Bomb, 343 g	631	32	44
Steak Tip, 310 g	452	16	45
Steak, 164 g	305	12	24
Tuna, 238 g	664	49	33
Turkey Club, 284 g	332	7	32
Turkey, 202 g	256	2	33
Salads			
Antipasto, 389 g	284	18	17
Caesar, 326 g	474	39	25
Chicken Caesar, 404 g	533	38	19
Chicken Stir Fry, 366 g	168	3	11
Cobb, 333 g	292	17	11
Greek, 387 g	299	23	17
Lobster, 415 g	376	26	12
Roast Beef, 352 g	131	3	10
• Steak Tip Caesar, 383 g	661	50	21
• Tossed, 274 g	49	1	11
Turkey, 366 g	157	2	10
Soup (Small)			
Beef Stew, 227 g	220	8	23
Beef Stew, 227 g	220	8	23
Chicken Noodle, 227 g	110	3	14
Ex. Broc. & Cheddar Cheese, 227 g	270	21	11
• Hearty Vegetable, 227 g	40	0	7
Italian Wedding, 227 g	120	6	11
• Lobster Bisque, 227 g	360	29	16
NE Clam Chowder, 227 g	320	18	31
Portuguese Kale, 227 g	130	4	16
Subs: Small Subs			
Big Papi, 340 g	525	15	60
BLT & Cheese, 244 g	463	19	51
Capicola & Cheese, 225 g	408	13	48
Cheese, 244 g	589	28	55
Cheeseburger, 246 g	526	26	44
Chicken Club, 289 g	593	29	49
Chicken Honey Dijon, 316 g	575	22	53
Chicken Salad, 252 g	692	44	48

RESTAURANTS & FAST-FOOD CHAINS

D'Angelo (cont.)

Subs: Small Subs (cont.)

	Cal	Fat	Cbs
Chicken Stir Fry, 291 g	449	11	53
Classic Veggie, 364 g	462	15	64
Grilled Chicken, 254 g	369	7	48
Ham & Cheese, 236 g	395	11	52
Ham & Salami, 216 g	456	19	48
Ham, 208 g	302	5	49
Hamburger, 227 g	466	22	42
Italian, 253 g	614	31	54
Lobster, 255 g	598	33	48
Meatball, 360 g	644	33	66
Mortadella & Cheese, 219 g	479	23	49
Number 9, 263 g	450	19	41
Pastrami, 227 g	613	34	47
Peppercorn Steak, 230 g	508	39	7
Pepperoni, 226 g	603	33	49
Roast Beef, 234 g	320	5	48
• Salad, 397 g	281	3	57
Salami & Cheese, 230 g	579	32	47
Seafood Salad, 227 g	498	23	61
Steak & Cheese, 202 g	446	19	40
Steak Bomb, 343 g	670	33	52
Steak Tip, 333 g	545	18	63
Steak, 181 g	373	14	37
Toasted BBQ Steak, 273 g	623	25	62
Toasted Italian Bistro, 210 g	585	31	49
Toasted Pastrami Ruben, 298 g	750	47	55
Toasted Roast Beef & Cheddar, 234 g	564	26	51
• Toasted Spicy Meatball, 453 g	933	57	71
Toasted Tuna & Swiss, 283 g	796	54	49
Toasted Turkey & Ham, 255 g	532	24	49
Toasted Turkey Thanksgiving, 234 g	705	20	80
Tuna, 241 g	685	46	47
Turkey Club, 291 g	401	9	49
Turkey, 163 g	317	4	45

Toppings

	Cal	Fat	Cbs
Bacon, 14 g	64	5	0
Buffalo Sauce, 1 oz.	10	0	2
Cheese Cheddar, 28 g	114	9	1
Cucumber, 3 slices, 28 g	4	0	1
Fat Free Mayonnaise, 1 packet, 12 g	10	0	2
• Hot Peppers, 1 oz.	0	0	1
Lettuce, 1 oz.	4	0	1
Mayonnaise (2 tbsp.), 30 g	225	25	1
Mushrooms, 1 oz.	7	0	1
Mustard, Honey Dijon, 2 tbsp, 36 g	60	0	18
Mustard Yellow, 2 tbsp., 30 g	20	1	2
• Olive Oil Blend, 2 tbsp., 27 g	239	27	0
Onions, 0.5 oz.	6	0	1
Pickles 8 slices, 14 g	0	0	1
Processed American Cheese, 1 oz.	95	7	3
Provolone Cheese, 1 oz.	100	8	1
Sweet Peppers, 1 oz.	8	0	2
Swiss Cheese, 1 oz.	106	8	1
Tomato 3 slices, 60 g	11	0	2
Turkey Gravy, 85 g	84	5	4
Vinegar, 2 tbsp., 30 g	1	0	0

Wraps

	Cal	Fat	Cbs
Big Papi, 347 g	593	23	56
BLT & Cheese, 229 g	544	26	54
Buffalo Chicken Salad, 400 g	823	44	67
Caesar Salad, 329 g	711	44	65
Capicola & Cheese, 242 g	494	20	53
Cheese, 261 g	675	35	59
Cheeseburger, 263 g	609	33	48

D'Angelo (cont.)

Wraps (cont.)

	Cal	Fat	Cbs
Chicken Caesar Salad, 421 g	830	47	65
• Chicken Cobb, 433 g	931	55	71
Chicken Filet & Bacon, 342 g	639	28	58
Chicken Honey Dijon, 396 g	672	29	60
Chicken Salad, 286 g	782	51	53
Chicken Stir, 308 g	535	17	57
ChixSFry D'Lite, 439 g	422	5	56
Classic Veggie, 389 g	486	13	68
Greek, 436 g	765	61	44
Grilled Chicken, 349 g	422	6	59
Ham & Cheese, 251 g	435	10	60
Ham & Salami, 260 g	513	18	57
Hamburger, 258 g	509	21	50
Italian, 277 g	631	29	59
Lobster, 315 g	749	43	57
Meatball, 392 g	687	31	75
Mortadella & Cheese, 251 g	522	21	58
Number 9, 276 g	517	24	44
Pastrami, 230 g	550	25	55
Peppercorn Steak, 315 g	702	40	45
Pepperoni, 230 g	519	21	57
Roast Beef, 249 g	448	13	58
• Salad, 429 g	324	2	66
Salami & Cheese, 258 g	605	29	56
Seafood Salad, 258 g	541	22	69
Steak & Cheese, 222 g	464	18	43
Steak Bomb, 343 g	670	33	52
Steak Tip, 298 g	432	16	41
Steak, 200 g	392	13	41
Tuna, 284 g	731	44	56
Turkey Club, 284 g	415	7	52
Turkey, 249 g	369	3	51

Dairy Queen

Blizzard Treats

	Cal	Fat	Cbs
• Med. Banana Split Blizzard®, 382 g	580	17	97
• Med. Choc. Chip Cookie Dough Blizzard®, 446 g	1030	40	151
Med. Reese's® P. Butter Cup Blizzard®, 383 g	790	28	114
Med. Strawberry CheeseQuake™ Blizzard®, 376 g	730	29	105
Medium Oreo® Cookies Blizzard®, 334 g	690	26	103

Burgers

	Cal	Fat	Cbs
Bacon Cheddar GrillBurger™, 229 g	650	37	41
Classic GrillBurger™ with Cheese, 231 g	560	30	42
Classic GrillBurger™, 212 g	470	23	42
DQ Homestyle Burger, 142 g	350	14	33
DQ® Homestyle® Bacon Double, 245 g	730	41	35
DQ® Homestyle® Cheeseburger, 156 g	400	18	34
DQ® Homestyle® Double Cheeseburger, 226 g	640	34	34
DQ® Ultimate® Burger, 259 g	780	48	33
• FlameThrower® GrillBurger™, 1/2 lb.	1030	73	41
FlameThrower® GrillBurger, 1/4 lb.	780	54	41
GrillBurger™ with Cheese, 1/2 lb.	820	49	47
GrillBurger™, 1/2 lb.	670	37	42
Mushroom Swiss GrillBurger™, 210 g	630	40	39

Cones

	Cal	Fat	Cbs
DQ® Chocolate Soft Serve, 1/2 Cup, 94 g	150	5	22
• DQ® Vanilla Soft Serve, 1/2 Cup, 94 g	150	5	22
Medium Chocolate Cone, 199 g	340	10	54
• Medium Dipped Cone, 220 g	490	23	61
• Medium Vanilla Cone, 199 g	340	10	54

DQ® Blizzard® Cakes

	Cal	Fat	Cbs
• Chocolate Xtreme Blizzard® Cake, 249 g	660	31	85
• Oreo® Cookies Blizzard® Cake, 220 g	490	20	67
Reese's® PB Cup Blizzard® Cake, 220 g	490	20	67

Dairy Queen (cont.)

	Cal	Fat	Cbs
DQ® Blizzard® Cakes (cont.)			
DQ® Medium French Fries, 196 g	510	23	70
DQ® Regular Onion Rings, 113 g	470	30	45
Hot Dogs			
All-Beef Chili Cheese Dog, 150 g	380	24	24
All-Beef Hot Dog, 115 g	300	15	30
Malts, Shakes and Arctic Rush			
• Medium Arctic Rush™ Slush, 595 g	310	0	63
• Medium Chocolate Malt, 567 g	900	21	157
Medium Chocolate Shake, 550 g	780	20	133
MooLatté® Frozen Blended Coffee			
• Cappuccino MooLatté®, 16 oz.	500	18	73
• Caramel MooLatté®, 16 oz.	630	19	103
French Vanilla MooLatté®, 16 oz.	570	18	90
Mocha MooLatté®, 16 oz.	590	23	84
Novelties			
• Buster Bar®, 148 g	480	31	45
Chocolate Dilly® Bar, 87 g	240	15	24
• DQ® Fudge Bar – no sugar added, 66 g	50	0	13
DQ® Sandwich, 85 g	190	5	32
DQ® Vanilla Orange Bar – no sugar added, 66 g	60	0	17
StarKiss®, 85 g	80	0	21
Royal Treats®			
• Banana Split, 374 g	530	14	98
• Brownie Earthquake™, 304 g	740	28	149
Peanut Buster® Parfait, 304 g	710	30	96
Salad Dressings			
DQ® Blue Cheese Dressing, 57 g	210	20	4
DQ® Honey Mustard Dressing, 57 g	260	21	18
• DQ® Ranch Dressing, 57 g	310	33	3
• Fat Free Italian Dressing, 43 g	10	0	3
Salads			
• Crispy Chicken Salad – no dressing, 424 g	420	22	90
Grilled Chicken Salad – no dressing, 424 g	270	11	92
• Side Salad - no dressing, 182 g	45	0	27
Sandwiches/Baskets			
Chicken Strip Basket™, 4 pcs., 446 g	1030	54	105
• Chicken Strip Basket™, 6 pcs., 531 g	1270	67	121
Crispy Chicken Sandwich, 198 g	540	29	47
• Grilled Chicken Sandwich, 177 g	350	16	49
Sundaes			
Medium Chocolate Sundae, 234 g	410	10	72
Medium Strawberry Sundae, 248 g	370	10	63

Damon's Grill

	Cal	Fat	Cbs
Aloha Chicken	515	12	45
Chimi Chicken	450	9	37
• Maui Salmon	535	21	40
• Grilled Chicken Breast Salad	340	10	18

Del Taco

	Cal	Fat	Cbs
Breakfast			
5-Piece Hash Brown Sticks, 80 g	250	19	20
8-Piece Hash Brown Sticks, 128 g	410	30	32
Bacon & Egg Quesadilla, 175 g	450	23	40
Big Fat Breakfast Taco, 167 g	559	17	36
• Breakfast Burrito, 107 g	250	11	24
Egg & Cheese Burrito, 213 g	450	24	39
• Macho Bacon & Egg Burrito ™, 454 g	1030	60	82
Shredded Beef Breakfast Burrito, 297 g	785	33	41
Steak & Egg Burrito, 255 g	580	34	41
Burgers			
• Bacon Double Del Cheeseburger™, 212 g	610	39	35
Bun Taco, 191 g	440	0	37
Cheeseburger, 131 g	330	13	37
Del Cheeseburger ™, 161 g	430	25	35

Del Taco (cont.)

	Cal	Fat	Cbs
Burgers (cont.)			
Double Del Cheeseburger ™, 202 g	560	35	35
• Hamburger, 118 g	280	21	37
Burritos			
Bean & Cheese Cup, 220 g	415	9	47
Bean & Cheese Green Burrito, 142 g	280	8	38
• Bean & Cheese Red Burrito, 142 g	270	8	38
Chicken Works Burrito, 312 g	520	23	57
Del Beef Burrito ™, 227 g	550	30	42
Del Classic Chicken Burrito ™, 227 g	560	36	41
Del Combo Burrito, 269 g	530	22	61
Deluxe Combo Burrito™, 340 g	570	25	64
Deluxe Del Beef Burrito™, 298 g	590	33	45
Half Pound Green Burrito, 241 g	430	12	59
Half Pound Red Burrito, 241 g	430	12	65
• Macho Beef Burrito ™, 539 g	1170	62	89
Macho Chicken Burrito ™, 524 g	930	33	111
Macho Combo Burrito ™, 553 g	1050	44	113
Shredded Beef Combo Burrito, 297 g	815	30	61
Spicy Chicken Burrito, 290 g	510	17	68
Steak Works Burrito, 312 g	590	31	58
Veggie Works Burrito, 319 g	490	18	69
Fries			
Chili Cheese Fries, 298 g	670	46	51
• Deluxe Chili Cheese Fries ™, 340 g	710	49	53
• Medium Fries, 198 g	490	32	47
Nachos			
Macho Nachos ®, 468 g	1100	63	113
Nachos, 113 g	380	24	40
Quesadilla			
Cheddar Quesadilla, 151 g	500	27	39
• Chicken Cheddar Quesadilla, 194 g	580	31	41
Spicy Jack Chicken Quesadilla, 194 g	570	30	40
• Spicy Jack Quesadilla, 151 g	490	26	38
Salads			
Mexican Caesar Salad (Large) w/ Dressing, 306 g	557	47	16
w/o Dressing, 246 g	257	13	14
w/Dressing +Chicken, 418 g	677	51	24
w/o Dressing +Chicken, 358 g	377	17	32
Mexican Caesar Salad (Side) with Dressing, 155 g	415	40	9
• w/o Dressing, 95 g	115	6	7
Deluxe Chicken Salad, 526 g	740	34	77
• Deluxe Taco Salad ™, 541 g	780	40	76
Taco Salad, 177 g	350	30	10
Shakes			
• Chocolate Shake, 425 g	680	16	117
• Strawberry Shake, 425 g	540	8	100
Vanilla Shake, 425 g	550	10	97
Sides			
Beans 'n Cheese Cup, 220 g	415	9	47
• Large Chips and Salsa, 255 g	465	21	45
Medium Chips and Salsa, 170 g	310	14	43
Rice Cup, 113 g	140	2	27
• Side of Bacon (2 slices), 10 g	50	4	0
Small Chips and Salsa, 85 g	155	7	22
Tacos			
Big Fat Chicken Taco ™, 153 g	340	13	38
• Big Fat Steak Taco ™, 153 g	390	19	38
Big Fat Taco ™, 153 g	320	11	39
Carne Asada Taco, 142 g	237	8	22
Chicken Soft Taco, 106 g	293	11	18
Chicken Taco Del Carbon, 98 g	170	5	19
Crispy Fish Taco ™, 131 g	290	16	30
Macho Taco ®, 170 g	308	17	16
Shredded Beef Taco Del Carbon, 92 g	199	11	17

RESTAURANTS & FAST-FOOD CHAINS

Del Taco (cont.)

	Cal	Fat	Cbs
Tacos (cont.)			
• Soft Taco, 80 g	160	8	16
Steak Taco Del Carbon, 98 g	220	11	19
Taco, 63 g	160	10	11

Denny's

	Cal	Fat	Cbs
Appetizers and Entrees			
Applesauce Musselman's®, 3 oz.	60	0	15
Baked Potato, plain w/skin, 7 oz.	220	0	51
Bread Stuffing, plain, 3 oz.	110	5	13
Buffalo Chicken Strips (5), 10 oz.	734	42	43
Buffalo Wings (9), 19 oz.	974	72	11
Chicken Strips (5), 10 oz.	720	33	56
Chicken Strips, 10 oz.	635	25	55
Corn, 4 oz.	110	2	23
Cottage Cheese, 3 oz.	73	3	2
Country Fried Steak, 9 oz.	644	46	30
Fish & Chips, 17 oz.	958	54	83
Fried Shrimp Dinner, 5 oz.	260	12	18
Grilled Chicken Alfredo, 24 oz.	1290	67	111
Grilled Chicken Dinner, 10 oz.	280	5	4
Grilled Shrimp Skewers/Pilaf/garlic brd, 13 oz.	650	29	59
Grilled Tilapia Dinner, 11 oz.	530	18	33
Lemon Pepper Tilapia, 15 oz.	810	48	38
Mashed Potatoes, plain, 5 oz.	170	7	23
Meat Loaf Dinner, 11 oz.	930	60	51
• Mini Burgers (6) w/Onion Rings, 25 oz.	2180	133	173
Mozzarella Sticks (8), 8 oz.	710	41	49
Mushroom Swiss Chopped Steak, 13 oz.	930	76	13
Nacho, 23 oz.	1278	64	117
Roast Turkey & Stuffing (incl. gravy), 12 oz.	510	14	66
Sampler ™, 17 oz.	1405	80	124
• Sliced Tomatoes (3 slices), 2 oz.	13	0	3
Smothered Cheese Fries, 9 oz.	767	48	69
Steakhouse Strip Dinner, 8 oz.	390	14	0
T-bone Steak Dinner, 13 oz.	630	29	0
Vegetable Blend, 4 oz.	60	4	5
Vegetable Rice Pilaf, 5 oz.	173	3	33
Breakfast			
All American Slam ® w/ hashbrowns, 14 oz.	950	75	21
Belgian Waffle Platter, 8 oz.	619	45	28
Buttermilk Pancake, 9 oz.	420	5	82
Cntry Fried Steak & Eggs w/ hashbrwns, 19 oz.	740	46	49
Country Fried Potatoes, 5 oz.	394	20	23
Fabulous French Toast Platter, 13 oz.	1261	79	110
French Toast Slam®(2 sl.), 14 oz.	1180	75	74
Grand Slam Slugger ™ w/hash brown, 24 oz.	1040	55	97
• Grits, 4 oz.	80	0	18
H.B.'s w/Onions, Cheese, Gravy, 8 oz.	493	25	54
Ham & Cheddar Omel w/eggbeaters, 10 oz.	468	32	5
Ham & Cheddar Omelette, 10 oz.	595	47	5
Ham and Jalapeño Scramble, 25 oz.	1080	53	117
Hashed Browns w/ Cheddar Cheese, 6 oz.	280	19	21
Hashed Browns, 4 oz.	197	12	20
Heartland Scramble, 24 oz.	1190	59	118
Lumberjack Slam w/ hash browns, 22 oz.	1140	53	108
Meat Lover's Breakfast, 22 oz.	1230	66	109
Meat Lover's Scramble, 23 oz.	1280	71	103
Moons Over My Hammy ®, 13 oz.	760	40	52
Original Grand Slam ®, 13 oz.	740	43	56
• Smoked Sausage Scramble, 26 oz.	1480	88	118
Steakhouse Strip & Eggs, 11 oz.	560	37	3
T-bone Steak & Eggs, 14 oz.	991	77	1
Ultimate Omelette® w/hash browns, 16 oz.	830	62	26
Veggie-Cheese Omel w/eggbeaters, 12 oz.	346	22	11
Veggie-Cheese Omel w/hashbrowns, 17 oz.	670	48	28

Denny's (cont.)

	Cal	Fat	Cbs
Breakfast Menu - a la carte			
Bacon, 4 strips, 1 oz.	162	18	1
Bagel, dry (1), 4 oz.	310	1	65
Banana, whole, 4 oz.	110	0	29
Biscuit, 2 oz.	192	10	22
Cherry Topping, 3 oz.	86	0	21
Cinnamon Apple Filling, 3 oz.	90	2	19
Cream Cheese, 1 oz.	100	10	1
• Egg Beaters ® Egg Substitute, 4 oz.	56	0	2
English Muffin, dry (1), 2 oz.	150	2	27
Grapefruit, 5 oz.	60	0	16
Grapes, 3 oz.	55	1	15
Ham, grilled slice, Honey Smoked, 3 oz.	85	3	6
Maple-Flavored Syrup, 2 oz.	143	0	36
One Egg, 2 oz.	120	10	1
Sausage Patties (2) patties, 3 oz.	295	28	1
Sausage, 4 links, 3 oz.	354	32	0
Sugar-Free Maple-Flavored Syrup, 2 oz.	23	0	9
Toast, dry, (1), 1 oz.	90	1	17
• Two Eggs and More Breakfast, 11 oz.	630	47	21
Whipped Cream, dollop, 0.5 oz.	23	2	2
Whipped Margarine, 0.5 oz.	87	10	0
Condiments & Beverages			
BBQ Sauce, 2 oz.	47	1	11
Blue Cheese Dressing, 1 oz.	163	18	1
Butter Roll, 2 pcs.	260	9	38
Caesar Dressing, 1 oz.	133	14	1
Cherry Limeade, 15 oz.	240	0	62
Croutons, 1 oz.	112	6	12
• Fat Free Italian, 1 oz.	15	1	3
Fat Free Ranch Dressing, 1 oz.	25	0	6
French Dressing, 1 oz.	106	10	3
Garlic Dinner Bread, 2 pieces	170	11	15
Honey Mustard Dressing, 1 oz.	160	15	20
Island Fizz, 15 oz.	250	0	64
OJ Mango, 14 oz.	240	0	60
Pico de Gallo, 3 oz.	21	0	5
Pineapple Dream, 15 oz.	180	0	64
Ranch Dressing, 1 oz.	129	14	1
Razzdango, 15 oz.	220	0	59
Sour Cream, 2 oz.	91	9	2
Strawberry Mango Pucker, 15 oz.	200	0	51
Thousand Island Dressing, 1 oz.	118	11	5
• Very Double Berry, 14 oz.	280	0	69
Desserts			
Apple Crisp, a la mode, 12 oz.	723	21	133
Apple Pie, 7 oz.	470	21	68
Banana Split, 19 oz.	894	43	121
Carrot Cake, 8 oz.	799	45	99
Cheesecake, 7 oz.	580	38	51
Coconut Cream Pie, 7 oz.	701	32	100
Double Scoop/Sundae, 6 oz.	375	27	29
• Floats (Root beer or Cola), 12 oz.	280	10	47
French Silk Pie, 7 oz.	737	56	58
Hershey's Chocolate Cake, 5 oz.	631	33	79
Hot Fudge Brownie a la mode, 10 oz.	997	42	147
Malted Milkshake (van/choc), 12 oz.	583	26	82
Milkshake (van/choc), 12 oz.	560	26	76
Neutron Brownie (kids), 3 oz.	344	16	49
Oreo Blender Blast Off (Kids), 10 oz.	580	29	72
Oreo Blender Blaster, 15 oz.	895	46	112
Pecan Pie, 6 oz.	740	41	88
Pumpkin Pie, 7 oz.	499	11	77
Single Scoop/Sundae (Delicious Dip), 5 oz.	290	16	35

Denny's (cont.)

Fit Fare	Cal	Fat	Cbs
2% Milk, 5 oz.	87	5	7
Bagel, dry, 4 oz.	310	1	65
Baked Potato, plain w/skin, 7 oz.	220	0	51
Banana (1), 4 oz.	110	0	29
• Boca Burger w/ sm fruit bowl, 15 oz.	570	11	83
Cereal (average), 1 oz.	100	0	23
Chicken Noodle, 12 oz.	170	9	14
Choice: Oatmeal, 4 oz.	100	2	18
Corn, 4 oz.	110	2	23
English Muffin, dry, 2 oz.	150	2	27
Fruit Medley, 4 oz.	80	0	20
Grapes, 3 oz.	55	1	15
Grilled Chicken Breast Dinner w/ Vegetables, 11 oz.	390	11	12
Grilled Chicken Breast Salad, 16 oz.	320	13	15
Grits, 4 oz.	80	0	18
Mashed Potatoes, 5 oz.	170	7	23
Side Garden Salad (w/o dressing), 7 oz.	113	7	6
Skinny Moons w/ fruit, 14 oz.	560	12	73
Sliced Tomatoes, 2 oz.	13	0	3
Slim Slam ™ (w/ fruit topping), 15 oz.	530	9	76
Tilapia, w/ Rice & Vegetables., 14 oz.	420	13	40
Toast, dry, 1 oz.	92	1	17
Vegetable Beef, 12 oz.	140	5	11
• Vegetable Blend, 4 oz.	60	3	5
Veggie EB Omelette w/Eng. Muffin, 14 oz.	340	9	37
Kid's			
• Anti-Gravity Grapes, 3 oz.	60	0	15
Astronaut Applesauce, 3 oz.	84	0	19
Big Dipper French Toastix ™, 7 oz.	627	71	71
Cosmic Cheeseburger™, 4 oz.	341	20	24
Deep-Sea Salad™ w/ Ranch, 4 oz.	240	20	13
Delicious Dip Sundae, 5 oz.	413	19	59
Flying Saucer Pizza ™, 4 oz.	331	14	38
Galactic Grilled Cheese, 3 oz.	334	20	28
Goldfish® Galaxy, 2 oz.	284	3	0
Junior Grand Slam ®, 5 oz.	400	21	38
Little Dippers w/ Applesauce & Marinara, 10 oz.	566	27	50
• Little Dippers w/ Marinara & Fries, 12 oz.	860	43	80
Macaroni & Cheese, 7 oz.	353	13	48
Moon Crater Mashed ™ w/ Gravy, 5 oz.	145	6	20
Moons & Stars Chicken Nuggets, 2 oz.	190	13	9
Neutron Brownie, 3 oz.	344	16	49
Smiley-Alien Hotcakes w/ Meat, 6 oz.	340	12	49
Smiley-Alien Hotcakes w/o Meat, 4 oz.	230	3	47
Promotionals			
Apple Strudel French Toast Slam, 18 oz.	1060	54	92
Cherry Danish French Toast Slam, 18 oz.	1070	54	96
• Grilled Chicken (2 pcs.), 10 oz.	280	4	4
Grilled Shrimp Skewers w/ rice pilaf, 11 oz.	450	18	39
Mushroom Swiss Chopped Steak 4, 13 oz.	930	76	13
Slam Burger, 17 oz.	720	40	69
Southwestern Chicken Sandwich, 15 oz.	1020	50	81
Steak & Cheese Omelette w/ Hash Brown, 24 oz.	1190	56	107
• Supreme French Toast 1, 18 oz.	1380	84	113
Sandwiches/Salads/Soups			
Bacon Cheddar Burger, 13 oz.	970	70	33
Bacon, Lettuce & Tomato, 7 oz.	570	37	36
Boca Burger®, 11 oz.	510	16	64
Broccoli & Cheddar, 12 oz.	270	17	17
Chef's Salad 3, 18 oz.	360	17	17
Chicken Noodle, 12 oz.	170	9	14
Chicken Ranch Melt, 13 oz.	920	42	79
Clam Chowder, 12 oz.	170	11	13
Classic Burger w/ Cheese, 13 oz.	940	59	56

Denny's (cont.)

Sandwiches/Salads/Soups (cont.)	Cal	Fat	Cbs
Classic Burger, 11 oz.	780	45	56
Club Sandwich, 11 oz.	658	34	55
Coleslaw, 5 oz.	260	22	15
Crispy Onion Burger w/ Fries, 21 oz.	1820	119	127
Fish Sandwich, 12 oz.	589	30	30
French Fries, unsalted, 5 oz.	423	20	57
Fried Chicken Strip Salad, 15 oz.	438	26	26
Grilled Chicken Breast Salad, 13 oz.	259	11	10
Grilled Chicken Sandwich w/o Dressing, 12 oz.	490	13	57
Jalapeño Burger w/ Fries, 19 oz.	1560	104	99
• Mini Burgers (6) w/ Onion Rings, 25 oz.	2180	133	173
Mushroom Swiss Burger, 16 oz.	900	55	62
Onion Rings, 4 oz.	381	23	38
Philly Melt, 17 oz.	740	43	51
Seasoned Fries, 5 oz.	460	28	46
Side Caesar (w/ dressing), 6 oz.	362	26	20
• Side Garden Salad (w/o dressing), 7 oz.	113	7	6
Spicy Buffalo Chicken Melt 1, 14 oz.	930	46	79
The Super Bird® Sandwich, 10 oz.	570	27	43
Turkey Breast Salad w/o dressing, 13 oz.	248	8	12
Vegetable Beef, 12 oz.	140	5	17
Western Burger w/ Fries, 21 oz.	1580	95	122
Seniors			
Grilled Cheese Sandwich, 7 oz.	540	30	50
Senior Belgian Waffle Slam ®, 9 oz.	580	41	29
Senior Chicken Strip Dinner, 5 oz.	285	10	31
Senior Club, 10 oz.	570	33	40
Senior Country Fried Steak, 5 oz.	341	23	18
Senior French Toast Slam, 7 oz.	591	43	37
• Senior Fried Shrimp Dinner, 4 oz.	149	6	14
Senior Grilled Chicken Breast, 6 oz.	200	5	15
Senior Grilled Tilapia, 6 oz.	248	10	0
Senior Lemon Pepper Tilapia, 9 oz.	509	41	6
Senior Pot Roast w/ Vegetables, 7 oz.	180	8	8
• Senior Scram. Egg & Cheddar, 13 oz.	790	46	56
Senior Turkey & Stuffing, 9 oz.	430	12	58
Sr. Bacon Cheddar Burger w/ Fries, 7 oz.	433	25	27
Sr. Fish & Chips w/ Slaw & Fries 13 oz.	756	47	64
Sr. Omelette w/ Hashbrowns, 12 oz.	760	55	36
Sr. Starter w/ Biscuit, 8 oz.	410	42	23
Toppings			
Cherry Topping, 2 oz.	57	0	14
Chocolate Topping, 2 oz.	133	1	34
• Fudge Topping, 2 oz.	201	10	30
Strawberry Topping, 2 oz.	77	1	17
• Whipped Cream (2 tbsp.), 0.5 oz.	23	2	2

Dippin' Dots

Cups: Flavored Ice	Cal	Fat	Cbs
Cherry Berry Ice, 75 g	90	0	23
Liberty Ice, 75 g	90	0	23
Pink Lemonade Ice, 75 g	90	0	23
Rainbow Ice, 75 g	90	0	23
Watermelon Ice, 75 g	90	0	23
Cups: Ice Cream			
Banana Split, 85 g	170	10	16
Bubble Gum, 85 g	165	10	15
Candy Bar Crunch, 85 g	208	13	34
Caramel Brownie Sundae, 85 g	170	10	16
Chocolate Chip Cookie Dough, 85 g	213	11	26
Chocolate, 85 g	165	10	15
Cookies 'n Cream w/ Oreo, 85 g	203	11	22
Cotton Candy, 85 g	170	10	16
Horchata, 85 g	170	10	16
Java Delight, 85 g	170	10	16

Dippin' Dots (cont.)

	Cal	Fat	Cbs
Cups: Ice Cream (cont.)			
Mint Chocolate, 85 g	165	10	15
• Moose Tracks, 85 g	218	13	21
Peanut Butter Chip, 85 g	165	10	15
• Root Beer Float, 85 g	111	3	20
Strawberry, 85 g	170	10	16
Tropical Tie Dye, 85 g	170	10	16
Vanilla, 85 g	170	10	16
Cups: No Sugar Added			
No Sugar Added Fat Free Fudge, 85 g	92	0	18
No Sugar Added Reduced Fat Vanilla, 85 g	123	6	13
Cups: Sherbet			
Lemon Lime Sherbet, 85 g	97	1	22
Orange Sherbet, 85 g	97	1	22
Raspberry Sherbet, 85 g	97	1	22
Yogurt			
Strawberry Cheesecake, 85 g	100	0	21

Domino's Pizza

	Cal	Fat	Cbs
12" Medium Feast Pizzas			
America's Favorite Feast, 59 g	130	10	4
Bacon Cheeseburger Feast, 55 g	140	11	3
Barbecue Feast, 51 g	130	8	8
Cheese Deep Dish, 23 g	60	5	2
• Cheese HT & TC, 18 g	45	4	1
Classic Hand-Tossed, 55 g	160	3	28
Crunchy Thin Crust, 22 g	80	4	12
Deluxe Feast, 56 g	100	8	4
Extra Cheese, 9 g	25	2	1
ExtravaganZZa, 81 g	160	12	5
Hawaiian Feast, 58 g	90	6	5
MeatZZa Feast, 65 g	150	11	4
Pepperoni Feast, 54 g	130	11	4
Philly Cheese Steak Feast, 44 g	100	7	1
Pizza Sauce, 15 g	10	1	1
• Ultimate Deep Dish, 56 g	160	6	24
Vegi Feast, 58 g	80	6	4
12" Medium, 1 topping pizza			
American Cheese, 11 g	40	3	0
Anchovies, 2 g	0	0	0
Bacon, 9 g	40	3	0
Banana Peppers, 8 g	0	0	0
Beef, 12 g	40	3	0
Black Olives, 8 g	10	1	1
Cheddar Cheese, 7 g	30	3	0
Cheese Deep Dish, 23 g	60	5	2
Cheese HT & TC, 18 g	45	4	1
Chicken Grilled, 12 g	15	0	0
Classic Hand-Tossed, 55 g	160	3	28
Crunchy Thin Crust, 22 g	80	4	12
Extra Cheese, 9 g	25	2	1
Garlic, 4 g	10	0	1
Green Chile Peppers, 8 g	0	0	0
Green Olive, 8 g	15	2	0
Green Peppers, 8 g	0	0	0
Ham, 10 g	10	0	0
Jalapeño, 8 g	0	0	0
• Mushrooms, 12 g	0	0	0
Onions, 8 g	0	0	1
Pepperoni, 8 g	40	4	0
Philly Meat, 9 g	10	0	0
Pineapple, 12 g	10	0	2
Pizza Sauce, 15 g	5	0	1
Provolone Cheese, 12 g	45	4	0
Sausage, 12 g	45	4	1
Tomatoes, 18 g	5	0	1

Domino's Pizza (cont.)

	Cal	Fat	Cbs
12" Medium, 1 topping pizza (cont.)			
• Ultimate Deep Dish, 56 g	160	6	24
12" Medium, 2-3 topping pizza			
American Cheese, 11 g	40	3	0
Anchovies, 2 g	0	0	0
Bacon, 6 g	25	2	0
Banana Peppers, 5 g	0	0	0
Beef, 9 g	25	3	0
Black Olives, 5 g	5	1	1
Cheddar Cheese, 7 g	30	3	0
Cheese Deep Dish, 23 g	60	5	2
Cheese HT & TC, 18 g	45	4	1
Chicken Grilled, 9 g	10	0	0
Classic Hand-Tossed, 55 g	160	3	28
Crunchy Thin Crust, 22 g	80	4	12
Extra Cheese, 9 g	25	2	1
Garlic, 3 g	10	0	1
Green Chile Peppers, 5 g	0	0	0
Green Olive, 5 g	10	1	0
• Green Peppers, 5 g	0	0	0
Ham, 7 g	10	0	0
Jalapeño, 5 g	0	0	0
Mushrooms, 9 g	0	0	0
Onions, 5 g	0	0	0
Pepperoni, 6 g	40	4	0
Philly Meat, 9 g	10	0	0
Pineapple, 9 g	5	0	1
Pizza Sauce, 15 g	10	1	1
Provolone Cheese, 12 g	45	4	0
Sausage, 9 g	30	3	1
Tomatoes, 12 g	0	0	1
• Ultimate Deep Dish, 56 g	160	6	24
14" Large Feast Pizzas			
America's Favorite Feast, 82 g	170	14	6
Bacon Cheeseburger Feast, 77 g	200	15	4
Barbecue Feast, 70 g	170	11	11
Cheese Deep Dish, 32 g	80	7	2
• Cheese HT & TC, 25 g	60	5	2
Classic Hand-Tossed, 75 g	220	4	38
Crunchy Thin Crust, 30 g	110	5	16
Deluxe Feast, 76 g	130	10	5
Extra Cheese, 12 g	30	3	1
ExtravaganZZa, 107 g	200	16	7
Hawaiian Feast, 82 g	130	8	7
MeatZZa Feast, 94 g	210	17	6
Pepperoni Feast, 74 g	180	15	5
Philly Cheese Steak Feast, 58 g	130	9	2
Pizza Sauce, 21 g	10	0	2
• Ultimate Deep Dish, 83 g	230	7	36
Vegi Feast, 79 g	120	8	6
14" Large, 1 topping pizza			
American Cheese, 12 g	45	4	0
Anchovies, 2 g	0	0	0
Bacon, 13 g	60	4	0
Banana Peppers, 11 g	0	0	1
Beef, 18 g	50	5	0
Black Olives, 7 g	10	1	1
Cheddar Cheese, 9 g	35	3	0
Cheese Deep Dish, 32 g	80	7	2
Cheese HT & TC, 25 g	60	5	2
Chicken Grilled, 18 g	20	1	0
Classic Hand-Tossed, 75 g	220	4	38
Crunchy Thin Crust, 30 g	110	5	16
Extra Cheese, 12 g	30	3	1
Garlic, 4 g	15	0	1

Domino's Pizza (cont.)

	Cal	Fat	Cbs
14" Large, 1 topping pizza (cont.)			
Green Chile Peppers, 11 g	0	0	0
Green Olive, 11 g	20	2	1
Green Peppers, 11 g	0	0	1
Ham, 13 g	15	1	0
• Jalapeño, 11 g	0	0	0
Mushrooms, 18 g	0	0	1
Onions, 11 g	0	0	1
Pepperoni, 11 g	50	5	0
Philly Meat, 12 g	15	1	0
Pineapple, 18 g	15	0	3
Pizza Sauce, 21 g	10	0	2
Provolone Cheese, 18 g	60	5	0
Sausage, 18 g	60	6	2
Tomatoes, 21 g	0	0	1
• Ultimate Deep Dish, 83 g	230	7	36
14" Large, 2-3 topping pizza			
American Cheese, 12 g	45	4	0
• Anchovies, 2 g	0	0	0
Bacon, 10 g	40	3	0
Banana Peppers, 7 g	0	0	0
Beef, 12 g	35	3	0
Black Olives, 7 g	10	1	1
Cheddar Cheese, 9 g	35	3	0
Cheese Deep Dish, 32 g	80	7	2
Cheese HT & TC, 25 g	60	5	2
Chicken Grilled, 12 g	15	0	0
Classic Hand-Tossed, 75 g	220	4	38
Crunchy Thin Crust, 30 g	110	5	16
Extra Cheese, 12 g	30	3	1
Garlic, 4 g	10	0	1
Green Chile Peppers, 7 g	0	0	0
Green Olive, 7 g	10	1	0
Green Peppers, 7 g	0	0	0
Ham, 11 g	10	1	0
Jalapeño, 7 g	0	0	0
Mushrooms, 12 g	0	0	0
Onions, 7 g	0	0	0
Pepperoni, 11 g	50	5	0
Philly Meat, 12 g	15	1	0
Pineapple, 12 g	10	0	2
Pizza Sauce, 21 g	10	0	2
Provolone Cheese, 18 g	60	5	0
Sausage, 12 g	45	4	1
Tomatoes, 16 g	0	0	1
• Ultimate Deep Dish, 83 g	230	7	36
Brooklyn Style Pizza			
• 14" Brooklyn Style w/ Pepperoni, 127 g	330	17	30
14" Brooklyn Style w/ Sausage, 136 g	350	18	31
16" Brooklyn Style w/ Pepperoni, 174 g	460	22	43
• 16" Brooklyn Style w/ Sausage, 187 g	480	25	44
Crispy Melt Pizza			
12" Plain Crispy Melt Pizza, 95 g	310	18	25
14" Plain Crispy Melt Pizza, 129 g	430	24	35
Dessert Pizza			
10" OREO® Dessert Pizza, 44 g	120	4	20
Side Items			
Barbecue Buffalo Wings, 87 g	230	14	6
Blue Cheese Dipping Cup, 43 g	210	22	2
Blue Cheese Dressing, 43 g	230	24	2
Breadsticks, 33 g	130	7	14
Buffalo Chicken Kickers™, 50 g	90	3	6
Buttermilk Ranch Dressing, 43 g	220	24	2
Cheesy Bread, 38 g	140	7	14
Cinna Stix, 35 g	140	7	17

Domino's Pizza (cont.)

	Cal	Fat	Cbs
Side Items (cont.)			
Creamy Caesar Dressing, 43 g	210	22	2
• Garlic Dipping Sauce, 50 g	440	49	0
Golden Italian Dressing, 43 g	220	23	2
Hot Buffalo Wings, 84 g	210	14	5
Hot Dipping Cup, 43 g	120	12	3
• Light Italian Dressing, 43 g	20	1	2
Marinara Dipping Sauce, 57 g	25	0	5
Ranch Dipping Cup, 43 g	190	21	2
Salad, Garden Fresh, 120 g	70	4	5
Salad, Grilled Chicken Caesar, 159 g	100	5	6
Sweet Icing Dipper Cup, 71 g	250	3	57

Don Pablo's

	Cal	Fat	Cbs
Appetizers			
• Beef Taquitos, 6 taquitos	561	34	36
Chicken Flautas, 6 flautas	507	31	39
Single Flauta, 1 flauta	65	4	6
• Single Taquito, 1 taquito	63	3	5
Carnitas			
Carnitas Cold Set	187	14	19
Traditional Pork Carnitas	1050	38	118
Classic Fajitas			
7" Flour Tortilla, each	124	4	20
Chicken	851	29	90
Lettuce Wraps, 3-4 wraps	0	0	1
• Onions and Peppers, 7 oz.	186	13	17
• Steak	1174	68	106
Steak and Chicken Combo	1013	48	98
Classic Quesadillas			
Cheese - Large, 8 slices	1597	99	105
Cheese - Small, 4 slices	812	50	52
Mesquite Grilled Chicken - Large, 8 slices	1332	65	110
• Mesquite Grilled Chicken - Small, 4 slices	665	32	55
Mesquite Grilled Steak - Large, 8 slices	1561	91	122
Mesquite Grilled Steak - Small, 4 slices	780	45	61
• The Don's Sampler, 1 order	2002	118	129
Cool Amigos			
Chicken Nachos	745	46	42
Chicken Sandwich	1068	52	108
Cool Amigo Chicken Quesadilla	1507	85	137
Cool Amigo Fajitas - Beef	1272	63	134
Cool Amigo Fajitas - Chicken	1099	44	125
• Cool Amigo Steak Quesadilla	1622	98	143
• Fried Ice Cream (Small)	424	18	58
Hamburger	1145	57	106
Steak Nachos	859	59	48
Create Your Own Combo			
Beef Enchilada, 1 enchilada	263	18	4
Beef Relleno, 1 relleno	299	17	20
Cheese Enchilada, 1 enchilada	232	16	5
• Cheese Relleno, 1 relleno	396	26	19
• Chicken Enchilada, 1 enchilada	210	13	9
Chicken Relleno, 1 relleno	235	11	21
Chicken Tamale, 1 tamale	222	10	25
Crispy Beef Taco, 1 taco	291	18	21
Crispy Chicken Taco, 1 taco	257	14	22
Pork Tamale, 1 tamale	270	14	24
Soft Beef Taco, 1 taco	327	18	29
Soft Chicken Taco, 1 taco	293	14	30
Spinach & Poblano Enchilada, 1 enchilada	258	13	30
Desserts			
Chocolate Volcano Cake	1380	77	161
• Fried Ice Cream, adult serving	827	35	116
• Sopapillas	1402	78	160

Don Pablo's (cont.)

	Cal	Fat	Cbs
Dos Tacos			
Don Diego	758	38	58
• Dos Beef Tacos - Soft	851	37	92
Dos Beef Tacos -Crispy	820	41	81
Dos Chicken Tacos - Crispy	766	34	83
Dos Chicken Tacos - Soft	780	29	94
• Mamma's Skinny Enchiladas	476	14	51
Rico's Lunch	794	39	70
Fajita Cold Set			
• Combo Cheese Topping, 1 oz.	108	8	0
Guacamole (optional), 1 oz.	52	5	2
Pico de Gallo, 1 oz.	8	0	2
• Shredded Lettuce, 1 oz.	0	0	0
Sour Cream, 1 oz.	77	7	2
Fajita Enchiladas			
Chicken, 3 enchiladas	872	51	21
• Mama's Skinny Enchiladas, 3 enchiladas	368	14	18
• Steak, 3 enchiladas	1101	77	33
Three Amigos, 3 enchiladas	697	46	18
Fajita Nachos			
Chicken Nacho	1396	87	73
Steak Nacho	1430	99	71
Little Amigos			
• Beef Taco Dinner	483	24	50
Cheese Enchilada Dinner	515	29	33
Chicken Stix	739	46	75
Corn Dog	724	40	80
• Dogs in a Blanket	1248	78	98
Grilled Cheese Crisp	884	48	92
Lunch			
Don Pablo's Lunch	755	39	54
Dos Beef Enchiladas	754	39	53
Dos Cheese Enchiladas	755	39	55
Dos Chicken Enchiladas	729	35	63
• El Favorito	982	52	81
Lunch-Sized Fajitas			
• Classic Chicken	600	20	74
• Classic Steak	772	39	83
Combo Fajita	685	29	78
Nachos			
Cheese	1317	98	48
Taco Beef	1625	113	85
Numero Uno Favorito			
• Chicken	1168	56	93
• Conquistador	1893	88	156
El Matador	1409	76	110
Steak and Chicken	1200	63	90
Quesadillas & Salads			
• Cheese	903	55	61
• Mesquite-Grilled Chicken	773	39	63
Mesquite-Grilled Steak	888	52	69
Salad Dressing			
Bleu Cheese, 3 oz.	451	48	3
• Cilantro Ranch Dressing, 3 oz.	494	46	20
Don's House Vinaigrette, 3 oz.	357	31	10
Honey Mustard, 3 oz.	315	27	17
• Low Fat French, 3 oz.	150	4	30
Ranch, 3 oz.	318	34	3
Salads			
Caesar Salad (Plain)	1388	114	79
Chicken Caesar Salad	1563	118	85
Flour Tortilla Taco Shell	486	27	50
• Steak Caesar Salad	1792	144	97
• Tortilla Salad	549	29	59

Don Pablo's (cont.)

	Cal	Fat	Cbs
Sides, Sauces & Garnishes			
Black Beans, 4 oz.	119	2	20
Charro Beans, 5 oz.	96	2	16
Chile-Mashed Potatoes, 3 oz.	108	6	12
• Chips and Salsa	338	17	43
Combo Cheese Topping, 1/4 oz.	27	2	0
Combo Cheese, 1 oz.	109	9	0
Guacamole, 1 oz.	52	5	2
Mexican Rice, 3 oz.	107	1	21
Pico de Gallo, 1 oz.	8	0	2
Ranchero Sauce, 5 oz.	44	0	9
Red Sauce, 2 oz.	17	0	4
Refritos, 5 oz.	262	10	31
Salsa, Spicy Chili Macho, 2 oz.	14	0	3
• Salsa, 1 oz.	6	0	1
• Seasoned Vegetables, 6 oz.	98	5	13
Seasoned Vegetables, 6 oz.	98	5	13
Side Salad	108	7	8
Sour Cream Sauce, 2 oz.	66	4	5
Sour Cream, 1.5 oz.	77	7	2
Sour Crema, 1 oz.	57	5	1
Spoon Bread, 4 oz.	250	12	32
Sizzling Fajitas & Enchilada Combos			
Chicken Fajitas & Chicken Enchilada	986	34	105
• Shrimp Fajitas & Shrimp Enchilada	981	63	65
• Steak Fajitas & Steak Enchilada	1255	66	119
Soup			
• Tortilla Soup - Bottomless Bowl, 12 oz.	258	12	26
• White Chicken Chili - Bottomless Bowl, 12 oz.	541	32	48
White Chicken Chili - Cup, 6 oz.	234	13	23
The Don's Dips			
• Dip Sampler, 4 dips, 2 oz.	519	39	27
• Guacamole, 2 oz.	83	8	4
Prairie Fire Bean Dip, 2 oz.	126	8	8
Queso Blanco, 2 oz.	113	9	4
Queso, 2 oz.	105	8	3
Prairie Fire Bean Dip Cup, 6 oz.	378	25	23
Queso Blanco Cup, 6 oz.	339	27	13
Queso Cup, 6 oz.	315	23	10
Traditional Favorites			
• Chicken Burrito, 1 burrito	878	48	70
Chicken Chimichanga, 1 burrito	1099	42	114
• Spicy Ground Beef and Bean Burrito, 1 burrito	1389	73	123
Spicy Ground Beef Chimi De Oro, 1 burrito	1349	68	131

Donatos Pizza

	Cal	Fat	Cbs
Desserts			
Apple Dessert Thin Crust Pizza, 368 g	773	21	134
• Cherry Dessert Thin Crust Pizza, 368 g	799	21	140
• Chocolate Chunk Cookie, 85 g	430	21	57
Dressings & Croutons			
Apple Cider Vinaigrette, 2 oz.	140	12	8
Blue Cheese, 2 oz.	230	24	2
Buttermilk Ranch, 2 oz.	230	24	2
• Chicken Bacon Ranch Pizza Dip, 3 oz.	450	47	4
Dijon Honey Mustard, 2 oz.	200	18	8
Fat Free Ranch, 2 oz.	45	0	10
Honey French, 2 oz.	220	18	14
House Italian, 2 oz.	230	24	1
• Light Italian, 2 oz.	20	1	2
Roasted Red Pepper Croutons, 0.5 oz.	50	3	5
Thousand Island, 2 oz.	220	21	7
Tuscan Caesar, 2 oz.	180	18	3
Oven Baked Subs			
Big Don Italian, 318 g	720	34	67
w/Pizza Sauce, 325 g	654	26	69

Donatos Pizza (cont.)

	Cal	Fat	Cbs
Oven Baked Subs (cont.)			
Big Don Sausage Italian, 417 g	1000	56	68
w/Pizza Sauce, 424 g	934	48	70
• Big Ham and Cheese, 316 g	620	22	68
Big Steak Hoagie w/ Mushroom Gravy, 337 g	800	39	68
Big Steak Hoagie w/ Pizza Sauce, 340 g	804	39	68
Grilled Chicken Club, 414 g	899	44	71
• Meatball, 407 g	1137	64	78
Roasted Vegy, 355 g	731	37	74
Steak and Cheese, 340 g	778	34	69
Pizza No Dough			
Chicken Spinach Mozzarella, 212 g	574	42	16
Chicken Vegy Medley™, 285 g	495	29	20
Classic Trio®, 220 g	532	37	18
Founder's Favorite®, 238 g	558	38	18
Hawaiian™, 200 g	436	26	22
Margherita, 231 g	589	46	16
Mariachi™ Beef, 283 g	528	34	23
Mariachi™ Chicken, 287 g	495	30	21
Pepperoni Zinger, 217 g	584	42	17
Pepperoni™, 175 g	499	35	17
Philly Cheesesteak, 224 g	521	33	19
Serious Cheese™, 170 g	457	31	17
• Serious Meat™, 256 g	653	46	19
The Works™, 260 g	547	37	21
• Vegy™, 261 g	418	25	23
Pizza Thicker Crust			
BBQ Chicken, 325 g	810	31	90
Chicken Spinach Mozzarella, 307 g	791	38	73
Chicken Vegy Medley, 328 g	657	24	75
Classic Trio, 336 g	832	41	78
Founder's Favorite®, 349 g	858	42	78
Hawaiian, 318 g	758	32	82
Margherita, 294 g	766	39	72
Mariachi Beef, 362 g	796	36	81
Mariachi Chicken, 373 g	806	35	81
Pepperoni Zinger, 308 g	827	41	76
Pepperoni, 285 g	798	39	76
Philly Cheesesteak, 296 g	728	31	74
Serious Cheese, 291 g	798	38	77
• Serious Meat, 348 g	907	47	78
The Works, 375 g	847	41	81
• Vegy, 374 g	715	29	83
Pizza Thin Crust			
• BBQ Chicken, 270 g	792	26	66
Chicken Spinach Mozzarella, 253 g	631	33	49
• Chicken Vegy Medley™, 273 g	497	20	51
Classic Trio®, 288 g	674	37	52
Founder's Favorite®, 302 g	702	38	52
Hawaiian™, 265 g	588	27	56
Margherita, 239 g	606	35	48
Mariachi™ Beef, 312 g	630	32	55
Mariachi™ Chicken, 324 g	639	30	56
Pepperoni Zinger, 254 g	656	36	50
Pepperoni, 230 g	627	34	50
Philly Cheesesteak, 255 g	596	29	51
Serious Cheese™, 237 g	627	34	51
Serious Meat™, 293 g	736	42	52
Spinach, 256 g	611	34	51
The Works™, 329 g	689	37	56
Vegy™, 319 g	544	24	57
White, 217 g	690	42	49
Salads			
• Caesar Side Salad, 104 g	87	6	3
• Entree Chicken Harvest Salad, 336 g	514	32	29

Donatos Pizza (cont.)

	Cal	Fat	Cbs
Salads (cont.)			
Italian Chef Entree Salad, 362 g	314	22	10
Italian Garden Side Salad, 142 g	108	8	4
Tuscan Chicken Caesar Entree Salad, 296 g	198	8	6
Starters			
3 Cheese Garlic Bread, 51 g	174	9	16
Breadsticks w/Nacho Cheese Sauce, 154 g	398	22	39
Breadsticks w/Pizza Sauce, 113 g	261	9	38
Buffalo Wings - BBQ, 232 g	595	43	10
Buffalo Wings - Garlic, 222 g	669	56	12
Buffalo Wings - Hot, 232 g	597	48	11
Buffalo Wings - Mild, 232 g	618	48	13
Buffalo Wings - Plain, 204 g	552	43	10
• Buffalo Wings - Spicy Garlic, 251 g	713	60	23
Buffalo Wings, 204 g	429	31	4
• Chicken Breast Strips, 74 g	125	4	12
Wedge Fries, 159 g	261	13	34
Stromboli			
3 Meat, 309 g	689	31	67
Cheese, 299 g	693	31	66
Deluxe, 304 g	613	25	68
• Pepperoni, 300 g	716	34	67
• Vegy, 310 g	606	24	69

Dunkin' Donuts

	Cal	Fat	Cbs
Bagels			
Blueberry Bagel, 1 bagel	330	3	66
Cinnamon Raisin Bagel, 1 bagel	330	3	65
Everything Bagel, 1 bagel	370	6	67
Multigrain Bagel, 1 bagel	380	6	68
Onion Bagel, 1 bagel	320	4	61
• Plain Bagel, 1 bagel	320	3	62
Poppyseed Bagel, 1 bagel	370	7	65
• Reduced Carb Bagel with Cheese, 1 bagel	380	12	45
Salt Bagel, 1 bagel	320	3	62
Sesame Bagel, 1 bagel	380	8	64
Wheat Bagel, 1 bagel	330	4	62
Bakery: Cookies			
Chocolate Chunk Cookie, 5 oz.	540	23	80
• Oatmeal Raisin Cookie, 5 oz.	480	14	83
• Peanut Butter Cup Cookie, 5 oz.	590	29	73
Bakery: Danish			
Apple Danish, 1 danish	330	20	32
• Cheese Danish, 1 danish	340	22	30
• Strawberry Cheese Danish, 1 danish	320	20	31
Bakery: Muffins			
Banana Walnut Muffin, 1 muffin	540	25	69
Blueberry Muffin, 1 muffin	470	17	73
• Chocolate Chip Muffin, 1 muffin	630	26	89
Coffee Cake Muffin, 1 muffin	580	19	78
Corn Muffin, 1 muffin	510	18	77
Cranberry Orange Muffin, 1 muffin	440	17	66
• English Muffin, 3 oz.	160	2	31
Honey Bran Raisin Muffin, 1 muffin	480	15	79
Lemon Raspberry Muffin, 1 muffin	460	15	75
Pumpkin Muffin, 1 muffin	560	24	82
Reduced Fat Blueberry Muffin, 1 muffin	400	5	78
Bakery: Other			
• Biscuit, 1 biscuit	440	22	51
• Plain Croissant, 1 croissant	270	14	30
Breakfast Flat Bread			
• Ham & Swiss Flat Bread	350	12	41
• Three Cheese Flat Bread	460	24	42
Turkey Cheddar & Bacon Flat Bread	360	13	41
Breakfast Sandwiches			
Bacon Egg Cheese Bagel Sandwich	540	18	69

Dunkin' Donuts (cont.)	Cal	Fat	Cbs
Breakfast Sandwiches (cont.)			
Bacon Egg Cheese Croissant Sandwich	440	25	33
Bacon Egg Cheese English Muffin Sandwich	360	16	36
Bacon Lover's Supreme Breakfast Sandwich	640	43	36
Egg Cheese Bagel Sandwich	470	15	65
Egg Cheese Biscuit Sandwich	540	29	53
Egg Cheese Croissant Sandwich	430	26	33
Egg Cheese English Muffin Sandwich	280	9	34
Ham Egg Cheese Bagel Sandwich	510	16	65
Ham Egg Cheese Croissant Sandwich	460	27	33
Ham Egg Cheese English Muffin Sandwich	310	10	34
• Hash Browns, 9 pieces	180	9	22
Sausage Egg Cheese Bagel Sandwich	660	35	63
• Sausage Egg Cheese Biscuit Sandwich	800	52	54
Sausage Egg Cheese Croissant Sandwich	630	45	34
Sausage Egg Cheese English Muffin Sandwich	530	32	37
Supreme Omelet on a Croissant	530	33	35
Coffee			
• Coffee, 10 fl.oz.	15	0	3
• with Cream and Sugar, 10 fl.oz.	120	6	15
with Cream, 10 fl.oz.	70	6	3
with Milk and Sugar, 10 fl.oz.	80	1	16
with Milk, 10 fl.oz.	35	1	4
with Skim Milk and Sugar, 10 fl.oz.	70	0	16
with Skim Milk, 10 fl.oz.	25	0	4
with Sugar, 10 fl.oz.	60	0	15
Coolatta®			
Cherry Lime SoBe® Coolatta®, 16 fl.oz.	250	0	62
Coffee Coolatta® with 2% Milk, 16 fl.oz.	190	2	41
with Cream, 16 fl.oz.	350	22	40
with Milk, 16 fl.oz.	210	4	42
• with Skim Milk, 16 fl.oz.	170	0	41
Lemonade Coolatta®, 16ozs.	240	0	59
Strawberry Fruit Coolatta®, 16 fl.oz.	290	0	72
Tropicana Orange Coolatta®, 16 fl.oz.	370	0	92
• Vanilla Bean Coolatta®, 16 fl.oz.	500	17	85
Cream Cheese			
Chive Cream Cheese, 2oz.	170	17	4
Garden Vegetable Cream Cheese, 2oz.	170	15	4
Lite Cream Cheese, 2oz.	120	9	5
• Lite Garden Vegetable Cream Cheese, 2oz.	100	8	5
Plain Cream Cheese, 2oz.	190	17	4
Salmon Cream Cheese, 2oz.	170	17	2
• Strawberry Cream Cheese, 2oz.	190	17	9
Deli Classics: Sandwiches			
• Ham and Swiss Sandwich	360	11	44
Roast Beef and Swiss Sandwich	530	25	45
• Tuna (Albacore) Sandwich	550	26	44
Turkey and Cheese Sandwich	510	22	45
Vegetarian Sandwich	420	21	51
Donuts			
Apple Crumb Donut, 1 donut	320	13	46
Apple N' Spice Donut, 1 donut	260	11	35
Bavarian Kreme Donut, 1 donut	250	11	35
Black Raspberry Donut, 1 donut	270	10	40
Blueberry Cake Donut, 1 donut	290	16	35
Blueberry Crumb Donut, 1 donut	330	13	48
Boston Kreme Donut, 1 donut	270	12	38
• Chocolate Coconut Cake Donut, 1 donut	370	21	42
Chocolate Frosted Cake Donut, 1 donut	330	19	36
Chocolate Frosted Donut, 1 donut	230	11	29
Chocolate Glazed Cake Donut, 1 donut	340	19	39
Chocolate Kreme Filled Donut, 1 donut	300	14	39
Cinnamon Cake Donut, 1 donut	310	18	34
Double Chocolate Cake Donut, 1 donut	340	20	36

Dunkin' Donuts (cont.)	Cal	Fat	Cbs
Donuts (cont.)			
• French Cruller, 1 donut	150	8	17
Glazed Cake Donut, 1 donut	330	18	38
Glazed Donut Jelly Filled Donut, 1 donut	270	10	39
Glazed Donut, 1 donut	230	10	30
Maple Frosted Donut, 1 donut	240	10	31
Marble Frosted Donut, 1 donut	230	11	30
Old Fashioned Cake Donut, 1 donut	280	18	26
Powdered Cake Donut, 1 donut	310	18	34
Pumpkin Glazed Donut, 1 donut	280	6	52
Strawberry Frosted Donut, 1 donut	240	10	32
Sugar Raised Donut, 1 donut	210	10	27
Vanilla Kreme Filled Donut, 1 donut	320	16	39
Wheat Glazed Cake Donut, 1 donut	310	19	32
Donuts: Fancies			
Apple Fritter, 1 fritter	290	13	35
Bow Tie Donut, 1 donut	300	17	34
• Chocolate Frosted Coffee Roll, 1 roll	340	20	36
Chocolate Iced Bismark, 1 donut	340	15	50
Coffee Roll, 1 roll	340	20	33
Eclair, 1 donut	300	15	39
• Glazed Fritter, 1 fritter	250	13	31
Maple Frosted Coffee Roll, 1 donut	340	20	36
Vanilla Frosted Coffee Roll, 1 donut	340	20	36
Donuts: Munchkins			
Cinnamon Cake Munchkin, 4 munchkins	260	15	29
Glazed Cake Munchkin, 4 munchkins	300	15	38
• Glazed Chocolate Cake Munchkin, 4 munchkins	300	15	39
Glazed Munchkin, 4 munchkins	300	15	38
Jelly Filled Munchkin, 5 munchkins	240	8	37
Plain Cake Munchkin, 4 munchkins	230	15	21
Powdered Cake Munchkin, 4 munchkins	260	15	29
• Sugar Raised Munchkin, 5 munchkins	190	8	26
Donuts: Sticks			
Cinnamon Cake Stick, 1 stick	340	20	36
Glazed Cake Stick, 1 stick	360	20	41
Glazed Chocolate Cake Stick, 1 stick	370	21	41
• Jelly Stick, 1 stick	420	20	53
• Plain Cake Stick, 1 stick	310	20	29
Powdered Cake Stick, 1 stick	340	20	37
Dunkin' Deli: Cravings Sandwiches			
Chicken Bruschetta Sandwich	580	25	48
Chipotle Chicken Sandwich	620	26	49
• Pastrami Supreme Sandwich	760	42	47
• Turkey Pesto Sandwich	530	23	46
Dunkin' Deli: Favorites Sandwiches			
• Avocado and Turkey Sandwich	500	22	49
Chicken Cordon Bleu Sandwich	550	19	51
Steak and Cheese Sandwich	510	23	45
• Toasted Italian Sandwich	630	34	49
Turkey and Bacon Club Sandwich	510	22	44
Dunkin' Deli: Salads			
Caesar Salad, 8 oz.	390	33	14
Chicken Caesar Salad, 11 oz.	520	36	16
Garden Salad, 14 oz.	240	12	24
• Mediterranean Salad, 15 oz.	220	11	23
• Oriental Salad, 14 oz.	580	35	39
Dunkin' Deli: Soups			
Broccoli Cheese Soup, 240 ml	180	13	10
• Chicken Noodle Soup, 240 ml	140	4	20
Clam Chowder, 240 ml	230	11	20
• Lasagna Soup, 240 ml	250	13	21
Timberline Chili with Beans, 240 ml	230	8	26
Flavored Coffee			
• Blueberry Coffee, 10 fl.oz.	20	0	4

Dunkin' Donuts (cont.)

	Cal	Fat	Cbs
Flavored Coffee (cont.)			
Caramel Cinnamon Coffee, 10 fl.oz.	20	0	4
Caramel Coffee, 10 fl.oz.	20	0	4
Chocolate Coffee, 10 fl.oz.	20	0	4
Cinnamon Coffee, 10 fl.oz.	20	0	4
Coconut Coffee, 10 fl.oz.	20	0	4
French Vanilla Coffee, 10 fl.oz.	20	0	4
Hazelnut Coffee, 10 fl.oz.	20	0	4
• Pumpkin Spice Coffee Medium, 14 fl.oz.	240	8	39
Raspberry Coffee, 10 fl.oz.	20	0	4
Toasted Almond Coffee, 10 fl.oz.	20	0	4
Hot Espresso Drinks			
Cappuccino with Soy Milk, 10 fl.oz.	70	3	6
with Soy Milk and Sugar, 10 fl.oz.	120	3	20
Cappuccino, 10 fl.oz.	80	5	7
with Sugar, 10 fl.oz.	130	5	21
Caramel Creme Hot Latte, 10 fl.oz.	260	9	40
Caramel Swirl Latte w/ Soy Milk, 10 fl.oz.	210	4	34
Caramel Swirl Latte, 10 fl.oz.	230	6	36
• Espresso, 2 fl.oz.	0	0	1
with Sugar, 2 fl.oz.	30	0	7
• Gingerbread Latte, 10 fl.oz.	400	9	68
Hot Latte Lite, 10 fl.oz.	70	0	10
Latte with Soy Milk, 10 fl.oz.	90	4	8
with Soy Milk and Sugar, 10 fl.oz.	150	4	22
Latte, 10 fl.oz.	120	4	0
with Sugar, 10 fl.oz.	160	6	22
Mocha Almond Hot Latte, 10 fl.oz.	290	10	46
Mocha Swirl Latte with Soy Milk, 10 fl.oz.	210	5	35
Mocha Swirl Latte, 10 fl.oz.	230	7	37
Pumpkin Spice Latte Medium, 16 fl.oz.	340	9	52
Turbo Hot™, 10 fl.oz.	130	6	20
Vanilla Latte Lite, 10 fl.oz.	80	0	12
Iced Coffee			
Berry Berry Iced Coffee, 16 fl.oz.	120	6	16
• Iced Coffee, 16 fl.oz.	15	0	3
with Cream and Sugar, 16 fl.oz.	120	6	16
with Cream, 16 fl.oz.	70	6	4
with Milk and Sugar, 16 fl.oz.	80	1	16
with Milk, 16 fl.oz.	35	1	4
with Skim Milk and Sugar, 16 fl.oz.	70	0	16
with Skim Milk, 16 fl.oz.	25	0	4
with Sugar, 16 fl.oz.	60	0	15
• Pumpkin Spice Iced Coffee, 24 fl.oz.	240	8	37
Turbo Ice™, 16 fl.oz.	120	7	14
Vanilla Iced Latte Lite, 16 fl.oz.	80	0	13
Iced Espresso Drinks			
Caramel Creme Iced Latte, 16 fl.oz.	260	9	40
Iced Caramel Swirl Latte, 16 fl.oz.	240	7	37
with Skim Milk, 16 fl.oz.	180	0	36
Iced Latte Lite, 16 fl.oz.	80	0	13
Iced Latte, 16 fl.oz.	120	7	11
Skim Milk and Sugar, 16 fl.oz.	120	0	23
with Skim Milk, 16 fl.oz.	70	0	11
with Sugar, 16 fl.oz.	170	7	23
Iced Mocha Swirl Latte, 16 fl.oz.	240	8	38
with Skim Milk, 16 fl.oz.	180	1	37
Mocha Almond Iced Latte, 16 fl.oz.	290	10	46
• Pumpkin Spice Iced Latte, 24 fl.oz.	340	9	52
Turbo Ice™, 16 fl.oz.	120	7	14
Other Beverages			
Dunkaccino®, 10 fl.oz.	230	11	35
• Hot Chocolate, 10 fl.oz.	230	7	39
Vanilla Chai, 10zs.	230	8	40
• White Hot Chocolate, 14 fl.oz.	340	13	55

Dunkin' Donuts (cont.)

	Cal	Fat	Cbs
Personal Pizza			
• Cheese Pizza, 1 pizza	400	19	46
Pepperoni Pizza, 1 pizza	410	19	45
• Supreme Pizza, 1 pizza	430	21	46
Smoothie			
• Mango Passion Fruit Smoothie, 24 fl.oz.	550	4	118
Strawberry Banana Smoothie, 24 fl.oz.	550	4	118
• Tropical Fruit Smoothie, 24 fl.oz.	540	4	117
Wildberry Smoothie, 24 fl.oz.	550	4	118

Dunn Bros. Coffee

	Cal	Fat	Cbs
Brewed Coffee			
• Brewed Coffee, 16 oz.	10	0	2
• Coffee with Steamed 2% Milk, 16 oz.	70	3	8
Coffee with Steamed Skim Milk, 16 oz.	55	0	8
Coffee with Steamed Soy Milk, 16 oz.	60	2	7
Depth Charge, 16 oz.	10	0	2
Chai Tea Latte			
• Chai Tea Latte, 16 oz.	165	4	27
• Skim Milk Chai Tea Latte, 16 oz.	140	0	27
Soy Milk Chai Tea Latte, 16 oz.	140	0	27
Espresso Drinks			
• Americano, 16 oz.	0	0	0
Caffe Latte, 16 oz.	142	5	14
Caramel Latte Macchiato, 16 oz.	230	5	38
Caramel Mocha Latte, 16 oz.	275	5	50
Mocha Latte, 16 oz.	275	5	50
Skim Milk Caffe Latte, 16 oz.	110	0	17
Skim Milk Cappuccino, 16 oz.	80	0	13
Skim Milk Caramel Latte Macchiato, 16 oz.	240	1	48
Skim Milk Caramel Mocha Latte, 16 oz.	240	1	50
Skim Milk Mocha Latte, 16 oz.	260	3	50
Skim Milk Vanilla Latte, 16 oz.	170	0	31
Skim White Mocha Latte, 16 oz.	260	5	46
Soy Cappuccino, 16 oz.	90	2	12
Soy Milk Caffe Latte, 16 oz.	140	4	16
Soy Milk Caramel Latte Macchiato, 16 oz.	260	4	47
Soy Milk Mocha Latte, 16 oz.	280	6	49
Soy Milk Vanilla Latte, 16 oz.	180	4	28
• Soy Milk White Mocha Latte, 16 oz.	290	8	45
Vanilla Latte, 16 oz.	210	5	30
White Mocha Latte, 16 oz.	270	9	52
Whole Milk Cappuccino, 16 oz.	110	5	12
Favorites			
Chocolate Steamed Nirvana, 16 oz.	325	5	63
• Hot Chocolate, 16 oz.	380	6	71
• Hot Spiced Apple Cider, 16 oz.	215	0	51
Skim Chocolate Steamed Nirvana, 16 oz.	290	3	61
Skim Hot Chocolate, 16 oz.	340	3	68
Soy Chocolate Steamed Nirvana, 16 oz.	300	5	60
Fruit Smoothies			
Mango, 16 oz.	250	0	58
• Strawberry Pink Freeze, 16 oz.	360	7	70
• Strawberry, 16 oz.	250	0	58
Wildberry, 16 oz.	250	0	58
IceCremas™			
Caramel IceCrema, 16 oz.	450	11	65
• Caramel Mocha IceCrema, 16 oz.	400	11	74
Chai IceCrema, 16 oz.	410	11	74
Coffee IceCrema, 16 oz.	260	10	41
Mocha IceCrema, 16 oz.	420	10	79
Skim Caramel Mocha IceCrema, 16 oz.	370	5	77
Skim Milk Caramel Mocha IceCrema, 16 oz.	370	5	77
Skim Milk Chai IceCrema, 16 oz.	350	4	75
• Skim Milk Coffee IceCrema, 16 oz.	210	3	41
Skim Milk Mocha IceCrema, 16 oz.	370	3	80

RESTAURANTS & FAST-FOOD CHAINS

Dunn Bros. Coffee (cont.)

	Cal	Fat	Cbs
IceCremas™ (cont.)			
Soy Milk Chai IceCrema, 16 oz.	360	5	75
Iced Drinks			
• Cold Press Coffee, 16 oz.	10	0	2
Iced Caramel Latte Macchiato, 16 oz.	200	4	35
Iced Chai, 16 oz.	130	6	23
Iced Latte, 16 oz.	90	4	9
Iced Mocha, 16 oz.	230	3	45
Iced White Mocha, 16 oz.	230	7	47
Italian Cream Soda, 16 oz.	190	2	42
Italian Soda, 16 oz.	170	0	42
Skim Milk Iced Chai, 16 oz.	140	0	30
Skim Milk Iced Latte Macchiato, 16 oz.	170	1	35
Skim Milk Iced Latte, 16 oz.	80	0	12
Skim Milk Iced Mocha, 16 oz.	220	3	45
Skim Milk Iced White Mocha, 16 oz.	210	5	47
Soy Milk Iced Chai, 16 oz.	150	2	30
Soy Milk Iced Latte, 16 oz.	100	3	11
• Soy Milk Iced Mocha, 16 oz.	240	5	45
Soy Milk Iced White Mocha, 16 oz.	210	6	46
Vanilla Iced Nirvana, 16 oz.	210	16	17

Eat N' Park

	Cal	Fat	Cbs
Appetizers			
Breaded Zucchini	415	23	39
Buffalo Chicken Tenders	434	21	24
Cheese Sticks	411	25	17
• Onion Rings	209	13	19
• Southwest Quesadilla	853	50	56
Stuffed Mushrooms	217	15	7
Bakery			
Bagel (Plain), 1 piece	312	2	61
Bagel (Raisin), 1 piece	320	2	65
• Bear Claw, 1 piece	515	24	66
Biscuit (Cheese), 1 piece	127	6	15
Biscuit, 1 piece	214	13	22
Boston Brown Bread, 2 slices	279	9	43
Bun (Hoagie), 1 piece	178	2	34
Bun (Hot Dog), 1 piece	128	3	21
Bun (Superburger), 1 piece	183	3	32
Bun (Three Cheese Hoagie), 1 piece	470	26	44
Cookie (Chocolate Chip), 1 piece	207	9	28
Cookie (Christmas), 1 piece	250	8	42
Cookie (Easter), 1 piece	251	8	42
Cookie (Halloween), 1 piece	250	8	42
Cookie (Macadamia Nut), 1 piece	240	16	22
Cookie (Shamrock), 1 piece	250	8	42
Cookie (Smiley®), 1 piece	250	8	42
Cookie (Steeler/Penguin/Pirate), 1 piece	250	8	42
Cookie (Valentine), 1 piece	250	8	42
Cornbread, 1 piece	108	4	16
Croissant, 1 piece	258	15	27
Crumby Buns, 1 piece	193	9	24
English Muffin, 1 piece	133	1	26
Garlic Toast, 1 slice	465	19	61
Honey Bun, 1 piece	172	8	22
• Italian Bread, 1 slice	54	1	10
Muffin (Apple Raisin), 1 piece	249	7	43
Muffin (Banana Nut), 1 piece	284	13	39
Muffin (Blueberry), 1 piece	242	8	39
Muffin (Chocolate Nut), 1 piece	313	13	45
Muffin (Corn), 1 piece	212	8	31
Muffin (Cranberry), 1 piece	266	10	41
Muffin (Mocha Java), 1 piece	222	9	34
Muffin (Oat Bran Apple Raisin), 1 piece	296	10	46
Muffin (Oat Bran), 1 piece	333	13	47

Eat N' Park (cont.)

	Cal	Fat	Cbs
Bakery (cont.)			
Muffin (Pumpkin Raisin), 1 piece	259	8	44
Muffin (Strawberry Créme), 1 piece	273	9	43
Muffin (Strawberry Filled), 1 piece	280	9	45
Pastry Bite, 1 piece	114	7	11
Raisin Bread, 1 slice	71	1	14
Roll (Kaiser), 1 piece	179	3	32
Rye Bread, 1 slice	83	1	15
SnoTop, 1 piece	111	4	16
Sourdough Bread, 1 slice	68	1	13
Sticky Loaf, 1 piece	293	13	40
Toast (Buttered), 1 slice	262	14	30
Toast (Dry), 1 slice	134	2	25
Toast (Raisin, Buttered), 1 slice	244	14	27
Toast (Rye, Buttered), 1 slice	267	14	31
Toast (Sourdough, Buttered), 1 slice	237	13	25
Toast (Whole Wheat, Buttered), 1 slice	259	14	30
White Bread, 1 slice	67	1	12
Whole Wheat, 1 slice	79	1	15
Yellow Bread, 1 slice	114	2	21
Breakfast			
• Bacon, 1 slice	37	3	0
Bacon, 2 Slices	73	6	0
Bacon, 3 Slices	111	9	0
Banana Foster French Toast, 1	598	18	96
Cereal (with Milk)	363	5	82
Cornbeef Hash, 7 1/2 oz.	341	23	16
Eat'n Smart Smile	230	3	32
Egg Beaters	76	0	6
Eggs (2 Poached w/toast & Promise®)	352	20	26
Eggs Benedict	590	34	37
Eggs, 1 Fried	102	8	1
Eggs, 1 Poached	77	5	1
French Toast	128	5	14
Fruit Cup	60	0	15
Ham, 3 oz.	110	4	1
Hash Browns, 6 oz.	237	12	24
Homefries, 6 oz.	208	12	24
Oatmeal (Plain)	154	3	27
Oatmeal (with Bananas)	317	6	58
Oatmeal (with Fruit)	424	10	68
Oatmeal (with Milk)	224	5	34
Omelette (Bacon and Cheese)	500	39	2
Omelette (Cheese)	390	30	2
Omelette (Ham and Cheese)	463	32	3
Omelette (Meat Lovers)	716	55	4
Omelette (Supreme)	418	30	9
Omelette (Western)	344	21	7
Pancake (Blueberry), 1 pancake	286	4	55
Pancake, 1 pancake	223	3	43
Sausage, 1 link	132	12	0
Scrambler	619	29	55
• Strawberry Waffle, 1 waffle	724	29	100
Waffles (Belgian), 1 waffle	623	32	69
Burgers			
American Grill Burger, 6 oz.	617	37	32
Bacon Cheeseburger	591	31	33
BBQ Bacon Cheddar Burger, 6 oz.	886	55	53
• Black Angus Superburger®	1086	73	28
Cheeseburger, 6 oz.	522	26	33
• Classic Gardenburger	250	6	41
Hamburger, 6 oz.	477	22	32
Mushroom and Onion Burger	706	40	45
Original Superburger®	707	49	38

Eat N' Park (cont.)

Condiments	Cal	Fat	Cbs
Butter (Whipped Blend)	96	11	0
Butter, 5 g	36	4	0
Cheese (Cream)	99	10	1
• Cheese (Mozzarella)	226	17	2
Honey	43	0	12
Honey Mustard	81	6	7
Jelly	34	0	9
Ketchup	23	0	6
• Lettuce (Leaf)	1	0	0
Lettuce (Shredded)	3	0	1
Margarine (Promise®)	32	4	0
Mayonnaise, 3/4 oz.	201	22	1
Mustard, 3/4 oz.	23	1	2
Onions (Grilled), 1 oz.	21	1	2
Onions (Raw)	11	0	2
Pickle Chips, 3 chips	3	0	1
Pickle Spear	4	0	1
Relish, 3/4 oz.	40	0	11
Salsa, 2 oz.	14	0	3
Sauce (BBQ), 2 oz.	84	0	22
Sauce (Cheese), 2 oz.	151	12	4
Sauce (Chipotle BBQ), 2 oz.	170	1	41
Sauce (Cocktail), 2 oz.	71	0	19
Sauce (Lite Soy), 1 tbsp.	8	0	1
Sauce (Supreme), 2 oz.	151	16	2
Sauce (Sweet'n Sour), 2 oz.	81	2	16
Sauce (Teriyaki), 2 tbsp.	15	0	3
Sour Cream, 2 oz.	40	2	4
Syrup (Maple), 2 oz.	221	0	60
Syrup (Reduced Maple), 2 oz.	34	0	9
Syrup (Sugar-Free), 2 oz.	43	0	11
Tomatoes, 2 slices	6	0	1
Tomatoes, 2 wedges	5	0	1
Desserts			
Cheesecake (with Strawberries), 1 piece	751	36	105
Cheesecake, 1 piece	507	36	40
Dulce de Leche Cheesecake, 1 piece	720	49	64
Grilled Stickies à la Mode Loaf, 1 piece	487	28	53
Grilled Stickies à la Mode, 1 piece	728	39	81
Ice Cream, 2 Scoops	285	16	33
NSA Lactose-Free Lo-Carb Vanilla Ice Cream, 4 oz.	130	8	15
Pie (Apple Cranberry), 1 slice	655	36	78
Pie (Apple), 1 slice	489	24	66
Pie (Apple, No Sugar Added), 1 slice	341	10	61
Pie (Banana Crème), 1 slice	439	22	55
Pie (Blackberry), 1 slice	510	23	73
Pie (Blueberry), 1 slice	439	23	55
Pie (Cherry), 1 slice	457	24	58
Pie (Chocolate Peanut Butter), 1 slice	566	39	49
Pie (Coconut Crème), 1 slice	480	26	55
Pie (Dutch Apple), 1 slice	528	26	73
Pie (Lemon Meringue), 1 slice	262	13	31
Pie (Orchard Fresh, 1 slice	500	24	67
Pie (Oreo Cream, 1 slice	495	28	60
Pie (Peach, No Sugar Added), 1 slice	298	10	50
Pie (Peachberry), 1 slice	389	19	52
Pie (Pecan), 1 slice	679	40	79
Pie (Pumpkin), 1 slice	395	19	49
Pie (Shell, Baked), 1 piece	195	14	16
Pie (Strawberry), 1 slice	360	18	49
Pumpkin Cranberry Cheesecake, 1 piece	450	24	53
• Sherbet (Plain), 1 piece	98	1	22
Sundae (Apple), 1 piece	569	21	96
Sundae (Apple, Junior), 1 piece	305	12	50

Eat N' Park (cont.)

Desserts (cont.)	Cal	Fat	Cbs
Sundae (Chocolate), 1 piece	525	22	85
Sundae (Chocolate, Junior), 1 piece	283	12	44
Sundae (Hot Fudge), 1 piece	625	31	85
Sundae (Hot Fudge, Junior), 1 piece	333	17	45
Sundae (Oreo), 1 piece	503	21	73
Sundae (Strawberry), 1 piece	606	21	106
• Sundae (Turtle), 1 piece	935	49	111
Dinners			
Baked Lemon Sole	282	17	11
• Breaded Fish	926	45	56
Chargrilled Chicken, 10 oz.	350	9	0
Chargrilled Chicken, 5 oz.	175	5	0
Chesapeake Crab Stuffed Cod	286	9	20
Chicken Broccoli Alfredo	604	19	61
Chicken Fillets, 5	529	26	28
Chicken Parmigiana Marinara	842	33	90
Chicken Parmigiana Meat Sauce	898	38	86
Chicken Stir-Fry	554	25	47
Ground Sirloin	422	25	0
Liver	283	12	12
Nantucket Cod	290	17	7
Pork Chops (Sesame)	320	18	2
Rosemary Chicken, 10 oz.	370	10	2
Salisbury Steak	442	24	28
Salmon (Alaskan Stockeye)	287	15	0
Scrod (Baked), 8 oz.	434	25	6
• Scrod (Floridian), 4 oz.	120	2	4
Scrod (Floridian), 8 oz.	240	3	8
Scrod (Maryland)	445	32	11
Spaghetti (Marinara)	621	8	120
Spaghetti (Meat Sauce)	820	19	140
T-Bone	568	39	1
Turkey	433	18	31
Dressing			
Bleu Cheese, 2 tbsp.	92	7	7
• Caesar, 2 tbsp.	245	25	8
French Fat-Free, 2 tbsp.	70	0	17
Fruit Salad, 2 tbsp.	143	14	5
House, 2 tbsp.	115	11	2
• Italian Fat-Free, 2 tbsp.	12	0	3
Italian, 2 tbsp.	122	12	4
Poppyseed, 2 tbsp.	240	16	24
Thousand Island, 2 tbsp.	95	9	3
Kids Menu			
Burger	285	15	21
• Cereal (Milk)	615	16	115
Cheeseburger	365	21	22
Chicken (Fillet)	317	16	17
Fish Plank	315	15	20
French Toast (Bacon)	355	16	35
French Toast (Sausage)	546	34	35
Giggle (Bacon)	380	27	20
Giggle (Sausage)	571	45	20
Grilled Cheese	524	39	21
Hot Dog	361	24	24
• Macaroni & Cheese	171	3	31
Peanut Butter & Jelly Sandwich	439	20	55
Pizza	413	13	49
Spaghetti	355	5	69
Salads			
• Buffalo Chicken	606	42	42
Chicken and Strawberry	216	6	13
Chicken Portabella	320	11	23
Fruit with Sherbet	308	3	73

Eat N' Park (cont.)

	Cal	Fat	Cbs
Salads (cont.)			
• Garden	95	3	16
Grilled Chicken	439	19	30
Napa Valley	504	25	18
Spinach and Chicken	376	17	9
Sandwiches			
Buffalo Chicken Sandwich	786	41	71
Chicken (Chargrilled), 5 oz.	350	7	39
Chicken (Fiesta), 5 oz.	430	13	41
Chicken Portabella Hoagie	836	55	46
Croissant (Tuna)	582	39	35
Grilled Cheese	507	36	26
• Hot Turkey	260	5	27
Pot Roast Melt	972	53	66
Reuben	720	49	31
Santa Fe Turkey and Bacon	854	60	44
Shredded Pot Roast	532	30	28
• Steak and Cheese	1011	71	38
Turkey Club	769	44	49
Whale of a Cod Sandwich	866	40	76
Seniors			
Baked Lemon Sole	141	9	6
• Banana Foster French Toast	495	15	82
Breaded Fish, 4 oz.	463	23	28
Chargrilled Chicken, 5 oz.	175	5	0
Chicken Fillet, 4 Pieces	423	21	22
French Toast	399	12	79
Hot Turkey Sandwich	175	5	18
Pork Chop (Sesame), 4 oz.	160	9	1
Pot Roast Sandwich	262	15	13
Rosemary Chicken, 5 oz.	196	6	2
Scrod (Baked), 4 oz.	330	24	6
• Scrod (Floridian), 4 oz.	119	2	4
Spaghetti (Marinara)	311	4	60
Spaghetti (Meat Sauce)	410	9	70
Sides			
Applesauce	108	0	28
Banana (Medium)	109	1	28
Bean Soup, 1 cup	145	4	18
Beef Noodle Soup, 1 cup	111	5	11
Broccoli (Steamed)	40	1	8
Broccoli Soup, 1 cup	197	11	22
Buttered Noodles	247	14	26
Cheese Soup, 1 cup	215	11	27
Chicken Noodle Soup, 1 cup	130	5	16
Chicken Rice Soup, 1 cup	76	1	11
Chili, 1 cup	132	5	13
Clam Chowder, 1 cup	159	8	19
Coleslaw	200	18	10
Cottage Cheese	114	2	5
• French Fries	347	18	44
• Gravy (Beef)	21	0	3
Gravy (Turkey)	32	1	3
Harvest Grain Soup, 1 cup	225	9	35
Minestrone Soup, 1 cup	85	2	15
Mushroom Barley Soup, 1 cup	69	1	13
Onion Rings, 10 pcs.	105	6	10
Potato (Baked)	190	0	44
Potato (Scalloped)	230	8	34
Potato (Whipped)	280	23	17
Potato Soup, 1 cup	214	10	32
Rice (Mexican)	111	2	22
Rice (White)	148	2	28
Rice Pilaf	137	4	23
Rice Pudding	163	2	31

Eat N' Park (cont.)

	Cal	Fat	Cbs
Sides (cont.)			
Strawberries, Fresh Cup	51	1	12
Sugar Snap Peas	29	0	7
Vegetable Beef Barley Soup, 1 cup	103	3	13
Vegetarian Pasta Soup, 1 cup	44	1	9
Wedding Soup, 1 cup	110	3	12

Edo Japan

	Cal	Fat	Cbs
Bento Boxes			
Beef Yakisoba Bento, 575 g	830	30	102
Chicken and Beef Bento, 566 g	880	26	120
• Chicken Yakisoba Bento, 582 g	800	25	102
Seafood Grill Bento, 652 g	860	16	129
Sizzling Shrimp Bento, 625 g	800	16	122
• Sukiyaki Beef Bento, 571 g	900	28	120
Teriyaki Chicken Bento, 578 g	870	24	120
Edo Extras			
6 Extra Shrimp, 65 g	80	3	2
California Roll, 216 g	430	17	61
Extra Beef, 132 g	260	15	3
Extra Chicken, 139 g	220	11	3
• Rice Side Dish, 297 g	480	1	106
• Teriyaki Sauce, 60 ml	45	0	11
Tofu, 106 g	90	5	5
Vegetable Spring Roll, 45 g	120	6	14
Yakisoba Side Dish, 340 g	430	4	89
Teriyaki Dishes			
• Beef and Shrimp, 486 g	690	19	82
Beef Yakisoba, 425 g	540	18	62
Chicken and Beef, 416 g	590	14	80
Chicken and Shrimp, 493 g	660	15	82
Chicken Yakisoba, 432 g	510	14	62
• Curry Chicken Bowl, 375 g	500	21	27
Fresh Grilled Vegetables, 342 g	380	1	81
Ginger Pork, 414 g	650	23	82
Hawaiian Chicken, 440 g	590	12	85
Seafood Grill, 502 g	570	4	89
Sizzling Shrimp, 475 g	510	5	82
Sukiyaki Beef, 421 g	610	16	80
Teriyaki Chicken, 428 g	580	12	80
Tropical Teriyaki, 505 g	670	15	87
• Beef Udon, 947 g	580	17	72
Chicken Udon, 953 g	550	13	72
Shrimp Udon, 964 g	480	5	74
• Vegetable Udon, 909 g	370	2	77

Einstein Bros. Bagels

	Cal	Fat	Cbs
Bagel Pretzels			
Asiago Cheese Bagel Pretzel, 116 g	300	5	57
• Cinnamon Sugar Bagel Pretzel, 123 g	330	3	71
• Plain Bagel Pretzel, 109 g	270	3	57
Salt Bagel Pretzel, 112 g	270	3	57
Bagel Dogs			
Add Cheddar Cheese, 8 oz.	660	32	64
• Add Cheddar Cheese, 8 oz.	670	33	64
Original Asiago Bagel Dog, 7 oz.	590	26	64
• Original Bagel Dog, 7 oz.	570	25	64
Bagels			
Asiago Cheese Bagel, 120 g	320	5	58
Blueberry Bagel, 115 g	290	2	64
Chocolate Chip Bagel, 113 g	290	3	60
Cinnamon Raisin Swirl Bagel, 115 g	290	1	64
Cinnamon Sugar, Chicago Style, 117 g	310	3	66
Cranberry Bagel, 115 g	290	1	64
Egg Bagel, 108 g	300	6	52
Everything Bagel, 112 g	290	2	60

Einstein Bros. Bagels (cont.)

	Cal	Fat	Cbs
Bagels (cont.)			
Garlic Dip'd Bagel, 112 g	280	1	60
Good Grains Bagel, 112 g	290	3	62
Honey Whole Wheat Bagel, 108 g	270	1	61
Onion Bagel, 108 g	270	2	59
Onion Dip'd Bagel, 112 g	290	1	63
Plain Bagel, 108 g	270	1	59
Poppy Dip'd Bagel, 112 g	290	3	60
• Potato Bagel, 107 g	260	1	58
• Power Bagel, Fruit & Nut, 120 g	380	6	72
Pumpernickel Bagel, 108 g	270	2	58
Sesame Dip'd Bagel, 110 g	310	3	62
Sundried Tomato Bagel, 108 g	270	2	58
Bread, Specialty			
Braided Challah Roll, 78 g	220	4	41
• Ciabatta Bread, 113 g	290	3	60
• Multi Grain Bread, 49 g	130	3	23
Breakfast Sandwiches			
• Bacon & Spinach Panini, 13 oz.	860	49	69
Egg Way with Bacon, 10 oz.	610	25	63
Egg Way with Black Forest Ham, 11 oz.	580	21	63
Egg Way with Sausage, 11 oz.	610	24	64
Egg Way, Original, 9 oz.	540	20	63
Egg Way, Spinach, Mshrm & Swiss, 11 oz.	540	20	65
Sausage Ranchero Panini, 12 oz.	690	28	65
Vegetable Breakfast Panini, 15 oz.	730	35	70
Breakfast Wraps			
• Sante Fe, 13 oz.	720	37	59
• Spicy Elmo, 12 oz.	730	41	56
Coffee Extras			
Half & Half, 1 fl.oz.	40	3	1
Light Whipped Cream, 30 ml	35	3	2
On Top Reduced Fat Topping, 8 g	20	2	2
Skim Milk, 8 fl.oz.	80	0	15
Syrup, Blackberry, 30 ml	100	0	25
Syrup, Caramel, 1 fl.oz.	100	0	25
Syrup, Cherry, 30 ml	100	0	25
Syrup, Chocolate, 30 ml	0	0	4
Syrup, Hazelnut, 1 fl.oz.	100	0	25
Syrup, Vanilla, 1 fl.oz.	100	0	25
• Syrup, Vanilla, Sugar Free, 1 fl.oz.	0	0	4
• Whole Milk, 8 fl.oz.	150	8	11
Coffee, Specialty (Medium)			
• Americano Regular, 8 fl.oz.	1	0	0
Cafe Latte Nonfat, 16 fl.oz.	140	1	20
Café Latte Whole milk, 16 fl.oz.	250	12	21
Café Latte, 16 fl.oz.	200	8	20
Cappuccino Nonfat Milk, 15 fl.oz.	130	1	19
Cappuccino Whole Milk, 16 fl.oz.	190	9	17
Cappuccino, 16 fl.oz.	190	7	19
Espresso, Regular, 2 fl.oz.	1	0	0
Low Fat Mocha, 15 fl.oz.	350	15	42
• Mocha Whole Milk, 16 fl.oz.	400	10	67
Mocha, 15 fl.oz.	390	20	42
Condiments & Spreads			
Ancho Lime Salsa, 1 oz.	10	1	1
Ancho Mayo, 16 g	50	5	1
Creamy Mustard Spread, 2 oz.	270	29	1
Deli Mustard, 5 g	5	0	0
Feta Pinenut Spread, 1 oz.	70	5	2
Honey Butter, 28 g	170	18	0
Hummus, 2 oz.	110	7	9
• Peanut Butter, Creamy, 2 oz.	330	28	12
Roasted Garlic Horseradish Spread, 28 g	15	0	4
Spicy Roasted Tomato Spread, 30 g	140	14	3

Einstein Bros. Bagels (cont.)

	Cal	Fat	Cbs
Condiments & Spreads (cont.)			
Whole Kosher Pickle, 50 g	5	0	1
• Yellow Mustard, 5 g	0	0	0
Cream Cheese			
Whipped Garden Vegetable Red. Fat, 20 g	60	5	3
Whipped Garlic Herb Reduced Fat, 20 g	60	5	3
Whipped Honey Almond Red. Fat, 20 g	70	5	6
Whipped Jalapeño Salsa Reduced Fat, 20 g	60	5	3
Whipped Onion and Chive, 20 g	70	6	3
• Whipped Plain Reduced Fat, 20 g	60	5	2
• Whipped Plain, 20 g	70	7	1
Whipped Smoked Salmon, 20 g	60	6	2
Whipped Strawberry Reduced Fat, 20 g	70	5	5
Deli Melts			
Ham Deli Melt, 10 oz.	540	18	62
Pastrami Deli Melt, 10 oz.	560	19	64
Tuna Salad Deli Melt, 11 oz.	610	25	64
• Turkey Deli Melt, 10 oz.	530	17	62
• Veggie Deli Melt, 13 oz.	660	30	76
Deli Sandwiches			
Deli Bacon, 9 oz.	830	52	52
• Deli Chicken Salad, 10 oz.	970	79	51
Deli Ham, 11 oz.	590	32	45
Deli Pastrami, 11 oz.	650	34	53
• Deli Tuna Salad, 10 oz.	440	15	50
Deli Turkey & Swiss, 11 oz.	700	42	49
Frozen Blended Drinks			
Wildberry, 18 fl.oz.	270	0	63
Gourmet Bagels			
Dutch Apple Bagel, 142 g	350	4	71
• Green Chile Bagel, 163 g	370	9	60
• Six-Cheese Bagel, 127 g	340	6	58
Spinach Florentine Bagel, 141 g	360	9	59
Iced Specialty Coffee			
Iced Latte, 16 fl.oz.	120	5	12
Iced Mocha, 16 fl.oz.	210	6	33
• Iced Non Fat Latte, 16 fl.oz.	90	0	12
Low Fat Iced Mocha, 16 fl.oz.	180	5	32
Low Fat Mocha, 12 fl.oz.	190	3	34
Whole Milk Iced Latte, 16 fl.oz.	190	9	17
• Whole Milk Iced Mocha, 16 fl.oz.	390	9	66
Other Hot Beverages (Medium)			
Chai Tea Latte 2% Milk, 16 fl.oz.	290	3	63
• Chai Tea Latte Skim Milk, 16 fl.oz.	270	0	63
Chai Tea Latte Whole Milk, 16 fl.oz.	310	4	63
Hot Chocolate, 12 fl.oz.	290	11	39
• Hot Chocolate, Whole Milk, 12 fl.oz.	320	14	39
Pizza Bagels			
Andouille Sausage, 7 oz.	480	14	66
• Cheese, 6 oz.	440	11	66
Cheesy Garlic & Herb, 6 oz.	520	18	68
Pepperoni, 7 oz.	480	15	66
• Spinach and Mushroom, 10 oz.	620	26	73
Salad Dressings			
Caesar Dressing, 30 g	150	16	1
Chile Lime Dressing, 32 g	60	4	5
• Raspberry Vinaigrette Dressing, 32 g	160	14	8
Salads (and Half Salads)			
• Bros Bistro Salad with Chicken, 15 oz.	960	72	39
Bros Bistro Salad, 11 oz.	820	68	38
Chicken Chipotle Salad, 14 oz.	670	41	53
Chipotle Salad, 12 oz.	600	39	53
Half Bros Bistro Salad with Chicken, 7 oz.	480	36	19
Half Bros Bistro Salad, 5 oz.	410	34	19
Half Caesar Salad with Chicken, 7 oz.	340	27	9

Einstein Bros. Bagels (cont.)

	Cal	Fat	Cbs
Salads (and Half Salads) (cont.)			
• Half Caesar Salad, 5 oz.	270	25	8
Half Chicken Chipotle Salad, 8 oz.	370	22	27
Half Chipotle Salad, 6 oz.	300	19	26
Sandwich Fillings			
Cheese Provolone, 1 oz.	80	6	0
Cheese, American, 1 oz.	80	6	1
Cheese, Gorgonzola, 1 oz.	100	9	0
Cheese, Medium Cheddar, 1 oz.	90	7	0
Cheese, Monterey Jack w/ Jalapeños, 1 oz.	80	6	1
Cheese, Monterey Jack, 1 oz.	80	6	0
Cheese, Swiss, 1 oz.	80	7	0
Chicken Breast, 4 oz.	140	5	1
• Chicken Salad, 4 oz.	700	74	2
Cold Smoked Salmon, 2 oz.	80	5	0
Ham, 3 oz.	100	4	0
Pastrami, 3 oz.	120	4	2
Thick Cut Bacon, 0.5 oz.	70	5	1
Tuna Salad, 4 oz.	170	10	2
• Turkey Sausage, 1 oz.	70	4	1
Sandwiches, Panini			
• Italian Chicken Panini, 13 oz.	830	42	67
• Turkey Club Panini, 14 oz.	790	39	68
Sides			
Bagel Croutons, 1 oz.	100	4	16
Fruit and Yogurt Parfait, 12 oz.	180	1	36
Fruit Salad, 11 oz.	140	0	36
• Kettle Classic Natural Potato Chips, 1 oz.	100	10	11
• Traditional Potato Salad, 140 g	355	29	20
Soups			
• Chicken Noodle (Cup), 9 oz.	120	4	14
Corn Crab Chowder (Cup), 9 oz.	280	18	18
Seafood Minestrone (Cup), 9 oz.	130	5	16
Turkey Chili (Cup), 9 oz.	220	7	24
• Vegetarian Broccoli Cheese (Cup), 9 oz.	290	20	16
Specialty Sandwiches			
Club Mex on Challah, 11 oz.	600	30	48
Grilled Chicken, Bacon and Swiss, 11 oz.	770	48	45
Lox & Bagel, 10 oz.	520	21	6
• Rachel (Overstuffed Size), 14 oz.	1050	71	53
Rachel (Regular Size), 10 oz.	930	66	51
Reuben (Overstuffed Size), 14 oz.	800	44	49
Reuben (Regular Size), 10 oz.	670	40	47
Roasted Turkey and Swiss, 11 oz.	700	42	49
Tasty Turkey on Asiago Bagel, 13 oz.	570	20	68
Turkey Rachel (Overstuffed Size), 14 oz.	970	65	50
Turkey Rachel (Regular Size), 10 oz.	890	64	50
Turkey Reuben (Overstuffed Size), 14 oz.	720	39	45
Turkey Reuben (Regular Size), 10 oz.	630	37	45
• Veg Out on Sesame Seed Bagel, 10 oz.	450	14	70
Sweets			
Apple Cinnamon Coffee Cake, 7 oz.	700	28	108
Blueberry Muffin, 5 oz.	480	22	65
Chocolate Chip Coffee Cake, 6 oz.	760	34	110
Chocolate Mudslide Cookie, 3 oz.	320	17	46
Cinnamon Stix, 4 oz.	370	21	41
Cinnamon Walnut Strudel, 5 oz.	630	42	56
English Toffee Snickerdoodle Cookie, 3 oz.	420	18	59
Fudge Brownie, 4 oz.	510	25	74
Heavenly Chocolate Chunk Cookie, 3 oz.	360	18	48
Iced Chocolate Hazelnut Croissant, 3 oz.	430	21	49
Iced Lemon Croissant, 3 oz.	371	17	46
Iced Sugar Cookie, 3 oz.	460	15	76
Lemon Pound Cake, 5 oz.	440	16	69
• Marshmallow Crispy Treat, 2 oz.	220	4	48

Einstein Bros. Bagels (cont.)

	Cal	Fat	Cbs
Sweets (cont.)			
• Mixed Berry Coffee Cake, 7 oz.	710	29	109
Oatmeal Raisin Cookie, 3 oz.	320	11	54
Strawberry White Chocolate Muffin, 6 oz.	550	25	78
Wraps			
• California Chicken Wrap, 13 oz.	630	29	63
• Chipotle Turkey Wrap, 13 oz.	740	37	70

El Pollo Loco

	Cal	Fat	Cbs
Bowls & Salads			
Caesar Bowl, 12 oz.	520	25	45
Caesar Pollo Salad, 11 oz.	520	38	17
Caesar Pollo Salad, w/o dressing, 9 oz.	220	7	15
Chicken Tostada without Shell, 15 oz.	410	11	42
Chicken Tostada, 17 oz.	840	40	76
• Garden Salad, 5 oz.	120	7	9
Loco Salad with Creamy Cilantro Dressing, 3 oz.	170	14	7
The Original Pollo Bowl®, 18 oz.	540	4	85
• Ultimate Pollo Bowl®, 24 oz.	880	26	90
Burritos			
• BRC Burrito, 8 oz.	390	10	61
Classic Chicken Burrito®, 10 oz.	500	14	63
Pollo Asado Burrito, 12 oz.	600	23	58
• Twice Grilled Burrito™, 15 oz.	830	37	58
Ultimate Grilled Burrito, 14 oz.	650	20	80
Desserts			
Caramel Flan, 6 oz.	290	12	41
Churros, 2 each	300	18	32
• Vanilla Kid Cone, 1 each	200	5	33
• Vanilla Large Cone, 1 each	510	14	84
Vanilla Regular Cone, 1 each	330	8	55
Vanilla Soft Serve - cup, 5 oz.	300	8	48
Dining			
BRC Burrito, 8 oz.	390	10	61
Caesar Pollo Salad w/o dressing, 9 oz.	220	7	15
Chicken Breast, Skinless, 4 oz.	180	4	0
Chicken Tortilla Soup (w/o Tortilla Strips), 10 oz.	140	6	8
Chicken Tortilla Soup, 11 oz.	210	9	18
Chicken Tostada w/o Shell, 15 oz.	410	11	42
• Fresh Vegetables (w/o margarine), 4 oz.	35	0	8
Garden Salad (w/o Tortilla Strips), 5 oz.	80	5	5
Garden Salad, 5 oz.	120	7	9
Pinto Beans, 6 oz.	140	0	25
Skinless Breast Meal, 12 oz.	310	12	17
Skinless Breast Meal, Special Request, 12 oz.	270	10	12
Spanish Rice, 5 oz.	160	1	34
Taco al Carbon, 3 oz.	150	5	17
• The Original Pollo Bowl®, 18 oz.	540	4	85
Dressings			
Creamy Cilantro, 2 oz.	220	23	1
Light Creamy Cilantro, 1 pkt.	70	5	6
• Light Italian, 1 pkt.	20	1	2
• Ranch, 1 pkt.	230	24	2
Thousand Island, 1 pkt.	220	21	6
Flame Grilled Chicken			
• Chicken Breast, 4 oz.	220	9	0
Chicken Breast, Skinless, 4 oz.	180	4	0
Chopped Breast Meat, 3 oz.	100	2	0
• Leg, 2 oz.	90	4	0
Thigh, 3 oz.	220	15	0
Wing, 1 oz.	90	5	0
Kids Meal			
BBQ Sauce, 1 oz.	44	0	11
• Cheese Quesadilla, 5 oz.	420	23	35
French Fries - Kid Size, 3 oz.	240	11	31
• Leg, 2 oz.	90	4	0

El Pollo Loco (cont.)

	Cal	Fat	Cbs
Kids Meal (cont.)			
Popcorn Chicken, 3 oz.	200	12	10
Loco Value Menu			
BRC Burrito, 8 oz.	390	10	61
• Cheese Quesadilla, 5 oz.	420	23	35
Chicken Taquito, 1 each	190	9	18
• Leg, 2 oz.	90	4	0
Loco Nachos, 3 oz.	310	18	31
Loco Salad w/ Creamy Cilantro Dressing, 3 oz.	170	14	7
Taco al Carbon, 3 oz.	150	5	17
Two Churros, 2 each	300	18	32
Mexican Favorites			
Chicken Soft Taco, 5 oz.	270	13	19
Chicken Tortilla Soup (with Tortilla Strips), 11 oz.	210	9	18
Chicken Verde Quesadilla, 9 oz.	590	27	53
• Crunchy Chicken Taco, 3 oz.	190	8	16
• Grilled Chicken Nachos, 17 oz.	1090	55	99
Salsas & More			
Avocado Salsa (Hot), 1 oz.	30	3	1
Chipotle Salsa (Hot), 1 oz.	5	0	1
Fried Serrano Pepper, 0 oz.	15	2	0
Guacamole, 1 oz.	45	4	4
• House Salsa (Mild), 1 oz.	5	0	1
• Jack & Poblano Queso, 2 oz.	100	8	4
Jalapeño Hot Sauce (Packet), 0 oz.	5	0	1
Ketchup (Packet), 0 oz.	10	0	2
Pico de Gallo (Medium), 1 oz.	10	1	1
Sour Cream, 1 oz.	60	5	1
Sides			
BBQ Black Beans, 6 oz.	200	3	36
Cole Slaw, 6 oz.	120	9	8
Corn Cobbette, 5 oz.	90	1	19
• French Fries, 6 oz.	440	21	57
Fresh Vegetables (w/o margarine), 4 oz.	35	0	8
Fresh Vegetables (with margarine), 4 oz.	60	3	8
Garden Salad, 5 oz.	120	7	9
Gravy, 1 oz.	10	0	2
Macaroni & Cheese, 6 oz.	280	17	28
Mashed Potatoes, 5 oz.	100	1	20
Pinto Beans, 6 oz.	140	0	25
Refried Beans (with Cheese), 6 oz.	270	7	36
Spanish Rice, 5 oz.	160	1	34
Tortillas & Chips			
6.5" Flour Tortillas, 2 each	210	7	30
• 6" Corn Tortillas, 2 each	120	2	24
• Tortilla Chips, 2 oz.	210	10	28

Famous Dave's

	Cal	Fat	Cbs
Entrees			
Char-Grilled Chicken Sandwich	510	10	53
• Dave's Sassy BBQ Chicken Salad	540	25	50
Georgia Chopped Pork Sandwich	510	15	62
• Sweet and Sassy Grilled Salmon Platter	450	26	11
Side Dish			
Drunkin' Apples, 4 oz.	140	5	26
• Firecracker Green Beans, 6 oz.	60	3	7
• Wilbur Beans, 4 oz.	150	4	26

Fatburger

	Cal	Fat	Cbs
Add-Ons			
American Cheese, 19 g	70	6	1
• Bacon, 15 g	70	6	0
Cheddar Cheese, 28 g	110	9	0
Chili Cup, 217 g	270	15	13
Fat Fries, 226 g	550	26	72
Homemade Onion Rings, 158 g	510	29	57

Fatburger (cont.)

	Cal	Fat	Cbs
Add-Ons (cont.)			
• Skinny Fries, 158 g	490	20	71
Shakes			
• Chocolate Shake, 495 g	880	38	120
• Strawberry Shake, 439 g	700	32	91
Vanilla Shake, 453 g	730	30	103
Signature Items			
Baby Fat, 155 g	300	15	24
• Fat Salad Wedge, 156 g	70	5	4
Fatburger, 255 g	520	29	32
Grilled Chicken Sandwich, 209 g	360	13	32
Hot Dog, 126 g	380	22	31
• Kingburger, 400 g	820	41	64
Sausage & Egg Sandwich, 155 g	620	44	33
Turkeyburger, 261 g	550	31	38
Veggieburger, 276 g	430	12	45

Fazoli's

	Cal	Fat	Cbs
Choose A Topping			
• Broccoli	25	0	5
Broccoli and Tomatoes	30	0	6
Garlic Shrimp	160	12	3
Italian Sausage	240	21	3
• Meatballs	250	18	6
Peppery Chicken	70	1	1
Desserts			
• Chocolate Chunk Cookie	510	26	68
• Original Cheesecake	290	22	17
Turtle Cheesecake	450	28	43
Drinks			
Lemon Ice - Peach	360	0	90
Lemon Ice - Pomegranate	360	0	90
Lemon Ice - Strawberry	320	0	81
• Lemon Ice - Triple Berry	360	0	91
• Original Lemon Ice - Regular	180	0	45
Extras			
Breadstick, Dry, 1 each	100	2	20
Garlic Breadstick, 1 each	150	7	20
Kids Meals			
Cheese Pizza	270	11	31
Fettuccine Alfredo	290	5	50
Meat Lasagna	260	13	21
Pepperoni Pizza	310	14	31
Ravioli with Marinara Sauce	290	7	43
Ravioli with Meat Sauce	300	8	42
Spaghetti with Marinara Sauce	270	2	53
Spaghetti with Meat Sauce	300	4	53
• Spaghetti with Meatballs	350	7	55
• Ziti with Meat Sauce	190	6	25
Oven-Baked Pastas			
Baked Spaghetti	680	22	90
Baked Spaghetti with Meatballs	940	40	100
Chicken Parmesan	960	33	117
Meat Lasagna	510	25	43
Rigatoni Romano	1090	54	101
Panini			
• Four Cheese & Tomato	510	22	53
Grilled Chicken	540	18	56
• Smoked Turkey	620	29	54
Pasta Bowls			
Fettuccine with Alfredo - Regular	780	18	125
Fettuccine with Alfredo - Small	520	12	83
• Fettuccine with Marinara - Small	450	3	88
Fettuccine with Marinara - Regular	670	4	132
Fettuccine with Meat Sauce - Regular	750	10	131
Fettuccine with Meat Sauce - Small	500	7	87

RESTAURANTS & FAST-FOOD CHAINS

Fazoli's (cont.)

	Cal	Fat	Cbs
Pasta Bowls (cont.)			
Penne with Alfredo - Regular	780	18	125
Penne with Alfredo - Small	520	12	83
Penne with Marinara - Small	450	3	88
Penne with Marinara- Regular	670	4	132
Penne with Meat Sauce - Regular	750	10	131
Penne with Meat Sauce - Small	500	7	87
Ravioli with Marinara Sauce	500	15	71
Ravioli with Meat Sauce	550	20	71
Spaghetti with Alfredo - Regular	780	18	125
Spaghetti with Alfredo - Small	520	12	83
Spaghetti with Marinara - Small	450	3	88
Spaghetti with Marinara- Regular	670	4	132
Spaghetti with Meat Sauce - Regular	750	10	131
Spaghetti with Meat Sauce - Small	500	7	87
Ziti with Meat Sauce - Regular	700	22	95
Ziti with Meat Sauce - Small	480	15	65
Pizza			
• Cheese, 1 slice	270	11	31
• Pepperoni, 1 slice	310	14	31
Salad Dressings & Croutons			
• Caesar, 2 oz.	230	25	1
Croutons, pack	70	3	8
Fat Free Honey Mustard, 2 oz.	60	0	15
• Fat Free Italian, 2 oz.	25	0	6
Honey French, 2 oz.	220	18	14
Italian, 2 oz.	160	14	7
Lite Ranch, 2 oz.	120	12	2
Ranch, 2 oz.	220	24	2
Salads			
Caesar Side Salad	40	2	4
Chicken & Fruit	220	2	28
• Chicken & Pasta Caesar	440	15	41
Chicken BLT Ranch	270	10	13
• Garden Side Salad	25	0	4
Parmesan Chicken	360	15	31
Pasta Side Salad	320	12	41
Sampler Platters			
Classic Sampler	810	25	110
Ultimate Sampler	980	29	134
Submarinos			
Club	730	34	65
Ham n' Swiss	680	30	65
• Italian Beef	660	24	68
• Original	940	58	68

Firehouse Subs

	Cal	Fat	Cbs
Chili & Salads			
• Chief's Salad w/ Chicken Salad, 16 oz.	690	54	16
Chief's Salad w/ Grilled Chicken, 16 oz.	340	15	12
Chief's Salad w/ Ham, 16 oz.	360	8	16
Chief's Salad w/ Turkey, 16 oz.	300	15	12
Chiefs Salad w/ Tuna Salad, 16 oz.	540	35	16
Chili, 8 oz.	320	18	20
Desserts			
• Brownies, 4 oz.	420	18	63
• Chocolate Chip Cookie, 3 oz.	290	14	37
Oatmeal Raisin Cookie, 3 oz.	310	16	35
Peanut Butter Cookie, 3 oz.	360	26	25
Large Subs			
• Chicken Salad (10 oz), 20 oz.	1380	90	99
Club on A Sub, 19 oz.	810	23	94
Corned Beef, 16 oz.	600	25	84
Engine Company, 18 oz.	670	19	88
Engineer, 20 oz.	620	26	94
Grilled Chicken (8 oz), 18 oz.	680	12	90

Firehouse Subs (cont.)

	Cal	Fat	Cbs
Large Subs (cont.)			
Ham, 16 oz.	630	10	94
Hero, 18 oz.	680	15	93
Hook & Ladder, 18 oz.	660	18	94
Italian, 9 oz.	1000	45	98
Meatball, 7 oz.	1220	69	98
NY Steamer, 14 oz.	750	38	86
Pastrami, 16 oz.	640	13	88
Roast Beef, 16 oz.	600	11	85
Steak, 17 oz.	830	27	93
Tuna Salad (10 oz), 20 oz.	1090	53	98
Turkey, 16 oz.	560	8	88
• Veggie (no meat), 14 oz.	500	20	92
Medium Subs			
Chicken Salad (5 oz.), 12 oz.	760	46	63
Club on A Sub, 11 oz.	490	13	60
Corned Beef, 11 oz.	400	17	55
Engine Company, 11 oz.	410	11	57
Engineer, 12 oz.	380	14	61
Grilled Chicken, 11 oz.	410	7	58
Ham, 11 oz.	430	7	62
Hero (6 oz. meat), 13 oz.	460	12	61
Hook & Ladder, 11 oz.	400	10	60
Italian, 11 oz.	660	33	60
• Meatball, 11 oz.	800	45	65
NY Steamer, 8 oz.	520	20	56
Pastrami, 11 oz.	420	9	58
Roast Beef, 11 oz.	400	8	56
Steak, 10 oz.	490	15	60
Tuna Salad (5 oz), 12 oz.	610	28	62
• Turkey, 11 oz.	370	4	58
Veggie (no meat), 10 oz.	370	11	60

Five Guys Famous Burgers and Fries

	Cal	Fat	Cbs
Famous Burgers			
• Bread, 77 g	260	9	39
Hamburger Beef, 94 g	280	19	0
• Hebrew National Hotdog, 90 g	285	26	1
Sides			
Five Guys Fries, 122 g	310	15	39
Toppings			
A.1. Original Steak Sauce, 17 g	15	0	3
Cattlemen's BBQ Sauce, 17 g	60	0	16
Frank's Original Hot Sauce, 5 g	0	0	0
• French's Yellow Mustard, 17 g	0	0	0
Green Peppers, 25 g	5	0	2
Jalapeños, 11 g	3	0	1
Ketchup, 17 g	15	0	4
Kraft American Cheese, 19 g	70	6	1
Lettuce, 30 g	4	0	1
• Mayonnaise, 14 g	100	11	N/A
Mt. Olive Fresh Kosher Dill Pickles, 28 g	5	0	1
Mt. Olive Special Sweet Green Relish, 15 g	15	0	4
Onions, 26 g	10	0	3
Patrick Cudahy Bacon, 14 g	80	7	0
Sautéed Mushrooms, 25 g	10	0	1
Tomatoes, 52 g	9	0	2

Fox's Pizza Den

	Cal	Fat	Cbs
Pizza			
12 Cheese Pizza, 1 pizza	1244	37	170
12 Pepperoni Pizza, 1 pizza	1420	53	170
14 sq. Cheese Slice, 1 slice	155	5	21
14 sq. Pepperoni Slice, 1 slice	178	7	21
16 Cheese Pizza, 1 pizza	2214	66	302
• 16 Pepperoni Pizza, 1 pizza	2484	90	302

Fox's Pizza Den (cont.)

	Cal	Fat	Cbs
Pizza (cont.)			
16" Round Pizza, 1 slice	226	7	31
20 sq. Cheese Slice, 1 slice	221	7	30
20 sq. Pepperoni Slice, 1 slice	248	9	30

Freshens

	Cal	Fat	Cbs
Smoothie			
All That Razz, 21 oz.	360	0	79
Berry Breeze, 21 oz.	306	0	77
Blueberry Bay, 21 oz.	376	0	81
Caribbean Craze, 21 oz.	288	0	73
Jamaican Jammer, 21 oz.	355	0	78
Mango Beach, 21 oz.	90	0	48
Maui Mango, 21 oz.	292	0	74
Mystic Mango, 21 oz.	357	3	82
Orange Shooter, 21 oz.	334	3	77
Orange Sunrise, 21 oz.	353	3	81
Peach Passion, 21 oz.	152	0	32
Peach Sunset, 21 oz.	268	0	67
Peachy Pineapple, 21 oz.	327	0	69
• Pina Collider, 21 oz.	429	4	88
Pineapple Paradise, 21 oz.	331	4	77
Raspberry Royale, 21 oz.	270	0	67
• Strawberry Oasis, 21 oz.	89	0	49
Strawberry Shooter, 21 oz.	246	0	64
Strawberry Squeeze, 21 oz.	313	0	68
Strawberry Sunrise, 21 oz.	153	0	35

Fuddruckers

	Cal	Fat	Cbs
Extras			
American Cheese, 1 slice	50	5	1
• Cheese Sauce, 2 fl.oz.	40	3	6
• Fuddruckers Spud Spice, 100 g	267	5	49
Mild Cheddar Cheese, 1 slice	80	7	0
Monterey Jack w/ Peppers, 1 slice	110	9	1
Monterey Jack, 1 slice	80	7	0
Signature Spread, Garlic & Herb, 1 tbsp.	90	10	0
Swiss, 1 slice	80	6	1
Hamburger Bun			
• Bun Dough, 3 oz.	240	5	40
• Bun Mix, 100 g	410	10	67
Meat Products			
• Ground Beef 76/24, 4 oz.	330	28	0
Turkey Patty, Approx. 1/3 lb.	240	17	0
• Veggie Patty, Approx. 1/4 lb.	150	4	22
Sides			
Beer Battered Onion Rings, 4 pcs.	150	8	18
Potato Wedges, 3 oz.	120	3	20

Giordano's

	Cal	Fat	Cbs
• Small Cheese Stuffed Pizza, 7 oz.	550	25	57
Small Spinach Stuffed Pizza, 7 oz.	500	21	54
• Small Vegetarian Stuffed Pizza, 7 oz.	470	19	55

Gloria Jean's

	Cal	Fat	Cbs
Blended Tea Lattes (Regular)			
• Chai Tea Latte, 24 oz.	174	3	31
• Green Tea Latte, 24 oz.	359	14	54
Mango Tea Latte, 24 oz.	316	12	55
Chillers (Regular)			
Chai Chiller, 24 oz.	416	14	66
• Crème Brulee Espresso Chiller, 24 oz.	319	9	52
Mocharetto Espresso Chiller, 24 oz.	405	13	66
Swiss Orange Mocha Espresso Chiller, 24 oz.	365	13	57
Vanilla Caramel Chiller, 24 oz.	634	21	100
• Very Vanilla Chiller, 24 oz.	839	38	114

Gloria Jean's (cont.)

	Cal	Fat	Cbs
Chillers (Regular) (cont.)			
White Caramel Oreo Chiller, 24 oz.	821	26	133
White Chocolate Oreo Chiller, 24 oz.	666	26	95
Cold Coffee Drinks (Regular)			
• Butter Rum Chiller, 24 oz.	656	19	112
Iced Café au Lait, 24 oz.	65	2	6
Iced Café Mocha, 24 oz.	397	17	51
Iced Cappuccino Chiller, 24 oz.	484	16	66
Iced Coffee, 24 oz.	5	0	0
Iced Latte, 24 oz.	200	8	19
• Iced Toddy, 24 oz.	2	0	0
Iced Toddy Supreme, 24 oz.	537	47	19
Iced White Chocolate Mocha, 24 oz.	410	19	50
Cold Drinks (Regular)			
Bulk Iced Tea, 24 oz.	5	0	1
• Italian Cream Soda, 24 oz.	441	13	83
Italian Cream Soda, Sugar-Free Syrup, 24 oz.	145	13	6
Italian Soda, 24 oz.	296	0	77
• Italian Soda, Sugar-Free Syrup, 24 oz.	0	0	0
Fruit Chillers (Regular)			
• Banana Chiller, 24 oz.	371	0	91
Banana Cream Chiller, 24 oz.	394	1	87
• Bananaberry Split Chiller, 24 oz.	709	26	123
Raspberries 'N Cream Chiller, 24 oz.	394	1	87
Raspberry Fruit Chiller, 24 oz.	371	0	91
Strawberries 'N Cream Chiller, 24 oz.	394	1	87
Strawberry Fruit Chiller, 24 oz.	371	0	91
Wildberries 'N Cream Fruit Chiller, 24 oz.	394	1	87
Wildberry Fruit Chiller, 24 oz.	371	0	91
Holiday Drinks (Regular)			
Butter Rum Latte, 16 oz.	580	17	100
• Noel Nog, 16 oz.	516	29	52
• Sleigh Ride Chiller, 16 oz.	586	19	92
Sleigh Ride Mocha, 16 oz.	538	17	87
White Chocolate Sleigh Ride, 16 oz.	582	19	91
Hot Coffee Drinks (Regular)			
Cafe Americano, 16 oz.	2	0	0
Cafe au Lait, 16 oz.	109	4	10
Cafe Breve, 16 oz.	314	28	10
Cafe Latte, 16 oz.	154	6	14
Cafe Mocha, 16 oz.	388	16	51
Cappuccino, 16 oz.	124	5	11
Creme Brulee Latte, 16 oz.	352	11	54
Espresso Con Pana, Double	21	2	1
Espresso Con Pana, Single	20	2	1
Espresso Macchiato, Double	9	0	1
Espresso Macchiato, Single	9	0	1
Espresso, Double	2	0	0
• Espresso, Single	1	0	0
Mocha Truffle, 16 oz.	320	13	43
• Mocharetto, 16 oz.	506	16	81
Swiss Orange Mocha, 16 oz.	447	16	66
Vanilla Caramelatte, 16 oz.	376	10	64
White Chocolate Mocha, 16 oz.	401	18	49
Hot Drinks (Regular)			
Hot Chai, 16 oz.	213	3	40
Hot Chocolate, 16 oz.	431	18	55
• Hot Tea, 16 oz.	0	0	0
Irish Nut Crème, 16 oz.	403	13	60
Mocha Caramelatte, 16 oz.	416	12	65
• Mon Cheri Mocha, 16 oz.	450	14	70
Steamers, 16 oz.	358	11	56
Steamers, Sugar-Free Syrup, 16 oz.	210	11	17
White Hot Chocolate, 16 oz.	445	20	51

Gloria Jean's (cont.)

Kids Drinks	Cal	Fat	Cbs
• BananaBerry Chiller	330	13	47
• Grapple Fruit Chiller	330	13	45
Strawbical Fruit Chiller	330	13	47
WaterBerry Chiller	330	13	47
Mocha Chillers (Regular)			
Banana Ana Mocha Chiller, 24 oz.	619	13	118
Banana Split Mocha Chiller, 24 oz.	701	13	138
• Coco Loco Mocha Chiller, 24 oz.	536	13	97
Cookies 'N Cream Mocha Chiller, 24 oz.	588	19	94
Cookies 'N Mint Mocha Chiller, 24 oz.	756	20	135
• English Toffee Twist Mocha Chiller, 24 oz.	776	27	124
Malted Mocha Chiller, 24 oz.	722	17	131
Mint Choco Bomb Mocha Chiller, 24 oz.	596	13	112
Nutty Mocha Frost Chiller, 24 oz.	750	22	130
Raspberry Dazzle Mocha Chiller, 24 oz.	619	13	118
Strawberry Supreme Mocha Chiller, 24 oz.	619	13	118
Promotional Drinks (Regular)			
• Chocolate Fudge Chiller, 24 oz.	664	28	108
• Iced Chai with Skim Milk, 24 oz.	193	0	41
Java Chiller, 24 oz.	459	18	70
Java Light Chiller, 24 oz.	255	6	41
Lite Mocha Chiller, 24 oz.	195	3	42
Madagascar Vanilla Chiller, 24 oz.	662	35	91
Strawberry Vanilla Chiller, 24 oz.	550	13	101

Godfather's Pizza

Desserts	Cal	Fat	Cbs
Apple Dessert (Alum Pan), 1/6	139	2	28
Apple Dessert (Large), 1/10	229	5	42
Apple Dessert (Medium), 1/8	206	4	39
Apple Dessert (Small), 1/6	202	5	37
• Breadsticks, 1 piece	80	2	14
Cheesesticks, 1/6	130	4	18
Cherry Dessert (Alum Pan), 1/6	142	2	29
Cherry Dessert (Large), 1/10	233	5	44
Cherry Dessert (Medium), 1/8	210	4	40
Cherry Dessert (Small), 1/6	206	5	38
Chocolate Chip Cookie, 1/6	195	8	30
Cinnamon Streusel (Alum Pan), 1/6	161	3	30
Cinnamon Streusel (Large), 1/10	258	7	45
Cinnamon Streusel (Medium), 1/8	228	6	40
Cinnamon Streusel (Small), 1/6	226	6	39
M&M Streusel Dessert (Alum Pan), 1/6	173	4	31
• M&M Streusel Dessert (Large), 1/10	300	8	51
M&M Streusel Dessert (Medium), 1/8	263	7	45
M&M Streusel Dessert (Small), 1/6	249	7	42
Monkey Bread (Alum Pan), 1/6	120	2	23
Potato Wedges, 4 oz.	192	9	24
Jumbo Original			
All Meat Combo, 1/10 pizza	610	27	56
Bacon Cheeseburger, 1/10 pizza	580	27	55
• Cheese, 1/10 pizza	430	13	53
Combo, 1/10 pizza	580	24	57
Hawaiian, 1/10 pizza	460	13	58
Hot Stuff, 1/10 pizza	590	26	56
Humble Pie, 1/10 pizza	620	30	56
Pepperoni, 1/10 pizza	490	18	54
Super Combo, 1/10 pizza	630	28	58
Super Hawaiian, 1/10 pizza	500	18	57
• Super Taco, 1/10 pizza	640	31	57
Taco, 1/10 pizza	590	27	56
Veggie, 1/10 pizza	450	14	56
Large Golden			
All Meat Combo, 1/10 pizza	350	17	29
Bacon Cheeseburger, 1/10 pizza	330	16	29

Godfather's Pizza (cont.)

Large Golden (cont.)	Cal	Fat	Cbs
• Cheese, 1/10 pizza	250	9	28
Combo, 1/10 pizza	330	15	30
Hawaiian, 1/10 pizza	270	10	31
Hot Stuff, 1/10 pizza	340	17	29
Humble Pie, 1/10 pizza	350	18	29
Pepperoni, 1/10 pizza	290	13	28
Super Combo, 1/10 pizza	370	18	31
Super Hawaiian, 1/10 pizza	291	12	30
• Super Taco, 1/10 pizza	380	20	30
Taco, 1/10 pizza	350	17	30
Veggie, 1/10 pizza	260	10	30
Large Original			
All Meat Combo, 1/10 pizza	410	18	38
Bacon Cheeseburger, 1/10 pizza	390	18	36
• Cheese, 1/10 pizza	290	9	36
Combo, 1/10 pizza	390	16	39
Hawaiian, 1/10 pizza	310	9	38
Hot Stuff, 1/10 pizza	400	18	38
Humble Pie, 1/10 pizza	420	20	38
Pepperoni, 1/10 pizza	330	12	36
Super Combo, 1/10 pizza	430	19	39
Super Hawaiian, 1/10 pizza	340	12	38
• Super Taco, 1/10 pizza	450	22	38
Taco, 1/10 pizza	420	19	38
Veggie, 1/10 pizza	310	10	38
Large Thin			
All Meat Combo, 1/10 pizza	310	17	20
Bacon Cheeseburger, 1/10 pizza	290	17	20
• Cheese, 1/10 pizza	220	10	19
Combo, 1/10 pizza	290	16	21
Hawaiian, 1/10 pizza	240	10	22
Hot Stuff, 1/10 pizza	300	17	20
Humble Pie, 1/10 pizza	310	19	20
Pepperoni, 1/10 pizza	250	13	19
Super Combo, 1/10 pizza	330	19	22
Super Hawaiian, 1/10 pizza	250	12	21
• Super Taco, 1/10 pizza	340	21	21
Taco, 1/10 pizza	310	18	21
Veggie, 1/10 pizza	230	10	21
Medium Golden			
All Meat Combo, 1/8 pizza	300	14	27
Bacon Cheeseburger, 1/8 pizza	270	12	26
• Cheese, 1/8 pizza	220	8	26
Combo, 1/8 pizza	290	13	28
Hawaiian, 1/8 pizza	240	8	29
Hot Stuff, 1/8 pizza	290	14	27
Humble Pie, 1/8 pizza	310	15	27
Pepperoni, 1/8 pizza	260	11	26
Super Combo, 1/8 pizza	320	15	27
Super Hawaiian, 1/8 pizza	250	10	27
• Super Taco, 1/8 pizza	330	17	28
Taco, 1/8 pizza	300	14	27
Veggie, 1/8 pizza	230	8	27
Medium Original			
All Meat Combo, 1/8 pizza	370	16	35
Bacon Cheeseburger, 1/8 pizza	330	13	35
• Cheese, 1/8 pizza	260	7	34
Combo, 1/8 pizza	350	14	37
Hawaiian, 1/8 pizza	280	8	38
Hot Stuff, 1/8 pizza	360	6	35
Humble Pie, 1/8 pizza	380	18	35
Pepperoni, 1/8 pizza	290	10	34
Super Combo, 1/8 pizza	390	17	37
Super Hawaiian, 1/8 pizza	280	8	37

Godfather's Pizza (cont.)

	Cal	Fat	Cbs
Medium Original (cont.)			
• Super Taco, 1/8 pizza	390	18	36
Taco, 1/8 pizza	360	16	36
Veggie, 1/8 pizza	270	9	36
Medium Thin			
All Meat Combo, 1/8 pizza	280	15	20
Bacon Cheeseburger, 1/8 pizza	250	13	20
• Cheese, 1/8 pizza	180	8	16
Combo, 1/8 pizza	250	13	18
Hawaiian, 1/8 pizza	200	9	19
Hot Stuff, 1/8 pizza	270	15	20
Humble Pie, 1/8 pizza	270	16	17
Pepperoni, 1/8 pizza	220	11	16
Super Combo, 1/8 pizza	300	16	21
Super Hawaiian, 1/8 pizza	230	11	21
• Super Taco, 1/8 pizza	310	18	21
Taco, 1/8 pizza	260	15	17
Veggie, 1/8 pizza	190	9	18
Mini Original			
All Meat Combo, 1/4 pizza	220	10	21
Bacon Cheeseburger, 1/4 pizza	210	10	21
• Cheese, 1/4 pizza	150	4	20
Combo, 1/4 pizza	210	8	22
Hawaiian, 1/4 pizza	160	4	23
Hot Stuff, 1/4 pizza	210	9	21
• Humble Pie, 1/4 pizza	230	11	21
Pepperoni, 1/4 pizza	160	5	20
Super Combo, 1/4 pizza	220	9	22
Super Hawaiian, 1/4 pizza	180	6	21
Super Taco, 1/4 pizza	230	10	22
Taco, 1/4 pizza	210	9	22
Veggie, 1/4 pizza	160	5	21

Gold Star Chili

	Cal	Fat	Cbs
Burritos			
Chili Beef Burrito with Topper, 383 g	710	32	78
• Chili Beef Burrito with Topper, 292 g	570	20	75
Crispy Chicken Burrito with Topper, 334 g	790	36	84
• Crispy Chicken Burrito, 277 g	840	22	62
Grilled Chicken Burrito with Topper, 325 g	730	33	72
Grilled Chicken Burrito, 268 g	580	19	59
Chili by the Bowl			
Chili, 8 oz.	213	12	8
Veggie Chili Bowl, 255 g	160	2	29
Fries and Garlic Bread			
Cheese Fries, 184 g	520	32	42
Chili Cheese Fries, 269 g	596	36	46
Fries, 149 g	366	19	44
Garlic Bread w/ Cheese, 68 g	271	18	19
• Garlic Bread, 54 g	213	13	19
Gold Star Chili			
Regular 2-Way bean, 425 g	489	12	71
Regular 2-Way onion bean, 468 g	505	12	75
Regular 2-Way onion, 383 g	436	11	62
Regular 2-Way, 340 g	420	11	58
Regular 3-Way, 397 g	648	30	59
Regular 4-Way, 439 g	665	30	63
Regular 5-Way, 525 g	733	30	76
• Super 5-Way, 794 g	1141	51	109
Gold Star Coney			
Cheese Coney, 160 g	343	18	31
Chili Cheese Sandwich, 132 g	288	12	30
• Chili Sandwich, 132 g	211	5	32
Coney, 146 g	286	14	30
• Low Carb Coney Bowl, 298 g	570	47	7

Gold Star Chili (cont.)

	Cal	Fat	Cbs
Sensational Entree Sized Salads			
• Caesar Salad, 105 g	90	5	6
Cafe Salad, 134 g	110	7	8
Burritos			
Crispy Chicken Caesar Salad, 238 g	280	11	22
Crispy Chicken Cafe Salad, 238 g	210	8	12
• Grilled Chkn Spring Harvest Salad, 315 g	300	13	23
Half Cafe Salad, 238 g	280	11	22
Low Carb Chili Salad, 230 g	160	7	23

Golden Corral

	Cal	Fat	Cbs
Brass Bell Bakery®			
Apple Pie, 1/10 pie	320	13	49
• Banana Pudding, 1/2 cup	466	19	70
Bread Pudding, 1/2 cup	200	5	37
Brownies, 1	240	9	40
Carrot Cake, 4 oz.	390	19	52
Cherry Pie, 1/10 pie	310	13	46
Chocolate Chip Cookies, 1	100	5	13
Chocolate White Chip Cookies, 1	100	5	13
Cinn-a-Gold Rolls®, 1	320	10	52
Coconut, 1	100	5	13
Key Lime Cheesecake, 1/10 pie	360	19	42
• Oatmeal Raisin Cookies, 1	90	4	14
Peanut Butter with Nuts Cookies, 1	100	6	12
Breads/Muffins			
• Corn Muffins, 3 oz.	204	5	32
Kaiser Rolls, 1	160	2	31
• Skillet Cornbread, 1 Portion	120	3	22
Yeast Rolls (without butter), 1	195	2	42
Cold Buffet			
• Cajun Potato Salad, 1 cup	330	23	22
Carrot & Raisin Salad, 1/2 cup	113	5	17
Chicken Salad, 1/2 cup	210	15	9
Coleslaw, 1 cup	250	19	19
Macaroni Salad, 1/2 cup	190	8	26
Marinated Mushroom, 1/2 cup	103	7	6
• Marinated Vegetables, 1/2 cup	47	2	5
Seafood Salad, 1 cup	270	17	18
Sliced Yellow Peaches, 1/2 cup	70	0	17
Tuna Salad, 1/2 cup	237	12	8
Condiments			
Cocktail Sauce, 1/4 cup	70	2	13
• Honey Butter (indiv. cup), 10 g	60	6	2
• Tartar Sauce, 2 tbsp.	150	16	1
Hot Buffet			
Asian Pork Roast, 1 cup	510	34	10
Awesome Pot Roast, 4 oz.	206	12	1
Barbecue Chicken (Leg Quarter), 1	480	22	20
Barbecue Pork Spareribs, 82 g	230	16	3
Barbecue Pork, 3 oz.	170	8	5
Bourbon Street Chicken, 4 oz.	210	11	5
Broccoli & Rice, 1/2 cup	220	5	36
Brown Gravy, 1 oz.	100	4	16
Buttered Noodles, 1/2 cup	163	4	24
Chicken & Pastry Noodles, 4 oz.	94	4	9
Chicken Breast Fillet, Marinated, 5 oz.	120	2	2
Chicken Tenders, 3 oz.	190	9	7
Country Fried Steak, 3 oz.	152	7	12
Creamy Chicken & Pasta, 1 cup	210	6	25
Fresh Fried Chicken (Leg/Thigh), 3 oz.	250	19	2
Grilled Pork Chop or Loin Slices, 3 oz.	119	4	0
Grilled Pork Chops (with bone), 1	200	13	0
Ham (Pit Style, Smoked), 2 oz.	80	2	1

Golden Corral (cont.)

Hot Buffet (cont.)	Cal	Fat	Cbs
Macaroni & Beef, 1 cup	260	11	26
Macaroni & Cheese, 1 cup	400	18	42
Mashed Potatoes (Scratch), 4 oz.	120	6	14
Meatloaf, 4 oz.	190	10	10
Pizza, 1 slice	230	8	28
Pork Roast, 3 oz.	220	17	0
Pork Steaks, 3.5 oz.	250	14	0
Potato Casserole, 1 cup	280	9	40
Poultry Gravy, 1 oz.	104	3	16
Roast Beef, 3 oz.	180	10	1
Roasted Herb Pork Chop, 3 oz.	334	17	6
Rotisserie Chicken (Breast/Wing), 6 oz.	320	15	1
Sirloin Steak, 3 oz.	219	13	0
Spaghetti Pasta, 2 oz.	210	1	42
Spaghetti Sauce, 1/2 cup	110	0	25
• Steakburgers, 6 oz.	859	55	0
Tamales, Beef, 85 g	240	16	18
Tortillas, 2	325	7	56
• Turkey Breast w/ Wing, 2 oz.	70	3	1
White Rice, 1/2 cup	178	5	27
Ice Cream/Toppings			
Caramel Topping, 100 g	318	4	67
Chocolate Soft Serve, 1/2 cup	100	2	18
Chocolate Syrup, 100 g	249	1	62
Hot Fudge Topping, 100 g	320	10	54
Sherbet, 1/2 cup	90	1	23
Strawberry Topping, 100 g	192	0	49
• Turtle Coating, 100 g	633	50	46
Vanilla Soft Serve, 1/2 cup	100	2	17
No Sugar Added/Sugar Free			
Blueberry Pie, 1/10 pie	270	8	48
Cheesecake, 1	220	14	18
Chocolate Chocolate Chip Cookies, 1	90	5	12
Oatmeal Bar, 1 Square	90	3	11
• Red Gelatin, 1/2 cup	10	0	0
Vanilla Cake, 1	130	7	19
Salad Bar Meats			
• Turkey - Dark, Julienne, 2 oz.	70	2	2
• Turkey - White, Julienne, 2 oz.	90	5	2
Salad Dressing			
• Blue Cheese Dressing, 2 tbsp.	190	20	2
Creamy Caesar Dressing, 2 tbsp.	110	11	2
Dijon Honey Mustard Dressing, 2 tbsp.	130	11	7
• Fat Free Ranch Dressing, 2 tbsp.	35	0	2
Fat Free Red French Dressing, 2 tbsp.	40	0	10
Fat Free Thou Island Dressing, 2 tbsp.	40	0	9
French Dressing, 2 tbsp.	120	11	5
Hot Bacon Dressing, 2 tbsp.	140	14	5
Lite Olive Oil Vinaigrette, 2 tbsp.	60	6	3
Poppy Seed Dressing, 2 tbsp.	130	10	8
Ranch Dressing, 2 tbsp.	120	12	2
Red French Dressing, 2 tbsp.	120	11	7
Sesame Oriental Dressing, 2 tbsp.	160	15	6
Thousand Island Dressing, 2 tbsp.	130	11	6
Seafood			
Battered Pollock Fish Fillet, 4 oz.	210	9	18
Breaded Butterflied Shrimp, 4 oz.	210	2	37
• Breaded Jumbo Shrimp, 4 oz.	230	2	36
Breaded Shrimp, 4 oz.	200	2	32
Cajun Style Fish Fillet, 3.5 oz.	210	9	19
Cajun Whitefish, 3 oz.	110	7	0
Cracker Crumb Fish Fillet, 3.5 oz.	229	13	17
Hot Steamed Shrimp, 1 cup	160	2	0
Kentucky Style Fish Fillet, 4 oz.	130	5	14

Golden Corral (cont.)

Seafood (cont.)	Cal	Fat	Cbs
Salmon Fillet, Carved, 2 oz.	138	9	0
Salmon Steaks w/Lemon Hrb Bttr, 3.5 oz.	208	14	4
• Steamed Whitefish, 3 oz.	82	3	0
Soup & Potato Bar			
Baked Potato (small, plain), 1	109	0	25
Broccoli Florets with Cheese, 1/2 cup	140	9	8
• Chicken Gumbo, 1/2 cup	70	2	10
Chicken Noodle, 1/2 cup	100	3	12
Clam Chowder, 1/2 cup	140	6	17
Potato with Bacon, 1/2 cup	120	5	17
Sweet Potato (Small), 1	137	0	32
• Timberline Chili, 1 cup	270	12	23
Vegetable Beef, 1/2 cup	100	2	17
Sunrise Breakfast Buffet			
• Bacon, 1 piece	60	5	1
• Corned Beef Hash, 1 cup	420	30	22
Creamed Chipped Beef, 1/2 cup	75	11	9
Eggs, Scrambled, 4 oz.	160	11	2
French Toast, 1 slice	241	8	23
Hash Brown Casserole, 1/2 cup	155	7	17
Hash Browns, 1/2 cup	102	7	8
Sausage Gravy, 1 oz.	41	3	2
Sausage Links, 3 Links	160	14	1
Sausage Patties, 1	247	21	0
Split Smoked Sausage, 1	250	23	2
Vegetables			
Asian Beans, 1 cup	140	2	26
Black-eyed Peas, 1/2 cup	149	1	28
Brussels Sprouts, 6 g	35	0	5
Cheese Sauce, Cheddar, 1/4 cup	110	9	4
Collard Greens, 3.5 oz.	60	4	4
Corn-on-the-Cob, 1	106	2	22
Creamed Corn, 3.5 oz.	90	1	20
Creamed Spinach, 1/2 cup	180	13	11
• Cut Corn, 1 cup	310	9	52
Escalloped Apples, 2/3 cup	180	2	40
Fresh Steamed Broccoli, 1/2 cup	25	1	5
Fresh Steamed Cabbage, 1/2 cup	60	5	1
Fresh Steamed Carrots, 1/2 cup	79	5	6
• Fresh Steamed Cauliflower, 1/2 cup	13	0	2
Fresh Vegetable Trio, 1/2 cup	25	0	5
Glazed Sesame Carrots, 1 cup	260	16	27
Green & Yellow Beans, 1/2 cup	71	5	4
Green Beans, 1/2 cup	34	0	6
Green Peas, 1/2 cup	109	6	10
Northern Beans, 1/2 cup	149	1	28
Pinto Beans, 1/2 cup	149	1	28
Ranch Style BBQ Beans, 1/2 cup	130	3	20
Southern Style Cabbage, 1/2 cup	26	1	4
Spinach, 1/3 cup	20	0	2
Squash Medley, 1/2 cup	66	5	3
Steamed Zucchini, 1/2 cup	60	5	1
Turnip Greens, 2/3 cup	18	0	3
Yams & Apples, 1/2 cup	160	2	35

Great Steak & Potato

Baked Potatoes	Cal	Fat	Cbs
Broccoli & Cheese, 238 g	295	12	35
Cheese & Bacon, 209 g	427	23	29
Potato Skins, 202 g	438	30	26
• Single, 6 g	158	0	36
Sour Cream & Chive, 170 g	198	7	31
• The Great Potato - Chicken, 360 g	519	24	37
The Great Potato - Ham, 360 g	503	26	43
The Great Potato - Steak, 374 g	542	29	37

Great Steak & Potato (cont.)

	Cal	Fat	Cbs
Baked Potatoes (cont.)			
The Great Potato - Turkey, 360 g	473	23	39
The King, 241 g	497	30	31
Breads/Tortillas			
• Bread, 12" White, 170 g	420	4	82
Bread, 7" Wheat, 113 g	310	4	56
Bread, 7" White, 113 g	290	3	55
• Pita, serving, 79 g	220	5	38
Tortilla, Low-Carb, Whole Wheat, 102 g	273	6	42
Cheese			
• Cheese, Mild Cheddar, serving, 2 oz.	223	18	0
Cheese, Provolone, serving, 2 oz.	202	16	2
• Cheese, Swiss, serving, 2 oz.	200	16	2
Kids Meals			
Nuggets, Kids, 78 g	165	9	10
Meats			
Chicken, serving, 4 oz.	138	3	0
Corned Beef, serving, 3 oz.	137	8	0
• Gyro Meat, serving, 4 oz.	205	12	5
Ham, serving, 4 oz.	122	4	6
Steak, serving, 5 oz.	160	7	0
• Turkey, serving, 4 oz.	91	1	2
Salads			
Chef, 398 g	244	11	13
• Garden, 256 g	37	0	8
Grilled Chicken, 464 g	389	21	13
Grilled Ham, 464 g	371	22	20
• Grilled Steak, 464 g	395	25	13
Grilled Turkey, 464 g	336	19	15
Sandwiches			
Buffalo Chicken Sandwich, Regular, 467 g	841	41	67
• Chicken Bacon Ranch, Regular - LTO, 432 g	995	56	66
Chicken Philly, Regular, 417 g	938	53	63
Chicken Philly, Wrap, 406 g	921	57	50
Chicken Teriyaki, Regular, 446 g	962	53	66
Chicken Teriyaki, Wrap, 435 g	945	57	53
Great Steak, Regular, 432 g	963	58	63
Great Steak, Wrap, 421 g	946	62	50
Ham Delight, Regular, 417 g	929	55	72
Ham Delight, Wrap, 406 g	912	58	58
Ham Explosion, Regular, 460 g	931	55	71
Ham Explosion, Wrap, 449 g	914	58	58
Reuben, Regular, 383 g	848	48	64
Reuben, Wrap, 372 g	831	51	51
Super Steak, Regular, 474 g	972	58	65
Super Steak, Wrap, 463 g	955	62	52
Turkey Philly, Regular, 417 g	892	52	65
Turkey Philly, Wrap, 406 g	875	55	52
Veggie Delight, Regular, 389 g	831	53	67
• Veggie Delight, Wrap, 378 g	814	56	54
Sauces/Dressings			
Dressing, Ranch, 1 oz.	171	12	1
Dressing, Thousand Island, 1 oz.	125	0	4
• Mayonnaise, Dijon, 28 g	205	22	0
Mayonnaise, Regular, 28 g	202	18	0
Oil, serving, 0.5 oz.	80	9	0
• Sauce, Buffalo, 1 oz.	10	0	2
Sauce, Dipping - Tomato, 2 oz.	14	0	3
Sauce, Teriyaki, 1 oz.	24	4	3
Sauce, Tzatziki, 1 oz.	46	0	2
Sides			
Cheese Sticks, Small, 97 g	286	17	23
Fresh Style Fry, Regular, 397 g	668	37	80
Fried Onion Petals, 86 g	190	11	22

Great Steak & Potato (cont.)

	Cal	Fat	Cbs
Toppings - Baked Potato			
Bacon, 1 oz.	76	18	0
• Cheddar Cheese, 2 oz.	223	12	0
Cheese Sauce, 2 oz.	155	0	3
• Chives, 1 oz.	0	4	0
Ham, 4 oz.	122	7	6
Sour Cream, 32 g	691		
Steak, 5 oz.	160	1	0
Turkey, 4 oz.	91	7	2
Toppings - Sandwich			
Broccoli, serving, 4 ea.	12	0	2
• Cucumber, serving, 1 oz.	4	0	1
Dill Pickle, serving, 1 ea.	5	0	1
Green Pepper, serving, 1 oz.	4	0	1
Lettuce, serving, 2 oz.	9	0	2
Mushrooms, serving, 1 oz.	5	2	1
Olives, serving, 1 oz.	16	0	1
Onion, serving, 2 oz.	19	0	4
• Pineapple, serving, 2 oz.	26	5	7
Sauerkraut, serving, 2 oz.	11	0	2
Tomato, serving, 1 oz.	5	0	1

Great Wraps

	Cal	Fat	Cbs
Breads			
• Croutons, 1 oz.	75	10	9
• Flour Tortilla, 12 oz.	320	10	47
Pita, 7 oz.	220	3	43
Spinach Tortilla, 12 oz.	290	9	43
Tomato Basil Tortilla, 12 oz.	320	9	49
Cheese			
• Cheddar Mix, 2 oz.	220	18	2
Crumbled Feta, 1 oz.	120	5	2
• Parmesan, 1 oz.	20	2	0
Pepper Jack, 2 oz.	220	18	2
Provolone, 2 oz.	200	16	2
Swiss, 2 oz.	160	12	0
Dressings			
• Balsamic Vinaigrette, 1 oz.	60	5	4
• Caesar, 2 oz.	300	32	4
Cuban Sauce, 1 oz.	170	16	2
Feta, 2 oz.	160	16	4
Lite Ranch, 2 oz.	200	3	2
Mayo, 1 oz.	100	11	2
Zeke, 2 oz.	90	10	4
Fresh Veggies			
• Black Olives, 1 oz.	60	3	1
Chopped Cucumber, 1 oz.	3	0	1
Chopped Onion, 1 oz.	10	0	2
Chopped Pepperoncini, 1 oz.	5	0	0
Chopped Tomatoes, 2 oz.	10	0	2
Jalapeños, 1 oz.	17	1	1
Red Pepper, 1 oz.	20	1	2
Romaine, 2 oz.	10	N/A	1
• Shredded Lettuce, 2 oz.	0	0	0
Spinach, 2 oz.	5	0	1
Sprouts, 1 oz.	2	0	0
Meats			
Bacon, 2 Slices	80	7	0
Chicken, 4 oz.	79	1	N/A
• Gyro, 4 oz.	350	32	4
Ham, 2 oz.	80	2	2
Large Chicken Tenderloin, 4 oz.	90	3	N/A
• Pork, 2 oz.	73	3	0
Steak, 4 oz.	110	4	1
Tuna, 4 oz.	105	0	0
Turkey, 4 oz.	80	0	4

Great Wraps (cont.)

	Cal	Fat	Cbs
Roasted Veggies			
Garlic Mushrooms, 1 oz.	5	2	1
• Green Pepper, 1 oz.	4	0	1
• Portabella Mushrooms, 3 oz.	81	14	5
Sauteed Onion, 1 oz.	27	1	3

Green Burrito

	Cal	Fat	Cbs
Burritos			
• Bean & Cheese Burrito - Chicken, 340 g	660	28	67
Bean & Cheese Burrito - Grnd Beef, 340 g	760	39	69
Bean & Cheese Burrito - Steak, 340 g	690	30	70
Bean & Cheese Burrito, 407 g	830	38	99
Carne Asada Burrito, 333 g	690	31	65
• Grilled Chicken Burrito, 506 g	1080	54	91
The Green Burrito™ - Chicken, 633 g	920	33	120
The Green Burrito™ - Steak, 633 g	950	35	122
Sides			
• Chips & Cheese, 142 g	690	40	65
Chips, 57 g	300	15	37
• Guacamole, 40 g	45	4	3
Pinto Beans & Cheese, 241 g	320	16	43
Rice, 198 g	340	10	58
Sour Cream, 40 g	50	4	3
Specialities			
Enchiladas (2) - Cheese, 220 g	430	28	30
Super Nachos - Chicken, 454 g	1020	55	96
• Super Nachos - Ground Beef, 465 g	1150	68	99
Super Nachos - Steak, 456 g	1050	58	99
Taco Salad - Chicken, 587 g	820	44	73
Taco Salad - Ground Beef, 587 g	940	57	75
Taco Salad - Steak, 587 g	850	47	76
• Taquitos (2) - Chicken, 92 g	150	7	16
Taquitos (5) - Chicken, 208 g	350	15	39
Tacos			
• Fish Taco, 171 g	300	12	36
• Hard Taco - Chicken, 110 g	200	10	14
Hard Taco - Ground Beef, 110 g	250	15	15
Hard Taco - Steak, 110 g	220	11	15
Soft Taco - Chicken, 123 g	210	7	18
Soft Taco - Ground Beef, 123 g	260	13	19
Soft Taco - Steak, 123 g	260	13	19

Hardee's

	Cal	Fat	Cbs
Breakfast			
Bacon Biscuit, 120 g	430	28	35
Bacon, Egg & Cheese Biscuit, 174 g	560	38	37
Big Country Brkfast - Bacon, 355 g	980	56	90
Big Country Brkfast - Chicken, 458 g	1140	61	105
Big Country Brkfast - Ham, 377 g	970	53	90
• Big Country Brkfast - Pork Chop, 455 g	1220	68	102
Big Country Brkfast - Sausage, 374 g	1060	64	91
Big Country Brkfast - Steak, 412 g	1150	68	98
Biscuits 'N' Gravy, 251 g	530	34	47
Breaded Chicken Fillet Biscuit, 226 g	600	34	50
Breaded Country Steak Biscuit, 180 g	620	41	44
Breaded Pork Chop Biscuit, 222 g	690	42	48
Country Ham Biscuit, 144 g	440	26	36
Country Steak & Egg Biscuit, 223 g	690	47	44
Egg Biscuit, 152 g	450	29	35
Frisco Breakfast Sandwich, 185 g	420	20	37
Ham, Egg & Cheese Biscuit, 220 g	560	35	37
Hash Rounds - medium, 114 g	350	22	34
Hash Rounds - small, 83 g	260	16	25
Loaded Biscuit 'N' Gravy Breakfast Bowl, 326 g	770	54	49
Loaded Breakfast Burrito, 258 g	780	51	38
Loaded Omelet Biscuit, 198 g	640	44	37

Hardee's (cont.)

	Cal	Fat	Cbs
Breakfast (cont.)			
Loaded Omelet, 89 g	270	21	2
Low Carb Breakfast Bowl, 208 g	620	50	6
Made from Scratch Biscuit, 109 g	370	23	35
Monster Biscuit, 212 g	710	51	37
Pancake Platter, 135 g	300	5	55
Sausage & Egg Biscuit, 185 g	610	44	36
Sausage Biscuit, 142 g	530	38	36
Sunrise Croissant with Bacon, 138 g	450	29	28
Sunrise Croissant with Ham, 164 g	430	26	28
Sunrise Croissant with Sausage, 161 g	550	38	29
• Sunrise Croissant, 57 g	210	10	26
Desserts			
Apple Turnover, 85 g	290	15	36
Chocolate Chip Cookie, 68 g	290	11	44
• Chocolate Malt (Hand-Dipped), 16 fl.oz.	780	35	97
Chocolate Shake (Hand-Dipped) (reg), 16 fl.oz.	700	34	85
• Single Scoop Ice Cream Bowl, 113 g	235	13	27
Single Scoop Ice Cream Cone, 126 g	285	13	37
Strawberry Malt (Hand-Dipped), 16 fl.oz.	775	35	98
Strawberry Shake (Hand-Dipped) (reg), 16 fl.oz.	700	33	86
Vanilla Malt (Hand-Dipped), 16 fl.oz.	770	35	97
Vanilla Shake (Hand-Dipped) (reg), 16 fl.oz.	710	33	87
Kids Meal			
• 2 Chicken Strips, 175 g	501	25	50
• Cheeseburger, 210 g	600	27	68
Hamburger, 197 g	560	24	67
Lunch & Dinner (Sandwiches & Burger)			
1/2 lb. Grilled Sourdough Thickburger, 381 g	1030	77	42
1/2 lb. Six Dollar Burger, 412 g	1060	73	58
1/3 lb. Bacon Cheese Thickburger, 334 g	910	64	50
1/3 lb. Cheeseburger, 254 g	680	39	52
1/3 lb. Low Carb Thickburger, 245 g	420	32	5
1/3 lb. Mushroom 'N' Swiss Thickburger, 276 g	720	42	48
1/3 lb. Thickburger, 349 g	910	64	53
1/4 lb. Double Cheeseburger, 186 g	510	26	38
1/4 lb. Double Hamburger, 161 g	420	19	37
2/3 lb. Double Bacon Cheese Thickburger, 463 g	1300	97	50
2/3 lb. Double Thickburger, 471 g	1250	90	54
• 2/3 lb. Monster Thickburger, 413 g	1420	108	46
3 Piece Chicken Strips, 145 g	380	21	27
5 Piece Chicken Strips, 241 g	630	34	45
Big Chicken Fillet Sandwich, 351 g	800	37	76
Big Hot Ham 'N' Cheese, 244 g	520	24	40
Big Roast Beef, 199 g	470	23	38
Charbroiled BBQ Chicken Sandwich, 242 g	340	4	40
Charbroiled Chicken Club Sandwich, 277 g	560	30	32
Cheeseburger, 131 g	350	16	36
• Hamburger, 118 g	310	12	36
Hot Dog, 152 g	420	30	22
Hot Ham 'N' Cheese, 191 g	420	18	39
Low Carb Charbroiled Chkn Club Sandwich, 250 g	370	21	10
Regular Roast Beef, 137 g	330	16	29
Spicy Chicken Sandwich, 159 g	470	25	46
Sides			
American Cheese slice (large), 16 g	60	5	1
Au Jus Sauce, 85 g	10	0	2
Bacon - 2 strips, 9 g	45	4	0
BBQ Sauce Dipping Sauce, 28 g	45	0	10
Chicken Gravy, 43 g	20	1	3
Cole Slaw small, 113 g	170	10	20
Crispy Curls - Medium, 132 g	410	20	52
• French Fries-Medium, 166 g	520	24	67
Fried Chicken Breast, 148 g	370	15	29
Fried Chicken Leg, 69 g	170	7	15

Hardee's (cont.)

Sides (cont.)	Cal	Fat	Cbs
Fried Chicken Thigh, 121 g	330	15	30
Fried Chicken Wing, 66 g	200	8	23
Honey Mustard Dipping Sauce, 28 g	110	9	6
Horseradish Sauce, 7 g	25	2	1
• Hot Sauce, 7 g	0	0	0
Ketchup, 9 g	10	0	2
Mashed Potatoes small, 142 g	90	2	17
Mayonnaise, 12 g	90	9	1
Peach Cobbler, 180 g	280	7	56
Ranch Dressing Dipping Sauce, 28 g	160	16	2
Sweet N Sour Dipping Sauce, 28 g	45	0	10
Swiss Cheese slice, 16 g	50	4	0

Harvey's

Breakfast	Cal	Fat	Cbs
• Bacon (3 Strips), 8 g	38	2	0
• Breakfast Club Deluxe, 264 g	478	24	33
Breakfast Club, 256 g	440	22	33
Extra Egg, 50 g	90	6	0
Homefries, 116 g	300	19	29
Sausage, 45 g	130	9	3
Toast (2 Slices White), 71 g	180	2	35
Toast (2 Slices Whole Wheat), 71 g	170	2	32
Dipping Sauces			
Creamy Caesar Dressing, 43 g	90	0	21
• Creamy Garlic Peppercorn Ranch Dressing, 43 g	160	12	13
Fat Free Honey Dijon Dressing, 43 g	80	1	17
• Light Italian Dressing, 43 g	80	0	21
Garnishes			
Bacon (Approx. 2 Slices), 5 g	25	2	0
Barbecue Sauce, 28 g	50	0	12
• Hot Peppers, 14 g	0	0	1
Ketchup, 8ml	10	0	0
Lettuce, 28 g	4	0	1
Light Mayonnaise, 15 g	45	5	1
Mustard, 7ml	5	0	0
Onions, 50 g	10	0	5
Pickle (Approx. 2 Slices), 40 g	5	0	0
• Real Canadian Cheddar Cheese Slice, 14 g	60	5	0
Relish, 20 g	20	0	5
Spicy Buffalo Sauce, 28 g	50	4	5
Tomato (Approx. 2 Slices), 50 g	10	0	2
Kids Combos			
• Cheeseburger Meal	830	35	112
• Chicken Strip Meal – 3 pcs.	610	21	92
Hamburger Meal	780	28	110
Hot Dog Meal	720	24	110
Main Menu Items			
Angus Burger w/ Cheese, 160 g	430	20	36
Angus Burger w/ Cheese, bacon, 183 g	540	29	36
Angus Burger, 146 g	370	16	36
Angus Patty only, 91 g	200	13	4
Chicken Strips – 3 Pieces, 114 g	310	16	24
Entrée Chicken Salad, 429 g	140	2	16
Entrée Garden Salad, 366 g	70	1	16
Grilled Chicken only, 117 g	170	4	1
Grilled Chicken, 183 g	340	6	32
Hot Dog only, 57 g	160	12	3
Hot Dog with Bun, 117 g	320	14	34
• Original Bacon Cheeseburger, 175 g	540	31	36
Original Cheeseburger, 160 g	440	23	35
Original Hamburger, 146 g	380	18	35
Original Patty only, 80 g	210	16	4
• Side Garden Salad, 198 g	40	0	8
Veggieburger, patty only, 73 g	150	7	7

Harvey's (cont.)

Main Menu Items (cont.)	Cal	Fat	Cbs
Veggieburger, 142 g	317	9	39
Salad Dressings			
• Creamy Caesar Dressing, 29 ml	140	14	2
Creamy Garlic Peppercorn Ranch Dressing, 29 ml	140	14	2
• Fat Free Honey Dijon Dressing, 28 ml	50	0	12
Light Italian Dressing, 28 ml	60	4	6
Side Orders			
Fries – Regular, 120 g	320	13	46
Gravy, 92 g	35	1	5
• Onion Rings – Regular, 81 g	280	14	34
• Poutine, 284 g	630	37	52

Heavenly Ham

Bone-In Hams	Cal	Fat	Cbs
• All Glaze and Visible Signs of Fat Removed, 3 oz.	159	3	4
• Glazed, 3 oz.	190	11	4
Boneless Hams			
• All Glaze and Visible Signs of Fat Removed, 3 oz.	89	1	4
• Glazed, 3 oz.	120	4	4
Classic Sandwiches			
• Dill-ectable Tuna	830	50	67
Heavenly's Famous Ham Salad	620	13	94
Perfect Turkey Salad	670	37	59
Swiss Philly	640	39	44
The Classic Roast Beef	650	39	52
The Divine Chicken Salad	790	62	36
The Heavenly Original	810	46	63
The Turkey Classic	790	36	86
• Veggie Heaven	610	37	48
Desserts			
Chocolate Chip, 1 cookie	270	12	40
• Fudge Brownie, 1 brownie	430	23	50
Heath Bar Crunch, 1 cookie	280	14	37
• Oatmeal Raisin Nut, 1 cookie	260	12	35
Peanut Butter, 1 cookie	290	18	29
White Chocolate Macadamia Nut, 1 cookie	290	15	35
Extras			
• Spinach Dip, 2 tbsp	130	14	2
• Tomato & Cucumber, 1/2 cup	60	5	5
Signature Sandwiches			
• Paradise Club	860	51	65
The Smokehouse	760	46	53
The Turkey Bistro	730	47	50
Turkey Ranch Wrangler	730	41	56
• Zesty Roast Beef	590	30	53
Soups & Salads			
Chef Salad	170	6	10
Chicken Salad	210	15	7
Chicken Salad Salad	260	17	14
• Garden Delight	35	0	6
Ham Salad	240	6	26
Ham Salad Salad	300	8	35
Heavenly Seven Bean Soup	150	2	24
• Taste of Italy Salad	490	35	14
Tuna Salad	290	25	0
Tuna Salad Salad	360	29	6
Turkey Salad	330	26	15
Spreads			
That Mustard, 1 tsp.	25	0	5
Turkeys			
Breast Whole Smoked Turkey, 3 oz.	146	8	1
• Glazed Boneless Smoked Turkey, 3 oz.	60	0	3
• Whole Roasted Turkey, 3 oz.	160	10	0

High Tech Burrito	Cal	Fat	Cbs
Asian Pan Seared Shrimp	325	13	N/A
Braised Tofu	467	10	N/A
California	475	11	N/A
Fresh Veggie	460	6	N/A
• Grilled Chicken Breast	237	8	N/A
Grilled Steak Fiesta	259	12	N/A
• Low Fat Chicken	532	10	N/A
Yellow Curry Shrimp	399	6	N/A

Hometown Buffet	Cal	Fat	Cbs

For nutritional information please see Country Buffet on pg. 122

Hooters	Cal	Fat	Cbs
Entrees			
Dozen Raw Oysters	115	4	7
• Garden Salad	115	2	22
• Grilled Big Fish Sandwich	435	5	46
Grilled Chicken Garden Salad	265	4	23
Grilled Chicken Sandwich	420	4	51
Snow Crab Legs, 1 lb	300	4	1
Steamed Shrimp	230	3	1
Side Dish			
Baked Beans	115	1	24
• Coleslaw	120	9	9
• Side Garden Salad	60	1	12

Hot Dog On A Stick	Cal	Fat	Cbs
Cheese on a Stick			
American Cheese on a Stick, 1 pc	240	13	22
Pepper Jack Cheese on a Stick, 1 pc	240	13	21
French Fries			
Fries, 7 oz.	700	37	83
Fresh Lemonade			
Cherry Lemonade, 18 oz.	230	0	58
• Lime Lemonade, 18 oz.	250	0	63
Original Lemonade, 18 oz.	210	0	52
• Sugar Free Lemonade, 18 oz.	15	0	3
Hot Dogs			
• Hot Dog on a Bun	470	26	41
Hot Dog on a Stick™	250	14	23
• Veggie Dog	180	3	24

Hungry Howie's Pizza	Cal	Fat	Cbs
Chicken Tenders			
Chicken Tenders, 2 pcs	140	5	11
Dressings			
Blue Cheese, 1 oz.	150	3	1
Creamy Italian, 1 oz.	120	2	2
Fat Free Italian, 2 oz.	25	0	5
Fat Free Ranch, 2 oz.	45	0	10
• French Style, 1 oz.	30	0	7
Greek, 1 oz.	110	2	2
Italian, 1 oz.	80	1	2
• Ranch, 1 oz.	180	3	1
Thousand Island, 1 oz.	140	2	4
Large Pizza			
Cheese Only Large Pizza, 1 slice	208	5	25
• Anchovies Topping only, 1 slice	55	3	0
Bacon Topping only, 1 slice	42	1	1
Banana Peppers Topping only, 1 slice	8	0	1
Beef Topping only, 1 slice	29	2	0
Black Olives Topping only, 1 slice	10	0	1
Green Olives Topping only, 1 slice	10	0	1
• Green Peppers Topping only, 1 slice	2	0	1
Ham Topping only, 1 slice	7	0	0
Mushroom Topping only, 1 slice	2	0	1

Hungry Howie's Pizza (cont.)	Cal	Fat	Cbs
Large Pizza (cont.)			
Onions Topping only, 1 slice	3	1	1
Pepperoni Topping only, 1 slice	22	2	0
Pineapple Topping only, 1 slice	5	1	1
Sausage Topping only, 1 slice	26	2	0
Large Thin Pizza			
Cheese Only Large Thin Pizza, 1 slice	124	6	11
• Anchovies Topping only, 1 slice	55	3	0
Bacon Topping only, 1 slice	42	1	1
Banana Peppers Topping only, 1 slice	8	0	1
Beef Topping only, 1 slice	29	2	0
Black Olives Topping only, 1 slice	10	0	1
Green Olives Topping only, 1 slice	10	0	1
• Green Peppers Topping only, 1 slice	2	0	1
Ham Topping only, 1 slice	7	0	0
Mushroom Topping only, 1 slice	2	0	1
Onions Topping only, 1 slice	3	1	1
Pepperoni Topping only, 1 slice	22	2	0
Pineapple Topping only, 1 slice	5	1	1
Sausage Topping only, 1 slice	26	2	0
Medium Pizza			
Cheese Only Medium Pizza, 1 slice	191	6	23
• Anchovies Topping only, 1 slice	44	3	0
Bacon Topping only, 1 slice	32	1	0
Banana Peppers Topping only, 1 slice	6	0	1
Beef Topping only, 1 slice	30	2	0
Black Olives Topping only, 1 slice	7	0	0
Green Olives Topping only, 1 slice	7	0	0
Green Peppers Topping only, 1 slice	2	1	0
Ham Topping only, 1 slice	7	0	0
• Mushroom Topping only, 1 slice	2	0	0
Onions Topping only, 1 slice	2	1	0
Pepperoni Topping only, 1 slice	22	2	0
Pineapple Topping only, 1 slice	5	1	2
Sausage Topping only, 1 slice	27	2	0
Medium Thin Pizza			
Cheese Only Medium Thin Pizza, 1 slice	111	5	10
• Anchovies Topping only, 1 slice	44	3	0
Bacon Topping only, 1 slice	32	1	0
Banana Peppers Topping only, 1 slice	6	0	1
Beef Topping only, 1 slice	30	2	0
Black Olives Topping only, 1 slice	7	0	0
Green Olives Topping only, 1 slice	7	0	0
Green Peppers Topping only, 1 slice	2	1	0
Ham Topping only, 1 slice	7	0	0
• Mushroom Topping only, 1 slice	2	0	0
Onions Topping only, 1 slice	2	1	0
Pepperoni Topping only, 1 slice	22	2	0
Pineapple Topping only, 1 slice	5	1	2
Sausage Topping only, 1 slice	27	2	0
Oven Baked Subs			
Deluxe Italian Sub, 1/2 sub	506	18	61
Ham & Cheese Sub, 1/2 sub	475	15	61
Pizza Special Sub, 1/2 sub	606	24	68
• Pizza Sub, 1/2 sub	689	34	67
Steak & Cheese Sub, 1/2 sub	491	15	64
Turkey Club Sub, 1/2 sub	556	15	63
• Turkey Sub, 1/2 sub	466	13	63
Vegetarian Sub, 1/2 sub	530	21	64
Salads			
Large Antipasto, 1/4 salad	101	7	3
Large Chef, 1/4 salad	99	6	4
• Large Garden, 1/4 salad	17	0	3
Large Greek, 1/4 salad	109	7	7
Small Antipasto, 1/2 salad	115	7	3

RESTAURANTS & FAST-FOOD CHAINS

Hungry Howie's Pizza (cont.)

	Cal	Fat	Cbs
Salads (cont.)			
Small Chef, 1/2 salad	114	7	4
Small Garden, 1/4 salad	20	0	3
• Small Greek, 1/2 salad	126	7	8
Sauces			
Blue Cheese Dressing, 1 oz.	152	16	1
• Dipping Sauce, 3 oz.	45	1	9
• Ranch Dressing, 1 oz.	175	19	1
Small Pizza			
Cheese Only Pizza, 1 slice	161	4	20
• Anchovies Topping only, 1 slice	34	3	0
Bacon Topping only, 1 slice	23	0	0
Banana Peppers Topping only, 1 slice	5	0	0
Beef Topping only, 1 slice	21	1	0
Black Olives Topping only, 1 slice	5	0	0
Green Olives Topping only, 1 slice	5	0	0
• Green Peppers Topping only, 1 slice	1	0	0
Ham Topping only	6	0	0
Mushroom Topping only	2	0	0
Onions Topping only	1	0	0
Pepperoni Topping only	20	2	0
Pineapple Topping only, 1 slice	4	0	1
Sausage Topping only, 1 slice	20	1	0
Wings			
Howie Wings, 5 wings	180	13	0
X-Large Pizza			
Cheese Only Extra Large Pizza, 1 slice	395	9	395
• Anchovies Topping only, 1 slice	88	5	88
Bacon Topping only, 1 slice	52	1	52
Banana Peppers Topping only, 1 slice	12	0	12
Beef Topping only, 1 slice	37	3	37
Black Olives Topping only, 1 slice	11	1	11
Green Olives Topping only, 1 slice	11	1	11
• Green Peppers Topping only, 1 slice	2	0	2
Ham Topping only, 1 slice	8	1	8
Mushroom Topping only, 1 slice	3	0	3
Onions Topping only, 1 slice	3	1	3
Pepperoni Topping only, 1 slice	26	2	26
Pineapple Topping only, 1 slice	6	1	6
Sausage Topping only, 1 slice	33	2	33

In-N-Out Burger

	Cal	Fat	Cbs
Burgers			
Cheeseburger w/Onion, 268 g	480	27	39
Protein® Style (no bun), 300 g	330	25	11
with mustard & ketchup, no spread, 268 g	400	18	41
• Double-Double® w/ Onion, 330 g	670	41	39
Protein® Style (no bun), 362 g	520	39	11
with mustard & ketchup, no spread, 330 g	590	32	41
Hamburger w/ Onion, 243 g	390	19	39
• Protein® Style (no bun), 275 g	240	17	11
with mustard & ketchup, no spread, 243 g	310	10	41
Shakes			
• Chocolate Shake, 15 oz.	690	36	83
Strawberry Shake, 15 oz.	690	33	91
• Vanilla Shake, 15 oz.	680	37	78
Sides			
French Fries, 125 g	400	18	54

Islands Restaurants

	Cal	Fat	Cbs
Appetizers			
Cheddar Fries, 4 oz.	310	20	27
• Chips & Salsa, 4 oz.	290	12	43
Island Fries, 5 oz.	420	31	32
Nachos, 4 oz.	400	29	20
Onion Rings, 4 oz.	380	15	55

Islands Restaurants (cont.)

	Cal	Fat	Cbs
Appetizers (cont.)			
Quesadilla, 4 oz.	290	20	18
Spinach-Artichoke Dip w/ Chips, 4 oz.	290	19	25
Tiki Tenders, 5 oz.	360	21	15
• Wings - Buffalo Style, 11 oz.	780	60	10
Burgers			
Big Wave w/ Cheese, 17 oz.	1220	75	69
Big Wave, 15 oz.	990	57	63
Bleunami, 16 oz.	1290	88	65
Hawaiian, 19 oz.	1450	91	85
Hula, 20 oz.	1390	90	70
• Kilauea, 20 oz.	1650	115	80
Maui, 18 oz.	1430	96	72
Pipeline, 20 oz.	1430	91	72
Sunset, 18 oz.	1250	75	75
• Veggie, 11 oz.	630	24	90
Dessert			
Chocolate Lava Dessert, 5 oz.	480	29	50
Kona Pie, 4 oz.	350	23	34
Gremmie			
Gremmie Fries, 4 oz.	290	17	32
Jr. Quesadilla w/ applesauce/carrots, 10 oz.	560	26	72
• Jr. Sundae, 3 oz.	220	15	17
Jr. Tiki Tenders w/ applesauce/carrots, 12 oz.	630	24	69
Jr. Wave w/chz, w/ applesauce/carrots, 14 oz.	760	40	65
Lil Chili Chz Dogger w/ applesauce/carrots, 16 oz.	1050	71	66
Lil Dogger w/ applesauce/carrots, 11 oz.	630	36	62
Sandcastle w/ applesauce/carrots, 10 oz.	520	21	66
Salads			
• Caesar - small, 5 oz.	270	20	14
China Coast, 25 oz.	1130	73	75
Garden salad, 8 oz.	300	27	3
Jungle Caesar - w/ chicken, 18 oz.	760	43	25
• Kaanapali Kobb, 30 oz.	1520	116	21
Wiqui Waqui, 29 oz.	960	53	47
Sandwiches & Other Items			
Moa kai (Tuna), 14 oz.	1310	101	65
• Rotisserie Chicken, 35 oz.	1650	80	148
Sandpiper, 18 oz.	1020	51	70
• Shorebird, 14 oz.	990	50	69
Toucan, 15 oz.	1050	52	79
Wedge, 12 oz.	1320	100	62
Soup			
Tortilla Soup - bowl, 12 oz.	320	20	20
Tortilla Soup - Large, 23 oz.	630	39	40
Tacos			
Baja, 23 oz.	870	35	70
• Cabo Loco, 19 oz.	1480	104	65
Islands Fish, 19 oz.	1320	84	100
• Northshore, 19 oz.	790	30	67
Yaki, 20 oz.	960	34	85

Jack in the Box

	Cal	Fat	Cbs
Breakfast			
Bacon Breakfast Jack®, 113 g	300	14	29
Bacon, Egg & Cheese Biscuit, 149 g	430	25	34
Blueberry French Toast Sticks, 121 g	450	20	59
Breakfast Jack®, 125 g	290	12	29
Chicken Biscuit, 154 g	450	24	42
Ciabatta Breakfast Sandwich, 278 g	710	36	63
Extreme Sausage® Sandwich, 213 g	670	48	31
• Hash Brown, 57 g	150	10	12
Meaty Breakfast Burrito, 183 g	480	29	29
Original French Toast Sticks, 121 g	470	23	58
Sausage Biscuit, 131 g	440	29	32
Sausage Breakfast Jack®, 154 g	450	28	29

Jack in the Box (cont.)

	Cal	Fat	Cbs
Breakfast (cont.)			
Sausage Croissant, 174 g	580	39	37
Sausage, Egg & Cheese Biscuit, 234 g	740	55	35
Sirloin Steak & Egg Burrito no Salsa, 289 g	790	48	52
• Sirloin Steak & Egg Burrito w/ Salsa, 312 g	790	48	54
Spicy Chicken Biscuit, 169 g	460	22	44
Supreme Croissant, 151 g	450	25	36
Ultimate Breakfast Sandwich, 249 g	570	27	49
Burgers & More			
Bacon 'n' Cheese Ciabatta Burger, 395 g	1120	76	66
Bacon Ultimate Cheeseburger, 338 g	1090	77	53
BBQ Bacon Sirloin Burger, 336 g	1010	49	91
Hamburger deluxe, 169 g	370	21	31
with Cheese, 194 g	460	28	33
• Hamburger, 118 g	310	14	30
with Cheese, 131 g	350	17	31
Jumbo Jack®, 261 g	600	35	51
with Cheese, 286 g	690	42	54
Junior Bacon Cheeseburger, 131 g	430	25	30
• Sirloin Bcn Chz Burger w/ Onions, 422 g	1160	76	61
Sirloin Chz Brgr w/ Grilled Onions, 421 g	1070	71	61
Sirloin Steak Melt, 277 g	640	40	34
Sngle Bacon Chz Ciabatta Burger, 308 g	870	54	66
Sourdough Jack®, 245 g	710	51	36
Sourdough Ultimate Cheeseburger, 291 g	950	73	36
Ultimate Cheeseburger, 323 g	1010	71	53
Chicken & Fish			
Bacon Chicken Sandwich, 152 g	440	24	39
Chicken Breast Strips (4), 201 g	500	25	36
• Chicken Fajita Pita - no salsa, 185 g	280	9	30
Chicken Sandwich, 145 g	400	21	38
Chipotle Chkn Ciabatta™ with Grilled Chkn, 312 g	690	28	65
w/ Spicy Crispy Chkn, 297 g	750	34	75
Fish & Chips - medium, 250 g	660	34	70
Jack's Spicy Chicken®, 270 g	620	31	61
w/ Cheese, 294 g	700	37	62
• Sirloin Steak 'n' Cheddar Ciabatta, 325 g	770	38	65
Sourdough Grilled Chicken Club, 266 g	530	28	34
Kids Meal			
• Applesauce (1 portion cup), 113 g	100	0	25
Chicken Breast Strips (2), 100 g	250	12	18
Grilled Cheese, 94 g	330	18	31
Hamburger, 118 g	310	14	30
w/ cheese, 131 g	350	17	31
• Natural Cut Fries kids portion, 82 g	220	11	27
Salads			
Asian Chkn Salad (w/ Grilled Chkn), 365 g	160	2	18
(w/ Crispy Chicken), 394 g	330	13	34
Chkn Club Salad (w/ Grilled Chkn), 373 g	320	16	11
(w/ Crispy Chicken), 402 g	480	27	28
• Side Salad, 123 g	50	3	5
SW Chkn Salad (w/ Grilled Chkn), 430 g	320	12	27
(w/ Crispy Chicken), 459 g	480	23	44
Sauces & Dressings			
Asian Sesame Dressing, 71 g	230	17	20
Bacon Ranch Dressing, 71 g	320	33	4
Barbecue Dipping Sauce, 28 g	45	0	11
Buttermilk House Dipping Sauce, 25 g	130	13	3
Creamy Southwest Dressing, 71 g	270	27	4
Franks® Red Hot® Buffalo Dipping Sauce, 28 g	10	0	2
Lite Ranch Dressing, 71 g	190	18	3
Log Cabin® Syrup, 62 g	190	0	49
Low Fat Balsamic Dressing, 71 g	40	2	6
Mayo-Onion Sauce (0.5 oz), 14 g	90	10	1
• Ranch Dressing, 71 g	390	41	4

Jack in the Box (cont.)

	Cal	Fat	Cbs
Sauces & Dressings (cont.)			
Soy Sauce, 9 g	5	0	1
Sweet & Sour Dipping Sauce, 28 g	45	0	11
• Taco Sauce, 9 g	0	0	0
Tartar Sauce, 43 g	210	22	2
Zesty Marinara Dipping Sauce, 25 g	15	0	4
Shakes & Desserts			
Cheesecake, 103 g	310	16	34
Chocolate Ice Cream Shake, 16 oz.	880	45	107
• Chocolate Overload Cake, 93 g	300	7	57
Egg Nog Shake, 16 oz.	870	44	103
• OREO® Cookie Ice Cream Shake, 16 oz.	910	49	102
Strawberry Ice Cream Shake, 16 oz.	880	44	105
Vanilla Ice Cream Shake, 16 oz.	790	44	83
Snacks & Extras			
Bacon Cheddar Potato Wedges, 257 g	720	48	52
Beef Monster Taco®, 112 g	240	14	20
Egg Roll (1), 57 g	130	6	15
Egg Rolls (3), 170 g	400	19	44
• Fruit Cup, 198 g	90	0	22
Mozzarella Cheese Sticks (3), 71 g	240	12	21
Natural Cut Fries - medium, 166 g	450	23	54
Onion Rings (8), 119 g	500	30	51
Regular Beef Taco, 76 g	160	8	15
• Sampler Trio, 236 g	750	39	65
Seasoned Curly Fries - medium, 125 g	400	23	45
Spicy Chicken Bites (7), 93 g	290	14	21
Stuffed Jalapeños (3), 72 g	230	13	22

Jack's

	Cal	Fat	Cbs
Breakfast Items			
Bacon Biscuit	290	15	31
Biscuit	250	11	31
Biscuit w/butter	350	23	31
• Egg and Cheese Biscuit	550	34	35
• Eggs	190	13	3
Sausage Biscuit	400	25	31
Chicken & Sides			
Chicken Breast	321	19	9
• Chicken Fingers, 3 Pieces	470	24	33
Chicken Leg	150	10	5
Chicken Thigh	260	19	9
Chicken Wings	170	12	6
• Mashed Potatoes, 4 oz.	70	1	15
Healthy Choice			
• Crispy Chicken	430	26	22
Grilled Chicken	260	12	7
Grilled Chicken Sandwich	410	15	44
Grits	100	8	8
• Side Salad	70	5	3
Spring Salad	170	11	7
Low Carb Items			
• 4 oz. Burger Patty w/cheese & 4 oz. green beans	670	48	10
• Eggs & Bacon Platter w/ 2 eggs & 3 slices bacon	250	18	3
Grilled Chkn w/ 4 oz. Green Beans & Cole Slaw	320	16	22
Sandwiches & Fries			
Big Bacon	700	42	45
Big Jack	500	27	40
Cheeseburger	380	17	35
• Double Big Jack Cheese	930	60	43
Double Cheeseburger	590	33	37
• Hamburger	270	8	35

Jamba Juice

	Cal	Fat	Cbs
All Fruit			
Mega Mango, 24 fl.oz.	340	1	85

RESTAURANTS & FAST-FOOD CHAINS

Jamba Juice (cont.)

All Fruit (cont.)	Cal	Fat	Cbs
Peach Perfection, 24 fl.oz.	320	1	78
• Pomegranate Paradise, 24 fl.oz.	340	1	86
• Strawberry Whirl, 24 fl.oz.	310	1	76
Baked Goods			
Apple Cinnamon Pretzel, 5 oz.	380	4	76
Blueberry Oatcake, 3 oz.	280	10	42
• Omega-3 Choc. Brownie Cookie, 1.5 oz.	150	4	30
Omega-3 Oatmeal Cookie, 2 oz.	150	6	26
Reduced-Fat Blueberry Lemon Loaf, 3 oz.	290	8	53
Reduced-Fat Cranberry Orange Loaf, 3 oz.	310	9	52
• Sourdough Parmesan Pretzel, 5 oz.	410	10	67
Zucchini Walnut Loaf, 3 oz.	270	9	43
Blended with A Purpose			
• 3 g Energizer, 24 fl.oz.	470	2	110
Acai Super-Antidoxidant, 24 fl.oz.	420	6	86
Coldbuster, 24 fl.oz.	410	3	95
• Fit n' Fruitful, 24 fl.oz.	370	4	84
Pomegranate Heart Defender, 24 fl.oz.	440	1	103
Protein Berry w/ Soy Protein, 24 fl.oz.	430	2	88
Protein Berry w /Whey, 24 fl.oz.	390	1	80
Boosts			
• 3 g Charger Super Boost, 3 g	5	0	2
Green Caffeine Boost, 2.7 g	5	0	2
Omega-3 Super Boost, 10 g	30	2	7
Soy Protein Boost, 8.9 g	30	N/A	N/A
Weight Burner Super Boost, 3.5 g	30	3	N/A
• Whey Protein Super Boost, 12 g	45	0	1
Creamy Indulgences			
• Matcha Green Tea Blast, 24 fl.oz.	440	1	97
Orange Dream Machine, 24 fl.oz.	490	2	107
• Peanut Butter Moo'd, 24 fl.oz.	840	21	139
Fresh Squeezed Juices			
Carrot Juice, 16 fl.oz.	90	1	22
Orange Juice, 16 fl.oz.	220	1	52
Jamba Classic			
Aloha Pineapple, 24 fl.oz.	470	2	111
Banana Berry, 24 fl.oz.	450	2	106
Caribbean Passion, 24 fl.oz.	420	2	97
Citrus Squeeze, 24 fl.oz.	440	2	104
Mango-a-go-go, 24 fl.oz.	470	2	110
• Orange a Peel, 24 fl.oz.	400	1	93
Peach Pleasure, 24 fl.oz.	440	2	104
Razzmatazz, 24 fl.oz.	440	2	102
Strawberries Wild, 24 fl.oz.	400	1	94
Strawberry Surf Rider, 24 fl.oz.	490	2	119
Jamba Light			
Berry Fulfilling, 24 fl.oz.	260	1	57
• Mango Mantra, 24 fl.oz.	280	1	64
• Strawberry Nirvana, 24 fl.oz.	250	1	55
Juices			
Orange Carrot Banana, 16 fl.oz.	170	1	40
Orange Mango Passion, 16 fl.oz.	180	1	43
Shots			
Matcha Green Tea Shot-OJ, 4 fl.oz.	60	0	13
• Matcha Green Tea Shot-Soy Milk, 4 fl.oz.	80	0	16
• Wheatgrass Shot, 1 fl.oz.	5	0	1
Wheatgrass Shot, 2 fl.oz.	15	0	1
Smoothies with Organic Granola			
• Berry Topper, 16 fl.oz.	490	10	89
• Chunky Strawberry, 16 fl.oz.	570	17	91
Mango Peach Topper, 16 fl.oz.	500	10	95
Yogurt & Fruit Blends			
• Bright Eyed & Blueberry, 16 fl.oz.	220	1	43
Bright Eyed & Blueberry, 24 fl.oz.	350	1	70

Jamba Juice (cont.)

Yogurt & Fruit Blends (cont.)	Cal	Fat	Cbs
Sunrise Strawberry, 16 fl.oz.	240	1	49
• Sunrise Strawberry, 24 fl.oz.	380	1	78

Jimboy's Tacos

Burritos	Cal	Fat	Cbs
Bean, 255 g	530	28	55
• Chicken, 213 g	590	29	45
• Ground Beef, 213 g	610	32	50
Shredded Beef, 213 g	540	24	45
Combo Burritos			
• Chicken, 284 g	580	28	52
• Ground Beef, 284 g	620	33	57
Shredded Beef, 284 g	580	28	53
Dessert			
ChocoTaco, 113 g	390	21	47
Dinner Plates			
Bean Burrito, 255 g	530	28	55
Bean Taco, 112 g	190	12	16
Cheese Enchilada, 168 g	390	27	16
Chicken Combo Burrito, 284 g	580	28	52
Chicken Enchilada, 168 g	320	18	16
Chicken Taco, 106 g	200	11	12
Chile Relleno, 128 g	300	24	8
Combination Plate Base, 354 g	470	15	71
• Ground Beef Combo Burrito, 284 g	620	33	57
Ground Beef Enchilada, 168 g	330	20	19
Ground Beef Taco, 106 g	220	14	14
Shredded Beef Combo Burrito, 284 g	580	28	53
Shredded Beef Enchilada, 168 g	300	17	16
• Shredded Beef Taco, 106 g	190	11	13
El Gordos			
Chicken, 208 g	400	20	29
• Ground Beef, 208 g	460	25	35
Shredded Beef, 208 g	400	19	30
• Steak, 222 g	400	18	33
Enchiladas			
Cheese (Includes Rice), 168 g	350	20	28
Chicken (Includes Rice), 253 g	460	21	42
• Ground Beef (Includes Rice), 253 g	470	23	45
• Shredded Beef (Includes Rice), 168 g	300	17	16
Kid's Meals			
• Cheese Quesadilla & Chips, 166 g	690	40	63
Ground Beef Taco & Chips, 170 g	510	29	51
• Kid-Size Bean Burrito & Chips, 179 g	480	25	54
Quesadillas			
• Cheese, 109 g	400	25	27
Chicken, 144 g	450	26	28
• Ground Beef, 144 g	480	29	31
Shredded Beef, 144 g	450	26	28
Side Orders			
6" Corn Tortilla, 27 g	60	1	12
8" Flour Tortilla, 52 g	170	4	28
Corn Chips, 69 g	280	15	36
• French Fries, 250 g	700	34	89
Side Cheese Sauce, 2 oz.	70	4	7
Side Guacamole, 2 oz.	90	8	4
• Side Salsa Cruda, 2 oz.	10	0	2
Side Sour Cream, 2 oz.	110	11	2
Super Burritos			
Chicken, 406 g	630	31	58
• Ground Beef, 392 g	670	35	63
Shredded Beef, 392 g	610	29	58
• Steak, 401 g	600	28	59
Super Nachos			
• Chicken, 420 g	830	45	86

(• = most healthy   = least healthy)   **Restaurants & Fast-Food Chains   75**

RESTAURANTS & FAST-FOOD CHAINS

Jimboy's Tacos (cont.)

	Cal	Fat	Cbs
Super Nachos (cont.)			
• Ground Beef, 393 g	780	40	78
Shredded Beef, 420 g	830	44	87
Taco Salads			
• Bean, 513 g	530	29	50
• Ground Beef, 584 g	660	37	56
Chicken, 584 g	610	31	50
Shredded Beef, 584 g	610	31	51
Tacoburger			
Ground Beef (Patty), 183 g	370	27	17
Tacos			
Bean, 112 g	190	12	16
Chicken, 106 g	200	11	12
Ground Beef, 106 g	220	14	15
• Jimboy's Fish Taco, 129 g	233	15	16
Shredded Beef, 106 g	190	11	13
• Steak, 134 g	190	10	15
Taquitos			
Ground Beef (3 in a serving), 90 g	230	17	16
The Works			
• Guacamole & Sour Cream, 61 g	90	8	4
• Guacamole, 34 g	35	3	2
Sour Cream, 42 g	50	5	2
Tostadas			
• Bean, 241 g	290	20	23
Chicken, 276 g	330	21	23
• Ground Beef, 276 g	360	24	26
Shredded Beef, 276 g	330	21	23
Vegetarian			
Bean Burrito, 255 g	530	28	55
Bean Taco, 112 g	190	12	16
Bean Tostada, 241 g	290	20	23
Cheese Enchilada & Rice, 168 g	350	20	28
Cheese Quesadilla, 109 g	400	25	27
• Chile Relleno & Rice, 304 g	530	32	40
Reg.Nachos (Chips & Cheese), 162 g	360	19	43
• Side Pinto Beans, 213 g	180	11	16
Side Spanish Rice, 164 g	260	5	48
Veggie Burrito, 354 g	500	17	72

Jimmy John's

	Cal	Fat	Cbs
8" Sub Sandwiches			
Big John®, 270 g	564	27	54
J.J.B.L.T.™, 238 g	662	35	54
• Pepe®, 298 g	684	37	55
• Totally Tuna™, 357 g	507	20	58
Turkey Tom®, 282 g	555	26	54
Vegetarian, 302 g	640	36	57
Vito®, 289 g	579	25	56
Giant Club Sandwiches			
Beach Club®, 409 g	796	37	78
Billy Club®, 416 g	867	40	77
• Bootlegger Club®, 377 g	720	28	74
Club Lulu™, 339 g	790	34	74
Club Tuna®, 429 g	724	29	79
Country Club®, 405 g	840	38	75
Gourmet Smoked Ham Club, 399 g	851	37	76
Gourmet Veggie Club®, 374 g	856	46	77
Hunter's Club®, 411 g	854	38	76
• Italian Night Club®, 422 g	975	52	77
Low-Carb Options			
Hunter's Club® Unwich, 357 g	520	38	8
The J.J. Gargantuan™ Unwich, 488 g	769	55	11
Low-Fat Options			
Slim 4 Turkey Breast, 207 g	407	1	70
Turkey Tom®, 282 g	555	26	54

Jimmy John's (cont.)

	Cal	Fat	Cbs
Plain Slims			
Slim 1 Ham & Cheese, 235 g	539	12	72
Slim 2 Roast Beef, 207 g	419	2	71
Slim 3 Tuna Salad, 272 g	582	19	74
• Slim 4 Turkey Breast, 207 g	407	1	70
Slim 5 Salami, Capicola, Cheese, 232 g	624	21	72
Slim 6 Double Provolone, 206 g	588	19	71
• The J.J. Gargantuan™, 504 g	1008	55	60
Side Items			
BBQ Jimmy Chips, 30 g	160	9	17
• Chocolate Chunk Cookie, 99 g	421	18	62
Jalapeño Chips, 30 g	150	7	18
• Pickle, Spear, 25 g	4	0	1
Pickle, Whole, 100 g	15	0	3
Raisin Oatmeal Cookie, 105 g	421	16	65
Regular Chips, 30 g	160	8	18
Sea Salt & Vinegar Chips, 30 g	140	8	16

Johnny Rockets

	Cal	Fat	Cbs
Chicken & Salads			
• Chicken Club Sandwich, 371 g	1068	39	126
Chicken Tenders, 213 g	520	22	47
Crispy Chicken Club Salad, 434 g	651	40	46
• Garden Salad, 305 g	271	19	21
Grilled Chicken Breast Sandwich, 271 g	632	33	52
Grilled Chicken Club Salad, 420 g	529	33	23
Desserts			
• A La Mode, 113 g	260	16	26
• Apple Pie, 293 g	930	59	88
Hot Fudge Sundae, 290 g	830	47	93
Fountain			
Add Malt, 14 g	60	2	10
• Big Apple Shake, 670 g	1585	90	175
Butterfinger® Shake, 517 g	1020	58	114
Chocolate Peanut Butter Shake, 510 g	1000	62	80
• Float, 411 g	420	26	42
Hershey's® Chocolate Shake, 574 g	1100	60	120
Mocha Fudge Shake, 488 g	870	52	89
Oreo® Cookies & Cream Shake, 517 g	1040	60	114
Strawberry Shake, 574 g	810	48	82
Strawberry-Banana Shake, 573 g	890	49	102
Vanilla Shake, 574 g	1120	60	131
Kids Fountain			
Add Malt, 8 g	36	1	6
• Big Apple, 402 g	951	36	79
Butterfinger® Shake, 310 g	612	35	68
Chocolate Peanut Butter Shake, 306 g	600	37	48
• Float, 247 g	252	16	25
Hershey's® Chocolate Shake, 344 g	660	36	72
Kids Jr. Sundae, 226 g	580	32	65
Mocha Fudge Shake, 293 g	522	31	53
Oreo® Cookies & Cream Shake, 310 g	624	36	68
Strawberry Shake, 344 g	486	29	49
Strawberry-banana Shake, 344 g	534	29	61
Vanilla Shake, 344 g	672	36	79
Kids Menu			
American Fries, 114 g	266	12	39
• Kids Chicken Tenders, 107 g	260	11	24
Kids Grilled Cheese, 87 g	386	18	40
Kids Hamburger, 121 g	378	17	38
Kids Hot Dog, 133 g	422	24	38
• Kids Peanut Butter & Jelly, 138 g	457	17	64
Original Hamburgers			
#12, 349 g	880	57	58
• Chili, 464 g	1254	84	67
Patty Melt, 261 g	786	48	48

RESTAURANTS & FAST-FOOD CHAINS

Johnny Rockets (cont.)

	Cal	Fat	Cbs
Original Hamburgers (cont.)			
Rocket Double®, 406 g	1192	79	58
Rocket Single®, 296 g	832	52	57
Route 66, 301 g	911	63	53
Smoke House, 294 g	972	60	60
St. Louis, 313 g	991	68	53
• Streamliner®, 299 g	422	11	60
The Original, 322 g	790	50	57
Turkey Single, 287 g	732	42	56
Other Favorites			
Bacon, Lettuce & Tomato, 201 g	491	30	42
• Chili Dog, 289 g	815	55	46
Egg Salad Sandwich, 313 g	688	49	41
Grilled Cheese, 151 g	542	30	40
Grilled Ham & Cheese, 243 g	514	24	40
• Hot Dog, 133 g	422	24	38
Philly Cheese Steak, 361 g	715	30	58
Tuna Melt, 300 g	754	45	40
Tuna Salad Sandwich, 313 g	708	46	41
Starters			
American Fries, 227 g	531	23	77
Cheese Fries, 284 g	759	42	78
• Chili Bowl, 369 g	872	69	24
Half Fries & Half Rings, 264 g	720	36	92
Onion Rings, 193 g	500	34	22
Rocket Wings® – Large Order, 276 g	538	20	33
• Rocket Wings® – Regular Order, 138 g	323	10	17

Kentucky Fried Chicken

	Cal	Fat	Cbs
Chicken			
• Extra Crispy Breast, 162 g	440	27	15
Extra Crispy Drumstick, 60 g	160	10	6
Extra Crispy Thigh, 114 g	370	28	12
Extra Crispy Whole Wing, 52 g	170	11	6
Original Breast w/o skin, breading, 108 g	140	2	1
Original Breast, 161 g	360	21	7
• Original Drumstick, 59 g	130	8	2
Original Thigh, 126 g	330	24	8
Original Whole Wing, 47 g	130	8	4
Desserts			
Apple Pie Mini's (3), 114 g	370	20	44
Double Choc. Chip Cake, 76 g	330	16	41
Lil' Bucket™ Chocolate Cream, 113 g	280	13	38
• Lil' Bucket™ Lemon Crème, 127 g	410	15	61
Lil' Bucket™ Strawberry Short Cake, 99 g	210	7	33
Sweet Life Chocolate Chip Cookie, 35 g	160	7	23
Sweet Life Oatmeal Raisin Cookie, 35 g	150	5	24
Sweet Life Sugar Cookie, 35 g	160	6	23
• Teddy Grahams®, Cinnamon, 21 g	90	3	15
Popcorn Chicken			
Popcorn Chicken-Individual, 116 g	400	26	22
• Popcorn Chicken-Kids, 85 g	290	19	16
• Popcorn Chicken-Large, 160 g	550	35	30
Pot Pie / Bowls			
• Chicken and Biscuit Bowl, 481 g	870	44	88
Chicken Pot Pie, 423 g	770	40	70
KFC Bowls™-Mshd Potato w/ Gravy, 531 g	740	35	80
• KFC Bowls™-Rice w/ Gravy, 384 g	620	28	67
Salads & More			
Caesar Side Salad w/o Dressing/croutons, 82 g	50	3	2
Crispy BLT Salad w/o Dressing, 360 g	330	17	18
• Crspy Caesar Salad w/o Dressing/croutons, 315 g	350	19	16
Hidden Valley® Ranch Dressing, 57 g	200	20	3
Hidden Valley® Golden Italian Light Dressing, 43 g	45	3	6
Hidden Valley® Ranch Fat Free Dressing, 43 g	35	0	8
• House Side Salad w/o Dressing, 90 g	15	0	2

Kentucky Fried Chicken (cont.)

	Cal	Fat	Cbs
Salads & More (cont.)			
KFC® Creamy Parmesan Caesar Dressing, 57 g	260	26	4
KFC® Parmesan Garlic Croutons Pouch, 14 g	60	3	8
Roasted BLT Salad w/o Dressing, 347 g	200	6	8
Rsted Caesar Salad w/o Dressing/croutons, 301 g	220	8	6
Sandwiches			
• Crispy Twister®, 252 g	550	28	49
Double Crunch Sandwich, 213 g	470	23	38
Honey BBQ Sandwich, 147 g	280	4	40
KFC Snacker®, 119 g	290	13	29
Buffalo, 118 g	260	8	31
Fish w/o Sauce, 108 g	290	12	29
Fish, 120 g	330	15	31
• Honey BBQ, 101 g	210	3	32
Ultimate Cheese, 120 g	280	11	30
Oven Roasted Twister®, 269 g	420	17	40
w/o Sauce, 247 g	330	7	39
Tender Roast® Sandwich, 236 g	380	13	29
w/o Sauce, 217 g	300	5	28
Sides (Individual)			
Baked Beans, 136 g	220	1	45
Biscuit, 57 g	220	11	24
Cole Slaw, 130 g	180	10	22
Corn on the Cob (3"), 82 g	70	2	13
Corn on the Cob (5.5"), 162 g	150	3	26
• Green Beans, 96 g	50	2	7
Macaroni and Cheese, 136 g	180	8	18
Mashed Potatoes with Gravy, 151 g	140	5	20
Mashed Potatoes without Gravy, 108 g	110	4	17
Potato Salad, 128 g	180	9	22
• Potato Wedges, 102 g	260	13	33
Seasoned Rice, 99 g	150	1	32
Strips			
Crispy Strips, 2 strips	240	13	11
Crispy Strips, 3 strips	350	19	16
Wings			
Boneless Fiery Buffalo Wings, 5 wings	420	20	33
Boneless Honey BBQ Wings, 5 wings	450	20	41
Boneless Sweet & Spicy Wings, 5 wings	440	19	38
• Boneless Teriyaki Wings, 5 wings	500	21	50
• Fiery Buffalo Wings, 5 wings	380	24	19
HBBQ Wings, 5 wings	390	24	23
Hot Wings®, 5 wings	350	24	14
Sweet & Spicy Wings, 5 wings	400	24	24
Teriyaki Wings, 5 wings	480	25	40

Kilwin's

	Cal	Fat	Cbs
Almond Bark, Milk Chocolate, 40 g	221	14	22
Almond Bark, White Chocolate, 40 g	221	13	24
Almond Butter Brickle, 40 g	218	14	23
Almond Cluster - Dark Chocolate, 40 g	221	16	18
Almond Cluster - Milk Chocolate, 40 g	226	16	18
Almond Toffee Crunch Bar, 40 g	192	13	18
Almond Toffee Crunch, 40 g	220	15	20
Almonds rstd & salted, 40 g	210	12	23
Almonds, Dark Chocolate, 40 g	225	16	19
Almonds, Milk Chocolate, 40 g	219	15	20
Amaretto Truffle, 40 g	237	17	21
Apricots, Dark Chocolate, 40 g	140	5	24
Apricots, Milk Chocolate, 40 g	142	5	24
Bavarian Cream, 40 g	167	6	28
Black Licorice Twist, 40 g	143	0	39
Bombe' Truffle, 40 g	230	17	21
Brugg Truffle, 40 g	230	17	21
Butter Pecan Fudge, 40 g	242	17	22
Caramel Assortment, 40 g	184	9	26

Kilwin's (cont.)	Cal	Fat	Cbs
Caramel Assortment, 40 g	233	16	22
Caramel Corn, 40 g	207	13	22
Caramel Sucker, 40 g	163	9	20
Caramel Topping, 40 g	107	5	15
Caramellows, Dark Chocolate, 40 g	173	9	23
Caramellows, Milk Chocolate, 40 g	178	8	24
Caramels, Dark Chocolate, 40 g	182	9	26
Caramels, Milk Chocolate, 40 g	185	8	27
Cashew Brittle, 40 g	195	10	28
Cashew Cluster - Milk Chocolate, 40 g	228	17	16
Cashew Cluster, Dark Chocolate, 40 g	225	17	16
Cashew Tuttles, Dark Chocolate, 40 g	205	13	21
Cashew Tuttles, Milk Chocolate, 40 g	207	13	21
Cashews, Dark Chocolate, 40 g	252	21	15
Cashews, Milk Chocolate, 40 g	222	16	18
Cashews, rstd & salted, 40 g	246	23	9
Chausse' Truffle, 40 g	240	17	20
Cherri Suisse Truffle, 40 g	232	16	21
Cherry Coins, 40 g	205	9	16
Cherry Cordial Assortment, 40 g	175	7	28
Cherry Cordial Assortment, 40 g	184	9	26
Cherry Cordial, Dark Chocolate, 40 g	173	7	28
Cherry Cordials, Milk Chocolate, 40 g	177	7	28
Chocolate Berryblues, 40 g	170	9	21
Chocolate Blackberries, 40 g	220	16	18
Chocolate Bon Bon, 40 g	167	6	29
Chocolate Card "Thank You", 40 g	153	9	17
Chocolate Coffee Beans, 40 g	178	7	29
Chocolate Cream, Dark Chocolate, 40 g	166	6	28
Chocolate Cream, Milk Chocolate, 40 g	168	6	28
Chocolate Espresso Beans, 40 g	200	12	23
Chocolate Fudge, 40 g	174	5	31
Chocolate Ice Cream Suckers, 40 g	135	4	26
Chocolate Jordan Almonds, 40 g	220	15	18
Chocolate Peanut Butter Fudge, 40 g	176	6	29
Chocolate Pecan Fudge, 40 g	169	5	31
Chocolate Star Pop, 40 g	231	14	23
Chocolate Toffee Almonds, 40 g	220	15	18
Chocolate Walnut Fudge, 40 g	175	6	31
Cinnamon Roasted Almond, 40 g	137	0	34
Coconut Cluster, Dark Chocolate, 40 g	204	12	24
Coconut Cluster, Milk Chocolate, 40 g	209	12	24
Coconut Macaroon, Dark Chocolate, 40 g	233	13	26
Coffee Truffle, 40 g	233	16	21
Custom Coin Dark Mint Chocolate, 40 g	350	21	37
Custom Gold Coins Milk Chocolate, 40 g	229	14	25
Custom Silver Coins Milk Chocolate, 40 g	221	14	25
Dark Chocolate Almonds, 40 g	210	13	21
Dark Chocolate Bar, 40 g	310	21	28
Dark Chocolate Break-up, 40 g	210	13	23
Dark Chocolate Heart, 40 g	221	14	25
Dark Chocolate Sea Foam, 40 g	130	0	32
Family Assortment, 40 g	209	13	23
Family Assortment, 40 g	206	12	24
Family Assortment, 40 g	209	13	23
Family Assortment, 40 g	204	12	23
• Flavored Swizzle Stick, 40 g	50	0	14
Fontineau Truffle, 40 g	229	16	21
French Chocolate, 40 g	198	11	24
French Mint Truffle, 40 g	226	15	23
Gourmet Chocolate Nut Mix, 40 g	220	16	18
Gourmet Nut Mix, 40 g	220	15	18
Gummi Bears, 40 g	140	0	34
Gummi Pet Crocodile, 40 g	130	0	32
Gummy Bears, 40 g	158	0	40

Kilwin's (cont.)	Cal	Fat	Cbs
Hazelnut Truffle, 40 g	233	17	21
Heavenly Hash, 40 g	183	8	26
Holland Mints, 40 g	160	5	32
Irish Cream Truffle, 40 g	233	16	21
Jamaican Truffle, 40 g	232	16	21
Jaw Breaker 2.25", 40 g	160	0	40
Katy Cream Assort, 40 g	174	7	28
Katy Cream Assort, 40 g	182	8	28
Katy Kiss Cluster, 40 g	218	14	21
Kilwin's Dome Milk Chocolate, 40 g	231	14	24
Kilwin's Fudge Topping, 40 g	232	14	26
Kilwin's Square Mint, 40 g	231	14	24
Le Gran Truffle, 40 g	233	17	21
Licorice Bridge Mix, 40 g	130	1	31
Macadamia Nuts rstd & salted, 40 g	286	30	5
Macadamia Tuttles, Milk Chocolate, 40 g	222	16	20
Macadamia Tuttles, White Chocolate, 40 g	216	15	21
Maple Cream, Dark Chocolate, 40 g	163	6	29
Maple Walnut Fudge, 40 g	168	4	32
Marshmallow, Dark Chocolate, 40 g	181	9	25
Marshmallow, Milk Chocolate, 40 g	186	9	25
Marzipan Bar, 40 g	150	3	30
Marzipan Fruits, 40 g	196	0	48
Milk Chocolate Alligator, 40 g	223	13	25
Milk Chocolate Almond Bar, 40 g	336	21	37
Milk Chocolate Almonds, 40 g	200	15	19
Milk Chocolate Bar, 40 g	153	9	17
Milk Chocolate Bar, 40 g	153	9	17
Milk Chocolate Bar, 40 g	229	14	25
Milk Chocolate Bar, 40 g	330	18	39
Milk Chocolate Break-up, 40 g	218	13	24
Milk Chocolate Caramel Apple, 40 g	220	12	25
Milk Chocolate Cigar, 40 g	179	7	29
Milk Chocolate Cigar, 40 g	231	14	24
Milk Chocolate Cigar, 40 g	231	14	24
Milk Chocolate Coins, 40 g	153	9	17
Milk Chocolate Crayons, 40 g	76	5	8
• Milk Chocolate Crisp Rice Bar, 40 g	350	22	34
Milk Chocolate Doctor Kit, 40 g	229	14	25
Milk Chocolate Fish, 40 g	229	14	25
Milk Chocolate Golf Set, 40 g	218	13	24
Milk Chocolate Hairdresser, 40 g	218	13	24
Milk Chocolate Heart, 40 g	229	14	25
Milk Chocolate Malt Balls, 40 g	190	9	28
Milk Chocolate Maltballs, 40 g	190	9	26
Milk Chocolate Mini Car, 40 g	229	14	25
Milk Chocolate Pansie, 40 g	229	14	25
Milk Chocolate Peanut Dino, 40 g	240	16	22
Milk Chocolate Peanuts, 40 g	220	15	18
Milk Chocolate Peanuts, 40 g	180	12	23
Milk Chocolate Raisins, 40 g	181	8	26
Milk Chocolate Raisins, 40 g	190	9	26
Milk Chocolate Sea Foam, 40 g	180	10	26
Milk Chocolate Tool Kit, 40 g	218	13	24
Milk Moose Sucker, 40 g	150	8	18
Mint Cookie Malt Balls, 40 g	140	1	31
Mint Smoothie Assortment, 40 g	180	8	26
Mint Smoothies, Dark Chocolate, 40 g	226	16	22
Mint Smoothies, Milk Chocolate, 40 g	229	16	22
Mixed Nuts, rstd & salted, 40 g	271	20	13
Molasses Chips, Dark Chocolate, 40 g	191	9	29
Molasses Chips, Milk Chocolate, 40 g	191	8	30
Natural Pistachios, 40 g	286	30	5
Nutcracker Sweets, 40 g	181	8	26
Orange Cream, Dark Chocolate, 40 g	161	5	30

Kilwin's (cont.)

	Cal	Fat	Cbs
Orange Cream, Milk Chocolate, 40 g	161	5	30
Orange Jellies, Dark Chocolate, 40 g	182	7	29
Orange Jellies, Milk Chocolate, 40 g	187	7	30
Orange Peel, Dark Chocolate, 40 g	167	8	26
Orange Peel, Milk Chocolate, 40 g	171	7	26
Oreo Cookie, White Chocolate, 40 g	209	11	27
Oreo Cookies, Milk Chocolate, 40 g	210	11	25
Pastel Chocolate Cherries, 40 g	200	10	26
Peanut Butter Cup, 40 g	180	5	33
Peanut Butter Fudge, 40 g	168	4	32
Peanut Cluster, Dark Chocolate, 40 g	217	15	18
Peanut Cluster, Milk Chocolate, 40 g	223	15	18
Peanut Corn, 40 g	166	4	32
Peanuts, Roasted & Salted, 40 g	243	22	7
Pecan Bark, Dark Chocolate, 40 g	219	15	21
Pecan Bark, Milk Chocolate, 40 g	226	15	22
Pecan Brittle, 40 g	152	8	19
Pecan Cluster, Dark Chocolate, 40 g	235	18	17
Pecan Cluster, Milk Chocolate, 40 g	240	18	18
Pecan Streakers, 40 g	212	13	24
Pecan Turtle Assortment, 40 g	175	7	28
Pecan Tuttles, Dark Chocolate, 40 g	223	16	19
Pecan Tuttles, Milk Chocolate, 40 g	226	16	19
Pecans rstd & salted, 40 g	232	20	7
Pecans, Dark Chocolate, 40 g	232	19	12
Pecans, Milk Chocolate, 40 g	247	21	15
Peppermint Patties Dark Chocolate, 40 g	177	8	28
Peppermint Patty, 40 g	200	9	33
Peanut Brittle, 40 g	186	14	21
Pnt Butter Cruncher Dark Chocolate, 40 g	214	13	23
Pnt Butter Cruncher Milk Chocolate, 40 g	218	13	23
Pnt Butter Smoothie, Dark Chocolate, 40 g	218	14	22
Pnt Butter Smoothie, Milk Chocolate, 40 g	222	14	22
Pretzels, Milk Chocolate, 40 g	199	9	27
Pretzels, White Chocolate, 40 g	199	9	28
Raisin Cluster, Dark Chocolate, 40 g	180	9	26
Raisin Cluster, Milk Chocolate, 40 g	186	9	27
Rasp & Blackberries, 40 g	190	10	25
Raspberry & Blackberry 10# case, 40 g	152	2	35
Raspberry Cream, Dark Chocolate, 40 g	159	5	29
Raspberry Cream, Milk Chocolate, 40 g	162	5	30
Raspberry Jellies, Dark Chocolate, 40 g	184	8	29
Raspberry Jellies, Milk Chocolate, 40 g	187	7	30
Raspberry Truffle, 40 g	230	17	21
Red Licorice Ropes, 40 g	160	0	39
Red Licorice Twist, 40 g	140	0	36
Royal Nut Assortment, 40 g	231	17	18
Royal Nut Assortment, 40 g	245	19	18
Salt Water Taffy, 40 g	130	8	15
Salt Water Taffy, bulk 27# case, 40 g	232	17	21
Sanded Lemon Drops, 40 g	166	0	42
Sour Gummi Bears, 40 g	136	0	32
Star of David, 40 g	180	11	20
Strawberry Bon Bon, 40 g	161	4	31
Sugar Free Caramel Corn, 40 g	224	15	20
Sugar Free Chocolate Fudge, 40 g	160	10	27
Sugar Free Chocolates, 40 g	147	9	27
Sugar Free Dark Pnut Cluster, 40 g	199	17	16
Sugar Free Festival Mints, 40 g	180	15	22
Sugar Free Hard Candy, 40 g	138	3	35
Sugar Free Milk Cashew Tuttle, 40 g	190	14	22
Sugar Free Milk Pecan Turtles, 40 g	190	14	21
Sugar Free Milk Pnut Cluster, 40 g	187	16	16
Sugar Free Milk Squares, 40 g	159	14	21
Sugar Free Pnt Brittle, 40 g	154	7	36

Kilwin's (cont.)

	Cal	Fat	Cbs
Sugar Free Pnut Butter Fudge, 40 g	150	9	26
Sugar Free Pnut Cluster Asst, 40 g	190	16	18
Sugar Free Taffy, 40 g	160	0	40
Sugar Free Toffee Crunch, 40 g	164	8	27
Sugar Free Vanilla Fudge, 40 g	150	9	28
Sugar Free White Pnut Cluster, 40 g	197	15	18
Sugar Free White Squares, 40 g	175	13	26
Swedish Fish, 40 g	160	3	37
Tart Cherry Cluster, Milk Chocolate, 40 g	194	9	27
Truffle Assortment, 40 g	226	16	19
Tuxedo Espresso Beans, 40 g	190	9	26
Vanilla Butter Cream, Dark Chocolate, 40 g	166	6	28
Vanilla Butter Cream, Milk Chocolate, 40 g	168	6	28
White Chocolate Break-up, 40 g	218	12	26
White Chocolate Popcorn, 40 g	220	16	18
White Golf Ball, 40 g	223	12	27
White Golf Ball, 40 g	129	6	19
White Moose Sucker, 40 g	164	10	18

Kohr Bros.

	Cal	Fat	Cbs
• Chocolate, 80 g	140	6	18
• Orange Sherbet, 87 g	104	2	21
Vanilla, 80 g	130	6	16

Kolache Factory

	Cal	Fat	Cbs
Croissants			
• Fruit (Average), 5 oz.	510	24	67
• Ham & Cheese, 7 oz.	620	39	45
Ham & Egg, 7 oz.	610	38	46
Italian Chicken, 8 oz.	550	32	46
Kolaches			
Bacon & Cheese, 2 oz.	180	7	23
Bacon, Egg & Cheese, 5 oz.	360	16	35
BBQ Beef, 3 oz.	180	6	18
Club, 5 oz.	260	9	35
Cream Cheese, 3 oz.	180	7	25
Fruit (Average), 4 oz.	180	3	38
Ham & Cheese, 3 oz.	180	7	23
Italian Chicken, 3 oz.	190	7	23
Jalapeño & Cheese, 3 oz.	180	7	25
Pizza, 3 oz.	200	9	24
• Polish, 6 oz.	510	29	47
Ranchero, 6 oz.	380	18	35
Sausage & Cheese, 3 oz.	240	11	29
• Sausage, 2 oz.	130	5	17
Sausage, Egg & Cheese, 5 oz.	400	20	35
Specialties			
Cinnamon Roll, 5 oz.	460	14	74
Cinnamon Twist, 4 oz.	450	29	45
• Mini-Cinnamon Roll, 4 oz.	230	7	37
• Raisin Nut Roll, 3 oz.	600	24	89
Sticky Bun, 5 oz.	440	20	61

Koo Koo Roo

	Cal	Fat	Cbs
Buffalo Wings (w/o Sauce)			
• 12 Buffalo Wings	1212	55	84
• 6 Buffalo Wings	606	28	42
Burritos			
• California Chicken Burrito	810	41	60
Fajita Chicken Burrito	750	33	70
• Original Chicken Burrito	709	28	71
Chicken Bowls (w/o Sauce)			
Chargrilled Chicken Bowl	569	19	57
• Southwest Bowl	570	19	67
• Spicy Ginger Garlic Bowl	485	6	63
Tostada Bowl (w/o shell)	528	22	45

Koo Koo Roo (cont.)

	Cal	Fat	Cbs
Cold Side Dishes			
Cantaloupe & Honeydew, 5 oz.	50	0	12
• Creamy Coleslaw, 5 oz.	238	20	14
Cucumber Salad, 5 oz.	41	0	9
Tangy Tomato Salad, 5 oz.	60	4	6
• Tossed Salad (w/o dressing), 3 oz.	16	0	3
Dessert			
Chewy Chocolate Chip Cookie, 3 oz.	360	15	53
Chewy Oat Raisin Cookie, 3 oz.	370	15	54
Kellogg's® Rice Krispies Treats®, 3 oz.	340	7	68
• Peanut Butter Cup Cookie, 3 oz.	460	22	58
• Snickerdoodle Cookie, 3 oz.	330	16	43
Triple Chocolate Brownie, 3 oz.	334	9	57
Extras			
BBQ Vinaigrette Dressing, 2 oz.	101	4	14
Caesar Dressing, 2 oz.	235	26	1
• Celery Sticks, 6 pcs	8	0	2
Chinese Salad Dressing, 3 oz.	325	26	26
Chipotle Sauce, 1 oz.	130	14	0
Cilantro Ranch Dressing, 2 oz.	200	21	2
Cranberry Sauce, 1 oz.	45	0	11
• Curry Sauce, 3 oz.	630	69	3
Fruit by the Foot ®, 1	80	2	17
Gravy, 2 oz.	50	4	3
House Salad Dressing, 2 oz.	90	6	6
Lahvash, 1	60	0	12
Pico De Gallo, 2 oz.	8	0	2
Ranch Dressing, 1 oz.	140	15	1
Rudi Roll, Half	150	2	29
Salsa, 2 oz.	11	0	2
Sour Cream, 1 oz.	60	6	1
Spicy Ginger & Garlic Sauce, 4 oz.	320	28	8
Tostada Shell, 1	403	34	21
Wing Sauce, 1 oz.	28	2	2
Fresh Roasted Turkey			
Hand Carved Turkey Sandwich	599	32	31
• Sliced Turkey Breast	182	8	0
Traditional Turkey Dinner	692	29	67
• Turkey Pot Pie	883	44	83
Hot Side Dishes			
Baked Yam, 6 oz.	197	0	47
Black Beans, 6 oz.	125	3	23
Butternut Squash, 6 oz.	66	0	17
Creamed Spinach, 5 oz.	100	6	10
Green Beans, 4 oz.	62	3	9
Italian Vegetable, 6 oz.	47	2	7
Kernel Corn, 5 oz.	105	1	26
• Macaroni & Cheese, 6 oz.	340	17	32
Mashed Potatoes, 7 oz.	186	5	32
Roasted Garlic Potatoes, 5 oz.	133	5	21
Saffron Rice, 4 oz.	175	7	25
Spanish Rice, 5 oz.	145	3	27
• Steamed Vegetables, 4 oz.	38	0	8
Sticky Rice, 5 oz.	155	0	34
Stuffing, 5 oz.	111	7	11
Original Chicken			
1 Original Breast, 4 oz.	187	6	0
3 Piece Original Dark, 5 oz.	320	16	5
Rotisserie Chicken			
• Breast & Wing, 7 oz.	355	16	1
• Half Rotisserie Chicken, 11 oz.	655	34	2
Leg & Thigh, 5 oz.	300	18	1
Salads (w/o Dressing)			
BBQ Chicken Salad	365	14	22
Chicken Caesar Salad	286	11	13

Koo Koo Roo (cont.)

	Cal	Fat	Cbs
Salads (w/o Dressing) (cont.)			
• Chinese Chicken Salad	550	29	39
• House Salad	113	4	16
Sandwiches			
• BBQ Chicken Sandwich	562	12	71
• Chicken Caesar Sandwich	781	36	63
Original Chicken Sandwich	661	29	63
Soups			
• Chicken Noodle Soup, 5 oz.	71	3	4
• Chicken Tortilla Soup, 5 oz.	112	6	7
Ten Vegetable Soup, 5 oz.	94	2	16
Wraps			
Caesar Chicken Wrap	757	39	59
Chipotle Chicken Wrap	924	43	89

Krispy Kreme Doughnuts

	Cal	Fat	Cbs
Chillers			
Berries & Kreme Chiller, 20 oz.	960	40	150
• Chocolate Chiller, 20 oz.	1050	42	170
Lemon Sherbert Chiller, 20 oz.	980	40	155
Lotta Latte Chiller, 20 oz.	1050	40	79
Mocha Dream Chiller, 20 oz.	1050	41	171
Orange You Glad Chiller, 20 oz.	300	0	71
Oranges & Kreme Chiller, 20 oz.	970	40	150
• Very Berry Chiller, 20 oz.	290	0	71
Doughnut Holes			
• Glazed Blueberry Donut Holes, 56 g	220	12	27
Glazed Cake Donut Holes, 56 g	210	10	29
Glazed Chocolate Cake Donut Holes, 56 g	210	10	29
Glazed Pumpkin Spice Donut Holes, 56 g	210	10	29
• Original Glazed Donut Holes, 54 g	200	11	25
Doughnuts			
• Apple Fritter, 101 g	380	20	47
Caramel Kreme Crunch, 98 g	380	19	49
Chocolate Glazed Cruller, 69 g	290	15	37
Chocolate Iced Cake, 71 g	280	14	36
Chocolate Iced Custard Filled, 86 g	300	17	35
Chocolate Iced Glazed, 66 g	250	12	33
Chocolate Iced Kreme Filled, 86 g	350	20	39
Chocolate Iced w/Sprinkles, 71 g	270	12	38
Cinnamon Apple Filled, 81 g	290	16	32
Cinnamon Bun, 67 g	260	16	28
Cinnamon Twist, 59 g	240	15	23
Dulce De Leche, 75 g	300	18	31
Glazed Chocolate Cake, 80 g	300	15	42
Glazed Cinnamon, 54 g	210	12	24
Glazed Cruller, 54 g	240	14	26
Glazed Kreme Filled, 86 g	340	20	39
Glazed Lemon Filled, 85 g	290	16	35
Glazed Pumpkin Spice, 80 g	300	14	42
Glazed Raspberry Filled, 85 g	300	16	36
Glazed Sour Cream, 80 g	300	13	43
Maple Iced Glazed, 66 g	240	12	32
New York Cheesecake, 90 g	340	20	34
Original Glazed, 52 g	200	12	22
Powdered Cake, 71 g	290	14	37
Powdered Strawberry Filled, 81 g	290	16	33
• Sugar, 49 g	200	12	21
Traditional Cake, 57 g	230	13	25

Krystal

	Cal	Fat	Cbs
B.A. Burger			
• BA Double Bacon Cheese, 305 g	800	53	41
BA w/ Cheese, 218 g	530	32	40
• BA, 202 g	470	27	39

Krystal (cont.)

	Cal	Fat	Cbs
Breakfast			
4 Carb Scrambler (bacon), 6 oz.	370	29	4
4 Carb Scrambler (sausage), 8 oz.	600	51	3
Bacon Egg Cheese Biscuit, 137 g	390	23	33
Biscuit & Gravy, 200 g	280	14	34
Chik Biscuit, 137 g	360	15	40
• Country Breakfast, 230 g	660	42	46
• Kryspers, 51 g	190	13	17
Krystal Sunriser, 94 g	240	14	14
Plain Biscuit, 87 g	270	13	33
Sausage Biscuit, 144 g	480	33	33
Scrambler, 312 g	440	26	33
Chiks			
Krystal Chik, 81 g	240	11	24
Dessert			
Blueberry Freeze, 454 g	230	0	58
Cherry Freeze, 454 g	230	0	58
Fried Apple Turnover, 81 g	220	10	31
Grape Freeze, 454 g	230	0	57
Green Apple Freeze, 454 g	230	0	57
• Lemon Icebox Pie, 99 g	260	9	41
• Orange Freeze, 454 g	220	0	54
Pomegranate Freeze, 454 g	230	0	57
Pups			
Chili Cheese Pup, 76 g	210	12	17
• Corn Pup, 68 g	260	19	19
• Plain Pup, 57 g	170	9	15
Sides			
Chik'n Bites (sm), 113 g	310	19	16
Chik'n Bites Salad, 262 g	290	20	12
• Chili Cheese Fries, 207 g	540	28	59
• Krystal Chili, 217 g	200	7	22
Regular Fries, 119 g	470	20	53
The Famous Krystal			
Bacon Cheese Krystal, 65 g	190	10	16
Cheese Krystal, 68 g	180	9	17
• DBL Cheese Krystal, 121 g	310	16	26
Double Krystal, 108 g	260	13	24
• Krystal, 60 g	160	7	17

L&L Hawaiian Barbecue

	Cal	Fat	Cbs
• BBQ Beef, 5 oz.	330	11	25
BBQ Chicken, 5 oz.	380	20	22
BBQ Short Ribs, 5 oz.	460	37	5
Chicken Katsu, 5 oz.	350	24	12
Katsu Sauce, 2 oz.	45	0	11
• Macaroni Salad, 5 oz.	520	30	57

LaRosa's Pizzeria

	Cal	Fat	Cbs
Appetizers			
Barbecue Wings (12 wings), 549 g	1257	77	48
Barbecue Wings (18 wings), 823 g	1884	115	71
Blue Cheese Dipping Cup, 42 g	230	24	2
Chicken Tenders, 243 g	541	31	30
Diablo Sauce, 64 g	206	15	17
Four Taste Sampler, 669 g	1569	99	82
French Fry Basket w/ Provolone, 385 g	862	56	73
Garlic Sauce Dipping Sauce, 51 g	360	40	0
Mozzarella Cheese Sticks, 181 g	636	43	36
Onion Twists (Regular), 207 g	462	27	48
Pizza Sauce Dipping Cup, 57 g	50	2	7
Ranch Dipping Cup, 42 g	230	24	2
• Seasoned Kitchen Chips (Regular), 170 g	433	26	47
Special Recipe Wings (12 wings), 549 g	1261	87	21
• Special Recipe Wings (18 wings), 823 g	1890	130	32
Spicy Hot Wings (12 wings), 542 g	1247	85	26

LaRosa's Pizzeria (cont.)

	Cal	Fat	Cbs
Appetizers (cont.)			
Spicy Hot Wings (18 wings), 811 g	1864	128	38
Calzones			
• 3 Meat & 3 Cheese, 441 g	1080	55	102
3 Veggie & 3 Cheese, 438 g	860	34	105
Cheese & Pepperoni, 375 g	960	45	101
Cheese, 364 g	840	34	101
Philly Cheesesteak Calzone, 348 g	872	39	90
• Philly Chicken Calzone, 341 g	745	24	90
Pizza Sauce Dipping Cup, 57 g	50	2	7
Ranch Dipping Cup, 42 g	230	24	2
Sausage Pelucci Calzone, 425 g	1042	52	92
Desserts			
Greater's Big Scoop cup, 210 g	600	42	56
Hot Fudge Brownie, 1/2 portion	758	40	99
• Italian Crème Cake, 257 g	998	57	112
• Pizza Frite, 1/2 portion	342	6	64
Focaccia Style Pizza (Medium)			
• Cheese (1/10 pizza), 42 g	230	12	23
Florentine (1/10 pizza), 94 g	240	13	24
• Roma (1/10 pizza), 94 g	300	18	23
Fresh Baked Breads			
Breadsticks (5 pcs.), 309 g	998	13	190
• Breadsticks w/ Provolone (5 pcs.), 389 g	1293	35	193
• Garlic Bread (2 pcs.), 66 g	240	9	35
Garlic Bread w/ Provolone (2 pcs.), 104 g	390	21	35
Garlic Sauce Dipping Sauce, 51 g	360	40	0
Pizza Sauce Dipping Cup, 57 g	50	2	7
Fresh Salads and Soup			
Baked Onion Soup, 272 g	304	16	28
Grilled Chicken Salad, 318 g	296	12	11
JoJo BLT w/ Chkn Antipasto, 271 g	317	21	12
• JoJo's BLT Salad w/ dressing, 257 g	505	35	9
• Minestrone Soup, 336 g	130	2	22
Tossed Salad, 205 g	163	9	10
Tuna Salad, 350 g	458	30	19
Hand Tossed Pizzas (Medium)			
Blanca, 86 g	251	10	27
Buddy Topper, 124 g	309	14	29
• Cheese, 96 g	230	8	29
Deluxe Topper, 123 g	291	12	29
• Meat Topper, 122 g	320	15	29
Pelucci Topper, 120 g	288	13	29
Pepperoni Topper, 111 g	298	14	29
Veggie Topper, 120 g	264	10	29
Hoagies			
Baked Buddy Hoagy, 248 g	665	28	62
Baked Royal Hoagy, 254 g	601	22	62
Fillet of Haddock Hoagy, 302 g	630	15	81
Link Sausage Hoagy, 273 g	621	24	64
Meatball Hoagy, 334 g	689	26	77
• Original Steak Hoagy, 321 g	727	35	65
• Philly Chicken Hoagy, 264 g	451	4	64
Philly Steak Hoagy, 263 g	621	25	64
Ingredients and Dressings for Hoagies			
Italian Dressing, 57 g	320	34	3
Kitchen Chips, 28 g	150	9	15
• Mushroom Sauce Mayonnaise, 57 g	400	11	0
• Pickle Chips, 39 g	5	0	1
Pizza Sauce, 57 g	50	2	7
Provolone, 28 g	103	7	1
Red Onion Slices, 14 g	6	0	1
Sharp White Cheddar, 26 g	92	8	1
Tartar Sauce, 57 g	260	24	11
Tomato Slices, 51 g	11	0	2

RESTAURANTS & FAST-FOOD CHAINS

LaRosa's Pizzeria (cont.)

	Cal	Fat	Cbs
Kid's Meals (values include all components of kids meal)			
Cheese Sticks & Potatoes, 286 g	536	28	55
Chicken Tenders & Potatoes, 299 g	492	26	49
• Mac 'n Cheese, 310 g	378	12	58
Smiley Pizza – Cheese, 382 g	726	30	79
• Smiley Pizza – Pepperoni, 396 g	796	36	79
Spaghetti and Meatball, 311 g	515	10	86
Lite and Low Fat Menu Items			
Large Lite Deluxe Pizza, 1 slice	300	9	42
• Low Fat Grilled Chicken Hoagy, 347 g	520	9	56
Low Fat Grilled Chicken Salad Meal, 349 g	380	10	40
Medium Lite Deluxe Pizza, 1 slice	190	6	27
• Minestrone Soup, 1 bowl	80	1	15
Small Lite Deluxe Pizza, 1 slice	170	5	25
Pan Crust Pizzas (Medium)			
Blanca, 100 g	350	22	28
Buddy Topper, 126 g	312	14	29
Cheese, 105 g	300	16	30
Deluxe Topper, 134 g	370	21	31
• Meat Topper, 132 g	400	23	30
• Pelucci Topper, 123 g	295	12	29
Pepperoni Topper, 121 g	370	22	30
Veggie Topper, 141 g	320	16	32
Pasta Dinners			
Add Chicken Strips w/ Trad. Sauce, 283 g	284	10	21
Add Link Sausage w/ Trad. Sauce, 283 g	416	26	21
Add Meatballs (3) w/ Trad. Sauce, 264 g	381	23	25
Cheese Ravioli, 496 g	661	26	80
Lasagna w/ Meat Sauce, 599 g	735	38	61
Meat Ravioli, 496 g	621	22	102
• Minestrone Soup, 336 g	130	2	22
Spaghetti & Meatballs, 640 g	870	28	119
Spaghetti or Ziti w/ Alfredo Sauce, 546 g	976	50	104
Spaghetti or Ziti w/ Meat Sauce, 546 g	698	18	104
Spaghetti or Ziti w/ Trad. Sauce, 546 g	640	12	113
Tossed Salad w/o dressing, 205 g	163	9	10
• Ziti Chicken Alfredo, 596 g	982	42	102
Ziti Sausage Pelucci, 624 g	766	20	115
Salad Dressing (one packet)			
Blue Cheese, 43 g	220	24	2
Caesar, 29 g	160	17	1
Fat Free Honey Dijon, 43 g	70	0	16
• Fat Free Italian, 43 g	20	0	4
Fat Free Ranch, 43 g	40	0	10
Honey French, 43 g	210	18	14
LaRosa's Creamy Garlic, 43 g	250	26	3
LaRosa's Italian, 43 g	230	26	2
• Ranch, 43 g	260	29	1
Thousand Island, 43 g	220	21	7
Stuffed Pizza Pie			
• Cheese, 114 g	339	14	40
• Meat, 239 g	790	53	44
Veggie, 167 g	393	18	43
Traditional Crust Pizzas (Medium)			
Blanca, 73 g	260	16	17
Buddy Topper, 105 g	275	15	20
• Cheese, 76 g	200	10	19
Deluxe Topper, 105 g	270	16	20
• Meat Topper, 102 g	300	18	20
Pelucci Topper, 102 g	258	13	20
Pepperoni Topper, 94 g	280	16	20
Veggie Topper, 113 g	220	11	21

LaMar's

	Cal	Fat	Cbs
Donuts			
Apple Fritter	650	26	91

LaMar's (cont.)

	Cal	Fat	Cbs
Donuts (cont.)			
Apple Spice Cake Donut	340	17	44
Bavarian Cream Bizmark	620	22	101
Blueberry Cake Donut	350	17	47
Blueberry Filled Bizmark	520	20	81
Caramel Iced LaMar's Bar (Unfilled)	430	18	59
Cherry Filled Bizmark	550	19	88
Chocolate Iced Bar (Chocolate Fluff Filled)	800	35	118
Chocolate Iced Bar (Bavarian Cream Filled)	600	22	96
Chocolate Iced Bar (White Fluff Filled)	810	35	120
Chocolate Iced Cake Donut	330	18	37
Chocolate Iced LaMar's Bar (Unfilled)	540	22	81
Cinnamon Roll	690	25	106
Cinnamon Twist	770	26	120
German Chocolate Knot	480	27	54
Lemon Filled Bizmark	530	21	80
Old Fashioned Sour Cream Donut	420	18	60
• Raisin Nut Cinnamon Roll	850	27	137
Ray's Chocolate Glazed Donut	290	11	44
• Ray's Original Glazed Donut	220	10	31
White Iced Cake Donut	320	17	38

Little Caesar's

	Cal	Fat	Cbs
Caesar Dips®			
Buffalo Ranch, 43 g	230	24	3
• Buffalo, 43 g	140	14	4
• Buttery Garlic, 43 g	380	42	0
Cheezy, 43 g	210	21	3
Chipotle, 43 g	220	24	2
Ranch, 43 g	250	26	3
Pizza			
• 14" Hot-N-Ready® Pizza Cheese, 94 g	200	7	25
14" Hot-N-Ready® Pizza Pepperoni, 99 g	230	9	25
3 Meat Treat®, 113 g	280	14	25
Baby Pan! Pan! Cheese, 133 g	320	15	33
• Baby Pan!Pan! Cheese, Pepperoni, 140 g	360	18	33
Deep Dish Pizza Cheese, 138 g	320	13	38
Deep Dish Pizza Pepperoni, 145 g	360	16	38
Hula Hawaiian™, 123 g	230	8	28
• Ultimate Supreme, 124 g	260	11	26
Vegetarian, 125 g	220	9	27
Specialty Items			
Barbecue Caesar Wings, 33 g	70	4	3
Chocolate Churro Sauce, 28 g	90	3	16
Churros, 42 g	150	4	25
Crazy Bread®, 38 g	100	3	15
Crazy Sauce®, 113 g	45	0	10
Dulce De Leche Churro Sauce, 28 g	90	3	16
Hot Caesar Wings, 33 g	60	5	1
Italian Cheese Bread®, 46 g	130	7	13
Mild Caesar Wings, 30 g	60	4	1
• Oven Roasted Caesar Wings®, 26 g	50	4	0
• Pepperoni Cheese Bread® 10 pcs, 49 g	150	8	13

Long John Silver's

	Cal	Fat	Cbs
Chicken			
Chicken Plank®, 52 g	140	8	9
Desserts			
Chocolate Cream Pie, 74 g	310	22	24
• Pecan Pie, 95 g	370	15	55
Pineapple Cream Pie, 89 g	290	13	39
Dipping Sauces			
Cocktail Sauce, 1 oz.	25	0	6
Tartar Sauce, 1 oz.	101	9	4
Fish and Seafood			
Alaskan Flounder, 104 g	250	11	26

Long John Silver's (cont.)

Food	Cal	Fat	Cbs
Fish and Seafood (cont.)			
Baked Cod, 101 g	120	5	1
Battered Fish, 92 g	260	16	17
• Battered Shrimp, 14 g	45	3	3
• Breaded Clams, 85 g	320	19	29
Buttered Lobster Bites, 99 g	250	9	27
Popcorn Shrimp, 83 g	270	16	23
Salads & Dressings			
• Crispy Chicken Club Salad, 390 g	510	30	35
Garden Ranch Dressing, 43 g	230	24	2
• Lite Italian Dressing, 43 g	20	1	3
Shrimp & Seafood Salad, 356 g	260	12	22
Thousand Island Dressing, 43 g	220	21	7
Sandwiches			
• Chicken Sandwich, 137 g	360	15	40
Fish Sandwich, 177 g	470	23	48
• Ultimate Fish Sandwich ®, 199 g	530	28	49
Sides			
Cole Slaw, 4 oz.	200	15	15
• Hushpuppies, 23 g	60	3	9
• Large Fries, 5 oz.	390	17	56
Lobster Stuffed Crab Cake, 62 g	170	9	16
Regular Fries, 3 oz.	230	10	34
Starters			
Cheesesticks, 45 g	140	8	12
Clam Chowder, 245 g	170	8	19
• Corn Cobbette, 95 g	90	3	14
Crumblies®, 1 oz.	170	12	14
• Rice, 4 oz.	180	4	34

Macaroni Grill

Food	Cal	Fat	Cbs
Amore De La Grill			
Boursin Filet	930	63	39
Chicken Portobello	1020	66	61
Chicken Sorrentino	1050	46	85
Grilled Halibut	830	43	56
• Grilled Pork Chops	1940	111	93
Grilled Salmon (Teriyaki)	1230	74	79
Honey Balsamic Chicken	1190	59	94
• Pollo Magro "Skinny Chicken"	330	5	29
Simple Salmon	660	42	18
Tuscan Ribeye	1000	66	40
Antipasti			
Calamari Fritti	1210	78	66
Crab Stuffed Mushrooms	750	38	71
Mozzarella Fritta	880	63	54
Parmesan Crusted Artichokes	820	62	40
Peasant Bread, 1 Loaf	520	11	89
• Romano's Sampler (All 3)	1640	98	126
Fried Calamari only	670	29	59
Fried Mozzarella only	480	32	32
• Tomato Bruschetta only	450	33	31
Garnish only	60	4	4
Shrimp & Artichoke Dip w/ Croutons	980	52	88
Tomato Bruschetta	1000	70	75
Brick-Oven Pizzas			
• BBQ Chicken Pizza, whole pizza	970	24	135
• Pesto Chicken Pizza, whole pizza	1940	101	163
Pizza Margherita, whole pizza	1010	34	123
Sicilian Pizza, whole pizza	1450	70	124
Clasico Italian			
Chicken & Shrimp Scaloppine, Dinner	1380	97	68
Chicken & Shrimp Scaloppine, Lunch	1260	89	66
Chicken Marsala, Dinner	1090	66	76
Chicken Marsala, Lunch	980	59	73
Chicken Scaloppine, Dinner	1110	71	68

Macaroni Grill (cont.)

Food	Cal	Fat	Cbs
Clasico Italian (cont.)			
Chicken Scaloppine, Lunch	1010	64	65
Eggplant Parmesan, Dinner	1240	64	118
Eggplant Parmesan, Lunch	1080	57	102
Fettuccine Alfredo w/ Chicken, Lunch & Dinner	1370	97	68
Fettuccine Alfredo w/ Shrimp, Lunch & Dinner	1320	95	70
Fettuccine Alfredo, Lunch & Dinner	1130	81	68
Layers & Layers of Lasagna, Dinner	1680	87	120
Layers & Layers of Lasagna, Lunch	890	47	61
Mama's Trio, Lunch & Dinner	1290	69	81
Mushroom Ravioli, Lunch & Dinner	990	67	57
Primo Chicken Parmesan, Dinner	2220	148	126
Primo Chicken Parmesan, Lunch	1380	86	89
Spaghetti & Meat Sauce, Dinner	1110	63	87
• Spaghetti & Meat Sauce, Lunch	830	46	66
• Spaghetti & Mtballs w/ Meat Sauce, Dinner	2430	128	207
Spaghetti & Mtballs w/ Meat Sauce, Lunch	1290	79	84
Spaghetti & Mtballs w/ Tom. Sauce, Dinner	1430	81	119
Spaghetti & Mtballs w/ Tom. Sauce, Lunch	1080	63	89
Traditional Lasagna, Lunch & Dinner	1040	54	65
Twice Bkd Lasagna w/ Mtballs, Lunch & Dinner	1470	83	81
Veal Marsala, Lunch & Dinner	1320	66	132
Veal Parmesan, Lunch & Dinner	1270	64	116
Desserts			
Amaretto Apple Crispetti	1300	45	218
• Dessert Ravioli	1630	74	223
• Italian Sorbetto with Biscotti	330	4	71
Lemon Passion	1150	56	149
New York Cheesecake	980	69	75
New York Cheesecake w/ Caramel Fudge	1610	96	169
Smothered Chocolate Cake	1180	68	140
Tiramisu	1000	64	89
Dressings & Sauces			
Balsamic Vinaigrette Dressing, 1 fl.oz.	100	9	2
Basil Aioli Sauce, 1 fl.oz.	130	14	1
Caesar Dressing, 1 fl.oz.	160	16	1
Cider Vinaigrette Dressing, 1 fl.oz.	140	11	9
Creamy Italian Dressing, 1 fl.oz.	110	10	5
• Fat-Free Creamy Italian Dressing, 1 fl.oz.	30	0	5
Honey Mustard Dressing, 1 fl.oz.	130	12	6
Italian Dressing, 1 fl.oz.	90	8	2
Low-Fat Caesar Dressing, 1 fl.oz.	30	2	4
Parmesan Peppercorn Ranch, 1 fl.oz.	90	9	1
Pizzaiola Sauce, 1 fl.oz.	30	2	2
• Roasted Garlic Lemon Vinaigrette, 1 fl.oz.	170	17	4
Toscana Dressing, 1 fl.oz.	160	17	1
Insalata (Salads)			
Caesar della Casa (House)	260	21	13
w/o dressing	110	5	12
• Chicken Caesar	920	69	24
w/o dressing	462	20	20
Chicken Florentine	840	53	62
w/o dressing	490	19	50
Garden della Casa (House)	240	15	20
w/o dressing	130	5	15
Insalata Blu	640	53	13
w/o chicken	760	56	13
w/o chicken, w/o dressing	570	38	9
w/o dressing	440	36	9
Mozzarella Alla Caprese, half order	260	21	5
Mozzarella Alla Caprese, full order	450	36	9
Parmesan-Crusted Chicken	1190	63	60
w/o dressing	1060	49	59
• Seared Sea Scallops	1320	91	40
w/o dressing	1050	68	22

Macaroni Grill (cont.)

	Cal	Fat	Cbs
Insalata (Salads) (cont.)			
Steak & Arugula	890	71	11
w/o dressing	570	37	9
Kid's - Lunch & Dinner			
Chicken Fingerias	650	45	39
• Double Macaroni 'n' Cheese	1200	62	108
Fettuccine Alfredo	580	30	53
• Grilled Chicken & Broccoli	390	5	51
Mona Lisa's Cheese Masterpizza	840	20	120
Mona Lisa's Pepperoni Masterpizza	920	27	120
Spaghetti & Meatballs w/ Meat Sauce	550	24	56
Spaghetti & Meatballs w/ Tomato Sauce	500	20	58
Kid's Sides			
Caesar della Casa w/ Caesar Dressing	170	12	11
Garden della Casa w/ Creamy Italian Dressing	120	8	9
• Grilled Asparagus	40	2	4
Grilled Broccoli	80	3	11
Macaroni 'n' Cheese	350	18	30
Shoestring Fries	250	15	27
• Vanilla Ice Cream w/ Chocolate Sauce, 1 Scoop	400	23	43
Oven Stuffed Pasta			
Chicken Cannelloni, Dinner	1080	58	62
• Chicken Cannelloni, Lunch	720	39	42
Lobster Ravioli, Lunch & Dinner	1090	78	55
• Marsala Chicken Ravioli	1300	85	55
Mushroom Ravioli	820	59	42
Pasta Di Prima			
Carmela's Chicken Rigatoni, Dinner	1320	85	84
Carmela's Chicken Rigatoni, Lunch	1030	64	64
Pasta Milano, Dinner	1120	57	108
• Pasta Milano, Lunch	920	48	83
• Penne Rustica, Dinner	1540	80	101
Penne Rustica, Lunch	1300	71	76
Penne with Oven Roasted Chicken	1330	80	83
Seafood Linguine	1130	71	79
Shrimp Portofino, Dinner	1110	78	66
Shrimp Portofino, Lunch	1070	78	66
Sizzling Shrimp Scampi	1380	97	94
Vodka Rustica, Lunch & Dinner	1160	58	77
Sandwiches			
• Brick-Oven Meatball Sandwich	1890	115	149
• Chicken Caesar Calzonetto	1540	88	124
Roasted Chicken & Cheese Sandwich	1630	91	128
Signature Sides			
Garlic Mashed Potatoes	280	14	35
• Grilled Asparagus	30	1	4
Pasta Salad	460	16	69
• Romano's Parmesan Chips	660	51	39
Sautéed Broccoli	260	22	12
Signature Soups			
Chicken Toscana Soup, 1 cup	260	16	18
Italian Sausage & Tomato Soup, 1 cup	180	7	22

Maggie Moo's Icecream

	Cal	Fat	Cbs
• Fat Free, 72 g	80	0	18
Low-Carb NSA, 64 g	130	9	10
Sorbet, 85 g	90	0	22
• Udderly Cream, 80 g	180	11	18

Manchu Wok

	Cal	Fat	Cbs
BBQ Pork, 5 oz.	427	26	21
Beef & Broccoli, 5 oz.	271	23	10
Black Mushroom, 5 oz.	159	10	11
Black Pepper Beef, 5 oz.	286	25	8
Butterfly Shrimp, 5 oz.	235	7	30
Chicken & Mushrooms, 5 oz.	254	22	8

Manchu Wok (cont.)

	Cal	Fat	Cbs
Chicken Wings, 5 oz.	406	33	7
Chicken with Snow, 5 oz.	227	18	11
Dry Ribs, 5 oz.	339	22	18
Fried Rice, 8 oz.	310	14	39
• Garlic Green Bean, 5 oz.	117	7	12
General Tso's Chicken, 5 oz.	319	21	23
Ginger Beef, 5 oz.	318	16	31
Green Bean Chicken, 5 oz.	258	21	11
Honey Garlic Chicken, 5 oz.	326	15	39
Honey Garlic Ribs, 5 oz.	393	19	42
Hunan Beef, 5 oz.	290	24	13
Kung Pao Chicken, 5 oz.	242	19	10
Lemon Chicken, 5 oz.	331	23	21
Mixed Vegetables, 5 oz.	130	9	12
Noodles, 8 oz.	259	13	29
Orange Chicken, 5 oz.	279	15	29
Oriental Grilled, 5 oz.	255	9	21
Pineapple Chicken, 5 oz.	253	17	20
Satay Chicken, 5 oz.	211	16	11
Sesame Chicken, 5 oz.	415	17	55
Spicy Beef, 5 oz.	287	25	9
• Sweet & Sour Chicken, 5 oz.	450	32	26
Sweet & Sour Pork, 5 oz.	271	16	24
Sweet & Sour Sauce, 4 oz.	115	0	30

Max & Erma's

	Cal	Fat	Cbs
Appetizers			
Black Bean Rolls Up	577	10	95
Beverages			
Fruit Smoothie	124	0	29
Dressings			
• Bleu Cheese, 2 tbsp.	201	21	0
Fat-Free French, 2 tbsp.	126	0	31
Fat-Free Honey Mustard, 2 tbsp.	60	0	14
Italian, 2 tbsp.	110	12	1
• Low-Fat Tex Mex Dressings, 2 tbsp.	23	0	2
Ranch, 2 tbsp.	120	13	1
Entrees			
Caribbean Chicken, Lunch Portion	536	20	59
Salads			
• Baby Green Salad w/o breadstick	119	11	6
Half Hula Bowl	366	4	57
• Hula Bowl	576	7	79
Shrimp Stack Salad	322	12	33
Sides			
Fruit Salad, 5 oz.	54	0	17
Garlic Breadstick, 1 Bread	156	6	21

Mazzio's Pizza

	Cal	Fat	Cbs
Deep Pan Pizza Choices: One Topping Pizzas			
• Canadian Bacon, 137 g	330	14	38
Cheese, 130 g	332	15	38
Chicken, 144 g	338	14	38
Hamburger (Beef), 144 g	359	17	38
Pepperoni, 131 g	352	17	37
• Sausage, 144 g	374	19	38
Deep Pan Pizza Choices: Pricebuster Pizzas			
• Cheesebuster, 130 g	348	16	38
• Meatbuster, 146 g	385	20	38
Supremebuster, 144 g	356	17	38
Deep Pan Pizza Choices: Specialty Pizzas			
4 Meat, 151 g	403	21	38
California Alfredo, 144 g	383	19	38
Chicken Club, 150 g	355	16	38
Combo, 160 g	381	19	39
• Greek, 142 g	414	24	38

Mazzio's Pizza (cont.)

	Cal	Fat	Cbs
Deep Pan Pizza Choices: Specialty Pizzas (cont.)			
Lucky 7 Pizza, 162 g	353	17	39
Mazzio's "Works", 171 g	406	21	39
Mexican, 183 g	413	21	42
• Veggie, 152 g	331	15	39
Dippin Zone: Calzone Rings & Quesapizza			
Chicken Quesapizza w/o Sauce, 113 g	317	13	33
Four Meat/Four Cheese Calzone w/o Sauce, 96 g	274	11	33
Ham Bacon & Cheddar Calzone w/o Sauce, 90 g	244	8	32
Pepperoni Calzone w/o Sauce, 87 g	260	10	33
• Pepperoni Quesapizza w/o Sauce, 99 g	332	16	32
Dippin Zone: Dippin Ribs			
Rib Dippers (3/4 lb) Tossed w/ BBQ, 138 g	458	32	13
Dippin Zone: Dippin' Chicken			
• Boneless Dippin' Chicken (10 ct), 51 g	122	6	7
• Rstd & BBQ Tossed Wings (10 ct), 82 g	191	12	7
Wings of Fire (10 ct) w/o Sauce, 71 g	161	11	1
Dippin Zone: Dippin' Fries			
Cheese Fries, 179 g	432	26	35
• Fries w/ Sandwich, 266 g	558	29	67
• Full Order, 133 g	279	14	34
Dippin Zone: Dippin' Sauces			
BBQ, 2 oz.	140	N/A	34
Blue Cheese, 2 oz.	302	32	2
• Buffalo, 2 oz.	19	N/A	4
Chocolate, 2 oz.	177	1	43
• Cool Ranch, 2 oz.	372	39	2
Honey Mustard, 2 oz.	260	22	14
Ketchup, 2 oz.	50	N/A	13
Marinara, 2 oz.	29	1	5
Picante, 2 oz.	20	N/A	4
Southwestern Ranch, 2 oz.	321	34	2
Vanilla, 2 oz.	181	0	45
Dippin Zone: Italian Dippin'			
Toasted Ravioli w/o Sauce, 43 g	118	5	13
Artichoke Spin Dip w/ Bread, 87 g	245	16	18
• Breadsticks w/o Sauce, 52 g	150	3	26
• Cheese Dippers w/o Sauce, 128 g	405	18	47
Garlic Cheese Toast w/o Sauce, 54 g	205	13	16
Garlic Toast w/o Sauce, 40 g	160	10	15
Mozzarella Sticks w/o Sauce, 57 g	181	12	10
Dippin Zone: Southwestern Dippin'			
• Cheese Nachos w/ Jalapeños, 113 g	423	30	19
Nachos (Beef w/ Jalapeños), 142 g	484	34	20
Nachos (Chicken w/ Jalapeños), 135 g	448	30	20
Nachos (Sausage w/ Jalapeños), 142 g	504	37	20
Dippin Zone: Sweet Dippin'			
Cinnamon Sticks w/o Sauce, 145 g	626	36	70
French Bread			
Deli, 1 bread	480	20	60
• Greek, 1 bread	623	31	61
• Hawaiian, 1 bread	449	13	62
Pepperoni, 1 bread	495	21	58
Southwestern Chicken, 1 bread	532	20	61
Original Crust Pizza Choices: One Topping Pizzas			
• Canadian Bacon, 113 g	231	8	30
• Cheese, 105 g	234	9	30
Chicken, 120 g	239	7	31
Hamburger (Beef), 120 g	260	10	31
Pepperoni, 106 g	254	10	30
• Sausage, 120 g	276	12	31
Original Crust Pizza Choices: Pricebuster Pizzas			
• Cheesebuster, 105 g	249	9	30
• Meatbuster, 121 g	286	13	31
Supremebuster, 119 g	257	10	31

Mazzio's Pizza (cont.)

	Cal	Fat	Cbs
Original Crust Pizza Choices: Specialty Pizzas			
4 Meat, 126 g	305	15	31
California Alfredo, 119 g	285	13	30
Chicken Club, 125 g	257	9	31
Combo, 135 g	282	12	31
• Greek, 117 g	315	17	30
Lucky 7 Pizza, 137 g	255	10	32
Mazzio's "Works", 146 g	307	14	31
Mexican, 158 g	314	14	35
• Veggie, 127 g	232	8	31
Pasta Choices: Signature Pastas			
Chicken Parmesan, 614 g	947	27	135
Chicken Spinach Artichoke Pasta, 463 g	1005	38	113
Chicken-Fried Chicken Alfredo, 479 g	1290	69	120
Fettuccine Alfredo, 343 g	1061	56	107
Garlic Toast, 1 Piece	160	10	15
• Greek Pasta, 458 g	1456	94	107
Lasagna Red & White, 669 g	984	62	64
w/ Alfredo, 598 g	1264	94	55
w/ Marinara, 740 g	704	30	73
w/ Meat Sauce, 712 g	949	52	64
• Spaghetti w/ Marinara, 449 g	641	8	120
w/ Meat Sauce, 428 g	825	25	113
w/ Meatballs (4) & Marinara, 562 g	972	34	126
w/ Meatballs (4) & Meat Sauce, 541 g	1156	50	119
Sandwiches			
Chkn, Bacon & Swiss (Focaccia), 392 g	1021	70	48
• Chkn, Bacon & Swiss (Hoagie), 510 g	1362	72	120
Ham & Cheddar (Focaccia), 351 g	747	47	47
Ham & Cheddar (Hoagie), 470 g	1088	50	119
Kosher Pickle Spear, 28 g	5	N/A	1
Mazzio's Sub (Focaccia), 344 g	768	49	45
Mazzio's Sub (Hoagie), 462 g	1109	52	117
Turkey & Swiss (Focaccia), 376 g	718	38	46
Turkey & Swiss (Hoagie), 494 g	1059	40	118
• Tuscan Smash (Focaccia), 354 g	645	34	45
Tuscan Smash (Hoagie), 473 g	986	36	117
Thin Crust Pizza Choices: One Topping Pizzas			
• Canadian Bacon, 91 g	179	8	18
Cheese, 84 g	182	9	18
• Chicken, 98 g	187	8	19
Hamburger, 98 g	208	11	19
Pepperoni, 85 g	202	11	18
• Sausage, 98 g	224	12	19
Thin Crust Pizza Choices: Pricebuster Pizzas			
• Cheesebuster, 84 g	197	9	19
• Meatbuster, 100 g	234	13	19
Supremebuster, 98 g	205	11	19
Thin Crust Pizza Choices: Specialty Pizzas			
4 Meat, 105 g	253	15	19
California Alfredo, 98 g	233	13	18
Chicken Club, 104 g	205	9	19
Combo, 114 g	231	13	19
• Greek, 96 g	263	17	19
Lucky 7 Pizza, 116 g	203	10	20
Mazzio's "Works", 125 g	255	15	20
Mexican, 136 g	262	14	23
• Veggie, 105 g	180	8	19

McDonald's

	Cal	Fat	Cbs
Breakfast			
Bacon, Egg, Cheese Biscuit, 5 oz.	450	25	36
Bacon, Egg, Cheese McGriddles®, 4 oz.	460	21	48
Big Breakfast® 9 oz.	720	46	49
Biscuit (Large), 3.2 oz.	320	16	39
Biscuit (Regular), 2.7 oz.	250	11	32

McDonald's (cont.)

Breakfast (cont.)	Cal	Fat	Cbs
• Dlx Breakfast w/o Syrup/Margarine, 15 oz.	1070	55	109
• Egg McMuffin®, 5 oz.	300	12	30
English Muffin, 2 oz.	160	3	27
Grape Jam, 0.5 oz.	35	0	9
Hash Browns, 2 oz.	140	8	15
Hotcake Syrup, 60 g	180	0	45
Hotcakes & Sausage (w/o Syrup/Margarine), 7 oz.	520	24	61
Hotcakes (w/o Syrup/Margarine), 5 oz.	350	9	60
McSkillet Burrito w/ Sausage, 8 oz.	610	36	44
w/ Steak, 9 oz.	570	30	44
Sausage Biscuit w/ Egg, 6 oz.	500	32	35
Sausage Biscuit, 4 oz.	410	27	33
Sausage Burrito, 4 oz.	300	16	26
Sausage McGriddles®, 5 oz.	420	22	44
Sausage McMuffin®, 4 oz.	370	22	29
w/ Egg, 6 oz.	450	27	30
Sausage Patty, 1 oz.	170	15	1
Sausage, Egg, Cheese McGriddles®, 7 oz.	560	32	48
Scrambled Eggs (2), 3 oz.	170	11	1
Strawberry Preserves, 0.5 oz.	35	0	9
Whipped Margarine, 6 g	40	5	0
Chicken McNuggets®/Selects® Premium Breast Strips/Sauces			
Barbecue Sauce, 28 g	50	0	12
• Chicken McNuggets® (6 piece), 3 oz.	250	15	15
Creamy Ranch Sauce, 2 oz.	200	22	2
Honey, 14 g	50	0	12
Hot Mustard Sauce, 28 g	60	3	9
• Premium Breast Strips (3 pcs.), 5 oz.	380	20	28
Spicy Buffalo Sauce, 2 oz.	70	7	1
SW Chipotle Barbecue Sauce, 2 oz.	70	0	18
Sweet 'N Sour Sauce, 28 g	50	0	12
Tangy Honey Mustard Sauce, 2 oz.	70	3	13
Desserts/Shakes			
• Apple Dippers, 68 g	35	0	8
Baked Apple Pie, 3 oz.	270	12	36
Chocolate Chip Cookie, 33 g	160	7	22
Chocolate Triple Thick® Shake, 16 fl.oz.	580	14	102
Cinnamon Melts, 4 oz.	460	19	66
Fruit 'n Yogurt Parfait, 5 oz.	160	2	31
w/o Granola, 5 oz.	130	2	25
Hot Caramel Sundae, 6 oz.	340	8	60
Hot Fudge Sundae, 6 oz.	330	10	54
Kiddie Cone, 1 oz.	45	1	8
Low Fat Caramel Dip, 1 oz.	70	1	15
McDonaldland® Choco Chip Cookies, 2 oz.	270	11	39
McDonaldland® Cookies, 2 oz.	250	8	42
• McFlurry® w/ M&M'S® Candies, 12 fl.oz.	620	20	96
McFlurry® w/ OREO® Cookies, 12 fl.oz.	560	16	88
Oatmeal Raisin Cookie, 33 g	150	6	22
Peanuts (for Sundaes), 0.5 oz.	45	4	2
Strawberry Sundae, 6 oz.	280	6	49
Strawberry Triple Thick® Shake, 16 fl.oz.	560	13	97
Sugar Cookie, 32 g	150	6	21
Vanilla Reduced Fat Ice Cream Cone, 3 oz.	150	4	24
Vanilla Triple Thick® Shake, 16 fl.oz.	550	13	96
French Fries			
Ketchup Packet, 10 g	15	0	3
• Large French Fries, 6 oz.	570	30	70
Medium French Fries, 4 oz.	380	20	47
Salt Packet, 1 g	0	0	0
• Small French Fries, 3 oz.	250	13	30
Iced Coffee			
• Caramel (Medium), 24 fl.oz.	190	8	27
Hazelnut (Medium), 24 fl.oz.	190	8	29

McDonald's (cont.)

Iced Coffee (cont.)	Cal	Fat	Cbs
• Regular (Medium), 24 fl.oz.	200	8	30
Vanilla (Medium), 24 fl.oz.	190	8	29
Salad			
Asian Salad w/ Grilled Chicken, 13 oz.	300	10	23
w/ Crispy Chicken, 13 oz.	380	17	33
w/o Chicken, 9 oz.	150	7	15
Bacon Ranch Salad w/ Grilled Chkn, 11 oz.	260	9	12
w/ Crispy Chicken, 11 oz.	350	16	23
w/o Chicken, 8 oz.	140	7	10
Butter Garlic Croutons, 0.5 oz.	60	2	10
Caesar Salad w/ Grilled Chicken, 11 oz.	220	6	12
w/ Crispy Chicken, 11 oz.	300	13	22
w/o Chicken, 8 oz.	90	4	9
• Side Salad, 3 oz.	20	0	4
Snack Size Fruit & Walnut Salad, 163 g	210	8	31
Southwest Salad w/ Grilled Chkn, 12 oz.	320	9	30
• w/ Crispy Chicken, 12 oz.	400	16	41
w/o Chicken, 8 oz.	140	5	20
Salad Dressings: Newman's Own®			
• Creamy Caesar Dressing, 2 fl.oz.	190	18	4
Creamy Southwest Dressing, 2 fl.oz.	100	6	11
• Low Fat Balsamic Vinaigrette, 2 fl.oz.	40	3	4
Low Fat Family Recipe Italian, 2 fl.oz.	60	3	8
Low Fat Sesame Ginger Dressing, 2 fl.oz.	90	3	15
Ranch Dressing, 2 fl.oz.	170	15	9
Sandwiches			
Big Mac®, 8 oz.	540	29	45
Big N' Tasty®, 7 oz.	460	24	37
w/ Cheese, 8 oz.	510	28	38
Cheeseburger, 4 oz.	300	12	33
Chipotle BBQ Snack Wrap w/ Grilled Chkn, 4 oz.	260	8	28
Dble Cheeseburger, 6 oz.	440	23	34
• Dble Quarter Pounder® w/ Cheese, 10 oz.	740	42	40
Filet-O-Fish®, 5 oz.	380	18	38
• Hamburger, 4 oz.	250	9	31
Honey Mustard Snack Wrap w/ Crispy Chkn, 4 oz.	320	15	34
McChicken®, 5 oz.	360	16	40
McRib®†, 7 oz.	500	26	44
Premium Crispy Chkn Club Sandwich, 9 oz.	660	28	63
Premium Grilled Chkn Classic Sandwich, 8 oz.	420	10	51
Premium Grilled Chkn Ranch BLT Sandwich, 9 oz.	520	16	53
Ranch Snack Wrap w/ Grilled Chkn, 4 oz.	270	10	26
Quarter Pounder®+, 6 oz.	410	19	37
w/ Cheese, 7 oz.	510	26	40

Mr. Goodcents

Bread	Cal	Fat	Cbs
• Gold, 106 g	189	3	26
Wheat Bread, 128 g	279	4	54
• White Bread, 128 g	288	2	58
Cold Subs (Half Sub)			
Centsable Sub Wheat Bread, 227 g	493	20	57
Centsable Sub White Bread, 227 g	502	19	61
Cheese Mix Wheat Bread, 213 g	571	26	57
Cheese Mix White Bread, 213 g	580	25	61
Ham & Cheese Wheat Bread, 227 g	410	10	58
Ham & Cheese White Bread, 227 g	419	9	62
Italian Sub Wheat Bread, 213 g	622	34	57
Italian Sub White Bread, 213 g	631	33	61
Original, Wheat Bread, 213 g	512	23	56
Original, White Bread, 213 g	520	22	60
Oven Rstd Chicken, Wheat Bread, 213 g	355	6	54
Oven Rstd Chicken, White Bread, 213 g	364	5	58
Penny Club Wheat Bread, 213 g	364	7	56
Penny Club White Bread, 213 g	373	5	60

Mr. Goodcents (cont.)

	Cal	Fat	Cbs
Cold Subs (Half Sub) (cont.)			
Pepperoni & Cheese Wheat Bread, 227 g	709	43	57
• Pepperoni & Cheese White Bread, 227 g	718	41	61
Roast Beef Wheat Bread, 213 g	369	7	54
Roast Beef White Bread, 213 g	378	5	58
Tuna Salad Wheat Bread, 213 g	500	21	62
Tuna Salad White Bread, 213 g	509	20	66
Turkey Wheat Bread, 213 g	354	6	57
Turkey White Bread, 213 g	363	4	61
• Veggie Sub Wheat Bread, 212 g	295	4	57
Veggie Sub White Bread, 212 g	305	2	61
Desserts			
• Baked Brownie, 65 g	260	10	41
• Giant Chocolate Chip Cookie, 71 g	420	22	52
Giant Peanut Butter Cookie, 71 g	340	20	36
Dress Options			
American Cheese, 14 g	41	3	0
Bacon, 3 slices	61	5	0
Cheddar Cheese, 14 g	57	5	0
Jalapeños, 7 g	2	0	0
Mayonnaise, 7 g	51	6	0
Mozzarella, 14 g	40	3	0
• Mustard, 7 g	0	0	0
Olives, 7 g	28	2	2
Pepper Jack, 14 g	51	4	1
Pickles, 14 g	5	0	1
Provolone, 14 g	50	4	0
• Ranch Dressing, 14 g	83	9	1
Spicy Mustard, 7 g	7	0	0
Spicy Ranch, 14 g	67	7	1
Standard Dress, 21 g	26	2	2
Standard Dress, no oil, 14 g	11	0	2
Swiss, 14 g	53	4	0
Goodcents Gold "Premium" Sandwiches			
Cold Centsable Sub, 234 g	460	25	31
Cold Cheese Mix, 220 g	481	26	30
Cold Ham & Cheese, 234 g	350	11	32
Cold Italian Sub, 220 g	649	44	30
Cold Mr. Goodcent Original, 220 g	479	28	29
Cold Oven Roasted Chicken Breast, 220 g	290	6	26
Cold Penny Club, 220 g	304	7	29
• Cold Pepperoni & Cheese, 234 g	750	54	32
• Cold Roast Beef, 220 g	309	7	26
Cold Tuna Salad, 220 g	410	21	34
Cold Turkey, 220 g	289	6	30
• Cold Veggie Sub, 181 g	205	3	30
Hot Chkn Bacon Ranch w/ Cheddar, 291 g	580	31	28
Hot Chkn Parmesan w/ Mozzarella, 305 g	436	15	33
Hot Meatball w/ Mozzarella, 291 g	624	33	38
Pastrami & Swiss, 284 g	440	18	28
Philly Jack 'n Cheese, 248 g	430	16	32
Roast Beef 'n Cheddar, 263 g	452	17	28
Hot Subs (Half Sub)			
Chken Parmesan Wheat Bread w/ Mzzrella, 326 g	526	15	61
Chken Parmesan White Bread w/ Mzzrella, 326 g	535	14	65
Chkn Bacon Ranch Wheat Bread w/ Chddr, 297 g	670	31	55
Chkn Bacon Ranch White Bread w/ Chddr, 297 g	679	30	59
Meatball Wheat Bread w/Mozzarella, 312 g	714	33	65
• Meatball White Bread w/ Mozzarella, 312 g	723	32	69
Pastrami & Swiss, Wheat, 305 g	530	18	56
Pastrami & Swiss, White, 305 g	539	17	60
• Philly Jack 'n Cheese, Wheat, 269 g	520	17	59
Philly Jack 'n Cheese, White, 269 g	529	15	63
Roast Beef 'n Cheddar, Wheat, 284 g	542	17	56
Roast Beef 'n Cheddar, White, 284 g	551	16	60

Mr. Goodcents (cont.)

	Cal	Fat	Cbs
Pastas			
Alfredo Sauce on Mostaccioli, 397 g	1290	80	106
• Chicken Alfredo on Mostaccioli, 510 g	1423	85	106
Chicken Parmesan on Mostaccioli, 525 g	695	12	100
Lasagna, 400 g	524	22	54
Red Sauce on Mostaccioli w/Mtball, 482 g	747	19	105
• Red Sauce on Mostaccioli, 397 g	522	4	100
Salads			
Chef Salad, 440 g	195	8	19
Garden Salad, 369 g	98	3	15
Grilled Chicken Salad, 482 g	232	8	15
• Side Salad, 212 g	52	2	8
• Tuna Salad, 454 g	320	21	23
Sides			
• Breadstick (1), 43 g	90	0	19
• Meatballs (2), 114 g	225	15	5
Pasta Salad, 142 g	213	6	35
Potato Salad, 142 g	192	7	28
Soups			
• Broccoli Cheese Soup, 8 oz.	360	22	32
• Chicken Noodle Soup, 8 oz.	120	1	22
Cream of Potato Soup, 8 oz.	320	14	42

Mr. Pita

	Cal	Fat	Cbs
12" Jumbo Size			
• Cranberry Turkey	597	2	104
Grilled Chicken & Broccoli	541	6	79
Grilled Chicken Caesar	514	7	70
Grilled Hawaiian Chicken	546	6	80
Grilled Raspberry Chicken	495	5	78
Ultra Combo (Chicken/Turkey)	514	4	77
Ultra Grilled Chicken	553	6	78
Ultra Supreme	510	5	77
• Ultra Turkey	495	2	77
7" Value Size			
• Cranberry Turkey	275	1	50
Grilled Chicken & Broccoli	235	2	36
Grilled Chicken Caesar	224	3	31
Grilled Hawaiian Chicken	232	2	35
Grilled Raspberry Chicken	214	2	35
Ultra Combo (Chicken/Turkey)	221	2	34
Ultra Grilled Chicken	229	3	34
Ultra Supreme	223	2	34
• Ultra Turkey	214	1	34
9" Regular Size			
• Cranberry Turkey	424	1	77
Grilled Chicken & Broccoli	373	4	57
Grilled Chicken Caesar	353	4	50
Grilled Hawaiian Chicken	375	4	57
• Grilled Raspberry Chicken	342	3	56
Ultra Combo (Chicken/Turkey)	354	3	56
Ultra Grilled Chicken	367	4	56
Ultra Supreme	350	3	56
Ultra Turkey	343	1	56

Mr. Sub

	Cal	Fat	Cbs
6" Classic Subs			
Albacore Tuna, 174 g	280	8	36
Assorted, 180 g	280	8	38
BBQ Rib, 141 g	360	16	34
BLT, 133 g	260	8	34
Breaded Chicken, 203 g	370	13	45
Great Canadian Club, 184 g	300	8	38
Grilled Chicken, 181 g	260	5	37
Italian Salami, 158 g	280	10	35
Louisiana Chicken, 161 g	280	8	34

Mr. Sub (cont.)

	Cal	Fat	Cbs
6" Classic Subs (cont.)			
Maple Baked Ham, 174 g	240	4	39
Meatball, 146 g	360	14	38
Mediterranean Vegetables, 182 g	220	4	40
w/ Cheese, 210 g	300	10	41
Montreal Style Corned Beef, 154 g	270	6	33
Pizza Supremo, 110 g	270	10	33
Philly Style Steak w/o Cheese, 133 g	250	5	34
w/ Cheese, 145 g	300	8	35
Roast Beef, 154 g	280	7	34
• Santa Fe Spicy Chicken, 230 g	370	13	45
Seafood w/ Crab, 154 g	290	10	42
Smoked Turkey Breast, 160 g	230	4	35
• Veggie, 118 g	180	2	34
6" Grilled Subs			
Classic Reuben, 182 g	280	6	34
Grilled Buffalo Chicken, 181 g	260	5	37
• Tuna Melt, 126 g	230	3	32
w/ Cheese, 156 g	330	10	33
Ultimate Club w/o Cheddar, 188 g	270	5	38
• w/ Cheese, 216 g	380	14	38
Breads: 12" Tortillas			
Cheese, 106 g	300	7	50
• Spinach w/ Pesto & Garlic, 106 g	300	7	50
Tomato w/ Basil, 106 g	300	7	50
• Whole Wheat, 106 g	290	7	47
Breads: 6" Buns			
Greek Sub Bun, 75 g	190	3	35
• Mozza-Cheddar Sub Bun, 77 g	190	4	32
Multigrain Sub Bun, 70 g	170	2	32
White Sub Bun, 70 g	170	2	32
Whole Wheat Sub Bun, 70 g	170	2	32
Cheese			
• Cheddar Cheese for 6" Subs, 28 g	120	9	0
Cheese Shred for Salads, 22 g	75	5	1
Cheese Shred for Wraps, 15 g	50	4	1
Feta Cheese for Greek Salad, 30 g	85	7	1
Parmesan for Caesar Salad, 15 g	60	4	1
Process Slice for 6" Pizza Sub, 25 g	80	6	3
• Process Slice for 6" Subs, 12 g	40	3	2
Cookies			
Carnival, 37 g	170	7	24
Double Chocolate Chip, 37 g	170	8	23
Milk Chocolate Chunk, 37 g	170	8	23
• Oatmeal Raisin, 37 g	160	7	23
• Triple Chocolate Chip, 37 g	170	8	23
Dressings			
• Caesar, 36 g	200	21	2
French, 36 g	130	13	5
Greek Feta, 36 g	170	17	4
• Lite Italian, 36 g	80	9	1
Ranch, 36 g	190	20	2
Renee's Dressings			
Balsamic, 45 g	170	16	6
Buttermilk Ranch, 45 g	180	18	3
• Greek Feta, 45 g	280	30	2
Mighty Caesar, 45 g	280	30	2
• Spring Herb and Garlic, 45 g	110	11	3
Salads			
Albacore Tuna, 240 g	140	6	8
Classic Caesar, 122 g	70	5	2
• Garden, 185 g	35	1	6
• Grilled Chicken Caesar, 185 g	160	7	6
Maple Baked Ham, 225 g	85	2	10
Mediterranean Greek, 225 g	70	3	8

Mr. Sub (cont.)

	Cal	Fat	Cbs
Salads (cont.)			
Seafood w/ Crab, 240 g	150	8	15
Smoked Turkey Breast, 225 g	85	2	8
Sauces			
BBQ Sauce, 30 g	40	0	10
Buttermilk Ranch, 10 g	40	4	1
Honey Mustard, 10 g	20	0	4
• Hot Sauce, 10 g	4	0	0
Louisiana Sauce, 10 g	5	0	1
Mayo Lite, 10 g	35	4	2
Meatball Sauce, 30 g	15	0	9
• Mr Sub Secret Sauce, 10 g	40	5	0
Pizza Sauce, 10 g	5	0	1
Yellow Mustard, 10 g	5	0	1
Soups			
Chicken Noodle, 250 g	110	3	17
Chicken w/ Rice, 250 g	90	2	15
Chili W/ Beef, 250 g	198	1	34
Cream of Broccoli, 250 g	170	10	16
Cream of Mushroom, 250 g	170	10	16
Cream of Potato & Leek, 250 g	190	9	23
Cream of Tomato, 250 g	150	6	20
Creamy Tomato & Rstd Red Pepper, 250 g	110	3	19
• Garden Vegetable, 250 g	60	0	13
• Hearty Chili w/ Beef, 250 g	231	2	36
Italian Wedding, 250 g	140	4	24
Mediterranean Chicken, 250 g	110	4	15
Minestrone, 250 g	80	0	17
Pasta Fagioli, 250 g	150	2	28
Vegetable Beef & Barley, 250 g	90	1	18
Toppings			
Bacon, 2 strips	50	4	0
Banana Peppers, 10 g	2	0	0
• Croutons, 14 g	60	2	10
Cucumbers, 3 slices	2	0	0
• Dill Pickles, 3 slices	1	0	0
Green Olives, 10 g	10	1	1
Green Pepper, 10 g	2	0	1
Iceberg Lettuce, 28 g	15	0	3
Jalapeño Peppers, 10 g	2	0	0
Red Onions, 10 g	4	0	1
Sliced Mushrooms, 10 g	3	0	1
Tomatoes, 3 wheels	20	0	4
Wraps			
Albacore Tuna, 248 g	460	16	52
Louisiana Chicken, 190 g	430	15	48
Roast Beef, 218 g	440	14	50
Seafood w/ Crab, 218 g	470	19	61
Smoked Turkey Breast, 220 g	370	9	51
Veggie, 164 g	310	8	49

Mrs. Fields

	Cal	Fat	Cbs
Bite-Size Nibbler® Cookies			
Cinnamon Sugar, 37 g	170	8	22
• Debra's Special Nibbler, 38 g	170	7	23
• Peanut Butter, 38 g	180	10	20
Semi-Sweet Chocolate, 38 g	170	8	24
Triple Chocolate, 38 g	170	9	23
White Chunk Macadamia, 38 g	180	9	23
Brownies			
Butterscotch Blondie, 76 g	350	14	52
Double Fudge, 76 g	360	20	45
Pecan Fudge, 76 g	360	20	46
• Special Walnut Fudge & Blondie, 76 g	330	16	43
Toffee Fudge, 76 g	360	19	47
Walnut Fudge, 76 g	360	20	45

Mrs. Fields (cont.)	Cal	Fat	Cbs
Cakes			
Chocolate Chip, 83 g	350	17	45
Cookies			
• Butter, 44 g	200	8	29
• Cut Out, 90 g	400	19	56
Debra's Special, 44 g	200	9	28
Peanut Butter, 44 g	210	12	24
Semi-Sweet Chocolate, 44 g	210	10	29
w/ Walnuts, 44 g	220	11	29
Triple Chocolate, 44 g	210	11	28
White Chunk Macadamia, 44 g	230	12	27
Muffins			
Blueberry, 21 g	70	3	10
• Chocolate Chip, 21 g	80	4	11
Mandarin Orange, 21 g	80	3	9
• Raspberry, 21 g	70	3	10

Noah's Bagels	Cal	Fat	Cbs
Bagel Dogs			
Artichoke & Grlc Sasge Bagel Dog, 229 g	530	11	81
Asiago Bagel Dog, 239 g	730	32	84
Cajun Andouille Sausage Bagel Dog, 225 g	600	21	78
• Chicken Portobello Bagel Dog, 229 g	510	12	78
Everything Bagel Dog, 237 g	660	27	76
• Plain Bagel Dog, 232 g	740	34	78
Polish Bagel Dog, 236 g	680	30	78
Bagel Sandwiches			
Chicken Salad on Plain Bagel, 312 g	740	36	77
Corned Beef on Plain Bagel, 382 g	910	45	94
Egg Salad on Plain Bagel, 312 g	750	40	77
• Hummus on Plain Bagel, 297 g	530	10	94
N.Y. Lox on Plain Bagel, 299 g	590	19	81
Pastrami on Plain Bagel, 382 g	910	45	94
• Rachel on Plain Bagel, 397 g	1010	51	100
Reuben on Plain Bagel, 397 g	910	40	95
Roast Beef on Plain Bagel, 382 g	750	31	78
Tuna Salad on Plain Bagel, 326 g	610	19	77
Turkey on Plain Bagel, 382 g	760	29	76
Veggie Sandwich, 283 g	560	18	85
Whitefish on Plain Bagel, 340 g	930	52	83
Bagels			
Asiago Cheese Topped Bagel, 134 g	410	5	78
Blueberry, 120 g	360	1	79
Candy Cane Bagel, 118 g	340	4	69
Cheddar Bagel, 113 g	300	2	63
Chocolate Chip Bagel, 120 g	400	5	80
Chopped Garlic Bagel, 124 g	360	1	78
Cinnamon Raisin Bagel, 120 g	360	1	80
Cinnamon Sugar Bagel, 149 g	520	21	80
Cracked Pepper Bagel, 120 g	390	5	78
Cranberry Orange Bagel, 120 g	360	1	80
Egg Bagel, 120 g	360	2	76
Everything Bagel, 124 g	360	2	77
• Good Grains Powerbagel, 114 g	280	5	53
Irish Soda Bagel, 113 g	360	6	69
Onion Bagel, 120 g	360	2	77
Plain Bagel, 120 g	350	1	77
Poppyseed Bagel, 124 g	370	1	78
Potato Bagel, 106 g	350	5	69
• Power Bagel w/ Peanut Butter, 117 g	750	34	92
Power Bagel, 120 g	410	5	81
Pumpernickel Bagel, 120 g	350	1	76
Pumpkin Bagel, 120 g	330	2	69
Salt Bagel, 120 g	350	1	77
Sesame Seed Bagel, 124 g	370	3	77
Sun-Dried Tomato Bagel, 120 g	360	2	77

Noah's Bagels (cont.)	Cal	Fat	Cbs
Bagels (cont.)			
Whole Wheat Bagel w/ Seeds, 124 g	350	3	74
Whole Wheat Bagel, 120 g	330	1	73
Bialies			
Artichoke Spinach & Asiago Bialy, 260 g	660	18	94
Artichoke Tomato Red Onion & Asiago Bialy, 323 g	670	18	98
Cheese Pizza Bialy, 248 g	600	12	97
• Four Cheese Tomato & Rosemary Bialy, 277 g	670	19	97
Mushroom & Four Cheese Bialy, 267 g	660	18	94
• Traditional Bialy, 177 g	450	5	91
Blended Drinks			
Frozen Café Caramel, 18 oz.	600	16	110
Frozen Café Latte, 18 oz.	460	18	72
Frozen Café Mocha, 18 oz.	570	14	107
• Frozen Strawberry, 18 oz.	440	19	73
Frozen Vanilla, 18 oz.	580	31	86
• Mudslide Smoothie, 18 oz.	690	36	101
Breads			
Braided Challah, 2 oz.	150	3	26
Challah Roll, 4 oz.	270	5	51
• Ciabatta Bread, 4 oz.	320	3	64
Corn Meal Rye Bread, 1 slice	170	1	35
• Focaccia Wedge, 1 oz.	110	3	17
Marble Rye Bread, 1 slice	160	1	34
Multigrain Bread, 1 slice	160	2	32
Potato Bread, 1 slice	220	3	44
Coffee Extras			
Light Whipped Cream, 30ml	30	2	2
On Top Reduced Fat Topping, 8 g	20	2	2
• Syrup, Almond, 30ml	90	0	23
Syrup, Hazelnut, 30ml	80	0	20
Syrup, Premium, Sugar Free Caramel, 30ml	0	0	0
• Syrup, Premium, Sugar Free Vanilla, 30ml	0	0	0
Syrup, Vanilla, 30ml	80	0	19
Condiments			
Deli Mustard, 5	4	0	0
• Mayo, 14	110	12	0
Whole Kosher Pickle, 50	5	0	1
• Yellow Mustard, 5	0	0	0
Deli Sandwich			
California Chicken, 365 g	520	19	56
Chicken Salad Deli, 262 g	590	36	41
Cornbeef Deli, 227 g	540	22	53
Deli Beef Roast, 296 g	390	8	41
• Double Decker Club Sandwich, 398 g	920	33	104
Egg Salad Deli, 262 g	600	41	41
Grilled Chicken Caesar Sandwich, 334 g	740	44	54
Pastrami Deli, 227 g	540	22	53
Rachel Sandwich, 347 g	860	51	64
Reuben Sandwich, 347 g	750	40	59
Spicy Chicken Sandwich, 331 g	530	22	52
Tuna Salad Deli, 276 g	450	20	41
• Turkey Deli, 296 g	390	6	39
Ultimate Grilled Cheese, 306 g	870	50	77
White Fish on Corn Meal Rye, 276 g	750	52	41
Egg Sandwiches			
• Egg Mit Artichoke & Tomato, 332 g	550	15	79
Egg Mit Cheese & Tomato, 336 g	800	39	83
Egg Mit Lox & Cheese, 281 g	610	23	74
Egg Mit Lox & Chi, 313 g	800	39	81
Egg Mit Plain, 265 g	710	34	81
Egg Mit Spinach Mushrm & Swiss, 315 g	840	43	82
• Egg Mit Turkey Sausage, 353 g	900	46	82
Egg Mit w/Cheese, 294 g	790	39	81
Egg Spinach, Bacon Panini, 339 g	770	35	71

RESTAURANTS & FAST-FOOD CHAINS

Noah's Bagels (cont.)

	Cal	Fat	Cbs
Egg Sandwiches (cont.)			
Egg, Vegetarian Omelet Panini, 311 g	670	26	75
Eggs Sensations			
Egg Sensation, 341 g	430	25	18
Gourmet Bagels			
• Dutch Apple Bagel (plain), 155 g	400	3	86
Jalapeño Cheddar Bagel, 141 g	420	6	78
• Roasted Red Pepper Bagel, 170 g	440	7	79
Six-cheese Bagel, 141 g	420	6	78
Spinach Florentine Bagel, 148 g	430	7	78
Iced Specialty Coffee			
Iced Americano, 8 oz.	1	0	0
• Iced Coffee, 12 oz.	0	0	0
Iced Latte, 16 oz.	120	5	12
Iced Mocha, 16 oz.	210	6	33
Iced Non Fat Latte, 16 oz.	90	0	12
Low Fat Iced Mocha, 16 oz.	180	3	32
Low Fat Mocha, Regular, 12 oz.	190	3	34
• Reg Macchiato, 12 oz.	240	6	36
Kosher Melts			
Hummus Ammmus Melt, 304 g	660	20	95
• Pizza Melt, 276 g	550	13	86
Tuna Melt, 304 g	680	24	82
• Veggie Melt, 311 g	700	33	83
Panini Sandwiches			
Italian Chicken Panini, 329 g	760	33	68
• Kosher Vegetarian on Plain Bagel, 401 g	860	40	79
• Tuna Panini, 331 g	740	28	89
Turkey Club Panini, 318 g	760	27	86
Vegetarian Panini, 401 g	840	41	71
Salad Dressings			
Asian Sesame Dressing, 2 tbsp.	140	12	6
Caesar Dressing, 2 tbsp.	150	16	1
• Dressing, Raspberry Vinaigrette, 2 tbsp.	160	14	8
• Harvest Chicken, 2 tbsp.	90	8	3
Salad Extras			
Bagel Croutons, 1 oz.	25	1	4
Salads			
Coleslaw, 85 g	180	16	8
Traditional Potato Salad, 140 g	290	21	21
Salads			
Caesar Salad, 198 g	410	35	16
Chicken Caesar Salad, 376 g	660	50	24
Chinese Chicken Salad, 369 g	480	5	84
• City Salad, 326 g	810	68	37
• Tuna Salad, 326 g	260	15	10
Sandwich Fillings			
American Cheese, 1 oz.	70	6	1
Cheddar Cheese, 1 oz.	80	7	0
• Provolone Cheese, 1 oz.	70	6	0
• Smoked Salmon, 2 oz.	110	6	2
Swiss Cheese, 1 oz.	80	6	1
Sides			
Egg Salad, 4 oz.	200	17	5
• Tuna Salad, 4 oz.	150	6	3
• White Fish Salad, 2 oz.	225	20	1
Soups			
• Broccoli, Sharp Cheddar (Bowl), 14 oz.	540	35	31
Broccoli, Sharp Cheddar (Cup), 9 oz.	280	19	15
Chicken & Wild Rice (Bowl), 14 oz.	440	9	67
Chicken & Wild Rice (Cup), 9 oz.	150	4	23
Chicken Noodle (Bowl), 14 oz.	510	21	39
• Chicken Noodle (Cup), 9 oz.	100	5	9
Clam Chowda (Bowl), 14 oz.	370	25	25
Clam Chowda (Cup), 9 oz.	260	15	20

Noah's Bagels (cont.)

	Cal	Fat	Cbs
Soups (cont.)			
Cream of Asparagus Soup (bowl), 14 oz.	390	35	17
Cream of Asparagus Soup (cup), 9 oz.	240	22	10
Low Fat Minestrone (Bowl), 14 oz.	430	6	75
Low Fat Minestrone (Cup), 9 oz.	110	4	19
Split Pea Soup (Bowl), 14 oz.	210	13	14
Split Pea Soup (Cup), 9 oz.	130	8	9
Turkey Chili (Bowl, 14 oz.	330	11	34
Turkey Chili (Cup), 9 oz.	230	7	25
Specialty Coffee			
• Americano Regular, 8 oz.	1	0	0
Cafe Latte, Regular, 10 oz.	100	1	14
Caffe Latte Nonfat, Regular, 12 oz.	100	0	14
Cappuccino Nonfat, Regular, 12 oz.	60	0	9
Cappuccino, Regular, 12 oz.	90	4	9
Espresso, Regular, 15 oz.	1	0	0
Low Fat Mocha, Regular, 12 oz.	190	3	34
• Macchiato, Regular, 12 oz.	240	6	36
Mocha, Regular, 12 oz.	230	6	34
Spreads			
Butter, 14	100	11	0
Fruit Spread, Grape, 1 oz.	75	0	19
Hummus, 2 oz.	110	7	9
• Peanut Butter, Crunchy, 2 tbsp.	641	52	2
Raspberry Preserves, 1 oz.	71	0	18
• Strawberry Preserves, 1 oz.	71	0	18
Sweets			
Apple Cinnamon Coffee Cake, 7 oz.	660	25	106
Blueberry Coffee Cake, 6 oz.	610	25	97
Blueberry Muffin, 5 oz.	470	21	64
Cheesecake Brownie, 5 oz.	520	27	67
• Chocolate Chip Coffee Cake, 6 oz.	730	31	108
• Cinnamon Twists, 4 oz.	370	21	41
Trail Mix Cookie, 4 oz.	480	19	70
White Chocolate Raspberry Scone, 4 oz.	480	22	63
White Chocolate Walnut Cookie, 4 oz.	439	24	52
Whipped Cream Cheese			
Blueberry, 20 g	70	5	6
Cappuccino, 20 g	70	5	5
• Garden Vegetable, 20 g	60	5	2
Garlic Herb, 20 g	60	5	3
Gingerbread, 20 g	70	5	5
Honey Almond Red. Fat, 20 g	70	5	5
Jalapeño Salsa, 20 g	60	5	3
Maple Raisin Walnut, 20 g	60	5	4
Onion and Chive, 20 g	70	6	3
Plain Reduced Fat, 20 g	60	5	2
Plain, 20 g	70	7	1
• Pumpkin, 20 g	100	8	6
Smoked Salmon, 20 g	60	5	3
Strawberry, 20 g	70	5	5
Sundried Tomato & Basil, 20 g	80	5	2

Noodles & Company

	Cal	Fat	Cbs
American (Regular)			
Buttered Noodles	940	42	111
• Caesar Salad	310	27	10
Chicken Noodle Soup	350	11	35
House Marinara	660	17	102
Mushroom Stroganoff	920	47	96
• Wisconsin Mac & Cheese®	1050	47	113
Asian (Regular Size)			
Bangkok Curry	460	16	69
• Chinese Chop Salad	250	10	36
Indonesian Peanut Sauté	660	20	132
Japanese Pan Noodles®	630	9	125

Noodles & Company (cont.)

	Cal	Fat	Cbs
Asian (Regular Size) (cont.)			
• Pad Thai	750	17	136
Thai Curry Soup	400	19	49
Mediterranean (Regular Size)			
Pasta Fresca	720	18	106
Penne Rosa	810	37	91
• Pesto Cavatappi®	820	34	91
• The Med Salad	320	13	38
Tomato Basil Bisque	450	30	39
Whole Grain Tuscan Fettuccine	600	23	78

Nothing but Noodles

	Cal	Fat	Cbs
Add-Ons			
• Beef, 1/2 bowl	110	4	0
Chicken, 1/2 bowl	100	3	0
• Shrimp, 1/2 bowl	53	1	1
Tofu, 1/2 bowl	60	4	1
Desserts			
Cannoli, 1 bowl	374	17	44
• Cotton Candy, 1 bowl	65	0	17
Key Lime Pie, 1 bowl	590	33	67
• New York Cheesecake, 1 bowl	770	53	59
Triple Chocolate Cake, 1 bowl	710	33	106
Kids			
Alfredo, 1 bowl	719	55	39
• Buttery Noodles, 1 bowl	723	49	51
Macaroni & Cheese, 1 bowl	454	26	38
• Spaghetti, 1 bowl	291	6	47
Noodle Bowls - American			
• Beef Stroganoff, 1/2 bowl	508	31	33
Buttery Noodles, 1/2 bowl	651	44	46
Santa Fe Pasta, 1/2 bowl	705	54	40
• Southwest Chipotle, 1/2 bowl	713	58	41
Spicy Cajun Pasta, 1/2 bowl	660	50	44
Noodle Bowls - Asian			
• Pad Thai Noodles, 1/2 bowl	602	10	118
• Sesame Lo Mein, 1/2 bowl	411	11	64
Spicy Japanese Noodles, 1/2 bowl	419	8	74
Thai Peanut, 1/2 bowl	568	20	89
Noodle Bowls - Italian			
Basil Pesto, 1/2 bowl	574	42	36
Cappelini Primavera, 1/2 bowl	500	28	56
• Fettuccini Alfredo, 1/2 bowl	723	56	36
Margherita Pasta, 1/2 bowl	474	31	36
Marinara Pasta, 1/2 bowl	487	11	77
• Three-Cheese Macaroni, 1/2 bowl	446	21	45
Pasta-Less Bowls			
Cheesy Chicken & Vegetables, 1/2 bowl	318	21	6
• Chicken Pomodoro, 1/2 bowl	452	34	7
Primavera Chkn & Vegetables, 1/2 bowl	318	15	26
• Shrimp Pesto Florentine, 1/2 bowl	308	25	5
Thai Curry Beef & Vegetables, 1/2 bowl	443	30	16
Rice Dishes			
General Tso's Chicken, 1/2 bowl	760	44	69
• Kung Pao Chicken, 1/2 bowl	935	51	89
• Thai Peanut Stir Fry, 1/2 bowl	595	27	59
Salads			
BBQ Chicken Salad, 1/2 bowl	205	15	11
Caesar Salad, 1/2 bowl	247	19	14
Chopped Salad, 1/2 bowl	229	15	10
Cranberry Spinach Salad, 1/2 bowl	154	10	18
• Garden Fresh Salad, 1/2 bowl	110	5	12
• Greek Salad, 1/2 bowl	409	31	26
Hunk of Lettuce, 1/2 bowl	229	21	7
Mandarin Orange Salad, 1/2 bowl	205	14	13
Oriental Salad, 1/2 bowl	187	11	20

Nothing but Noodles (cont.)

	Cal	Fat	Cbs
Salads (cont.)			
Pear & Balsamic Spinach Salad, 1/2 bowl	395	28	38
Spicy Cucumber & Chkn Salad, 1/2 bowl	284	15	10
Steak Salad, 1/2 bowl	135	19	7
Sun-Dried Tomato, 1/2 bowl	271	12	32
Soups			
Tomato Bisque, 1/2 bowl	253	23	9
Starters			
Cucumber Side Salad, 1 bowl	193	16	13
• Fresh Mozzarella, 1 bowl	767	27	134
• Garlic Breadsticks, 1 bowl	106	4	0
Mozzarella Cheese Bread, 1 bowl	633	17	86
Potstickers, 1 bowl	479	33	39
Thai Lettuce Wraps, 1/2 bowl	361	23	15

O'Charley's

	Cal	Fat	Cbs
Appetizers & Sides			
• Buffalo Kickin' Wings, 10 pcs.	1830	147	43
Chckn O' Tenders- Create Your Own Combo, 6 pcs.	850	57	34
Chicken O' Tenders, 6 pcs.	850	57	34
Chips and Salsa, full order	520	18	82
Chkn O' Tenders w/ Buffalo Sauce, 6 pcs.	810	53	31
Chkn O' Tenders w/ Chipotle BBQ Sauce, 6 pcs.	690	32	47
Chkn O' Tenders w/ Honey Mustard, 6 pcs.	850	57	34
French Fries, full order	300	18	30
Island Cole Slaw, 1 side	250	19	19
Loaded Baked Potato, 1 side	480	29	54
Onion Rings w/ Sauce, full order	1800	139	119
Over-Loaded Potato Skins, full order	1340	99	48
Plain Potato, 1 side	420	24	52
• Rice Pilaf, 1 side	200	5	31
Smashed Potatoes, 1 side	370	12	47
Southwstrn Chkn Quesadilla, full order	990	59	53
Spicy Jack Cheese Wedges, 7 pcs.	880	60	55
Spinach & Artichoke Dip, full order	940	51	107
Steak House Quesadilla, full order	1330	95	56
Three-Cheese Shrimp Dip, full order	870	49	85
Top Shelf Combo Appetizer, full order	1830	130	81
Brunch			
• Brunch Bread with Jelly	260	10	38
Cajun Chicken Omelette	870	63	13
• Cranberry Pecan Waffle	1380	61	189
Eggs & Bacon	820	53	56
Eggs & Sausage	890	60	56
Ham & Cheese Omelette	1140	78	59
Spanish Omelette	1180	80	66
Steak & Eggs	1260	78	57
Strawberry Chocolate Chip Waffle	1290	50	196
Ultimate Omelette	1180	79	68
Chicken & Ribs			
Chicken Parmesan	860	42	70
Chipotle BBQ Ribs, full rack	1540	95	89
Chipotle BBQ Ribs, half rack	780	47	48
• Grilled Chicken	460	13	26
Prime Time Prime Rib, 10 oz.	1020	79	3
• Prime Time Prime Rib, 16 oz.	1630	127	4
Signature Baby Back Ribs, full rack	1480	96	76
Signature Baby Back Ribs, half rack	750	48	39
Teriyaki Chicken	500	6	57
Desserts			
• Blueberry Muffin, 1 piece	60	4	8
Caramel Pie Ice Cream Scoop - 1 scoop	160	7	23
Key Lime Pie, 1 slice	610	23	90
Ooey Gooey Caramel Pie, 1 slice	720	27	106
• Ultimate Choc. Chocolate Cake, 1 slice	1080	59	152

O'Charley's (cont.)

Dressings

	Cal	Fat	Cbs
Balsamic Dressing, 2 oz.	230	17	17
Bleu Cheese Dressing, 2 oz.	230	25	4
• Greek Feta Vinaigrette, 2 oz.	620	64	7
Honey Mustard Dressing, 2 oz.	330	32	11
Honey Mustard, Light, 2 oz.	120	4	21
• Italian Dressing, Light, 2 oz.	70	5	7
Ranch Dressing, 2 oz.	190	19	4
Ranch Dressing, Light, 2 oz.	70	5	7
Thousand Island Dressing, 2 oz.	210	19	8

Kid's Menu

	Cal	Fat	Cbs
Jr. Brunch	600	36	55
Jr. Cheeseburger	650	35	48
Jr. Chicken Tenders	310	17	12
Jr. Corn Dogs	500	38	32
Jr. French Toast	1100	56	117
Jr. Hamburger	540	25	47
Jr. Macaroni and Cheese	360	23	27
• Jr. Pasta	230	4	42
Jr. Shrimp	310	18	25
• Jr. Waffle	1150	55	149

Sandwiches & Burgers

	Cal	Fat	Cbs
Bacon & Cheese Trio Chkn Sandwich	800	40	53
Bacon & Cheese Trio Chkn Sandwich w/ Mayo	1110	75	54
Buffalo Kickin Sandwich	980	58	72
Club Sandwich	1020	59	83
Grilled Chicken Sandwich	610	27	52
• Half-Club Sandwich-Lunch	510	30	42
• Mushroom Swiss Burger	1490	111	56
Whiskey Sirloin Sandwich	930	48	65

Seafood & Pasta

	Cal	Fat	Cbs
Bayou Shrimp Pasta	1280	78	101
Blackened Rainbow Trout	690	52	5
Cajun Chicken Pasta	1260	69	88
Caribbean Coconut Shrimp	650	26	88
• Catfish Platter	1690	141	65
Catfish Platter - Lunch	1170	99	37
Cedar-Planked Salmon	590	35	2
Chipotle BBQ Salmon, 10 oz.	670	37	17
Fisherman's Platter	1410	85	108
• Fresh Atlantic Grilled Salmon - Lunch	370	22	2
Fried Shrimp Dinner	490	30	27
Grilled Shrimp Dinner	600	41	33
Whiskey Salmon, 10 oz.	760	44	23

Signature Soups & Salads

	Cal	Fat	Cbs
• Black & Bleu Caesar Salad	920	65	21
• Broccoli & Three Cheese Soup, 1 cup	100	5	10
Cajun Chicken Salad	740	49	17
California Chicken Salad	560	26	42
Chicken Harvest Soup, 1 cup	220	11	16
Chicken Tortilla Soup, 1 cup	120	7	11
Clam Chowder, 1 cup	170	10	11
Classic Chicken Caesar Salad	490	30	13
House Salad - Entree	230	11	19
House Salad - Side	210	11	15
O'riginal Southern Fried Chicken Salad	720	41	34
Pecan Chicken Tender Salad	840	54	46
Roasted Tomato Basil Soup, 1 cup	130	9	10
Southwestern Steak Soup, 1 cup	100	5	10

Steak

	Cal	Fat	Cbs
• Butcher's Cut Steak, 5 oz.	260	14	0
Filet Mignon	500	30	0
Flame-Grilled Top Sirloin, 10 oz.	580	35	0
Flame-Grilled Top Sirloin, 7 oz.	430	28	0
Louisiana Sirloin	670	38	3

O'Charley's (cont.)

Steak (cont.)

	Cal	Fat	Cbs
Our Favorite Ribeye Steak	810	55	0
• Steak Tips Monterey	1000	64	47

Old Spaghetti Factory

Appetizers

	Cal	Fat	Cbs
Bay Shrimp Crostini, 8 oz.	630	19	86
• Garlic Cheese Bread Starter, 14 oz.	1220	85	105
Meatballs Starter	910	61	23
Portuguese Linguica, 17 oz.	840	37	85
Sausage Starter, 284 g	690	56	7
• Shrimp, Spinach & Artichoke Dip, 298 g	580	9	103
Tapenade of Black Olives, 10 oz.	810	37	99
Tortellini Starter, 340 g	930	56	82

Desserts

	Cal	Fat	Cbs
• Caramel Turtle Pie Dessert, 9 oz.	660	29	93
Mud Pie Dessert, 9 oz.	680	32	90
• New York Cheese Cake w/ Berry Topping, 8 oz.	690	40	72

Dinner Menu Items

	Cal	Fat	Cbs
Baked Chicken (Orzo Pilaf/Broccoli), 17 oz.	740	48	20
Baked Chicken, 447 g	880	47	55
Chicken Fettuccine, 517 g	960	56	74
Chicken Marsala, 498 g	960	44	55
Chicken Parmigiana, 554 g	840	34	84
Eggplant Parmigiana, 532 g	670	32	75
• Fettuccine Alfredo, 439 g	1130	83	71
Lasagna, 454 g	630	33	36
Pot Pourri, 461 g	710	30	84
Salmon Tuscany, 17 oz.	680	43	21
• Spaghetti w/ Tomato Sauce, 425 g	440	5	84
w/ Clam Sauce & Mizithra, 439 g	960	54	81
w/ Clam Sauce, 425 g	690	28	84
w/ Meat & Clam Sauce, 425 g	580	17	84
w/ Meat Sauce & Mizithra, 439 g	850	42	80
w/ Meat Sauce & Sausage, 539 g	830	35	85
w/ Meatballs, 20 oz.	840	33	86
w/ Mizithra, 384 g	1010	64	74
w/ Mushroom & Clam Sauces, 425 g	570	18	83
w/ Mushroom & Meat Sauces, 425 g	460	6	83
w/ Mushroom Sauce & Mizithra, 439 g	850	43	80
w/ Mushroom Sauce, 425 g	460	7	83
w/ Rich Meat Sauce, 425 g	470	5	83
w/ Tomato & Meat Sauces, 425 g	460	5	84
w/ Tomato & Mizithra, 439 g	840	42	81
w/ Tomato Sauce & Clam Sauce, 425 g	560	17	84
Spinach & Cheese Ravioli, 319 g	480	15	59
Spinach Tortellini w/ Alfredo Sauce, 342 g	930	56	82

Dinner Specials

	Cal	Fat	Cbs
Angel Hair Florentine, 454 g	600	21	73
Chicken Penne w/ Tomato Alfredo, 17 oz.	760	32	74
• Coconut Shrimp Curry, 516 g	860	45	76
Meatloaf w/ Eggplant & Broccoli, 16 oz.	720	48	34
Pesto Basil Cream Sauce, 411 g	790	47	73
Rigatoni Bolognese, 398 g	620	32	48
• Shrimp & Artichoke Linguini, 13 oz.	590	18	78
Spaghetti Vesuvius, 425 g	590	18	82

Kids Meals

	Cal	Fat	Cbs
Grilled Cheese Sandwich, 102 g	360	22	28
Macaroni & Cheese, 284 g	350	9	57
• Spaghetti w/ Tomato Sauce & Meatballs, 333 g	440	13	59
• Spaghetti w/ Tomato Sauce, 284 g	300	4	56

Lunch Menu Items

	Cal	Fat	Cbs
Chicken Fettuccine, 404 g	830	55	56
Chicken Parmigiana, 554 g	840	34	84
Fettuccine Alfredo, 312 g	780	55	53
Lasagna, 369 g	520	27	29

Old Spaghetti Factory (cont.)

Lunch Menu Items (cont.)	Cal	Fat	Cbs
Pot Pourri, 284 g	480	22	54
• Spaghetti w/ Tomato Sauce, 284 g	300	4	56
w/ Brown Butter & Mizithra, 242 g	590	34	49
w/ Clam & Mizithra, 262 g	520	26	53
w/ Clam Sauce, 284 g	460	19	56
w/ Meat & Clam, 284 g	380	11	56
w/ Meat & Mizithra, 262 g	450	19	53
w/ Meat Sauce & Sausage, 390 g	620	29	57
w/ Meatballs, 383 g	610	24	62
w/ Mushroom & Clam, 284 g	380	12	56
w/ Mushroom & Meat, 284 g	310	4	55
w/ Mushroom & Mizithra, 262 g	450	19	52
w/ Mushroom Sauce, 284 g	310	5	55
w/ Rich Meat Sauce, 284 g	310	4	55
w/ Tomato & Clam Sauce, 284 g	380	11	56
w/ Tomato & Meat Sauce, 284 g	300	4	56
w/ Tomato & Mizithra, 262 g	440	18	53
Spinach & Cheese Ravioli, 319 g	480	15	59
• Spinach Tortellini w/ Alfredo Sauce, 342 g	930	56	82
Lunch Specials			
Angel Hair Florentine, 454 g	600	21	73
• Chicken Cacciatore, 19 oz.	1120	66	82
Manicotti, 326 g	510	21	55
• Shrimp & Artichoke Linguini, 354 g	440	14	58
Shrimp Newberg, 411 g	800	47	54
Platters			
• Hearty Platter #4 w/ Tomato Sauce, 709 g	740	9	140
w/ Clam Sauce, 709 g	1140	47	140
w/ Meat Sauce, 709 g	780	9	139
• w/ Mizithra, 624 g	1590	98	122
w/ Mushroom Sauce, 709 g	760	12	138
Lasagna & Chicken Marsala, 709 g	1000	42	42
Ravioli & Spaghetti w/ Meat Sauce, 602 g	790	19	115
Spaghetti w/ Sauce, Mtballs & Sausage, 687 g	1280	64	94
Salad Dressings			
1000 Island, 2 oz.	150	15	4
Balsamic Vinaigrette, 28 g	170	18	2
Blue Cheese, 2 oz.	190	21	1
• Caesar, 57 g	320	34	1
Creamy Pesto, 2 oz.	200	21	1
• Fat Free Honey Mustard, 2 oz.	60	0	13
Reduced Calorie French, 2 oz.	100	6	13
Salads			
BLT Salad, 14 oz.	760	59	30
Cobb Salad (no dressing), 19 oz.	700	44	15
• Dinner Chicken Caesar Salad, 20 oz.	1050	83	29
House Salad w/Caesar Dressing, 6 oz.	190	15	8
Lunch Chicken Caesar Salad, 15 oz.	780	60	21
Mango Macadamia Chicken Salad, 20 oz.	850	51	70
• Orzo Salad, 4 oz.	80	3	11
Shrimp Louie Salad, 15 oz.	680	56	19
Small Caesar Salad, 7 oz.	380	34	11
Sandwiches			
Brie & Arugula Sandwich, 13 oz.	1350	102	61
• Factory Burger, 20 oz.	1380	89	39
Meatball Sandwich, 447 g	900	50	64
• Sausage Sandwich, 411 g	830	49	57
Seafood Cheddar Melt, 15 oz.	980	56	74
Tuscan Chicken Sandwich, 496 g	1110	67	55
Sides			
• Broccoli Salad Garnish, 71 g	120	11	5
• Large Side of Broccoli, 424 g	630	58	18
Small Side of Broccoli, 212 g	320	29	9

Old Spaghetti Factory (cont.)

Soups	Cal	Fat	Cbs
Chicken Mulligatawny, 9 oz.	250	14	20
• Chicken Orzo, 9 oz.	90	3	9
• Clam Chowder, 9 oz.	380	29	25
Cream of Broccoli, 9 oz.	220	12	19
Mediterranean White Bean, 9 oz.	150	6	19
Minestrone, 10 oz.	120	5	15

Olive Garden

Appetizers	Cal	Fat	Cbs
Alfredo Dipping Sauce	380	N/A	N/A
• Breadstick w/ Garlic-Butter Spread	150	N/A	N/A
Bruschetta	440	N/A	N/A
Calamari	890	N/A	N/A
Add Marinara Sauce	70	N/A	N/A
Add Parmesan-Peppercorn Sauce	300	N/A	N/A
Caprese Flatbread	600	N/A	N/A
Create a Sampler Italiano			
Add Marinara Sauce	70	N/A	N/A
Add Parmesan-Peppercorn Sauce	300	N/A	N/A
Add Tomato Sauce	45	N/A	N/A
Calamari	440	N/A	N/A
Chicken Fingers	330	N/A	N/A
Fried Mozzarella	370	N/A	N/A
Fried Zucchini	370	N/A	N/A
Stuffed Mushrooms	410	N/A	N/A
Toasted Beef & Pork Ravioli	360	N/A	N/A
Grilled Chicken Flatbread	760	N/A	N/A
Hot Artichoke-Spinach Dip	660	N/A	N/A
Marinara Dipping Sauce	70	N/A	N/A
Mussels di Napoli	180	N/A	N/A
Sicilian Scampi	500	N/A	N/A
• Smoked Mozzarella Fondula	930	N/A	N/A
Stuffed Mushrooms	410	N/A	N/A
Beef & Pork			
Chianti Braised Short Ribs	1060	N/A	N/A
Mixed Grill	770	N/A	N/A
• Pork Filettino	640	N/A	N/A
Steak Gorgonzola-Alfredo	1310	N/A	N/A
Steak Toscana	880	N/A	N/A
Beverages			
Bellini Peach-Raspberry Iced Tea	70	N/A	N/A
Caffe Latte	130	N/A	N/A
Caffe le Toscana Coffee	3	N/A	N/A
Caffe Mocha	180	N/A	N/A
Cappuccino	150	N/A	N/A
Caramel Hazelnut Macchiato	220	N/A	N/A
Cream Sodas	200	N/A	N/A
• Frozen Cappuccino	320	N/A	N/A
Herbal and Flavored Hot Tea	3	N/A	N/A
Italian Sodas	120	N/A	N/A
• Lavazza Espresso	2	N/A	N/A
Raspberry Lemonade	145	N/A	N/A
Sicilian Splash	100	N/A	N/A
Chicken			
Chicken & Gnocchi Veronese	1030	N/A	N/A
• Chicken & Shrimp Carbonara	1440	N/A	N/A
Chicken Alfredo	1430	N/A	N/A
Chicken Marsala	770	N/A	N/A
Chicken Scampi	1020	N/A	N/A
Garlic-Herb Chicken con Broccoli	960	N/A	N/A
Stuffed Chicken Marsala	800	N/A	N/A
• Venetian Apricot Chicken	380	N/A	N/A
Classic Recipes			
Capellini Pomodoro	840	N/A	N/A
Chicken Parmigiana	1090	N/A	N/A

Olive Garden (cont.)

Classic Recipes (cont.)	Cal	Fat	Cbs
Eggplant Parmigiana	850	N/A	N/A
Fettuccine Alfredo	1220	N/A	N/A
Five Cheese Ziti al Forno	1050	N/A	N/A
Lasagna Classico	850	N/A	N/A
• Linguine alla Marinara	430	N/A	N/A
Spaghetti & Italian Sausage	1270	N/A	N/A
Spaghetti & Meatballs	1110	N/A	N/A
Spaghetti w/ Meat Sauce	710	N/A	N/A
• Tour of Italy	1450	N/A	N/A
Filled Pastas			
• Braised Beef & Tortellini	1020	N/A	N/A
Cheese Ravioli w/ Marinara Sauce	660	N/A	N/A
w/ Meat Sauce	790	N/A	N/A
Manicotti Formaggio	940	N/A	N/A
• Ravioli di Portobello	610	N/A	N/A
Fish & Seafood			
Grilled Shrimp Caprese	900	N/A	N/A
Herb-Grilled Salmon	610	N/A	N/A
• Parmesan Crusted Tilapia	590	N/A	N/A
• Seafood Alfredo	1020	N/A	N/A
Seafood Portofino	800	N/A	N/A
Shrimp & Asparagus Risotto	620	N/A	N/A
Shrimp Primavera	730	N/A	N/A
Pizza			
• Chicken Alfredo Pizza	1180	N/A	N/A
Create Your Own Pizza			
Add Bell Peppers	10	N/A	N/A
Add Black Olives	45	N/A	N/A
Add Italian Sausage	140	N/A	N/A
Add Mushrooms	6	N/A	N/A
Add Onions	15	N/A	N/A
Add Pepperoni	120	N/A	N/A
Add Roma Tomatoes	10	N/A	N/A
• Cheese Only	910	N/A	N/A
Soups & Salads			
Garden-Fresh Salad w/ dressing	350	N/A	N/A
w/out Dressing	120	N/A	N/A
• Grilled Chicken Caesar	850	N/A	N/A
• Minestrone, 1 bowl	100	N/A	N/A
Pasta e Fagioli, 1 bowl	130	N/A	N/A
Zuppa Toscana, 1 bowl	170	N/A	N/A

On the Border Mexican Grill

Appetizers	Cal	Fat	Cbs
Border Sampler, full	1970	121	114
Chicken Flautas w/ Queso, full	1060	68	64
• Chile Con Queso, 1 bowl	390	29	14
Chips & Salsa, full	500	25	58
Dble-Stacked Club Quesadillas, full	1860	123	88
Empanadas - Beef, full	1150	81	68
Empanadas - Chicken, full	1090	74	68
Fajita Chicken Con Queso w/ Tortillas	1480	93	61
Grande Fajita Nachos - Chicken, full	1890	113	109
Grande Fajita Nachos - Combo, full	1940	121	109
Grande Fajita Nachos - Steak, full	1970	127	109
Guacamole Live!, full	520	60	23
Guacamole, full	170	13	12
Queso Live! - Fajita Chicken w/ Chips	1320	84	77
Queso Live! - Fajita Steak w/ Chips	1390	94	77
Queso Live! - Taco Beef w/ Chips	1390	95	80
• Stacked Border Nachos, full	2740	166	191
Stffd Jalapeños w/ Chili con Queso, full	980	56	70
Ultimate Loaded Queso	900	59	46
Border Smart			
Chicken Salsa Fresca, full order	520	9	60

On the Border Mexican Grill (cont.)

Border Smart (cont.)	Cal	Fat	Cbs
Grilled Fajita Chicken Tacos, full order	570	9	78
• Jalapeño-BBQ Salmon, full order	590	21	45
• Pico Shrimp Tacos, full order	490	5	78
Burritos & Chimis			
Beef Burrito w/ Chili con Carne Sauce	930	49	57
• Big Beef Bordurrito w/ Side Salad	1600	103	119
Big Chicken Bordurrito w/ Side Salad	1420	87	121
Border Chimichanga - Fajita Chicken	1230	93	51
Border Chimichanga - Ground Beef	1310	98	49
Border Chimichanga- Spicy Chicken	1160	85	46
• Chicken Burrito w/ Sour Cream Sauce	850	54	55
Three Sauce Fajita Chicken Burrito	870	45	59
Three Sauce Fajita Steak Burrito	1050	61	57
Create Your Own Combo			
Cheese Chile Relleno, 1 each	880	61	60
Chicken Flautas w/ Chili con Queso, 1 each	300	19	17
Crispy Taco - Beef, 1 each	330	20	19
• Crispy Taco - Chicken, 1 each	240	12	16
Crispy Taco - Veggie, 1 each	250	16	20
• Dos XX® Fish Tacos, 1 serving	1590	113	100
Empanadas - Beef w/ Chili con Queso, 2 each	530	38	30
Empanadas - Chicken w/ Chili con Queso, 2 each	490	33	28
Enchilada - Beef, 1 each	340	17	27
Enchilada - Cheese & Onion, 1 each	410	24	27
Enchilada - Chicken, 1 each	350	23	21
Fish Taco, 1 each	530	38	33
Pork Tamale, 1 each	310	17	26
Soft Taco - Beef, 1 each	340	19	23
Soft Taco - Chicken, 1 each	250	11	20
Desserts			
• Border Brownie Sundae w/ Vanilla Ice Cream	1360	78	158
Chocolate Turtle Empanadas, 4 each	1280	81	131
Dulce De Leche Cheesecake	1160	72	122
Kahlua® Ice Cream Pie	850	44	100
Sizzling Apple Crisp	960	36	157
Sopapillas	1230	56	136
• Vanilla Ice Cream, 1 scoop	180	10	19
Fajita Grill			
Carnitas (roasted pork) Fajitas	830	62	19
• Chicken Chipotle Fajita Favorites	1160	86	46
Corn Tortillas, 3 each	230	4	43
• Grlld Vegetable Fajitas w/ Portobello Mushrooms	390	28	30
Homemade Flour Tortillas, 3 each	360	11	54
Lettuce, Sour Cream, Pico de Gallo, Cheese	200	16	5
Lettuce, Sour Cream, Pico de Gallo, Guacamole	160	13	9
Monterey Ranch Chicken Fajita Favorites	840	54	17
Original Mesquite-Grilled Chicken Fajitas	440	18	20
Original Mesquite-Grilled Shrimp Fajitas	750	63	18
Original Mesquite-Grilled Steak Fajitas	620	41	18
Parrilla Butter, 1 oz.	120	13	1
Smothered Steak Fajitas	860	57	20
Favoritos			
Brisket Tacos w/ Jalapeño BBQ Sauce, 3 each	1200	56	114
• Corona Extra Dinner	2040	126	136
Dos XX® Fish Tacos	1590	113	100
Enchilada Suizas w/ Sauce, 3 each	1110	71	70
Quesadillas - Double-Stacked Club w/ Dressing	1990	55	89
Quesadillas - Fajita Chicken	1430	91	59
Quesadillas - Fajita Chicken & Steak Combo	1450	98	59
Quesadillas - Fajita Steak	1530	107	59
Superior Dinner	1350	85	80
• Tacos - Buffalo Chicken w/ Dressing, 2 each	960	62	61
Tacos - Carne Asada w/ Dressing, 2 each	1250	83	56
Tacos - Southwest Chicken w/ Sauce, 3 each	1180	77	63

On the Border Mexican Grill (cont.)

Favoritos (cont.)	Cal	Fat	Cbs
Tres Enchilada Dinner - Beef, 3 each	1010	52	80
Tres Enchilada Dinner - Chicken, 3 each	1040	68	64
Tres Enchiladas Dinner - Cheese, 3 each	1150	68	79
Kids Menu			
Border Chicken Strips	570	36	38
Cheeseburger	500	32	23
Corn Dog	320	21	11
Crispy Taco Mexican Dinner - Beef	740	31	77
Crispy Taco Mexican Dinner - Chicken	740	28	85
Dessert - Sundae w /Chocolate Syrup	300	13	40
Dessert - Sundae w/ Strawberry Purée	340	13	52
Grilled Chicken	130	2	1
Grilled Chicken Sandwich	630	21	63
Hamburger	390	23	23
• Nachos - Bean & Cheese	980	57	71
Nachos - Cheese	670	47	28
Side - French Fries	240	13	31
Side - Mexican Rice	220	6	33
Side - Salad w/ Chipotle Honey Mustard Dressing	250	22	12
Side - Salad w/ Ranch Dressing	180	17	5
• Side - Sautéed Vegetables	70	4	9
Soft Taco Mexican Dinner - Beef	840	35	91
Soft Taco Mexican Dinner - Chicken	750	27	89
Off the Grill			
• Baja Chicken	610	43	50
Bandera Sirloin	640	43	13
Carne Asada & Shrimp	1040	74	22
Pico Chicken & Shrimp	730	51	9
• Ranchiladas	1360	86	53
Salad Dressings & Sauces			
Chili Con Carne Sauce, 2 oz.	70	3	6
Chipotle Honey Mustard Dressing, 2 oz.	310	29	11
• Chipotle Mayonnaise, 2 oz.	380	42	2
Fat-free Balsamic Vinaigrette, 2 oz.	50	0	10
Jalapeño BBQ Sauce, 2 oz.	100	1	20
Ranch Dressing, 2 oz.	220	23	2
• Ranchero Sauce, 2 oz.	18	1	3
Roasted Jalapeño Ranch Dressing, 2 oz.	180	19	2
Roasted Jalapeño Sauce, 2 oz.	240	26	2
Salsa Fresca, 2 oz.	20	0	3
Salsa, 2 oz.	25	1	3
Smoked Jalapeño Vinaigrette, 2 oz.	231	22	8
Sour Cream Sauce, 2 oz.	140	14	2
Tomatillo Cream Sauce, 2 oz.	120	11	3
Salads & Soup			
Blackened Chicken Fiesta Salad w/ Dressing	1150	75	54
Chicken Fiesta Salad w/ Dressing	1140	74	52
Chicken Tortilla Soup, 1 bowl	350	22	24
Grande Taco Salad w/ Spicy Chicken	1280	89	74
• Grande Taco Salad w/ Taco Beef	1450	102	78
Grilled Steak Ensalada w/ Vinaigrette	1120	75	54
• House Salad	170	10	15
Sizzling Fajita Salad - Chicken	760	48	23
Sizzling Fajita Salad - Steak	910	65	24
Side Items & Extras			
Beans - Black	180	7	19
Beans - Refried	290	11	36
Black Bean & Corn Relish, 2 oz.	70	4	6
• Cheesy Pepper Jack Mashed Potatoes	380	27	26
Guacamole, 1 scoop	60	5	4
Mexican Rice	220	6	33
• Pico de Gallo, 1 scoop	20	1	2
Sautéed Shrimp, 4 each	170	10	1
Sour Cream, 1 scoop	90	8	3

On the Border Mexican Grill (cont.)

Side Items & Extras (cont.)	Cal	Fat	Cbs
Vegetables - Grilled	50	1	8
Vegetables - Sautéed	70	4	9

Orange Julius

Add a Banana	Cal	Fat	Cbs
1/2 Banana, 3 oz.	60	N/A	13
1 Banana, 6 oz.	110	1	27
Beverages			
Bananarilla, 20 oz.	370	9	69
Cool Cappuccino, 20 oz.	480	13	86
• Orange Julius®, 20 oz.	270	1	68
Piña Colada, 20 oz.	410	9	87
Raspberry Julius, 20 oz.	300	2	76
Raspery, 20 oz.	400	10	78
• Strawberry Banana, 20 oz.	500	9	97
Strawberry Julius, 20 oz.	280	1	72
Tripleberry, 20 oz.	460	10	92
Tropical, 20 oz.	370	9	69
Fruit Smoothies			
3-Berry Blast, 20 oz.	610	10	144
Banana Chill, 20 oz.	550	10	134
Berry Lemon Lively, 20 oz.	450	10	101
Blackberry Storm, 20 oz.	630	70	129
Blackberry Toner, 20 oz.	440	10	96
Blueberrathon, 20 oz.	350	15	89
Blueberry Burst, 20 oz.	470	5	106
• Cocoa Latte Swirl, 20 oz.	640	80	122
Mango Passion, 20 oz.	360	0	80
Orange Swirl™, 20 oz.	490	90	96
Peaches & Cream, 20 oz.	500	0	116
Raspberry Créme, 20 oz.	540	70	107
• Raspberry Crush, 20 oz.	330	20	83
Strawberried Treasure, 20 oz.	550	70	103
Strawberry Sensation, 20 oz.	430	0	98
Strawberry Xtreme, 20 oz.	410	5	87
Tart 'N' Berry™, 20 oz.	450	10	102
Tropical Tango, 20 oz.	400	25	90
Tropi-Colada, 20 oz.	560	70	110
Wild Blue Twist™, 20 oz.	490	5	115
Nutrition Boost			
Fiber Plus, 6 g	5	0	4
Heart Health, 4 g	15	0	3
• Joint Care, 6 g	20	0	5

Outback Steakhouse

Add-on Mates	Cal	Fat	Cbs
Grilled Onions	130	N/A	N/A
Sauteed Mushrooms	160	N/A	N/A
Classics & Pasta			
• Alice Springs Chicken	2000	N/A	N/A
• Grilled Pork Chops	1340	N/A	N/A
No Rules Pasta	1390	N/A	N/A
Fresh Made Sides			
Aussie Chips	350	N/A	N/A
Classic Wedge Salad	490	N/A	N/A
Dressed Baked Potato	380	N/A	N/A
Fresh Steamed Broccoli	130	N/A	N/A
• w/o Butter	30	N/A	N/A
Fresh Steamed French Green Beans	150	N/A	N/A
Fresh Steamed Veggies	160	N/A	N/A
House Salad	570	N/A	N/A
Roasted Garlic Mashed Potatoes	350	N/A	N/A
• Sweet Potato	590	N/A	N/A
Walkabout Soup	480	N/A	N/A
Whole Grain Wild Rice	190	N/A	N/A

RESTAURANTS & FAST-FOOD CHAINS

Outback Steakhouse (cont.)

	Cal	Fat	Cbs
Prime Rib & Roasted Sirloin			
Prime Rib, 12 oz.	520	N/A	N/A
Prime Rib, 16 oz.	690	N/A	N/A
• Prime Rib, 8 oz.	350	N/A	N/A
• Slow Roasted Sirloin Medley	1150	N/A	N/A
Simply Grilled			
• Baby Back Ribs w/ Chips and Apples	2260	N/A	N/A
Baby Back Ribs, 1/2 rack	1520	N/A	N/A
Chicken Griller	1400	N/A	N/A
Chicken on the Barbie	860	N/A	N/A
Filet Griller	1100	N/A	N/A
• Rack of Lamb	820	N/A	N/A
Salmon Griller	1390	N/A	N/A
Scallop Griller	1250	N/A	N/A
Shrimp Griller	1880	N/A	N/A
Straight from the Sea			
Atlantic Salmon, 7 oz.	1540	N/A	N/A
• Atlantic Salmon, 9 oz.	1640	N/A	N/A
Boomerang Shrimp	1620	N/A	N/A
Fresh Tilapia	700	N/A	N/A
• Lobster Tail, 1 tail	550	N/A	N/A
Lobster Tails, 2 tails	670	N/A	N/A
Lobster Tails, 3 tails	800	N/A	N/A
USDA "Choice" Steaks			
New York Strip, 14 oz.	730	N/A	N/A
Outback Special , 12 oz.	860	N/A	N/A
Outback Special , 9 oz.	680	N/A	N/A
Ribeye, 14 oz.	1210	N/A	N/A
• The Melbourne, 22 oz.	1410	N/A	N/A
• Victoria's Center Cut Fillet, 7 oz.	600	N/A	N/A
Victoria's Center Cut Fillet, 9 oz.	740	N/A	N/A
Victoria's Crowned Fillet w/ Blue Cheese, 7 oz.	830	N/A	N/A
Victoria's Crowned Fillet w/ Blue Cheese, 9 oz.	970	N/A	N/A
Victoria's Crowned Fillet w/ Horseradish, 7 oz.	820	N/A	N/A
Victoria's Crowned Fillet w/ Horseradish, 9 oz.	960	N/A	N/A

P.F. Chang's China Bistro

	Cal	Fat	Cbs
Added Extras			
Chili Bean Sauce	81	1	12
• Crispy Green Bean Sauce	451	48	5
Mustard Vinaigrette	66	2	7
Potsticker Sauce	57	1	0
Rice Sticks	135	0	33
• Shrimp Dumpling Sauce	24	0	1
Special Sauce	55	1	9
Spicy Plum Sauce	110	0	28
Sweet and Sour Sauce	57	0	15
Chicken			
Chang's Spicy Chicken	923	37	88
Chicken with Black Bean Sauce	678	23	33
Dali Chicken	1091	52	53
• Ginger Chicken with Broccoli	656	26	45
Ginger Chicken with Broccoli - Gluten Free	677	30	43
Ground Chicken and Eggplant	792	40	73
• Kung Pao Chicken	1228	79	58
Mu Shu Chicken	715	38	49
Orange Peel Chicken	1151	46	127
Philip's Better Lemon Chicken	1051	42	113
Sweet and Sour Chicken	764	20	107
Desserts			
Apple Pie Mini Dessert	170	4	34
Banana Split Mini Dessert	167	6	28
Banana Spring Rolls	814	37	130
Carrot Cake Mini Dessert	295	14	42
• Coconut-pineapple Ice Cream	111	12	25
Creamy Strawberry Cheesecake Mini Dessert	239	20	14

P.F. Chang's China Bistro (cont.)

	Cal	Fat	Cbs
Desserts (cont.)			
Flourless Chocolate Dome - Gluten Free	572	26	84
Great Wall Of Chocolate Mini Dessert	336	26	24
S'mores Mini Dessert	323	12	50
• The Great Wall Of Chocolate Cake	2237	90	376
Tiramisu Mini Dessert	202	14	15
Tres Leche Lemon Dream Mini Dessert	216	8	32
Meat			
Beef A La Sichuan	1172	64	56
Chengdu Spiced Lamb	1056	75	34
Mongolian Beef	1178	73	29
• Mu Shu Pork	871	50	50
• Orange Peel Beef	1568	85	115
Sweet and Sour Pork	1095	46	106
Wok Charred Beef	941	63	33
Wok Seared Lamb	1081	80	29
Noodles, Meins, and Rice			
• Brown Rice - Cup	254	2	53
Cantonese Chow Fun with Chicken	1045	23	146
with Beef	1212	38	142
Chow Mein with Beef	793	26	84
with Chicken	689	16	84
with Pork	898	34	83
with Shrimp	625	13	84
Chow Mein Combo	912	34	86
Double Pan-fried Noodles with Beef	1186	56	112
with Chicken	1072	47	115
with Pork	1208	60	114
with Shrimp	1031	46	115
Dan Dan Noodles	1087	30	145
Double Pan-fried Noodles Combo	1384	69	118
Garlic Noodles	612	11	111
P.F. Chang's Fried Rice with Beef	1228	40	150
with Chicken	1208	44	151
with Pork	1360	57	150
with Shrimp	1154	41	149
P.F. Chang's Fried Rice Combo	1539	69	154
Singapore Street Noodles	572	16	81
Singapore Street Noodles - Gluten Free	566	15	81
• Tam's Noodles	1678	93	144
White Rice - Cup	295	1	64
Seafood			
Cantonese Scallops	408	16	26
• Cantonese Shrimp	330	12	21
Chang's Lemon Scallops	952	28	100
Crispy Honey Shrimp	1061	44	118
• Hot Fish	1338	71	111
Kung Pao Scallops	1136	57	66
Kung Pao Shrimp	977	58	58
Lemon Pepper Shrimp	701	36	59
Oolong Marinated Sea Bass	521	12	40
Orange Peel Shrimp	1010	41	118
Salt and Pepper Prawns	844	50	55
Shrimp with Candied Walnuts	1225	80	74
Sichuan from the Sea Calamari	1078	36	118
Sichuan from the Sea Scallops	1030	36	98
Sichuan from the Sea Shrimp	728	37	55
Wild Alaskan Sockeye Salmon Stmd w/ Ginger	646	36	23
Sides			
Asian Slaw	585	57	19
Garlic Snap Peas - Large	205	10	23
Garlic Snap Peas - Small	129	7	13
Shanghai Cucumbers	124	6	8
Sichuan-style Asparagus - Large	204	6	34
Sichuan-style Asparagus - Small	97	3	16

P.F. Chang's China Bistro (cont.)

	Cal	Fat	Cbs
Sides (cont.)			
• Spicy Green Beans - Large	602	40	48
Spicy Green Beans - Small	234	13	23
Spinach Stir-fried with Garlic - Large	140	6	16
• Spinach Stir-fried with Garlic - Small	77	3	9
Soups and Salads			
Bikini Shrimp Salad	192	6	30
with Watermelon Citrus Vinaigrette Add	240	23	7
Chang's Chicken Noodle Soup - 1 bowl	512	13	30
Chang's Wedge	244	19	12
with Chicken	595	35	12
with Creamy Wedge Dressing	443	43	8
Chicken Chopped Salad	401	14	21
with Our Signature Ginger Dressing	483	48	9
Egg Drop Soup - 1 bowl	367	14	51
• Egg Drop Soup - 1 cup	48	2	7
• Hot and Sour Soup - 1 Bowl	652	18	82
Hot and Sour Soup - 1 cup	85	2	11
Wonton Soup - 1 bowl	354	10	44
Starters			
Chang's Chicken Lettuce Wraps	377	12	35
Chang's Chicken Lettuce Wraps - Gluten Free	477	12	63
• Chang's Spare Ribs	1356	89	43
Chang's Vegetarian Lettuce Wraps	281	4	37
Crab Wontons	440	26	32
Crispy Green Beans	507	28	59
Harvest Spring Rolls	287	15	30
Northern Style Spare Ribs	720	54	6
Peking Dumplings - Pan Fried	367	23	21
Peking Dumplings - Steamed	327	18	21
Salt And Pepper Calamari	720	11	118
• Seared Ahi Tuna	210	9	9
Shrimp Dumplings - Pan Fried	305	13	25
Shrimp Dumplings - Steamed	265	8	25
Vegetable Dumplings - Pan Fried	307	11	43
Vegetable Dumplings - Steamed	267	7	43
The Grill			
• Asian Marinated New York Strip	1432	86	68
Citrus Soy Salmon - with Brown Rice	1000	59	42
Citrus Soy Salmon - with White Rice	1025	58	49
• Lemongrass Prawns	907	58	65
Sichuan Chicken Flatbread	1160	80	56
Traditional Lunch Bowls			
Almond And Cashew Chicken with Brown Rice	909	27	101
Almond And Cashew Chicken with White Rice,	955	26	112
Beef with Broccoli with Brown Rice	844	27	87
Beef with Broccoli with White Rice	890	26	99
• Buddha's Feast with Brown Rice	541	8	101
Buddha's Feast with White Rice	587	6	113
Citrus Soy Salmon with Brown Rice	1047	63	67
• Citrus Soy Salmon with White Rice	1093	62	79
Crispy Honey Chicken with Brown Rice	943	13	126
Crispy Honey Chicken with White Rice	989	12	138
Moo Goo Gai Pan with Brown Rice	545	8	76
Moo Goo Gai Pan with White Rice	591	6	88
Pepper Steak with Brown Rice	820	28	82
Pepper Steak with White Rice	968	39	94
Shrimp with Lobster Sauce with Brown Rice	686	25	75
Shrimp with Lobster Sauce with White Rice	732	23	87
Traditions			
Almond And Cashew Chicken	815	30	63
Beef with Broccoli	1118	65	38
Crispy Honey Chicken	867	11	121
Lo Mein with Beef	1374	80	94
with Chicken	1198	67	97

P.F. Chang's China Bistro (cont.)

	Cal	Fat	Cbs
Traditions (cont.)			
with Pork	1400	54	95
with Shrimp	1134	64	97
• Lo Mein Combo	1409	83	98
Moo Goo Gai Pan	661	34	32
Pepper Steak	971	48	32
• Shrimp with Lobster Sauce	480	22	24
Vegetarian Plates			
• Buddha's Feast - Steamed	137	1	29
Buddha's Feast - Stir Fried	367	5	66
Coconut Curry Vegetables	686	46	48
Stir-fried Eggplant	590	34	64
• Vegetable Chow Fun	878	8	181
Vegetarian Ma Po Tofu	537	19	51

Panda Express

	Cal	Fat	Cbs
Appetizers			
Chicken Egg Roll, 3 oz.	170	8	17
• Chicken Potsticker, 6 pieces.	440	25	49
Cream Cheese Rangoon, 3 pieces	190	8	24
• Veggie Spring Roll, 2 oz.	80	4	11
Beef			
Broccoli Beef, 6 oz.	150	7	11
Mongolian Beef, 6 oz.	180	11	15
Chicken			
Black Pepper Chicken, 6 oz.	200	12	11
Kung Pao Chicken, 6 oz.	240	15	12
Mandarin Chicken, 6 oz.	250	10	8
• Mushroom Chicken, 6 oz.	130	6	8
• Orange Chicken, 6 oz.	500	27	42
Potato Chicken, 6 oz.	200	10	21
String Bean Chicken Breast, 6 oz.	160	8	10
Pork			
BBQ Pork, 6 oz.	440	23	15
Sweet & Sour Pork, 6 oz.	400	23	35
Rice & Noodles			
Chow Mein, 8 oz.	390	12	59
• Fried Rice, 8 oz.	450	14	67
• Steamed Rice, 8 oz.	380	3	81
Sauces			
Mandarin Sauce, 2 oz.	70	0	17
• Potsticker Sauce, 2 oz.	35	0	8
• Sweet & Sour Sauce, 2 oz.	80	0	19
Shrimp			
• Crispy Shrimp, 100 g	260	13	26
Kung Pao Shrimp, 6 oz.	240	14	14
• Tangy Shrimp, 6 oz.	150	5	16
Soup			
Egg Flower Soup, 12 oz.	88	2	16
Hot & Sour Soup, 12 oz.	110	4	14
Veggies			
Eggplant and Tofu, 6 oz.	180	10	20
Mixed Veggies, 6 oz.	90	7	8

Panera Bread

	Cal	Fat	Cbs
Artisan Breads			
• Ciabatta, 6 oz.	460	5	98
Country Demi, 2 oz.	130	0	27
Country Loaf, 2 oz.	130	0	27
• Country Miche, 2 oz.	120	0	25
Focaccia, 2 oz.	160	3	29
French Baguette, 2 oz.	140	0	28
French Miche, 2 oz.	120	0	25
Sesame Semolina Demi, 2 oz.	130	1	27
Sesame Semolina Loaf, 2 oz.	130	1	27
Sesame Semolina Miche, 2 oz.	130	1	25

Panera Bread (cont.)

Artisan Breads (cont.)	Cal	Fat	Cbs
Stone-Milled Rye Loaf, 2 oz.	120	0	25
Stone-Milled Rye Miche, 2 oz.	120	0	24
Three Cheese Demi, 2 oz.	140	2	24
Three Cheese Loaf, 2 oz.	140	2	24
Three Cheese Miche, 2 oz.	130	2	23
Three Seed Demi, 2 oz.	140	3	25
Whole Grain Baguette, 2 oz.	140	1	28
Whole Grain Loaf, 2 oz.	130	1	26
Whole Grain Miche, 2 oz.	140	1	27
Artisan Pastries			
Caramel Apple, 4 oz.	400	19	51
Cheese, 4 oz.	380	22	38
Cherry, 5 oz.	420	21	51
• Chocolate Crumb, 4 oz.	470	21	64
Chocolate, 4 oz.	340	20	37
• Fresh Strawberries & Citrus, 4 oz.	310	16	37
Pecan Braid, 4 oz.	410	22	48
Baked Egg Soufflés			
Four Cheese, 6 oz.	470	30	35
Spinach & Artichoke, 6 oz.	490	32	36
• Spinach & Bacon, 6 oz.	530	34	36
• Turkey Sausage & Potato, 6 oz.	440	27	36
Brownies			
Caramel Pecan, 4 oz.	470	24	59
Very Chocolate, 4 oz.	460	22	61
Cafe Sandwiches - Half Portions			
Chicken Salad on Sesame Semolina	340	12	44
Chicken Salad on Whole Grain	290	14	33
Smoked Ham & Swiss on Rye	340	17	27
Smoked Ham & Swiss on Stn-Milled Rye	380	16	37
Smoked Turkey Breast on Country	300	9	39
• Smoked Turkey Breast on Sourdough	230	8	24
Tuna Salad on Honey Wheat	350	23	29
• Tuna Salad on Whole Grain	420	22	43
Cookies			
Chocolate Chipper, 3 oz.	410	20	55
Chocolate Duet with Walnuts, 3 oz.	400	22	52
• Nutty Chocolate Chipper, 3 oz.	430	24	51
• Nutty Oatmeal Raisin, 3 oz.	340	14	50
Shortbread, 3 oz.	350	21	36
Cream Cheese Spreads			
• Plain, 2 oz.	200	19	2
Reduced Fat Hazelnut, 2 oz.	150	12	6
Reduced Fat Honey Walnut, 2 oz.	160	11	10
Reduced Fat Plain, 2 oz.	140	13	2
Reduced Fat Raspberry, 2 oz.	150	11	8
Reduced Fat Sun-Dried Tomato Cream, 2 oz.	140	12	4
• Reduced Fat Veggie, 2 oz.	120	10	3
Crispani®			
BBQ Chicken, 5 oz.	380	15	42
Italian Meat Classic, 5 oz.	380	18	38
Pepperoni, 4 oz.	380	18	38
Roasted Wild Mushroom, 4 oz.	340	16	38
• Sausage & Roasted Peppers, 5 oz.	380	18	38
Three Cheese, 4 oz.	340	15	37
• Tomato & Fresh Basil, 4 oz.	320	13	37
Espresso Drinks			
• Caffe Latte, 9 oz.	120	5	12
Caffe Mocha, 12 oz.	370	15	60
Cappuccino, 9 oz.	120	5	12
Caramel Latte, 12 oz.	390	16	53
• Pumpkin Spice Latte, 13 oz.	410	10	68
Freshly Baked Bagels			
Asiago Cheese, 5 oz.	350	6	60

Panera Bread (cont.)

Freshly Baked Bagels (cont.)	Cal	Fat	Cbs
Blueberry, 5 oz.	330	1	69
• Cinnamon Crunch, 5 oz.	410	8	75
Cranberry Walnut, 5 oz.	370	5	71
Dutch Apple & Raisin, 5 oz.	370	3	78
Everything, 4 oz.	300	2	60
French Toast, 5 oz.	380	5	73
Gingerbread, 5 oz.	390	5	77
• Plain, 4 oz.	290	1	61
Sesame, 4 oz.	310	4	58
Whole Grain, 5 oz.	340	3	66
Frozen Drinks			
Caramel - Grande, 16 oz.	550	23	80
Mango - Grande, 16 oz.	350	10	60
• Mocha - Grande, 16 oz.	570	25	88
• Strawberry Smoothie - Grande, 18 oz.	250	2	53
Hand-Tossed Salads			
Asian Sesame Chicken, half portion	220	11	16
Caesar, half portion	220	16	13
• Classic Cafe, half portion	90	5	9
• Fuji Apple Chicken, half portion	290	15	19
Greek, half portion	260	24	7
Grilled Chicken Caesar, half portion	280	17	14
Grilled Salmon, half portion	170	7	16
Orchard Harvest, half portion	210	12	15
Hot Drinks			
Chai Tea Latte, 10 oz.	190	4	31
• Hot Chocolate, 11 oz.	370	15	60
Hot Panini			
• Half Chkn Pomodoro on French, 6 oz.	280	10	25
Half Chkn Pomodoro on Sesame Semolina, 7 oz.	350	10	43
• Half Frontega Chicken®, 6 oz.	400	16	40
Half Portobello & Mozzarella, 6 oz.	330	12	41
Half Smokehouse Turkey® on Focaccia, 6 oz.	360	12	39
Half Smokehouse Turkey® on Three Chz, 6 oz.	350	11	37
Half Turkey Artichoke, 7 oz.	350	11	44
Iced Drinks			
Iced Green Tea - Grande, 16 oz.	100	0	25
• Iced Chai Tea Latte, 16 oz.	150	4	25
• Home Style Lemonade - Grande, 16 oz.	90	0	22
Mini Bundt Cakes			
• Lemon Poppyseed, 5 oz.	460	20	63
• Pineapple Upside-Down, 6 oz.	520	25	74
Muffins & Muffies			
Carrot Walnut Muffin, 5 oz.	430	19	61
• Chocolate Chip Muffie, 3 oz.	240	10	36
Cranberry Orange Muffin, 5 oz.	400	15	59
Pumpkin Muffie, 3 oz.	310	7	49
• Pumpkin Muffin, 6 oz.	590	13	93
Reduced Fat Wild Blueberry Muffin, 5 oz.	360	10	61
Wild Blueberry Muffin, 5 oz.	400	16	59
Panera Kids™			
Deli Sandwich - Roast Beef, 6 oz.	370	13	36
Deli Sandwich - Smoked Ham, 6 oz.	360	14	35
Deli Sandwich - Smoked Turkey, 6 oz.	350	12	36
• Grilled Cheese Sandwich, 4 oz.	290	11	35
• Peanut Butter & Jelly Sandwich, 5 oz.	420	16	55
Salad Dressings			
Balsamic Vinaigrette, 2 oz.	130	10	9
Caesar Dressing, 2 oz.	150	15	3
Cherry Balsamic Vinaigrette, 2 oz.	130	12	7
• Fat-Free Raspberry Dressing, 2 oz.	35	0	8
Fuji Apple Vinaigrette, 2 oz.	150	12	11
• Greek Dressing, 2 oz.	220	24	0
Low-Fat Rstd Grlc Meyer Lemon Vinaigrette, 2 oz.	60	2	9

Panera Bread (cont.)

	Cal	Fat	Cbs
Salad Dressings (cont.)			
Reduced-Sugar Asian Sesame Vinaigrette, 2 oz.	90	8	4
Scones			
• Cinnamon Chip, 5 oz.	530	27	67
Orange, 5 oz.	430	21	54
• Tart Cherry, 4 oz.	380	16	58
Wild Blueberry, 4 oz.	410	15	63
Signature Sandwiches			
Asiago Roast Beef, half portion	350	16	28
Bacon Turkey Bravo®, half portion	370	13	42
Chicken Caesar on Focaccia, half portion	400	16	41
Chicken Caesar on Three Cheese, half portion	380	15	39
• Chicken Tomesto on French, half portion	240	7	27
Chicken Tomesto on Three Cheese, half portion	310	8	40
Chipotle Chicken on Artisan French, half portion	470	24	39
Chipotle Chicken on Specialty French, half portion	400	24	25
• Italian Combo, half portion	530	24	53
Mediterranean Veggie, half portion	300	6	50
Sierra Turkey, half portion	420	20	41
Soups			
Baked Potato, 8 oz.	230	14	21
Broccoli Cheddar, 8 oz.	230	16	13
Cream of Chicken & Wild Rice, 8 oz.	200	12	19
French Onion (with cheese & croutons), 8 oz.	220	10	23
• French Onion (without cheese & croutons), 8 oz.	80	3	12
Low-Fat Chicken Noodle, 8 oz.	100	2	15
Low-Fat Vegetarian Black Bean, 8 oz.	160	1	31
Low-Fat Vegetarian Garden Vegetable, 8 oz.	90	1	17
• New England Clam Chowder, 8 oz.	320	28	11
Parisian Chicken, 9 oz.	170	11	13
Vegetarian Fiesta Con Queso, 8 oz.	250	16	18
Specialty Breads			
Asiago Cheese Demi, 2 oz.	150	4	22
Asiago Cheese Loaf, 2 oz.	150	4	22
Cinnamon Raisin Loaf, 2 oz.	170	3	32
Cranberry Walnut Panettone, 2 oz.	210	10	27
French Baguette, 2 oz.	150	2	30
French Loaf, 2 oz.	140	2	28
French Roll, 2 oz.	170	2	34
Holiday, 2 oz.	150	2	29
Honey Wheat loaf, 2 oz.	160	3	30
Sourdough Baguette, 2 oz.	150	0	30
Sourdough Loaf, 2 oz.	140	0	28
Sourdough Roll, 3 oz.	190	1	38
• Sourdough Soup Bowl, 8 oz.	560	2	115
Sunflower Loaf, 2 oz.	180	6	26
• Tomato Basil Loaf, 2 oz.	130	1	27
White Whole Grain Wheat Loaf, 2 oz.	140	2	28
XL French Loaf, 2 oz.	140	2	28
Specialty Pastries			
• Bear Claw, 5 oz.	460	27	49
• Coffee Cake - Cherry Cheese, 2 oz.	210	11	26
French Croissant, 2 oz.	240	14	25
Sweet Rolls			
• Cinnamon Roll, 6 oz.	610	27	90
• Cobblestone, 7 oz.	590	12	107
Pecan Roll, 5 oz.	591	32	73

Papa Gino's

	Cal	Fat	Cbs
Appetizers & Snacks: Small			
BBQ Chick Tenders, 1/2 portion	259	9	28
Buff. Chick. Tender, 1/2 portion	199	7	20
• Cheese Breadsticks, 1/2 portion	535	24	58
• Chicken Tender, 1/2 portion	190	7	18
Cinnamon Sticks, 1/2 portion	309	10	50
French Fries, 1/2 portion	331	19	38

Papa Gino's (cont.)

	Cal	Fat	Cbs
Appetizers & Snacks: Small (cont.)			
Marinara Dip Sauce, 1/2 portion	57	1	13
Mozzarella Sticks, 1/2 portion	347	15	35
Toasted Ravioli, 1/2 portion	286	15	33
Appetizers & Snacks: Large			
BBQ Chicken Tender, 1/4 portion	259	9	28
Buff. Chick. Tender, 1/4 portion	199	7	20
• Cheese Breadsticks, 1/4 portion	535	24	58
Cheese Garlic Bread, 1/4 portion	222	5	36
• Chicken Tender, 1/4 portion	190	7	18
Cinnamon Stick Icing, 1/4 portion	240	1	57
French Fries, 1/4 portion	362	22	38
Mozzarella Sticks, 1/4 portion	347	15	35
Toasted Ravioli Small, 1/4 portion	286	15	33
Extras			
• Hot Peppers, 1 oz.	0	0	1
• Mayonnaise, 28 g	213	24	1
Mushrooms, 1 oz.	7	0	1
Onions, 0.5 oz.	6	0	1
Pickles, 1 oz.	0	0	1
Processed American Cheese, 1 oz.	95	7	3
Provolone Cheese, 1 oz.	100	8	1
Sweet Green Pepper, 1 oz.	6	0	1
Tomato, 60 g	11	0	2
Kids Meal			
Cheese Slice, 158 g	316	9	44
Chicken Tender Meal, 219 g	481	26	44
• Hot Dog Meal, 213 g	511	29	49
• Penne, 254 g	336	6	61
Pepperoni Slice, 172 g	388	16	44
Spaghetti & Meatball, 296 g	456	16	63
Large Thick Crust Pizza			
BBQ Chicken, 158 g	379	10	53
Buffalo Chicken, 153 g	350	10	47
Cheese, 155 g	365	12	47
Cheeseburger, 178 g	423	16	49
Chicken Pepper, 190 g	385	12	48
Fenway, 207 g	414	15	50
Garlic Chicken, 186 g	398	12	50
Hawaiian, 182 g	386	11	49
Meat Combo, 172 g	427	17	47
• PapaRoni, 169 g	428	18	48
Pepperoni, 148 g	360	11	49
• Super Veggie, 204 g	348	10	50
Works, 189 g	405	15	49
Large Thin Crust Pizza			
BBQ Chicken, 130 g	273	7	39
Buffalo Chicken, 125 g	244	7	32
• Cheese, 110 g	224	6	32
Chicken Pepper, 163 g	285	10	34
Garlic Chicken, 159 g	292	11	35
Meat Combo, 140 g	323	14	33
• PapaRoni, 138 g	323	15	33
Pepperoni, 122 g	269	10	32
Works, 156 g	300	12	34
Pasta Entrees			
• Broccoli Ravioli, 386 g	445	20	49
Papa Platter Penne, 641 g	1003	34	136
Papa Platter Spaghetti, 641 g	1003	34	136
Pasta Trio Plate, 563 g	916	30	130
Penne Alfredo Chix, 559 g	1021	42	119
Penne Alfredo, 417 g	901	37	111
Penne, 474 g	651	11	118
Spaghetti & Meatballs, 559 g	893	30	123
Spaghetti Alfredo Chix Broccoli, 559 g	1021	42	119

Papa Gino's (cont.)

	Cal	Fat	Cbs
Pasta Entrees (cont.)			
Spaghetti Alfredo, 417 g	901	37	111
• Spaghetti Chicken Parmesan, 656 g	1080	41	128
Spaghetti, 474 g	653	11	118
Pasta Sides			
• Meatballs, 128 g	270	18	9
Penne Alfredo, 209 g	450	18	55
Penne, 254 g	336	6	61
• Spaghetti Alfredo, 209 g	450	18	55
Spaghetti, 254 g	337	6	61
Pizza			
Cheese, 1 slice	316	9	44
Pepperoni, 1 slice	388	16	44
Salads			
Buffalo Chicken Tender, 325 g	319	15	32
Caesar, 234 g	191	8	20
Chicken Bacon Cheddar, 415 g	481	21	26
Chicken Caesar, 365 g	324	8	16
Chicken Tender, 308 g	282	10	30
• Garden, 289 g	176	6	27
Greek, 335 g	202	11	12
• Italian Chopped, 357 g	574	50	12
Single Breadstick, 82 g	215	10	23
Salads Dressing			
Bleu Cheese, 30 g	150	15	3
• Caesar, 85 g	397	43	0
• Fat Free Honey Dijon, 43 g	59	0	13
Honey Mustard, 30 g	150	14	7
Olive Oil Vinaigrette, 85 g	170	17	9
Ranch, 85 g	284	31	3
Small Thin Crust Pizza			
BBQ Chicken, 105 g	209	4	31
Buffalo Chicken, 93 g	176	4	24
• Cheese, 87 g	166	4	25
Chicken Pepper, 131 g	208	7	25
Garlic Chicken, 117 g	213	7	27
• Meat Combo, 113 g	257	11	25
PapaRoni, 105 g	235	10	25
Pepperoni, 95 g	203	8	25
Super Veggie, 144 g	186	5	28
Works, 127 g	219	8	27
Subs & Sandwiches: Large			
BLT, 430 g	1025	48	107
Chicken Cutlet, 358 g	743	18	107
Chicken Parm, 477 g	1082	44	114
Italian, 520 g	1243	62	106
• Meatball Parm, 576 g	1376	63	120
Meatball, 519 g	1174	54	120
Seafood Salad, 404 g	949	37	116
Steak & Cheese, 446 g	1168	53	106
Steak, 364 g	891	33	99
Super Steak, 673 g	1235	53	120
Tuna, 401 g	1086	56	100
Turkey Club, 487 g	842	21	105
• Turkey, 333 g	619	2	101
Vegetarian, 456 g	778	22	113
Subs & Sandwiches: Panini Sandwiches			
• Basil Chicken, 424 g	1117	62	89
• Eggplant, 376 g	768	30	101
Italian Deli, 374 g	950	52	72
Sausage & Pepper, 431 g	1106	68	76
Subs & Sandwiches: Small			
BLT, 312 g	683	31	72
• Hot Dog w/ Roll, 128 g	391	25	30
• Italian, 313 g	905	48	69

Papa Gino's (cont.)

	Cal	Fat	Cbs
Subs & Sandwiches: Small (cont.)			
Lobster Roll, 227 g	545	35	31
Meatball Parm, 327 g	832	36	76
Meatball, 299 g	731	33	76
Seafood Salad, 284 g	680	34	69
Steak & Cheese, 269 g	694	30	68
Steak, 241 g	600	23	65
Super Steak, 428 g	741	30	78
Tuna, 281 g	734	38	67
Turkey Club, 333 g	600	19	70
Turkey, 224 g	444	2	72
Toppings (per large slice)			
Bacon, 13 g	59	4	0
BBQ Chicken, 99 g	240	9	28
Black Olives, 11 g	13	1	1
Broccoli, 20 g	6	0	1
Buffalo Chicken, 96 g	219	9	24
Capicola, 6 g	7	0	0
Cheese, 86 g	208	9	24
Chicken Pepper, 121 g	247	11	25
Extra Cheese, 12 g	35	3	0
Garlic Chicken, 118 g	251	11	25
Green Pepper, 12 g	2	0	1
Hamburger, 19 g	59	4	0
• Meat Combo, 106 g	274	14	25
Mushrooms, 12 g	3	0	0
Naples, 116 g	273	14	25
Onions, 12 g	5	0	1
PapaRoni, 105 g	274	14	25
Pepperoni, 7 g	31	3	0
Pepperoni, 93 g	238	11	24
Saus Arrabbiata, 111 g	259	13	25
Sausage, 21 g	74	7	0
• Sliced Tomato, 7 g	1	0	0
Super Veggie, 128 g	222	9	26
Works, 116 g	258	12	25

Papa John's Pizza

	Cal	Fat	Cbs
10" Pizza			
• Cheese Pizza, 91 g	210	8	27
Pepperoni Pizza, 91 g	220	9	27
• Sausage Pizza, 95 g	240	11	26
14" Pizza			
• Cheese Pizza, 132 g	300	11	39
Pepperoni Pizza, 128 g	310	13	38
• Sausage Pizza, 134 g	330	15	37
BBQ Chicken & Bacon			
Original Crust Pizza, 150 g	340	11	44
• Pan Crust Pizza, 156 g	410	140	44
• Thin Crust Pizza, 114 g	290	14	29
Garden Fresh			
Original Crust Pizza, 160 g	280	9	40
• Pan Crust Pizza, 173 g	360	13	40
• Thin Crust Pizza, 134 g	210	11	23
Grilled Chicken Alfredo			
Original Crust Pizza, 132 g	310	12	36
• Pan Crust Pizza, 138 g	380	16	36
• Thin Crust Pizza, 96 g	240	13	20
Hawaiian BBQ Chicken			
Original Crust Pizza, 164 g	340	11	46
• Pan Crust Pizza, 170 g	420	16	46
• Thin Crust Pizza, 127 g	290	14	31
Italian Meats Trio			
Original Crust Pizza, 150 g	340	11	38
• Pan Crust Pizza, 164 g	440	20	40
• Thin Crust Pizza, 113 g	280	12	22

Papa John's Pizza (cont.)

	Cal	Fat	Cbs
Roma Meats			
Original Crust Pizza, 158 g	340	11	39
• Pan Crust Pizza, 170 g	430	20	40
• Thin Crust Pizza, 122 g	280	12	22
Six Cheese			
Original Crust Pizza, 133 g	320	13	38
• Pan Crust Pizza, 144 g	400	21	40
• Thin Crust Pizza, 96 g	250	14	21
Spicy Italian			
Original Crust Pizza, 147 g	370	11	39
• Pan Crust Pizza, 159 g	450	15	39
• Thin Crust Pizza, 110 g	320	14	24
Spinach Alfredo			
Original Crust Pizza, 116 g	280	11	36
• Pan Crust Pizza, 122 g	360	15	36
• Thin Crust Pizza, 79 g	220	13	19
Spinach Alfredo Chicken Tomato			
Original Crust Pizza, 144 g	290	11	37
• Pan Crust Pizza, 153 g	380	16	37
• Thin Crust Pizza, 110 g	230	13	21
The Meats			
Original Crust Pizza, 141 g	350	16	38
• Pan Crust Pizza, 152 g	420	19	38
• Thin Crust Pizza, 105 g	300	18	23
The Works			
Original Crust Pizza, 157 g	330	11	39
• Pan Crust Pizza, 167 g	400	15	39
• Thin Crust Pizza, 120 g	280	14	24

Papa Murphy's

	Cal	Fat	Cbs
Cheesy Bread			
Cheesy Bread, 75 g	220	8	31
Dessert Pizzas			
Apple, 97 g	245	5	46
• Cherry, 97 g	235	5	44
Chocolate Chip Cookies, 57 g	245	11	34
• Cinnamon Rolls, 111 g	344	10	58
Cinnamon Wheel, 82 g	250	7	42
Family Size (16") Original Crust Pizzas			
Barbecue Chicken, 144 g	334	12	36
• Cheese, 109 g	260	10	29
Cowboy, 151 g	340	17	31
Gourmet Chicken Garlic, 137 g	320	14	30
Gourmet Classic Italian, 146 g	352	18	31
Gourmet Vegetarian, 144 g	302	13	31
Hawaiian, 136 g	285	11	33
Herb Chicken Mediterranean, 128 g	338	15	35
Murphy's Combination, 158 g	355	18	31
• Papa's Favorite, 170 g	355	18	31
Papa-Roni Signature, 125 g	340	17	29
Pepperoni, 118 g	310	15	29
Rancher, 140 g	325	15	30
Specialty of the House, 145 g	310	14	31
Vegetarian Combo, 160 g	285	12	32
Veggie Mediterranean, 113 g	320	14	34
Family Size Calzones			
• Chicken Florentine, 218 g	457	19	46
Combo, 184 g	434	19	45
Italian, 209 g	449	20	46
• Veggie, 197 g	390	16	45
Family Size Stuffed Pizzas			
5-Meat, 143 g	365	16	38
• Big Murphy, 157 g	360	16	40
Chicago-Style, 149 g	365	16	38
• Chicken and Bacon, 151 g	373	15	38

Papa Murphy's (cont.)

	Cal	Fat	Cbs
Large (14") Original Crust Pizzas			
Barbecue Chicken, 134 g	308	11	35
• Cheese, 98 g	240	10	26
Cowboy, 137 g	310	16	28
Gourmet Chicken Garlic, 124 g	291	12	27
Gourmet Classic Italian, 129 g	315	16	27
Gourmet Vegetarian, 127 g	273	12	28
Hawaiian, 124 g	255	10	29
Herb Chicken Mediterranean, 114 g	300	13	31
• Murphy's Combination, 141 g	320	16	28
Papa's All Meat, 125 g	315	16	27
Papa's Favorite, 153 g	320	16	28
Pepperoni, 106 g	280	14	26
Rancher, 125 g	290	14	27
Specialty of the House, 154 g	290	14	28
Vegetarian Combo, 145 g	260	11	29
Veggie Mediterranean, 102 g	285	13	31
Large (14") Thin Crust deLITE Pizzas			
Barbecue Chicken deLITE, 79 g	181	8	17
• Cheese deLITE, 58 g	140	7	13
Cowboy deLITE, 86 g	190	11	13
Gourmet Chicken Bacon Artichoke deLITE, 78 g	181	9	13
Gourmet Chicken Garlic deLITE, 76 g	172	9	13
Gourmet Classic Italian deLITE, 85 g	180	10	13
Gourmet Vegetarian deLITE, 76 g	161	8	13
Hawaiian deLITE, 77 g	150	7	15
Herb Chicken Mediterranean deLITE, 68 g	180	9	16
Meat deLITE, 76 g	190	11	13
Murphy's Combination deLITE, 91 g	195	12	14
Papa's All Meat deLITE, 76 g	187	11	13
• Papa's Favorite deLITE, 96 g	195	11	14
Pepperoni deLITE, 64 g	165	9	13
Rancher deLITE, 77 g	175	9	13
Specialty of the House deLITE, 82 g	170	9	13
Vegetarian Combo deLITE, 92 g	150	8	14
Veggie deLITE, 71 g	152	8	13
Veggie Mediterranean deLITE, 59 g	165	9	15
Large Size Calzones			
• Chicken Florentine, 215 g	455	19	45
Combo, 182 g	440	20	44
Italian, 196 g	440	20	45
• Veggie, 186 g	390	16	44
Large Size Stuffed Pizzas			
5-Meat, 142 g	361	15	37
• Big Murphy, 152 g	355	15	38
Chicago-Style, 145 g	356	15	38
• Chicken and Bacon, 148 g	366	15	38
Medium (12") Original Crust Pizzas			
Barbecue Chicken, 117 g	273	10	30
Cheese, 90 g	215	9	24
Cowboy, 125 g	280	14	25
Gourmet Chicken Garlic, 112 g	263	12	24
Gourmet Classic Italian, 125 g	271	13	25
Gourmet Vegetarian, 113 g	248	11	25
• Hawaiian, 91 g	190	7	22
Herb Chicken Mediterranean, 103 g	272	12	28
Murphy's Combination, 131 g	290	15	26
Papa's All Meat, 113 g	280	14	24
• Papa's Favorite, 138 g	290	15	26
Pepperoni, 97 g	250	12	24
Rancher, 114 g	265	12	25
Specialty of the House, 97 g	210	10	20
Vegetarian Combo, 133 g	235	10	26
Veggie Mediterranean, 92 g	255	12	28

RESTAURANTS & FAST-FOOD CHAINS

Papa Murphy's (cont.)

	Cal	Fat	Cbs
Salads			
• Caesar, 120 g	47	2	4
Chicken Caesar, 163 g	108	3	5
Club, 189 g	145	9	6
Garden, 206 g	100	6	8
Italian, 186 g	136	10	7
• Lasagna, 201 g	255	14	17

Pei Wei Asian Diner

	Cal	Fat	Cbs
Dan Dan Noodles			
Chicken, 1/2 portion	390	7	54
First Tastes			
Crab Wontons, 2 pcs.	190	13	9
Crispy Potstickers, 2 pcs.	130	7	10
Edamame, 1/2 portion	156	8	12
• Hot & Sour Soup, 1 bowl	500	28	37
Hot & Sour Soup, 1 cup	150	9	11
Minced Chkn w/ Cool Lettuce Wraps, 1/2 portion	250	4	31
• Pei Wei Spring Rolls, 1 roll	90	5	11
Wonton Soup, 1 bowl	260	5	49
Wonton Soup, 1 cup	110	2	23
Fried Rice			
• Beef, 1/2 portion	580	21	56
Chicken, 1/2 portion	470	11	56
Pork, 1/2 portion	500	16	57
Scallops, 1/2 portion	410	9	56
Shrimp, 1/2 portion	420	10	55
• Vegetables & Tofu, 1/2 portion	380	7	60
Japanese Udon Noodles			
• Beef, 1/2 portion	600	26	57
Chicken, 1/2 portion	490	16	57
Pork, 1/2 portion	520	21	57
Scallops, 1/2 portion	450	16	58
Shrimp, 1/2 portion	460	16	57
• Vegetables & Tofu, 1/2 portion	440	16	63
Kid's Wei™			
Honey Seared Chicken, 1/2 portion	290	17	19
Teriyaki Chicken, 1/2 portion	240	5	20
Lo Mein Noodles			
• Beef, 1/2 portion	570	21	61
Chicken, 1/2 portion	460	11	61
Pork, 1/2 portion	490	16	62
• Scallops, 1/2 portion	390	8	61
Shrimp, 1/2 portion	400	8	60
Vegetables & Tofu, 1/2 portion	400	8	66
Pad Thai			
• Beef, 1/2 portion	670	30	63
Chicken, 1/2 portion	560	20	61
Pork, 1/2 portion	590	25	62
Scallops, 1/2	480	16	61
Shrimp, 1/2 portion	490	17	60
• Vegetables & Tofu, 1/2 portion	470	17	66
Rice & Noodles			
Brown Rice, 1/2 portion	170	2	37
• Egg Noodles, 1/2 portion	210	3	39
Rice Noodles, 1/2 portion	130	0	32
• Udon Noodles, 1/2 portion	101	0	20
White Rice, 1/2 portion	200	0	44
Salads			
Asian Chopped Chicken Salad, 1/2 portion	280	15	13
w/o Dressing	200	8	10
• Pei Wei Spicy Chicken Salad, 1/2 portion	350	16	28
w/o Dressing	210	3	23
• Vietnamese Chicken Salad Rolls, 3 rolls	80	4	9
Sauces & Sides			
Fortune Cookie	30	0	7

Pei Wei Asian Diner (cont.)

	Cal	Fat	Cbs
Sauces & Sides (cont.)			
Lettuce Wrap Sauce, 2 oz.	70	5	2
Lime Vinaigrette, 2 oz.	230	20	13
• Rice Sticks, 1 cup	130	0	33
Sesame Ginger Dressing, 2 oz.	170	16	5
Sweet Chile Sauce, 2 oz.	140	0	34
Thai Peanut Sauce, 2 oz.	168	11	15
• Sgntre Dishes: Asian Coconut Curry Beef, 1/2 portion	550	37	20
Chicken, 1/2 portion	380	19	23
Pork, 1/2 portion	420	26	24
Scallops, 1/2 portion	290	16	19
Shrimp, 1/2 portion	300	17	18
Vegetables & Tofu, 1/2 portion	220	14	19
Signature Dishes: Blazing Noodles			
• Beef, 1/2 portion	570	36	23
Chicken, 1/2 portion	420	22	22
Pork, 1/2 portion	460	29	23
Scallops, 1/2 portion	370	21	24
Shrimp, 1/2 portion	380	22	23
• Vegetables & Tofu, 1/2 portion	300	17	27
Signature Dishes: Ginger Broccoli			
• Beef, 1/2 portion	450	22	19
Chicken, 1/2 portion	300	9	19
Pork, 1/2 portion	340	16	20
Scallops, 1/2 portion	220	6	19
Shrimp, 1/2 portion	230	7	18
• Vegetables & Tofu, 1/2 portion	170	4	23
Signature Dishes: Honey Seared			
Chicken, 1/2 portion	420	15	45
• Pork, 1/2 portion	460	21	46
• Shrimp, 1/2 portion	370	14	43
Signature Dishes: Lemon Pepper			
• Beef, 1/2 portion	550	31	32
Chicken, 1/2 portion	440	20	34
Pork, 1/2 portion	480	28	35
Scallops, 1/2 portion	360	17	35
Shrimp, 1/2 portion	380	18	34
• Vegetables & Tofu, 1/2 portion	230	10	29
Signature Dishes: Mandarin Kung Pao			
• Beef, 1/2 portion	610	34	31
Chicken, 1/2 portion	450	21	28
Pork, 1/2 portion	500	29	28
Scallops, 1/2 portion	400	19	32
Shrimp, 1/2 portion	400	19	28
• Vegetables & Tofu, 1/2 portion	290	15	23
Signature Dishes: Mongolian			
• Beef, 1/2 portion	420	22	14
Chicken, 1/2 portion	280	9	14
Pork, 1/2 portion	320	16	15
Scallops, 1/2 portion	190	6	13
Shrimp, 1/2 portion	210	6	12
• Vegetables & Tofu, 1/2 portion	180	6	19
Signature Dishes: Orange Peel			
• Beef, 1/2 portion	660	31	52
Chicken, 1/2 portion	520	18	52
Pork, 1/2 portion	560	25	53
Scallops, 1/2 portion	440	15	52
Shrimp, 1/2 portion	460	16	51
• Vegetables & Tofu, 1/2 portion	330	10	46
Signature Dishes: Pei Wei Spicy			
• Beef, 1/2 portion	480	26	25
Chicken, 1/2 portion	330	13	25
Pork, 1/2 portion	380	20	26
Scallops, 1/2 portion	270	10	27
Shrimp, 1/2 portion	300	11	29

Pei Wei Asian Diner (cont.)

	Cal	Fat	Cbs
Signature Dishes: Pei Wei Spicy (cont.)			
• Vegetables & Tofu, 1/2 portion	250	16	21
Signature Dishes: Spicy Korean			
• Beef, 1/2 portion	490	24	26
Chicken, 1/2 portion	350	11	26
Pork, 1/2 portion	390	18	27
Scallops, 1/2 portion	270	8	25
Shrimp, 1/2 portion	280	9	24
• Vegetables & Tofu, 1/2 portion	240	9	27
Signature Dishes: Sweet & Sour			
Chicken, 1/2 portion	440	13	61
• Pork, 1/2 portion	480	18	61
• Shrimp, 1/2 portion	390	11	59
Soba Miso Bowl			
• Beef, 1/2 portion	530	18	53
Chicken, 1/2 portion	420	8	53
Pork, 1/2 portion	450	13	53
• Scallops, 1/2 portion	350	5	52
Shrimp, 1/2 portion	360	6	51
Vegetables & Tofu, 1/2 portion	360	7	57
Teriyaki Bowl with Brown Rice			
• Beef, 1/2 portion	580	17	66
Chicken, 1/2 portion	460	7	64
Pork, 1/2 portion	490	13	64
• Scallops, 1/2 portion	400	5	65
Shrimp, 1/2 portion	410	5	64
Vegetables & Tofu, 1/2 portion	410	6	71
Teriyaki Bowl with White Rice			
• Beef, 1/2 portion	560	16	62
Chicken, 1/2 portion	440	6	60
Pork, 1/2 portion	470	11	61
• Scallops, 1/2 portion	380	4	62
Shrimp, 1/2 portion	390	5	61
Vegetables & Tofu, 1/2 portion	390	5	68

Penn Station

	Cal	Fat	Cbs
Bread			
Small Bread, 7"	260	0	54
Cheeses			
• American, 1 oz.	100	5	1
• Provolone, 1 oz.	100	8	1
Swiss, 1 oz.	100	8	1
Condiments/Toppings			
Honey Mustard, 0.5 oz.	66	6	2
• Mayonnaise, 0.5 oz.	101	11	0
Olive Oil & Vinegar, 0.5 oz.	96	11	0
Oregano, 0.5 tbsp.	16	2	0
Parmesan Cheese, 0.5 oz.	25	2	0
Pizza Sauce, 1 oz.	18	0	4
• Sauerkraut, 4 oz.	16	0	4
Meats			
• Artichokes, 1 oz.	8	0	2
Bacon, 2 slices	55	4	0
Chicken Salad, 1 oz.	66	5	3
Chicken, 1 oz.	47	1	0
Corned Beef, 1 oz.	73	2	1
Ham, 1 oz.	33	1	0
• Pepperoni, 1 oz.	140	13	0
Salami, 1 oz.	120	11	0
Sausage, 1 oz.	90	7	1
Steak, 1 oz.	38	2	0
Tuna Salad, 1 oz.	60	4	3
Turkey (white), 1 oz.	25	0	0
Veggies			
• Banana Peppers (Grilled), 0.5 oz.	1	0	0
Green Peppers (Grilled), 0.5 oz.	4	0	1

Penn Station (cont.)

	Cal	Fat	Cbs
Veggies (cont.)			
Lettuce, 15 oz.	5	0	0
Mushrooms (Grilled), 0.5 oz.	3	0	0
Pickles, 0.5 oz.	1	0	0
Red Onions, 1 oz.	17	0	3
Tomato, 1 oz.	5	0	1
• Yellow Onions (Grilled), 2 oz.	22	0	5

Pepe's Mexican

	Cal	Fat	Cbs
Beef Menu			
• Beef & Bean Burrito Suizo, 314 g	640	34	55
Beef & Bean Burrito, 228 g	510	24	52
Beef & Bean Tostada Suiza, 184 g	440	29	26
Beef & Bean Tostada, 186 g	380	23	26
Beef Enchilada Suiza, 124 g	220	11	16
Beef Flauta - Plain, 57 g	160	9	10
Beef Flauta with Cheese and Sauce, 80 g	190	12	11
Beef Taco Crisp, 138 g	210	11	16
Beef Taco Salad with 4 oz Salsa, 536 g	550	26	52
Beef Taco Soft Corn, 161 g	250	10	28
Beef Taco Soft Flour, 146 g	250	11	24
Refried Beans with Mexican Cheese, 126 g	300	20	22
• Spanish Rice with Ranchera Sauce, 112 g	140	6	21
Taco Salad w/ 4 oz Salsa - no shell, 475 g	330	19	20
Burritos			
• Beef & Bean Burrito Suizo, 314 g	640	34	55
Beef & Bean Burrito, 228 g	510	24	52
Chicken & Bean Burrito Suizo, 314 g	610	31	54
Chicken & Bean Burrito, 228 g	480	21	51
Pork & Bean Burrito Suizo, 314 g	600	29	54
• Pork & Bean Burrito, 228 g	470	19	51
Chicken Menu			
• Chicken & Bean Burrito Suizo, 314 g	610	31	54
Chicken & Bean Burrito, 228 g	480	21	51
Chicken & Bean Tostada Suiza, 184 g	410	26	25
Chicken & Bean Tostada, 186 g	360	21	21
• Chicken Enchilada Suiza, 124 g	190	9	15
Chicken Flauta - Plain, 57 g	190	10	16
Chicken Flauta with Sauce & Cheese, 80 g	230	13	17
Chicken Taco Crisp, 138 g	190	9	15
Chicken Taco Salad with 4 oz Salsa - no shell, 475 g	300	16	19
Chicken Taco Salad with 4 oz Salsa, 536 g	520	23	51
Chicken Taco Soft Corn, 161 g	230	8	27
Chicken Taco Soft Flour, 146 g	230	9	23
Refried Beans with Mexican Cheese, 126 g	300	20	22
Spanish Rice with Ranchera Sauce, 112 g	140	6	21
Flautas			
Beef Flauta - Plain, 57 g	160	9	10
Beef Flauta with Cheese and Sauce, 80 g	190	12	11
Chicken Flauta - Plain, 57 g	190	10	16
• Chicken Flauta with Sauce & Cheese, 80 g	230	13	17
Pork Menu			
• Pork & Bean Burrito Suizo, 314 g	600	29	54
Pork & Bean Burrito, 228 g	470	19	51
Pork & Bean Tostada Suiza, 184 g	410	25	26
Pork & Bean Tostada, 186 g	350	20	26
Pork Enchilada Suiza, 124 g	190	8	15
• Pork Taco Crisp, 135 g	170	6	16
Pork Taco Salad with 4 oz Salsa - no shell, 475 g	290	13	19
Pork Taco Salad with 4 oz Salsa, 536 g	500	20	52
Pork Taco Soft Corn, 160 g	220	6	27
Pork Taco Soft Flour, 145 g	220	7	24
Refried Beans with Mexican Cheese, 126 g	300	20	22
Spanish Rice with Ranchera Sauce, 112 g	140	6	21
Salads			
Beef Taco Salad with 4 oz Salsa - no shell, 475 g	330	19	20

Pepe's Mexican (cont.)

	Cal	Fat	Cbs
Salads (cont.)			
• Beef Taco Salad with 4 oz Salsa, 536 g	550	26	52
Chicken Taco Salad with 4 oz Salsa - no shell, 475 g	300	16	19
Chicken Taco Salad with 4 oz Salsa, 536 g	520	23	51
• Pork Taco Salad with 4 oz Salsa - no shell, 475 g	290	13	19
Pork Taco Salad with 4 oz Salsa, 536 g	500	20	52
Taco			
Beef Taco Crisp, 138 g	210	11	16
Beef Taco Soft Corn, 161 g	250	10	28
• Beef Taco Soft Flour, 146 g	250	11	24
Chicken Taco Crisp, 138 g	190	9	15
Chicken Taco Soft Corn, 161 g	230	8	27
Chicken Taco Soft Flour, 146 g	230	9	23
• Pork Taco Crisp, 135 g	170	6	16
Pork Taco Soft Corn, 160 g	220	6	27
Pork Taco Soft Flour, 145 g	220	7	24
Tostadas			
• Beef & Bean Tostada Suiza, 184 g	440	29	26
Beef & Bean Tostada, 186 g	380	23	26
Chicken & Bean Tostada Suiza, 184 g	410	26	25
Chicken & Bean Tostada, 186 g	360	21	21
Pork & Bean Tostada Suiza, 184 g	410	25	26
• Pork & Bean Tostada, 186 g	350	20	26

Peter Piper Pizza

	Cal	Fat	Cbs
Appetizers & Desserts			
Breadsticks, 69 g	250	10	36
Chicken Strips, 138 g	300	9	26
Cinnamon Crunch Dessert, 86 g	220	2	49
• Garlic Cheese Bread, 92 g	310	14	37
• Wings, 48 g	110	8	0
Healthier Choices Made Easy			
California Veggie Crust Original, 1 slice	200	6	23
California Veggie Crust Ultra Thin, 1 slice	130	4	15
• Cheese Pizza Crust Original, 1 slice	300	6	23
• Cheese Pizza Crust Ultra Thin, 1 slice	130	4	15
Chicken Caesar Salad No Dressing	130	4	15
Cinnamon Crunch Dessert Pie, 1 slice	130	4	15
Garden Fresh Salad No Dressing	130	4	15
Mushroom Pizza Crust Original, 1 slice	200	6	23
Mushroom Pizza Crust Ultra Thin, 1 slice	130	4	15
Pizza: 14" Large Pizza			
Cheese Hand-tossed, 110 g	290	9	38
Cheese Original, 111 g	300	9	37
Cheese Pan, 110 g	290	9	38
Cheese Thin, 52 g	150	5	14
Ham & Pineapple Hand-tossed, 115 g	280	7	39
Ham & Pineapple Original, 116 g	280	7	38
Ham & Pineapple Pan, 129 g	310	7	46
• Ham & Pineapple Thin, 55 g	130	4	15
Pepperoni & Sausage Hand-tossed, 111 g	310	11	38
Pepperoni & Sausage Original, 112 g	310	11	37
Pepperoni & Sausage Pan, 125 g	340	11	45
Pepperoni & Sausage Thin, 53 g	150	7	14
Pepperoni Hand-tossed, 104 g	290	10	37
Pepperoni Original, 105 g	300	10	36
Pepperoni Pan, 118 g	330	10	44
Pepperoni Thin, 48 g	150	6	13
Sausage Hand-tossed, 115 g	310	10	39
Sausage Original, 116 g	310	10	38
• Sausage Pan, 129 g	340	11	46
Sausage Thin, 55 g	150	7	14
Pizza: 14" Large Specialty Pizza			
5 Meat Supreme Hand-tossed, 126 g	350	13	38
5 Meat Supreme Original, 127 g	350	13	38
5 Meat Supreme Pan, 140 g	380	13	46

Peter Piper Pizza (cont.)

	Cal	Fat	Cbs
Pizza: 14" Large Specialty Pizza (cont.)			
5 Meat Supreme Thin, 63 g	180	8	14
California Veggie Hand-tossed, 119 g	270	7	39
California Veggie Original, 91 g	200	6	23
California Veggie Pan, 134 g	300	7	47
• California Veggie Thin, 61 g	130	5	15
Chicago Classic Hand-tossed, 121 g	300	10	39
Chicago Classic Original, 121 g	300	10	38
Chicago Classic Pan, 135 g	340	10	46
Chicago Classic Thin, 59 g	150	6	15
NY 3 Chz w/ Pepperoni Hand-tossed, 127 g	380	16	39
NY 3 Chz w/ Pepperoni Original, 127 g	380	16	38
• NY 3 Chz w/ Pepperoni Pan, 141 g	410	16	46
NY 3 Chz w/ Pepperoni Thin, 63 g	200	10	14
Smoke House Hand-tossed, 129 g	370	15	39
Smoke House Original, 130 g	370	15	38
Smoke House Pan, 143 g	400	15	46
Smoke House Thin, 65 g	200	9	15
The Werax Hand-tossed, 139 g	310	11	39
The Werax Original, 140 g	320	11	38
The Werax Pan, 153 g	350	11	46
The Werax Thin, 71 g	160	7	14
Pizza: 16" Extra Large Pizza			
Cheese Hand-tossed, 98 g	260	8	33
Cheese Original, 98 g	260	8	32
Cheese Pan, 107 g	290	8	38
Cheese Thin, 51 g	140	5	13
Ham & Pineapple Hand-tossed, 103 g	250	6	35
Ham & Pineapple Original, 103 g	250	6	33
Ham & Pineapple Pan, 112 g	270	6	39
• Ham & Pineapple Thin, 55 g	130	4	14
Pepperoni & Sausage Hand-tossed, 99 g	280	10	33
Pepperoni & Sausage Original, 99 g	280	10	32
Pepperoni & Sausage Pan, 109 g	300	10	38
Pepperoni & Sausage Thin, 52 g	150	7	13
Pepperoni Hand-tossed, 92 g	260	8	33
Pepperoni Original, 92 g	260	8	32
Pepperoni Pan, 101 g	280	9	37
Pepperoni Thin, 47 g	140	6	13
Sausage Hand-tossed, 104 g	280	10	34
Sausage Original, 104 g	280	10	33
• Sausage Pan, 113 g	300	10	39
Sausage Thin, 56 g	150	7	14
Pizza: 16" Extra Large Specialty Pizza			
5 Meat Supreme Hand-tossed, 115 g	320	13	34
5 Meat Supreme Original, 115 g	320	13	33
5 Meat Supreme Pan, 125 g	340	13	39
5 Meat Supreme Thin, 64 g	190	9	14
California Veggie Hand-tossed, 106 g	240	6	34
California Veggie Original, 106 g	240	6	33
California Veggie Pan, 115 g	260	6	39
• California Veggie Thin, 57 g	130	4	14
Chicago Classic Hand-tossed, 111 g	270	9	34
Chicago Classic Original, 111 g	270	9	33
Chicago Classic Pan, 120 g	290	9	39
Chicago Classic Thin, 61 g	150	6	14
New York 3 Cheese with Pepperoni Hand-tossed, 113 g	340	14	34
New York 3 Cheese with Pepperoni Original, 112 g	340	14	32
• New York 3 Cheese with Pepperoni Pan, 122 g	360	15	39
New York 3 Cheese with Pepperoni Thin, 62 g	200	10	14
Smoke House Hand-tossed, 116 g	340	13	34
Smoke House Original, 116 g	340	13	33
Smoke House Pan, 126 g	360	14	39
Smoke House Thin, 65 g	200	10	14
The Werax Hand-tossed, 128 g	280	10	34

Peter Piper Pizza (cont.)

	Cal	Fat	Cbs
Pizza: 16" Extra Large Specialty Pizza (cont.)			
The Werax Original, 128 g	290	10	33
The Werax Pan, 137 g	310	10	39
The Werax Thin, 74 g	160	7	14
Salads			
Chicken Caesar, 229 g	200	8	10
• Family, 371 g	290	16	14
Garden, 250 g	50	0	10
Italian Chef, 114 g	20	0	4
• Side, 145 g	20	0	4

Petro's

	Cal	Fat	Cbs
Chili: Large			
• Chicken	375	6	58
Original	504	19	57
• Veggie	525	15	79
Chili: Medium			
• Chicken	275	4	43
Original	370	14	42
• Veggie	385	11	58
Chili: Small			
• Chicken	175	3	27
Original	235	9	26
• Veggie	245	7	37
Large Petro®			
• Chicken	969	52	88
Original	1073	63	87
• Veggie	1089	60	105
Lite Pasta Petro®			
• Large	678	5	108
Medium	494	4	80
• Small	333	2	53
Lite Petro®			
• Large	787	24	99
Medium	532	16	66
• Small	382	12	48
Medium Petro®			
• Chicken	665	36	59
Original	734	43	58
• Veggie	745	41	70
Miscellaneous: Baked Potatoes			
• #1 Lite	363	0	74
#2 Butter Sour Cream	482	18	74
#3 Loaded	679	33	78
• #4 Loaded w/ Chili	780	37	90
#5 Broccoli 3 Cheese	657	30	77
Miscellaneous: Hot Dogs			
Chili	315	17	28
Chili/cheese	347	19	29
• Loaded	352	19	30
• Plain	266	14	22
Slaw	352	16	23
Pasta Petro®			
• Large	848	37	91
Medium	627	27	68
• Small	406	17	46
Pee Wee Petro®			
• Chicken	259	14	23
Original	284	16	22
• Veggie	289	16	27
Salads: Garden Salads			
Large	86	1	16
Small	43	1	8
Salads: Petro Salads			
Grilled Chicken	742	41	42
Original	570	36	42

Petro's (cont.)

	Cal	Fat	Cbs
Small Petro®			
• Chicken	464	24	43
Original	516	30	43
• Veggie	524	28	52

Philly Connection

	Cal	Fat	Cbs
Original Cheesesteak Sandwich			
Regular, 10"	623	15	73
Small, 7"	455	11	55

Piccadilly

	Cal	Fat	Cbs
Low Carb Items			
Au Jus, 3 fl.oz.	6	0	1
Beans, Green, Fresh, 5 oz.	136	11	8
Beef, Chopped Steak, Fried Jumbo, 8 oz.	737	59	11
Beef, Chopped Steak, Fried Regular, 5 oz.	414	33	6
Beef, Roast Leg (Small), 4 oz.	352	22	2
Beef, Steak, Filet Mignon, 6 oz.	341	20	1
Beef, Steak, New Your Strip, 10 oz.	876	71	1
Beef, Steak, Ribeye or Sirloin Strip, 7 oz.	673	58	1
Beef, Steak, Ribeye, 10 oz.	1042	91	2
• Beef, Steak, Ribeye, 14 oz.	1353	116	2
Broccoli w/Cheese Sauce, full portion	106	7	9
Broccoli, Fresh Florets, 4 oz.	90	7	5
Brussel Sprouts, Buttered, full portion	91	6	8
Cabbage, Bacon Seasoned, Steamed, full portion	106	8	6
Cabbage, Buttered, Steamed, full portion	68	5	6
Cauliflower, Buttered, full portion	89	6	8
Cheese Sauce, 2 fl.oz.	35	1	5
Chicken Breast, Mesquite Smoke	212	8	1
Chicken Breast, Mesquite w BBQ sauce	240	9	6
Chicken, Baked (Quarters)	849	61	6
Chicken, Baked Cajun, Boneless Breast	431	27	9
Chicken, Baked Italian, Boneless Breast	548	41	8
Chicken, Barbecued (Quarters)	796	53	12
Chicken, Rotisserie- Herb Style (Dark), 1 quarter	827	65	12
Chicken, Rotisserie- Herb Style (Half), 1 half	1179	75	4
Chicken, Rotisserie- Herb Style (White), 1 quarter	521	31	2
Chicken, SW Chicken Breast, full portion	522	35	9
Cottage Cheese, Creamed, 4 oz.	117	5	3
Cucumbers and Sour Cream, 5 oz.	86	6	6
Fish, Basa, Blackened	408	32	2
Fish, Basa, Cajun Baked	263	15	4
Fish, Basa, Stuffed	438	30	9
Fish, Catfish Filet, Blackened	523	43	2
Fish, Catfish Filet, Stuffed	552	40	9
Fish, Catfish, Cajun Baked, full portion	404	28	6
Fish, Grouper Filet, Baked, 6 oz.	305	9	8
Fish, Tilapia, Cajun Baked, full portion	267	19	7
Fish, Trout Filets, Baked, full portion	464	19	10
Fish, Trout, Almondine, Baked, full portion	490	22	11
Gelatin, Plain Sugar- Free, full portion	58	0	1
Greens, Collard, Mustard, Turnip, 3 oz.	135	10	3
Greens, Turnip w/Diced Turnips, 3 oz.	150	12	4
Gumbo, Chicken (no rice), 10 oz.	98	2	11
Gumbo, Chicken and Sausage (no rice), 10 oz.	224	15	10
Okra, Creole, full portion	79	4	9
Peas, Sugar Snap, Mixed, 5 oz.	102	5	10
Pork Loin, Bone In, Roast, 5 oz.	373	13	10
Salad Dressing, Blue Cheese, 2 tbsp	160	18	1
Salad Dressing, French, 2 tbsp	130	13	5
Salad Dressing, Italian, 2 tbsp	160	17	1
Salad Dressing, Ranch, 2 tbsp	150	17	1
Salad Dressing, Ranch, Fat Free, 2 tbsp	36	0	7
Salad Dressing, Thousand Island, 2 tbsp	170	18	2
Salad, Asparagus and Tomato, full portion	88	5	10

Piccadilly (cont.)

	Cal	Fat	Cbs
Low Carb Items (cont.)			
Salad, Caesar, 3 oz.	143	11	7
Salad, Cauliflower, Fresh, 4 oz.	117	8	9
Salad, Chef's (Small), 6 oz.	143	9	4
Salad, Coleslaw, Italian, 4 oz.	163	16	5
Salad, Coleslaw, Kosher Style, 4 oz.	143	13	7
Salad, Combination, 4 oz.	73	5	5
Salad, Cucumber and Celery, 4 oz.	74	4	9
Salad, Cucumber and Tomato, 4 oz.	41	0	10
Salad, Cucumber Mix, 6 oz.	61	4	7
Salad, Louisianne Bowl, full portion	44	3	2
Salad, Mexican, 4 oz.	58	3	8
Salad, Piccadilly Bowl, full portion	27	0	6
• Salad, Spring Salad Bowl (Small), 3 oz.	15	0	3
Salad, Tomato, Cucumber and Onion, 4 oz.	44	0	10
Salad, Veggie Combination w/Cherry Tom, full portion	68	4	9
Spinach, Buttered, or Bacon Seasoned, 4 oz.	80	6	3
Turkey Breast, Carved, 6 oz.	267	10	5
Vegetables, Mixed, 4 oz.	137	7	17
Popular Items			
Beans, Green, Fresh, 5 oz.	136	11	8
Beef, Roast, 6 oz.	481	30	3
Blueberry Pie, Sugar- Free, 1 slice	314	17	42
Broccoli, Fresh Florets, 4 oz.	90	7	5
Cherry Pie, Sugar-Free, 1 slice	334	17	45
Chicken, Grilled Breast, 6 oz.	478	26	23
• Chocolate Almond Pie, Sugar Free, 1 slice	612	44	49
Corn, Fresh, 4 oz.	125	6	18
Fish, Tilapia, Baked, full portion	210	11	10
Okra, Fried, 3 oz.	242	13	26
Pork Loin, Marinated Boneless, 6 oz.	365	24	1
Rolls, White, Parker House, 1 each	147	5	22
Rolls, Whole Wheat, 1 each	231	8	37
Salad Dressing, Ranch, Fat-Free, 2 tbsp.	36	0	7
Salad, Piccadilly Fruit, 6 oz.	78	0	20
Salad, Shrimp Remoulade, 12 oz.	516	28	33
• Salad, Spring Bowl, 3 oz.	15	0	3
Shrimp, Fried, full portion	462	19	34

Pizza Hut

	Cal	Fat	Cbs
Appetizers			
Breadsticks, 1 bread	150	6	20
Cheese Breadsticks, 1 bread	200	10	21
Hot Wings, 2 pieces	120	7	1
• Mild Wings, 2 pieces	110	7	2
• Wing Blue Cheese Dipping Sauce, 2 oz.	220	23	3
Wing Ranch Dipping Sauce, 2 oz.	220	23	3
Desserts			
• Apple Dessert Pizza, 101 g	260	5	52
Cherry Dessert Pizza, 101 g	260	5	47
• Cinnamon Sticks, 55 g	170	5	27
White Icing Dipping Cup, 2 oz.	190	0	47
Dressings & Dipping Sauces			
• Breadstick Dipping Sauce, 3 oz.	40	0	8
• French Dressing, 30 g	150	13	9
Italian Dressing, 30 g	140	15	2
Lite Italian Dressing, 30 g	70	5	5
Lite Ranch Dressing, 30 g	60	6	1
Ranch Dressing, 30 g	100	10	2
Thousand Island Dressing, 30 g	120	11	5
Pizza: 12" Medium Hand-Tossed Style Pizzas			
Cheese Only, 98 g	230	10	25
Italian Sausage & Red Onion, 114 g	260	12	26
• Meat Lover's®, 129 g	340	19	25
Pepperoni & Mushroom, 104 g	230	9	25
Pepperoni, 96 g	240	11	24

Pizza Hut (cont.)

	Cal	Fat	Cbs
Pizza: 12" Medium Hand-Tossed Style Pizzas (cont.)			
Quartered Ham & Pineapple, 104 g	220	8	26
Supreme, 122 g	270	13	26
• Veggie Lover's®, 115 g	210	8	26
Pizza: 12" Medium Pan Pizzas			
Cheese Only, 104 g	270	13	27
Italian Sausage & Red Onion, 119 g	300	15	28
• Meat Lover's®, 135 g	370	22	28
Pepperoni & Mushroom, 109 g	260	13	27
Pepperoni, 102 g	280	14	27
Quartered Ham & Pineapple, 109 g	250	11	28
Supreme, 127 g	310	16	28
• Veggie Lover's®, 119 g	250	11	28
Pizza: 12" Medium Thin 'N Crispy Pizzas			
Cheese Only, 79 g	200	8	21
Italian Sausage & Red Onion, 97 g	230	11	23
• Meat Lover's®, 111 g	310	18	22
Pepperoni & Mushroom, 87 g	190	8	21
Pepperoni, 77 g	210	10	21
• Quartered Ham & Pineapple, 87 g	180	6	22
Supreme, 106 g	230	11	22
Veggie Lover's®, 101 g	180	7	23
Pizza: 14" Large Hand-Tossed Style Pizzas			
Cheese Only, 142 g	340	14	36
Italian Sausage & Red Onion, 163 g	370	17	38
• Meat Lover's®, 187 g	490	27	37
Pepperoni & Mushroom, 149 g	330	14	36
Pepperoni, 140 g	360	16	35
• Quartered Ham & Pineapple, 150 g	310	11	38
Supreme, 174 g	390	18	37
Veggie Lover's®, 163 g	310	12	37
Pizza: 14" Large Pan Pizza			
Cheese Only, 146 g	390	19	38
Italian Sausage & Red Onion, 165 g	420	22	39
• Meat Lover's®, 190 g	530	31	39
Pepperoni & Mushroom, 151 g	380	18	37
Pepperoni, 143 g	400	21	37
Quartered Ham & Pineapple, 152 g	360	16	39
Supreme, 176 g	440	23	39
• Veggie Lover's®, 163 g	350	16	39
Pizza: 14" Large Stuffed Crust Pizzas			
Cheese Only, 150 g	360	16	37
Italian Sausage & Red Onion, 174 g	410	20	39
• Meat Lover's®, 199 g	520	29	38
Pepperoni & Mushroom, 160 g	360	16	37
Pepperoni, 152 g	390	19	37
Quartered Ham & Pineapple, 161 g	350	14	39
Supreme, 185 g	420	21	39
• Veggie Lover's®, 173 g	340	14	38
Pizza: 14" Large Thin N' Crispy Pizza			
Cheese Only, 111 g	280	12	30
Italian Sausage & Red Onion, 136 g	320	15	32
• Meat Lover's®, 157 g	430	25	31
Pepperoni & Mushroom, 122 g	270	12	30
Pepperoni, 109 g	300	14	29
• Quartered Ham & Pineapple, 123 g	260	9	32
Supreme, 148 g	330	16	31
Veggie Lover's®, 141 g	260	10	31
Pizza: 6" Personal Pan Pizzas			
Cheese Only, 249 g	620	26	69
Italian Sausage & Red Onion, 286 g	690	33	71
• Meat Lover's®, 333 g	890	49	70
Pepperoni & Mushroom, 256 g	600	25	68
Pepperoni, 245 g	640	29	67
Quartered Ham & Pineapple, 258 g	570	21	70

Pizza Hut (cont.)

	Cal	Fat	Cbs
Pizza: 6" Personal Pan Pizzas (cont.)			
Supreme, 303 g	710	34	70
• Veggie Lover's®, 275 g	560	22	70
Pizza: XL Full House Pizza™			
Cheese Only, 114 g	280	12	30
Italian Sausage & Red Onion, 130 g	300	14	32
• Meat Lover's®, 143 g	370	20	31
Pepperoni & Mushroom, 121 g	270	11	30
Pepperoni, 111 g	280	13	30
Quartered Ham & Pineapple, 121 g	260	10	32
Supreme, 139 g	310	14	31
• Veggie Lover's®, 135 g	260	10	31

Pizza Pizza

	Cal	Fat	Cbs
Classic Pizza			
Beacon Double Cheeseburger, 97 g	220	7	29
Big Bacon Bonanza, 93 g	220	7	29
Canadian Eh!, 112 g	230	7	30
Cheese, 89 g	200	5	29
Classic Super, 110 g	210	6	30
• Deep Dish Pepperoni, 129 g	330	11	45
• Garden Veggie, 111 g	190	5	30
New York Pepperoni, 92 g	230	8	30
Pepperoni & Mushroom, 105 g	210	6	30
Pepperoni, 93 g	210	6	29
Silican, 108 g	240	9	30
Spicy BBQ Chicken, 104 g	200	5	30
Tropical Hawaiian, 100 g	220	7	30
Signature Pizza			
Bacon Chicken Mushroom Melt, 112 g	270	12	29
Chicken Bruschetta Parm, 94 g	180	6	22
Chicken Mango, 115 g	220	7	30
Garden Riviera, 107 g	220	6	31
• Meat Supreme, 120 g	290	13	30
Mediterranean Vegetarian, 125 g	210	6	31
Napa Valley, 86 g	200	8	22
Pesto Amore, 76 g	170	7	19
Philly Cheese Steak, 116 g	230	6	31
• Sweet Chili Chicken, 91 g	170	5	26
Trio Pomodoro, 91 g	180	6	22

Planet Smoothie

	Cal	Fat	Cbs
Smoothies			
2 Piece Bikini-Chocolate™, 22 oz.	321	1	80
2 Piece Bikini-Strawberry™, 22 oz.	286	1	72
Acai (Ah-SIGH-ee), 22 oz.	510	6	118
Berry Bada-Bing™, 22 oz.	362	0	88
Big Bang™, 22 oz.	347	1	80
Billy Bob Banana™, 22 oz.	312	1	78
• Captain Kid (12 oz)™, 22 oz.	194	2	47
Chocolate Chimp™, 22 oz.	400	1	93
Chocolate Elvis™, 22 oz.	522	9	109
Frozen Goat™, 22 oz.	358	1	85
Grape Ape™, 22 oz.	304	1	78
Hangover Over™, 22 oz.	312	1	78
Leapin' Lizard™, 22 oz.	209	0	55
Lunar Lemonade Raspberry™, 22 oz.	375	1	97
Lunar Lemonade™, 22 oz.	378	1	98
Mediterranean Monster™, 22 oz.	310	1	80
Merlin's Pineapple LB™, 22 oz.	413	2	57
Merlin's Pineapple Myoplex™, 22 oz.	392	2	53
Merlin's Strawberry LB™, 22 oz.	484	2	78
Merlin's Strawberry Myoplex™, 22 oz.	463	2	74
Mr. Mongo-Chocolate™, 22 oz.	516	1	117
Mr. Mongo-Strawberry, 22 oz.	421	1	92
• PBJ™, 22 oz.	560	17	97

Planet Smoothie (cont.)

	Cal	Fat	Cbs
Smoothies (cont.)			
Rasmanian Devil™, 22 oz.	265	1	66
Road Runner™, 22 oz.	279	1	72
Screamsicle™, 22 oz.	365	2	86
Shag-a-delic™, 22 oz.	430	1	104
Spazz™, 22 oz.	266	1	68
The Last Mango™, 22 oz.	354	3	83
Thelma & Louise™, 22 oz.	226	0	59
Twig & Berries™, 22 oz.	297	1	74
Vinnie del Rocco™, 22 oz.	385	4	92
Werewolf™, 22 oz.	261	1	67
Yo' Adriane™, 22 oz.	263	0	65
Zeus Juice™, 22 oz.	248	1	65

Pollo Tropical

	Cal	Fat	Cbs
Chicken			
• 1/4 Chicken dark meat w/o skin, 3 oz.	191	10	0
1/4 Chicken dark meat, 4 oz.	291	18	0
1/4 Chicken white meat w/o skin, 4 oz.	204	6	0
• 1/4 Chicken white meat, 6 oz.	323	16	0
Boneless Chicken Breast, 6 oz.	241	3	0
Condiments			
BBQ Sauce, 2 oz.	83	0	20
Caesar Dressing, 1 oz.	161	17	1
• Extra dressing is 1.75 oz, 2 oz.	281	30	2
Guacamole Sauce, 2 oz.	75	6	3
Guava BBQ Sauce, 2 oz.	83	0	22
Mojo Sauce, 1 oz.	97	9	3
Mustard Curry Sauce, 2 oz.	265	30	0
Salsa, 2 oz.	8	0	2
Desserts			
Flan, 5 oz.	390	13	59
• Key Lime, 4 oz.	210	9	25
Tres Leches (Caribbean Cream Cake), 5 oz.	410	9	76
Ribs			
1/4 Rack Ribs, 2 oz.	200	15	1
1/2 Rack Ribs, 4 oz.	400	31	2
Roast Pork			
Roast Pork, 6 oz.	392	23	0
Salads			
Chicken Caesar Salad, 14,45 oz.	669	41	13
Sandwiches			
• Chicken Caesar Sandwich, 13 oz.	881	34	71
Grilled Chicken Sandwich, 15 oz.	827	24	84
• Roast Pork Sandwich, 12 oz.	773	26	83
Shrimp			
Shrimp Skewer (One Skewer), 108 oz.	1	1	0
Sides			
• Balsamic Tomato, Combo Side, 4 oz.	88	1	7
Balsamic Tomato, Small Side, 8 oz.	176	2	14
Black Beans, Combo Side, 4 oz.	90	3	18
Black Beans, Small Side, 9 oz.	203	6	41
Black Beans/White Rice Combo side, 9 oz.	294	6	58
• Black Beans/White Rice Value side, 13 oz.	458	9	90
Boiled Yuca Combo Side, 8 oz.	188	0	51
Boiled Yuca Small Side, 10 oz.	251	0	68
Caesar Salad, Combo Side, 3 oz.	130	11	4
Caesar Salad, Small Side, 4 oz.	207	18	6
Caribbean Chicken Soup, Large Bowl, 16 oz.	237	3	40
Caribbean Chicken Soup, Small Bowl, 8 oz.	121	2	21
Corn, Combo Side, 4 oz.	121	4	19
Corn, Small Side, 8 oz.	225	8	37
French Fries, Combo Side, 4 oz.	311	15	40
French Fries, Small Side, 4 oz.	311	15	40
Tropical Shrimp Soup, Large Bowl, 16 oz.	280	5	38
Tropical Shrimp Soup, Small Bowl, 8 oz.	134	3	18

Pollo Tropical (cont.)

	Cal	Fat	Cbs
Sides (cont.)			
White Rice, Combo Side, 5 oz.	203	3	40
White Rice, Small Side, 8 oz.	339	6	66
Yellow Rice w/Veg, Combo Side, 5 oz.	163	3	31
Yellow Rice w/Veg, Small Side, 8 oz.	245	4	47
Steaks			
Beef skewers / Two Per Serving, 4 oz.	289	19	4
• Beef skewers, 1 oz.	77	5	1
• Steak & Chicken (dark meat), 6 oz.	437	28	2
Steak & Shrimp, 255 oz.	330	11	2
Tropical Favorites			
Bananas Tropical®, 7 oz.	437	11	89
Yucatan Fries®, 6 oz.	497	24	69
Tropichops®			
• Chkn w/ Yellow Rice & Veggies, 10 oz.	341	5	50
Chkn w/ Yellow Rice & Veggies, 23 oz.	864	21	93
Grilled Chicken Deluxe, 13 oz.	409	6	52
Grilled Chicken Deluxe, 25 oz.	753	11	91
Pork w/ White Rice & Black Beans, 20 oz.	714	23	97
• Pork w/ White Rice & Black Beans, 31 oz.	1273	50	147
Pork w/ Yellow Rice & Vegetables, 12 oz.	480	21	91
Pork w/ Yellow Rice & Vegetables, 30 oz.	1020	43	96
Ropa Vieja (shredded beef), 19 oz.	618	17	98
Ropa Vieja (shredded beef), 33 oz.	1160	41	161
Shrimp Creole TropiChop MAX, 26 oz.	1002	29	129
Shrimp Creole TropiChop, 14 oz.	506	11	75
Vegetarian TropiChop Max®, 31 oz.	950	21	177
Vegetarian TropiChop®, 19 oz.	580	13	109
Wraps			
Chx Caesar Wrap, 13 oz.	901	48	64
• Chx Classic Wrap, 13 oz.	694	26	68
Curry Chx Wrap, 14 oz.	930	43	94
• Steak Wrap, 15 oz.	993	48	106

Popeye's Chicken & Biscuits

	Cal	Fat	Cbs
Cajun Wings			
Cajun Wing segments, 244 g	595	43	19
Louisiana Legends			
• Chicken & Sausage Jambalaya, 453 g	660	33	60
• Chicken Etouffee, 453 g	480	30	18
Crawfish Etouffee, 453 g	540	15	75
Smothered Chicken, 453 g	630	24	72
Mild Chicken			
• Breast, 179 g	350	20	8
• Leg, 63 g	110	7	3
Strips, 116 g	250	10	16
Thigh, 111 g	280	20	7
Wing, 59 g	150	10	5
Mild Chicken (Skinless and Breading Removed)			
Breast, 123 g	120	2	0
Leg, 52 g	50	2	0
• Strips, 94 g	130	3	3
Thigh, 72 g	80	4	0
• Wing, 42 g	40	2	0
Sandwiches			
Deluxe w/ Mayo, 265 g	630	31	53
Deluxe w/o Mayo, 237 g	480	15	54
Seafood			
Popcorn Shrimp, 85 g	280	16	22
Sides			
Biscuits, 60 g	240	13	26
Cajun Rice, 117 g	170	6	22
Chicken Etouffee, 151 g	160	10	6
Cinnamon Apple Turnover, 86 g	250	12	34
Coleslaw, 138 g	260	23	14
Corn on the Cob, 284 g	190	2	37

Popeye's Chicken & Biscuits (cont.)

	Cal	Fat	Cbs
Sides (cont.)			
Crawfish Etouffee, 151 g	180	5	25
French Fries, 88 g	310	17	35
• Green Beans, 100 g	70	1	14
Jambalaya, 151 g	220	11	20
Mashed Potatoes w/ Gravy, 142 g	130	4	18
Mashed Potatoes w/o Gravy, 113 g	100	3	17
• Red Beans & Rice, 174 g	320	19	31
Smothered Chicken, 151 g	210	8	24
Spicy Chicken			
• Breast, 179 g	360	22	8
• Leg, 63 g	100	5	3
Strips, 116 g	270	11	21
Thigh, 111 g	300	24	7
Wing, 59 g	140	9	5
Spicy Chicken (Skinless and Breading Removed)			
Breast, 123 g	120	2	1
Leg, 52 g	50	2	0
• Strips, 94 g	150	4	5
• Thigh, 72 g	80	3	2
• Wing, 42 g	40	2	0

Port of Subs

	Cal	Fat	Cbs
Brownies			
Brownies, 5 oz.	300	10	48
Cold Submarine Sandwiches			
Bacon Lettuce & Tomato, 8 oz.	519	30	43
• Ham American, 10 oz.	382	20	45
• Ham Salami Capicolla Pepperoni Provolone, 10 oz.	532	26	45
Ham Salami Provolone, 9 oz.	469	21	45
Ham Turkey Provolone, 10 oz.	434	15	46
Peppered Pastrami Swiss, 9 oz.	439	17	44
Peppered Pastrami Turkey Swiss, 8 oz.	511	26	44
Roast Beef Provolone, 10 oz.	421	14	43
Roast Beef Turkey Provolone, 10 oz.	421	14	45
Roasted Chicken Breast Provolone, 10 oz.	410	13	45
Salami Pepperoni Provolone, 8 oz.	511	27	45
Salami Provolone, 8 oz.	479	25	45
Salami Turkey Provolone, 9 oz.	465	20	46
Smoked Ham Swiss, 10 oz.	447	17	45
Smoked Ham Turkey Cheddar, 10 oz.	431	15	47
Tuna (w/o cheese), 9 oz.	422	18	45
Turkey Provolone, 11 oz.	421	14	47
Fresh Salads			
Caesar Salad, 6 oz.	333	30	7
Chef Salad, 11 oz.	388	25	13
• Garden Salad, 8 oz.	93	5	10
• Grilled Chicken Caesar Salad, 13 oz.	541	34	15
Grilled Chicken Salad, 13 oz.	300	10	16
Macaroni Salad, 8 oz.	440	30	36
Potato Salad, 8 oz.	360	26	54
Tuna Salad, 8 oz.	311	23	12
Hot Sandwiches			
• Grilled Chicken, 9 oz.	563	11	68
• Hot Pastrami, 9 oz.	758	17	62
Meatball, 9 oz.	653	25	76
Kid's Meal Sandwich			
Ham, 3 oz.	200	3	4
• Salami, 3 oz.	254	9	4
• Turkey, 3 oz.	190	3	4
Sandwiches			
• Ham Turkey, 10 oz.	328	5	46
Peppered Pastrami, 8 oz.	293	4	44
Roast Beef Turkey, 9 oz.	315	4	45
Roast Beef, 9 oz.	315	4	43
Roasted Chicken Breast, 9 oz.	304	3	44

Port of Subs (cont.)

	Cal	Fat	Cbs
Sandwiches (cont.)			
Smoked Ham Turkey, 10 oz.	320	5	46
Smoked Ham, 8 oz.	301	4	44
Turkey, 10 oz.	315	4	47
• Vegetarian (w/o cheese), 7 oz.	238	2	44
Soup - Medium			
Boston Clam Chowder, 6 oz.	105	4	13
• Broccoli Cheese, 6 oz.	120	6	13
• Minestrone, 6 oz.	53	1	8
Roasted Chicken Noodle, 6 oz.	83	2	9
Wraps			
Chicken Caesar, 11 oz.	762	35	63
• Hot Grilled Chkn Smokey Cheddar, 11 oz.	661	23	63
Tortilla Only, 4 oz.	330	8	55
• Turkey & Bacon Ranch, 12 oz.	785	44	190

Pret a Manger

	Cal	Fat	Cbs
Bagels			
Cinnamon Bagel, 113 g	300	0	64
with Cream Cheese, 142 g	390	9	65
• Plain Bagel, 113 g	300	0	0
• with Cream Cheese, 160 g	460	16	65
Sesame Bagel, 113 g	300	8	64
with Cream Cheese, 142 g	390	17	65
Baguettes			
All Natural Smoked Ham & Swiss, 625 g	620	16	66
Bell & Evans Chicken & Mozzarella, 344 g	580	19	72
Cream Chz, Tomato & Basil Brkfst, 176 g	390	19	45
Just Made French Brie & Basil, 280 g	560	23	66
Organic Egg & Bacon Brkfst, 146 g	410	18	42
• Organic Egg & Tomato Brkfst, 153 g	340	12	43
Pret's Classic Tuna Salad, 295 g	580	20	67
• Slow-Roast Beef, Arugula & Parmegiano, 245 g	670	13	65
Chips & Popcorn			
Cracked Pepper Potato Chips, 1 oz.	150	9	16
Lightly Salted Potato Chips, 1 oz.	150	9	15
• New York Cheddar Potato Chips, 28 g	180	9	15
• Pret's Organic Popcorn, 32 g	131	6	19
Salt & Vinegar Potato Chips, 1 oz.	150	9	16
Spicy Thai Potato Chips., 28 g	150	9	15
Yogurt & Green Onion Potato Chips, 28 g	150	9	15
Cookies, Cakes & Treats			
Banana Cake, 128 g	420	24	48
Carrot Cake, 128 g	460	29	47
Chocolate Brownie, 96 g	390	20	51
Chocolate Cake, 128 g	470	19	71
Chocolate Chunk Cookie, 71 g	310	16	43
Fruit & Oat Slice, 96 g	410	18	55
Harvest Cookie, 43 g	180	8	24
Love Bar, 105 g	460	25	54
• Mini Brownie, 45 g	180	9	24
• Pecan Pie, 128 g	510	27	63
Raspberry Bar, 104 g	420	20	60
Croissants			
• Almond Croissant, 74 g	265	15	27
Pain au Chocolate, 62 g	221	12	24
• Plain Croissant, 34 g	130	7	13
Juices & Smoothies			
• Blueberry Pomegranate Smoothie, 240ml.	160	2	29
Carrot Juice, 236 ml.	72	0	15
Cranberry Apple Cider, 80 oz.	60	0	14
• Iced Tea & Lemonade, 8 oz.	40	0	12
Lemonade, 8 oz.	130	0	30
Mango Smoothie, 8 oz.	130	0	33
Organic Grapefruit Juice, 8 oz.	100	0	23
Organic Orange Juice, 8 oz.	110	0	27

Pret a Manger (cont.)

	Cal	Fat	Cbs
Juices & Smoothies (cont.)			
Raspberry Smoothie, 8 oz.	120	0	28
Muffins			
Banana Nut Muffin, 55 g	170	7	25
Blueberry Muffin, 55 g	150	4	26
Carrot & Zucchini Muffin, 55 g	190	10	24
• Hot Oatmeal, 149 g	530	10	99
Lemon Poppyseed Muffin, 55 g	180	8	24
• Raisin Bran Muffin, 55 g	120	3	3
Pret Yogurt Pots - Low Fat			
Blueberry & Granola PretPot, 283 g	350	16	43
• Honey & Banana PretPot, 337 g	530	18	84
Honey & Granola PretPot, 203 g	330	14	47
• Strawberry & Rhubarb PretPot, 197 g	170	6	28
Yoga Bunny PretPot, 187 g	240	12	28
Salad Dressing			
Balsamic Dressing Cup, 1 oz.	110	9	5
• Caesar Dressing Cup, 1 oz.	160	17	3
Honey Dijon Dressing Cup, 1 oz.	70	6	3
• Toasted Sesame Dressing Cup, 1 oz.	60	4	7
Salads			
• All Natural Cobb & Greens, 287 g	460	25	33
Bell & Evans Grilled Chicken Caesar, 338 g	390	15	24
• Pret's Salmon Sushi, 293 g	350	15	37
Pret's Tuna Sushi, 315 g	430	20	36
Chicken & Avocado Salad, 349 g	420	29	38
Sandwiches			
Bell & Evans Chicken and Bacon, 267 g	520	15	59
Bell & Evans Chicken Avocado, 257 g	580	23	62
• Bell & Evans Chicken Coronation, 303 g	320	27	78
Holiday Lunch, 288 g	490	13	70
Avocado Grana Padana Parmegiano, 293 g	560	27	59
Bacon, Lettuce & Tomato, 232 g	550	21	51
Murray's Natural Turkey Club, 341 g	530	21	59
• Organic Egg Salad, Spinach & Parmegiano, 301 g	580	27	54
Pret's Classic Tuna Salad, 282 g	430	19	43
Soups			
Angus Steak Chilli Medium, 12 oz.	345	14	29
Beef Stew Medium, 12 oz.	285	7	26
Broccoli & Cheddar Medium, 1 2 oz.	360	29	14
Butternut Squash Medium, 12 oz.	270	11	27
• Chicken Corn Chowder Medium, 12 oz.	375	24	27
Chicken Fajita Medium, 12 oz.	345	18	26
Chicken Noodle Medium, 12 oz.	180	3	21
Chicken Pot Pie Medium, 12 oz.	345	17	18
Italian Wedding w/ Meatball, 12 oz.	210	5	27
Leek and Potato Medium, 12 oz.	195	11	21
Loaded Potato Medium, 12 oz.	315	21	14
Mediterranean Eggplant & Zucchini, 12 oz.	120	8	9
Moroccan Lentil Medium, 12 oz.	345	17	36
Roasted Vegetable Medium, 12 oz.	225	14	21
Shrimp & Roast Corn Medium, 12	285	17	21
Thai Chicken with Curry Medium, 12 oz.	240	9	29
Tomato and Garden Vegetable, 12 oz.	150	4	21
• Tomato Basil Medium, 12 oz.	120	5	12
White Bean & Escarole Medium, 12 oz.	330	11	42
White Chicken Cilantro Medium, 12 oz.	375	14	35
Zesty Green Pea w/ Mint, 12 oz.	360	7	57
The Ridiculous No Bread Sandwich			
• No Bread Crayfish & Avocado, 228 g	200	14	11
No Bread Grilled Chicken Provencal, 318 g	240	16	20
No Bread Mezze, 238 g	410	17	51
• No Bread More Than Mozzarella, 376 g	420	35	16
No Bread Rock Shrimp Cocktail, 312 g	310	21	14

RESTAURANTS & FAST-FOOD CHAINS

Pret a Manger (cont.)

Wraps	Cal	Fat	Cbs
• Bell & Evans Chicken Jalepeño Hot Wrap, 374 g	550	24	57
• Marguerita Pizza Hot Wrap, 303 g	820	43	55
Natural Reuben Hot Wrap, 230 g	600	34	41

Pretzel Time

Bites	Cal	Fat	Cbs
Bites Cinnamon Sugar, 165 g	520	12	95
Bites Large, 165 g	510	13	88
• Bites Medium, 210 g	640	16	112
• Bites Small, 150 g	450	11	80
• PT Pretzel Dog, 167 g	440	27	34
Breezers			
Coffee, 20 fl.oz.	640	21	107
• Mochas, 20 fl.oz.	620	20	106
• Peach, 20 fl.oz.	650	20	117
Raspberry, 20 fl.oz.	650	20	117
Strawberry Banana, 20 fl.oz.	650	20	115
Pretzels			
• Caramel Nut, 129 g	390	7	74
Cinnamon Sugar, 122 g	370	8	68
Garlic, 118 g	350	7	64
Original, 114 g	340	7	61
Parmesan, 119 g	360	9	61
Plain, 108 g	290	2	61
• Ranch, 117 g	240	7	63
Sauces			
Caramel, 2 oz.	140	0	35
Cheddar Cheese, 2 oz.	70	5	6
Cream Cheese Icing, 2 oz.	180	9	22
• Cream Cheese, 2 oz.	200	20	4
Ketchup, 18 g	20	0	4
• Mustard, 10 g	5	0	1
Nacho Cheese, 2 oz.	80	5	7
Pizza Cheese, 2 oz.	30	1	6

Pretzelmaker

Bites	Cal	Fat	Cbs
Bites Cinnamon Sugar, 165 g	520	12	95
Bites Large, 165 g	510	13	88
• Bites Medium, 210 g	640	16	112
• Bites Small, 150 g	450	11	80
Breezers			
Coffee, 20 fl.oz.	640	21	107
• Mochas, 20 fl.oz.	620	20	106
• Peach, 20 fl.oz.	650	20	117
Raspberry, 20 fl.oz.	650	20	117
Strawberry Banana, 20 fl.oz.	650	20	115
Pretzels			
Caramel Nut, 129 g	390	7	74
Cinnamon Sugar, 122 g	370	8	68
Garlic, 118 g	350	7	64
Original, 114 g	340	7	61
Parmesan, 119 g	360	9	61
Plain, 108 g	290	2	61
• PT Pretzel Dog, 167 g	440	27	34
• Ranch, 117 g	240	7	63
Sauces			
Caramel, 2 oz.	140	0	35
Cheddar Cheese, 2 oz.	70	5	6
Cream Cheese Icing, 2 oz.	180	9	22
• Cream Cheese, 2 oz.	200	20	4
Ketchup, 18 g	20	0	4
• Mustard, 10 g	5	0	1
Nacho Cheese, 2 oz.	80	5	7
Pizza Cheese, 2 oz.	30	1	6

Qdoba Mexican Grill

Burritos	Cal	Fat	Cbs
• Fajita Ranchera Naked Burrito	530	23	35
• Grilled Vegetable Burrito	790	18	130
Naked Steak Burrito	610	18	69
Specialties			
Chicken Mexican Gumbo, 1 bowl	710	23	81
Tortilla Soup, 1 bowl	150	7	15
Tacos & Salad			
• 2 Grilled Vegetable Soft Tacos	340	16	40
• Grilled Veggie Naked Taco Salad	240	8	33
Naked Chicken Taco Salad	310	10	25

Quizno's Sub

Meals	Cal	Fat	Cbs
Small Traditional on wheat	490	N/A	N/A
Small Turkey Ranch & Swiss on wheat	470	N/A	N/A
Salads			
• Black & Bleu	380	N/A	N/A
Classic Cobb	400	N/A	N/A
• Raspberry Chipotle Salad	500	N/A	N/A
Sammies			
Alpine Chicken	310	N/A	N/A
Bistro Steak Melt	320	N/A	N/A
• Italiano	325	N/A	N/A
• Sonoma Turkey	300	N/A	N/A
Sides			
Cup of Chili	140	N/A	N/A
• Side Salad w/ Fat Free Blsmc Vinaigrette	130	N/A	N/A
• Side Salad with Raspberry Chipotle	220	N/A	N/A
Side Salad w/ Reduced Fat Bttrmlk Ranch	130	N/A	N/A
Subs			
• Baja Chicken, 6"	500	N/A	N/A
Black Angus Steak, 6"	480	N/A	N/A
• Honey Bourbon Chicken, 6"	320	N/A	N/A
Steakhouse Beef Dip, 6"	430	N/A	N/A
The Traditional, 6"	360	N/A	N/A
Turkey Bacon Guacamole, 6"	440	N/A	N/A
Turkey Ranch & Swiss, 6"	340	N/A	N/A
Tuscan Turkey, 6"	400	N/A	N/A

Ranch 1

Salads	Cal	Fat	Cbs
• Chicken on Gourmet Greens Salad, 15 oz.	350	11	31
Gourmet Greens Salad, 12 oz.	220	7	31
• Zesty Caesar Salad, 7 oz.	180	3	31
Zesty Chicken Caesar Salad, 9 oz.	290	6	31
Side Kicks			
• Fruit Cup, 8 oz.	90	1	18
• Ranch Fries (Large), 6 oz.	420	17	62
Ranch Fries (Regular), 5 oz.	350	14	51
Signature Sandwiches			
American Rancher, 9 oz.	390	10	51
• Club Sandwich, 9 oz.	470	16	53
Grilled Chicken Philly Sandwich, 9 oz.	450	14	53
• Ranch Classic, 9 oz.	370	5	53
Spicy Grilled Chicken Sandwich, 9 oz.	420	11	58
Specialities			
Baked Potato with Broccoli, 18 oz.	510	1	117
• Baked Potato with Cheese, 19 oz.	790	25	118
Baked Potato with Chicken, 14 oz.	610	4	114
Chicken Tenders (all white meat), 7 oz.	370	15	7
Grilled Chicken & Vegetable Platter, 25 oz.	790	7	129
• Grilled Chicken Fajita, 7 oz.	330	16	25
Grilled Chicken Hot Pasta, 19 oz.	590	10	86

Red Robin

	Cal	Fat	Cbs
Chicken Burgers			
Blackened Chicken Burger, 345 g	791	48	50
• California Chicken Burger, 406 g	982	62	50
Crispy Chicken Burger, 368 g	929	56	71
• Jamaican Jerk'd, 361 g	678	34	53
Teriyaki Chicken Burger, 435 g	900	47	65
Whiskey River BBQ Chicken Burger, 398 g	954	51	72
Classic Gourmet Burgers			
5 Alarm Burger, 372 g	907	58	50
• A.1. Peppercorn Burger, 378 g	1440	97	94
Blackened Bayou Burger, 364 g	858	57	44
Bleu Ribbon Burger, 393 g	1062	63	71
Guacamole Bacon Burger, 407 g	1151	76	52
Monster Burger, 485 g	1151	69	57
Red Robin Bacon Cheeseburger, 344 g	1030	70	47
• Red Robin Gourmet Cheeseburger	850	49	57
Royal Red Robin Burger, 408 g	1178	82	48
Santa Fe Burger, 384 g	1036	63	63
Sauteed Shroom Burger, 440 g	971	60	52
Sicilian Burger, 435 g	1070	66	46
The Banzai Burger, 421 g	1054	63	69
Whiskey River BBQ Burger, 402 g	1129	69	72
Desserts			
• Birthday Sundae, 138 g	312	17	49
Hot Apple Crisp, 497 g	784	13	165
Hot Fudge Sundae, 277 g	673	37	119
Kid's Sundae, 141 g	324	18	52
• Mountain High Mudd Pie , 441 g	1390	69	205
Entrees			
Arctic Code Fish & Chips, 446 g	991	60	76
Carnitas Fajitas, 676 g	1159	63	81
Chicken Fajitas, 634 g	1051	49	80
• Chicken Parmigiano Pasta, 968 g	1542	73	152
Clucks & Fries Buffalo Style, 545 g	1486	106	91
Clucks & Fries, 419 g	1261	80	90
• Ensenada Chicken Platter, 563 g	590	30	14
Jumbo Shrimp & Slaw Platter, 712 g	1235	58	120
Red's Rice Bowl, 839 g	1008	29	142
Shrimp & Cod Duo, 749 g	1407	83	107
Southwest Chicken Pasta, 875 g	1539	89	121
Insanely Delicious Burgers			
Bruschetta Chicken Burger, 375 g	876	54	54
Chili Chili Cheeseburger, 405 g	979	57	58
• Honky Tonk BBQ Pork Burger, 389 g	679	24	78
• Prime Rib Dip, 675 g	988	56	57
Kid's Menu: Kids			
Carnival Corn Dog, 197 g	490	20	62
• Cheesey Mac 'n Cheesey, 435 g	481	22	57
Chick-Chick-Chicken Fingers, 180 g	481	24	44
• Chick-n-Cheese Quesadilla, 306 g	763	35	60
Grilled Cheesewich, 242 g	635	38	56
Grilled Chick-N-Parmesan Noodles, 272 g	518	28	44
Red Robin Burger, 206 g	541	24	52
Red Robinetti Spaghetti, 522 g	614	15	95
Red's Pizzeria Pizza, 263 g	561	26	54
Lighten Up Burgers			
Crispy Fish Burger, 289 g	565	27	58
• Grilled Salmon Burger, 359 g	745	38	52
Grilled Turkey Burger, 273 g	704	43	51
• Lettuce-Wrapped Protein Burger, 387 g	439	27	10
The Garden Burger, 296 g	517	18	63
Salads			
Apple Harvest Chicken Salad, 512 g	603	34	39
Asian Chicken Salad, 610 g	488	6	70
Cobb Salad, 712 g	832	50	45

Red Robin (cont.)

	Cal	Fat	Cbs
Salads (cont.)			
• Crispy Chicken Tender Salad, 671 g	1326	87	84
Fajita Fiesta Pollo Salad, 756 g	1238	85	67
Mighty Caesar Salad, 436 g	784	51	60
Mighty Caesar-Blackened Chicken, 563 g	980	61	61
Mighty Caesar-Grilled Chicken, 557 g	980	61	61
Mighty Caesar-Salmon, 577 g	960	57	60
Side Caesar Salad, 281 g	611	31	65
• Side Dinner Salad, 212 g	217	13	15
Sandwiches			
BLTA Croissant, 673 g	1077	66	114
Shareable Starters			
Cheeseburger Con Queso, 456 g	1303	85	75
Chili Chili Nachos w/ Chicken, 634 g	1379	89	67
Chili Chili Nachos, 513 g	1183	80	66
Creamy Artichoke & Spanish Dip, 520 g	1201	73	101
Fresh-Fried Cheese Sticks, 415 g	1181	70	86
• Guacamole, Salsa & Chips, 344 g	800	47	88
Just-in-quesadilla, 574 g	1073	55	72
RR's Buzzard Wings, 427 g	1023	81	4
• Towering Onion Rings, 541 g	1837	124	160
Soups			
• Chicken Tortilla Soup, 1 cup	173	9	11
• Clamdigger's Clam Chowder, 1 cup	346	20	26
French Onion Soup Cup, 1 cup	280	11	27
Red's Homemade Chili, 1 cup	302	19	16
Wraps			
Caesar's Chicken Wrap, 677 g	1244	60	122
Whiskey River BBQ Chicken Wrap, 740 g	1526	81	138

Red Lobster

	Cal	Fat	Cbs
Appetizers			
Buffalo Chicken Wings	680	N/A	N/A
Chicken Breast Strips	690	N/A	N/A
Chilled Jumbo Shrimp Cocktail	121	N/A	N/A
• Crispy Calamari and Vegetables	1520	N/A	N/A
• Hand-Shucked Oysters on the Half Shell, 6 pcs.	50	N/A	N/A
Lobster Pizza	720	N/A	N/A
Lobster, Artichoke and Seafood Dip	1080	N/A	N/A
Lobster, Crab & Seafood-Stuffed Mshrms	380	N/A	N/A
Mozzarella Cheesesticks	680	N/A	N/A
New England Seafood Sampler	890	N/A	N/A
Pan-Seared Crab Cakes	360	N/A	N/A
Parrot Bay Jumbo Coconut Shrimp	588	N/A	N/A
Southwestern Lobster Rolls	780	N/A	N/A
Steamed Clams	430	N/A	N/A
Ultimate Fondue	1490	N/A	N/A
Condiments and Sauces			
Add Petite Shrimp to your Salad	15	N/A	N/A
Baked Potato	190	N/A	N/A
add Butter	90	N/A	N/A
add Sour Cream	30	N/A	N/A
Caesar Salad	270	N/A	N/A
Cheddar Bay Biscuit, 1 biscuit	150	N/A	N/A
Coleslaw	200	N/A	N/A
• Creamy Lobster Topped Baked Potato	370	N/A	N/A
Creamy Lobster Topped Mashed Potatoes	360	N/A	N/A
Fresh Asparagus	60	N/A	N/A
Fresh Broccoli	45	N/A	N/A
Fries	330	N/A	N/A
Garden Salad	90	N/A	N/A
Home-Style Mashed Potatoes	180	N/A	N/A
• Lemon Wedge	5	N/A	N/A
Wild Rice Pilaf	180	N/A	N/A
Create Your Own Appetizer Combo			
Chicken Breast Strips	414	N/A	N/A

Red Lobster (cont.)

	Cal	Fat	Cbs
Create Your Own Appetizer Combo (cont.)			
Clam Strips	370	N/A	N/A
• Crispy Calamari and Vegetables	775	N/A	N/A
Mozzarella Cheesesticks	340	N/A	N/A
• Stuffed Mushrooms	220	N/A	N/A
Create Your Own Feast			
Crab Linguini Alfredo	560	N/A	N/A
Garlic Shrimp Scampi	195	N/A	N/A
Garlic-Grilled Jumbo Shrimp	105	N/A	N/A
Grilled Salmon	210	N/A	N/A
Grilled Sirloin Steak	250	N/A	N/A
• Parrot Bay Jumbo Coconut Shrimp	784	N/A	N/A
Seafood-Stuffed Flounder	160	N/A	N/A
Shrimp Linguini Alfredo	550	N/A	N/A
• Steamed Snow Crab Legs	80	N/A	N/A
Walt's Favorite Shrimp	466	N/A	N/A
Dipping Sauces			
100% Melted Butter, 1 oz.	230	N/A	N/A
Cocktail Sauce, 1 oz.	50	N/A	N/A
• Honey Mustard Dipping Sauce, 1 oz.	240	N/A	N/A
Horseradish, 1 oz.	20	N/A	N/A
Ketchup, 1 oz.	30	N/A	N/A
Marinara Sauce, 1 oz.	30	N/A	N/A
• Pico de Gallo, 1 oz.	10	N/A	N/A
Piña Colada Sauce, 1 oz.	120	N/A	N/A
Remoulade, 2 oz.	150	N/A	N/A
Sweet and Spicy Glaze, 1 oz.	90	N/A	N/A
Tartar Sauce, 1 oz.	130	N/A	N/A
Dressings			
Balsamic Vinaigrette, 1 oz.	60	N/A	N/A
Blue Cheese, 1 oz.	170	N/A	N/A
• Caesar, 1 oz.	200	N/A	N/A
French, 1 oz.	120	N/A	N/A
Honey Mustard Dressing, 1 oz.	100	N/A	N/A
• Ranch (Fat-Free), 1 oz.	40	N/A	N/A
Ranch, 1 oz.	110	N/A	N/A
Thousand Island, 1 oz.	130	N/A	N/A
Lobster & Crab			
Chef's Signature Lobster & Shrimp Pasta	1020	N/A	N/A
• Crab Linguini Alfredo	1120	N/A	N/A
• Live Maine Lobster, 1 1/4 lb	45	N/A	N/A
Lobster & Seafood Mixed Grill	630	N/A	N/A
North Pacific King Crab Legs	390	N/A	N/A
Rock Lobster Tail	90	N/A	N/A
Snow Crab Legs, 1 lb	160	N/A	N/A
Other			
Steamed King Crab Legs, 1/2 lb	130	N/A	N/A
Steamed Snow Crab Legs, 1/2 lb	80	N/A	N/A
Shrimp			
Crunchy Popcorn Shrimp	560	N/A	N/A
• Garlic-Grilled Jumbo Shrimp	245	N/A	N/A
Maui Luau Shrimp and Salmon	790	N/A	N/A
• Parrot Bay Jumbo Coconut Shrimp	980	N/A	N/A
Shrimp Linguini Alfredo	550	N/A	N/A
Spicy Asian-Garlic Jumbo Shrimp	245	N/A	N/A
Tequila-Lime Jumbo Shrimp	360	N/A	N/A
Walt's Favorite Shrimp	700	N/A	N/A
Shrimp Your Way			
• Coconut Shrimp Bites	290	N/A	N/A
Fried Shrimp	190	N/A	N/A
Popcorn Shrimp	180	N/A	N/A
• Scampi	130	N/A	N/A
Signature Combinations			
• Admiral's Feast	1506	N/A	N/A
Seaside Shrimp Trio	1030	N/A	N/A

Red Lobster (cont.)

	Cal	Fat	Cbs
Signature Combinations (cont.)			
• Ultimate Feast	638	N/A	N/A
Soups & Salads			
• Apple-Walnut Chicken Salad	900	N/A	N/A
• Manhattan Clam Chowder, 1 cup	80	N/A	N/A
New England Clam Chowder, 1 cup	240	N/A	N/A
Seafood Caesar Salad	680	N/A	N/A
Specialty Drinks			
• Sail Away Smoothie - Banana Bay Choco	460	N/A	N/A
Sail Away Smoothie - Strawberry Banana	340	N/A	N/A
Sail Away Smoothie - Sunset Strawberry	250	N/A	N/A
• Tropical Freezes - Orange or Pineapple	250	N/A	N/A
Steak & Chicken			
Aztec Chicken	755	N/A	N/A
• Cajun Chicken Linguini Alfredo	1260	N/A	N/A
Grilled Center-Cut New York Strip	480	N/A	N/A
Grilled Chicken Breast	610	N/A	N/A
Honey BBQ Shrimp and Chicken	710	N/A	N/A
New York Steak and Rock Lobster Tail	570	N/A	N/A
New York Strip Steak and Shrimp	946	N/A	N/A
• Sirloin Steak and Rock Lobster Tail	340	N/A	N/A
Sirloin Steak and Shrimp	716	N/A	N/A
Steak Lobster-and-Shrimp Oscar	990	N/A	N/A
Traditional Favorites			
• Broiled Seafood Platter	280	N/A	N/A
• Classic Fried Seafood Platter	1090	N/A	N/A
Farm-Raised Catfish - Blackened	380	N/A	N/A
Farm-Raised Catfish - Golden-Fried	440	N/A	N/A
Golden-Fried Flounder	440	N/A	N/A
Oven-Broiled Flounder	280	N/A	N/A
Seafood-Stuffed Flounder	320	N/A	N/A

Rita's

	Cal	Fat	Cbs
Ice			
Cream Ice Regular, 12 oz.	312	4	70
Custard Regular, 7 oz.	385	21	43
Gelati w/ Choc. Cust. Regular, 10 oz.	351	11	60
Gelati w/ Van. Cust. Regular, 10 oz.	366	13	59
• Ice Regular, 12 oz.	263	0	69
Misto w/ Choc. Cust. Regular, 15 oz.	409	7	90
• Misto w/ Van. Cust. Regular, 15 oz.	420	7	90
Made with Cream Ice			
• Gelati w/ Choc. Cust. Regular, 10 oz.	368	13	60
Gelati w/ Van. Cust. Regular, 10 oz.	392	15	61
Misto w/ Choc. Cust. Regular, 15 oz.	463	11	90
• Misto w/ Van. Cust. Regular, 15 oz.	473	12	90

Robeks

	Cal	Fat	Cbs
Bowls			
Açai Energy Bowl™, 12 oz.	267	3	55
Super Açai Bowl™, 12 oz.	314	6	61
Frozen Yogurt			
Average, 12 oz.	250	0	58
Shakes & Freezes			
800 lb. Gorilla™, 12 oz.	375	9	50
Bananasplit Shake, 12 oz.	302	0	69
Lemon Freeze, 12 oz.	279	2	60
• Orange Freeze, 12 oz.	242	0	56
• P-Nut Power Shake, 12 oz.	422	18	52
Smoothies			
Açai Energizer™, 12 oz.	167	1	36
Awesome Açai™, 12 oz.	183	1	42
Banzai Blueberry™, 12 oz.	175	1	38
Berry Brilliance®, 12 oz.	194	1	45
Big Wednesday®, 12 oz.	172	1	40
Cardio Cooler™, 12 oz.	215	1	44

Robeks (cont.)

	Cal	Fat	Cbs
Smoothies (cont.)			
Citrus Stinger™, 12 oz.	194	1	40
Cranberry Quest™, 12 oz.	173	0	40
Dr. Robeks®, 12 oz.	181	1	40
Green Tea Sensation™, 12 oz.	222	1	42
Guava Lava™, 12 oz.	180	1	42
Hummingbird®, 12 oz.	185	1	44
Innite Orange®, 12 oz.	181	0	42
Mahalo Mango®, 12 oz.	174	1	42
• Malibu Peach™, 12 oz.	153	0	36
Outrageous Raspberry, 12 oz.	174	1	39
Passionfruit Cove®, 12 oz.	168	1	38
Pina Koolada™, 12 oz.	261	8	46
Polar Pineapple™, 12 oz.	164	1	38
Pomegranate Passion™, 12 oz.	196	0	48
Pomegranate Power™, 12 oz.	211	0	50
• Pro Arobek®, 12 oz.	265	1	54
Raspberry Romance®, 12 oz.	172	0	42
Robeks MuscleMax™, 12 oz.	202	1	38
Robeks Rejuvenator™, 12 oz.	193	1	43
South Pacific Squeeze®, 12 oz.	188	1	42
Strawnana Berry™, 12 oz.	179	0	44
Venice Burner®, 12 oz.	231	1	46
Zen Berry®, 12 oz.	190	1	45

Rockfish Seafood Grill

	Cal	Fat	Cbs
Be The Chef: Choose A Fish			
Ahi Tuna	248	N/A	N/A
Alaskan Flounder	255	N/A	N/A
• Chicken	188	N/A	N/A
North Atlantic Salmon	356	N/A	N/A
Shrimp	325	N/A	N/A
Tilapia	341	N/A	N/A
Trophy Rainbow Trout	355	N/A	N/A
• U.S. Farm- Raised Catfish	488	N/A	N/A
Be The Chef: Choose A Prep Style			
Blackened	17	N/A	N/A
Be The Chef: Choose A Sauce			
Ancho Cream	102	N/A	N/A
• Lemon-Butter	244	N/A	N/A
Maple Glaze	106	N/A	N/A
Pontchartrain	115	N/A	N/A
Roasted Red Pepper	34	N/A	N/A
• Tomatillo Salsa	18	N/A	N/A
Be The Chef: Choose A Side			
Mixed Veggies	17	N/A	N/A
• New Potatoes	152	N/A	N/A
• Steamed Spinach	17	N/A	N/A
Wild Rice	100	N/A	N/A
Salads			
Pacific Cove Crab Salad	423	18	33
• Roaring River Salmon Salad	462	19	30
Seared Ahi Tuna Salad	335	14	10
• Small Southwest Caesar Salad	251	34	17
Stream			
Ahi Tuna Ciabatta	516	17	41
Baked & Stuffed Shrimp	493	34	19
• Louisiana Gumbo	445	16	54
• Santa Fe Fish Tacos	564	18	101
Tilapia In The Bag	501	18	31
Tilapia Pontchartrain	493	24	9

Rocky Rococo

	Cal	Fat	Cbs
Bread			
• Breadsticks w/ Jalapeño Chz Sauce, 8 oz.	531	18	72
Breadsticks with Marinara Sauce, 8 oz.	420	7	72

Rocky Rococo (cont.)

	Cal	Fat	Cbs
Bread (cont.)			
• Wheat muffin, 1 muffin	200	4	38
Pasta			
Can't Decide, 14 oz.	464	9	77
Fettuccine with Alfredo Sauce, 14 oz.	459	14	66
• Light Fettuccine with Alfredo Sauce, 7 oz.	229	7	33
Light Spaghetti with Meat Sauce, 7 oz.	250	3	44
Light Spaghetti with Meatballs, 8 oz.	314	8	45
Light Spaghetti with Tomato Sauce, 7 oz.	235	2	44
Spaghetti with Meat Sauce, 14 oz.	499	7	87
• Spaghetti with Meatballs, 15 oz.	628	16	89
Spaghetti with Tomato Sauce, 14 oz.	470	4	87
Pizza			
• Cheese, 1 slice	380	9	54
Garden, 1 slice	391	10	56
Pepperoni, 1 slice	427	13	54
• Sausage Mushroom, 1 slice	499	19	55
Sausage, 1 slice	495	19	54

Roly Poly

	Cal	Fat	Cbs
Egg Items			
All American Egg Roly on Low-carb	441	26	24
All American Egg Roly on Wheat	458	26	27
• All American Egg Roly on White	468	26	29
Christo Melt on Low-carb	313	15	24
Christo Melt on Wheat	330	16	27
Christo Melt on White	340	16	30
Steak and Eggs on Low-carb	319	15	26
Steak and Eggs on Wheat	336	16	29
Steak and Eggs on White	346	16	31
• Veggie Scramble Egg Roly on Low-carb	296	15	26
Veggie Scramble Egg Roly on Wheat	314	16	29
Veggie Scramble Egg Roly on White	324	16	32
Western Egg Roly on Low-carb	310	17	26
Western Egg Roly on Wheat	328	17	29
Western Egg Roly on White	338	18	32
Kids Items			
Kids Cheese Dog on Low-carb	246	14	22
Kids Cheese Dog on Wheat	264	14	25
Kids Cheese Dog on White	274	15	28
• Kids Chicken Melt on Low-carb	193	7	22
Kids Chicken Melt on Wheat	210	7	25
Kids Chicken Melt on White	220	8	28
Kids Grilled Cheese on Low-carb	200	10	22
Kids Grilled Cheese on Wheat	218	10	24
Kids Grilled Cheese on White	228	10	27
Kids Meat and Cheese on Low-carb	193	7	22
Kids Meat and Cheese on Wheat	210	7	25
Kids Meat and Cheese on White	220	8	28
Kids Peanut Butter and Jelly on Low-carb	255	11	34
Kids Peanut Butter and Jelly on Wheat	272	11	36
• Kids Peanut Butter and Jelly on White	282	11	39
Salad			
Alpine Chef	412	24	14
• Chipotle Caesar	599	31	23
Cobb Salad	566	34	12
• Greek Salad	242	16	17
Las Olas Salad	349	14	12
Spa Salad	255	15	26
Walnut Spinach	515	43	15
Sandwich: Black Forest Ham & Roast Pork			
BarBQ Pork Melt Wheat	302	10	26
BarBQ Pork Melt White	315	10	27
Italian Classic Wheat	328	12	28
Italian Classic White	341	12	29
• Key West Cuban Mix Wheat	297	9	27

RESTAURANTS & FAST-FOOD CHAINS

Roly Poly (cont.)	Cal	Fat	Cbs
Sandwich: Black Forest Ham & Roast Pork (cont.)			
Key West Cuban Mix White	310	9	28
Peachtree Melt Wheat	327	11	28
Peachtree Melt White	340	11	29
Porky's Nightmare Wheat	312	12	26
Porky's Nightmare White	325	12	28
Southside Club Wheat	364	18	29
• Southside Club White	374	19	32
Sandwich: Chicken			
Basil Cashew Chicken Wheat	288	11	27
Basil Cashew Chicken White	301	11	28
Buffalo Chicken Melt Wheat	355	11	33
Buffalo Chicken Melt White	365	12	35
Buffalo Slim Wheat	279	6	26
Catalina Chicken Salad Wheat	305	12	27
Catalina Chicken Salad White	318	13	28
Chicken Caesar Wheat	312	12	28
Chicken Caesar White	325	12	30
Chicken Cordonbleu Wheat	303	11	27
Chicken Cordonbleu White	319	11	28
Chicken Fajita Wheat	279	8	27
Chicken Fajita White	292	8	28
• Chicken Popper Wheat	246	7	29
• Chicken Popper White	259	7	30
Cobb Salad Wheat	318	14	28
Cobb Salad White	331	14	29
Delhi Chicken Wheat	319	12	32
Delhi Chicken White	332	13	33
Hickory Chicken Wheat	336	11	27
Hickory Chicken White	349	11	29
Oriental Chicken Wheat	262	6	31
Oriental Chicken White	275	6	32
Pesto Chicken Wheat	410	18	31
• Pesto Chicken White	420	18	34
Santa Fe Chicken Wheat	272	8	27
Santa Fe Chicken White	285	8	28
Sandwich: Sliced Steak & Roast Beef			
Chipotle Cheesesteak Wheat	363	17	29
• Chipotle Cheesesteak White	373	17	32
• Pepper Steak Wheat	237	9	26
Pepper Steak White	250	9	28
Philly Melt Wheat	257	7	26
Philly Melt White	270	7	27
Ranch Roast Wheat	316	14	28
Ranch Roast White	329	14	29
Russian Beef Wheat	282	11	26
Russian Beef White	295	11	28
Santa Fe Steak Wheat	279	8	27
Santa Fe Steak White	292	8	28
Steak Fajita Wheat	283	8	27
Steak Fajita White	296	8	29
Sandwich: Tuna Salad			
• Popeye's Tuna Wheat	309	5	30
Texas Tuna Melt Wheat	309	13	26
Texas Tuna Melt White	322	14	27
Thai Hot Tuna Wheat	327	13	27
• Thai Hot Tuna White	340	13	28
Tuna Luau Wheat	323	15	29
Tuna Luau White	336	15	30
Sandwich: Turkey & Smoked Turkey			
California Turkey Wheat	319	14	34
California Turkey White	332	14	35
Cider House Melt Wheat	252	5	284
Greek Turkey Wheat	256	5	30
Hickory Christo Wheat	302	10	28

Roly Poly (cont.)	Cal	Fat	Cbs
Sandwich: Turkey & Smoked Turkey (cont.)			
Hickory Christo White	315	10	29
Hot Honey Wheat	291	9	28
Hot Honey White	304	9	30
Italian Turkey Wheat	320	12	31
Italian Turkey White	333	12	32
Pesto Turkey Club Wheat	382	20	31
• Pesto Turkey Club White	392	20	34
Smokehouse Turkey Wheat	319	11	28
Smokehouse Turkey White	332	11	29
Thanksgiving Wheat	276	8	30
Thanksgiving White	289	8	32
Turkey Applejack Wheat	311	13	27
Turkey Applejack White	324	13	28
Tuscan Turkey Wheat	228	4	31
• Tuscan Turkey White	241	4	32
Wild Turkey Wheat	275	12	29
Wild Turkey White	288	12	30
Sandwich: Veggie & Cheese			
California Hummer Wheat	305	14	29
California Hummer White	318	14	31
French Twist Wheat	264	11	28
French Twist White	277	11	29
Italian Veggie Wheat	246	9	29
Italian Veggie White	259	9	30
Monster Veggie Wheat	275	10	29
Monster Veggie White	288	10	31
Nut & Honey Wheat	360	18	35
• Nut & Honey White	373	19	37
Spinach Stuffer Wheat	229	8	31
Spinach Stuffer White	242	9	32
• Ultimate Veggie Wheat	196	4	31
Ultimate Veggie White	209	4	32
Veggie Fajita Wheat	229	8	28
Veggie Fajita White	242	9	30
Sandwiches Special			
Alpine Chicken Melt on Wheat	456	18	33
Alpine Chicken Melt on White	466	18	36
BBQ Veggie Ranchero on Wheat	321	5	31
Buffalo Chicken Melt on Low-carb	338	11	30
Buffalo Chicken Melt on Wheat	355	11	33
Buffalo Chicken Melt on White	365	12	35
Cajun Chicken Melt on Low-carb	378	15	28
Cajun Chicken Melt on Wheat	395	16	30
Cajun Chicken Melt on White	405	16	33
Cajun Club on Low-carb	343	16	30
Cajun Club on Wheat	361	17	33
Cajun Club on White	371	17	35
Caribbean Mix on Low-carb	454	19	42
Caribbean Mix on Wheat	472	20	44
Caribbean Mix on White	418	20	31
Carnita Chicken on Low-carb	373	13	32
Carnita Chicken on Wheat	391	13	35
Carnita Chicken on White	401	14	37
Carnita Steak on Low-carb	364	15	32
Carnita Steak on Wheat	382	15	34
Carnita Steak on White	392	16	37
Carolina Shrimp Melt on Low-carb	258	11	25
Carolina Shrimp Melt on Wheat	276	11	27
Carolina Shrimp Melt on White	286	12	30
Cherry Pecan Chicken Club on Low-carb	593	34	41
Cherry Pecan Chicken Club on Wheat	640	37	44
• Cherry Pecan Chicken Club on White	650	38	47
Chicken Bruschetta on Low-carb	339	11	30
Chicken Bruschetta on Wheat	357	11	33

Roly Poly (cont.)

Sandwiches Special (cont.)

	Cal	Fat	Cbs
Chicken Bruschetta on White	367	11	35
Chicken Pizza on Low-carb	392	16	29
Chicken Pizza on Wheat	409	16	31
Chicken Pizza on White	419	17	34
Chipotle Cheesesteak on Low-carb	346	16	26
Chipotle Cheesesteak on Wheat	363	17	29
Chipotle Cheesesteak on White	373	17	32
Chipotle Chicken on Low-carb	405	18	27
Chipotle Chicken on Wheat	423	18	30
Chipotle Chicken on White	433	19	33
Coney Island Melt on Low-carb	442	29	26
Coney Island Melt on Wheat	460	29	29
Coney Island Melt on White	470	30	31
Creole Chicken on Low-carb	231	5	27
• Creole Chicken on Wheat	218	5	27
Creole Chicken on Wheat	248	5	30
Creole Chicken on White	258	6	33
Extreme Veggie on Wheat	263	11	35
Extreme Veggie on White	273	12	38
Ginger Shrimp on Wheat	282	5	26
Grand Central on Low-carb	380	20	33
Grand Central on Wheat	398	20	36
Grand Central on White	408	20	38
Guilt Free Cobbler on Wheat	307	4	32
Harvest Melt on Wheat	223	4	30
Hawaiian Chicken on Wheat	284	6	29
Holiday Meltdown on Low-carb	384	19	30
Holiday Meltdown on Wheat	402	19	33
Holiday Meltdown on White	412	20	36
Huevos Rancheros on Low-carb	331	17	30
Huevos Rancheros on Wheat	349	17	33
Huevos Rancheros on White	359	18	35
Indian Chicken on Wheat	299	6	29
Longhorn Melt on Low-carb	402	20	27
Longhorn Melt on Wheat	419	21	30
Longhorn Melt on White	429	21	32
Mandarin Tuna on Low-carb	249	5	32
Mandarin Tuna on Wheat	266	5	34
Mandarin Tuna on White	276	6	37
Monster Fajita on Low-carb	373	17	29
Monster Fajita on Wheat	391	17	32
Monster Fajita on White	401	17	34
Monterey Chicken on Low-carb	419	18	32
Monterey Chicken on Wheat	437	18	35
Monterey Chicken on White	447	19	37
Moroccan Tofu on Low-carb	229	10	28
Moroccan Tofu on Wheat	246	10	31
Moroccan Tofu on White	256	10	33
Nantucket Lobster on Low-carb	310	16	31
Nantucket Lobster on Wheat	328	17	34
Nantucket Lobster on White	338	17	36
New Orleans Melt on Low-carb	276	11	26
New Orleans Melt on Wheat	293	11	29
New Orleans Melt on White	303	11	32
New Yorker on Low-carb	290	12	28
New Yorker on Wheat	308	12	31
New Yorker on White	318	13	33
Orange County Smoked Turkey on Lowcarb	493	30	31
Orange County Smoked Turkey on Wheat	511	30	34
Orange County Smoked Turkey on White	521	31	37
Palm Beach Tuna on Low-carb	293	11	30
Palm Beach Tuna on Wheat	311	11	33
Palm Beach Tuna on White	321	12	35
Peking Chicken on Wheat	230	6	28

Roly Poly (cont.)

Sandwiches Special (cont.)

	Cal	Fat	Cbs
Pesto Chicken on Low-carb	392	18	28
Pesto Chicken on Wheat	410	18	31
Pesto Chicken on White	420	18	34
Pesto Club on Low-carb	349	17	30
Pesto Club on Wheat	366	17	33
Pesto Club on White	376	17	36
Popeye's Tuna on Low- Carb	237	5	30
Popeye's Tuna on Wheat	254	5	33
Popeye's Tuna on White	264	6	35
Ranchero Chicken on Low-carb	364	12	32
Ranchero Chicken on Wheat	382	13	35
Ranchero Chicken on White	392	13	38
Ranchero Steak on Low-carb	356	14	32
Ranchero Steak on Wheat	373	15	35
Ranchero Steak on White	383	15	37
Roly Poly Pounder on Low-carb	425	20	30
Roly Poly Pounder on Wheat	443	20	33
Roly Poly Pounder on White	453	21	36
Roly Polynesian on Low-carb	372	16	29
Roly Polynesian on Wheat	390	17	31
Roly Polynesian on White	400	17	34
Roly Reuben on Low-carb	350	20	23
Roly Reuben on Wheat	367	20	26
Roly Reuben on White	377	21	29
Roma Chicken on Low-carb	340	10	30
Roma Chicken on Wheat	358	11	33
Roma Chicken on White	368	11	36
Shrimp Club on Low-carb	319	18	26
Shrimp Club on Wheat	336	18	28
Shrimp Club on White	346	19	31
Steak & Bearnaise on Low-carb	345	16	25
Steak & Bearnaise on Wheat	363	17	28
Steak & Bearnaise on White	373	17	31
Teriyaki Tuna on Low-carb	399	22	29
Teriyaki Tuna on Wheat	417	22	31
Teriyaki Tuna on White	427	22	34
Thai Peanut Chicken on Low-carb	378	15	27
Thai Peanut Chicken on Wheat	395	16	30
Thai Peanut Chicken on White	405	16	33
Thai Peanut Tofu on Low-carb	218	9	28
Thai Peanut Tofu on Wheat	236	9	31
Thai Peanut Tofu on White	246	9	34
Tofu Tahini on Low- Carb	220	9	28
Tofu Tahini on Wheat	238	9	30
Tofu Tahini on White	248	10	33
Tuna Club on Low-carb	385	21	26
Tuna Club on Wheat	403	21	29
Tuna Club on White	413	22	32
Turkey Saga on Low-carb	329	17	29
Turkey Saga on Wheat	348	17	32
Turkey Saga on White	357	17	35
Westport Club on Wheat	382	19	32
Westport Club on White	392	19	35
Soup: Classic Soups			
Baja Chicken Enchilada	210	14	12
Broccoli Cheddar	160	11	10
Clam Chowder	150	5	12
Classic Chili	160	5	18
Harvest Mushroom Bisque	90	5	11
Loaded Baked Potato	170	11	15
Mexican Style Chicken Tortilla	130	3	18
• Old Fashioned Chicken Noodle	70	2	11
Roasted Garlic Tomato	160	11	12
• Seafood Bisque	217	14	12

Roly Poly (cont.)

	Cal	Fat	Cbs
Soup: Classic Vegetarian Soups			
Corn & Green Chile Bisque	130	7	14
• Garden Vegetable	60	0	12
• Spring Asparagus	130	9	10
Sweet Items			
Apple Strudel	393	19	51
Chocolate Cheesecake	456	24	58
• Fruit Melt	289	14	36
Peach Granola	456	24	58
• Rock N Roll Sweet Roly	456	24	58

Round Table Pizza

	Cal	Fat	Cbs
Appetizers and Sandwiches			
Buffalo Wings, 12 wings	860	62	10
Buffalo Wings, 6 wings	420	28	2
Chicken Club, 353 g	760	34	67
Garlic Bread w/ Cheese, 189 g	630	33	59
Garlic Bread, 132 g	470	21	59
Garlic Parmesan Twists, 3 pcs.	500	14	73
• Garlic Parmesan Twists, 6 pcs.	1010	29	146
Ham Club, 375 g	810	37	76
Honey BBQ Wings, 12 wings	930	55	27
• Honey BBQ Wings, 6 wings	390	25	8
RT Pizza Sandwich, 271 g	690	34	65
RT Veggie Sandwich, 306 g	680	29	79
Turkey Club, 375 g	800	37	75
Turkey Sante Fe, 369 g	850	44	74
Large Cheese			
Original Crust, 1 slice	210	8	25
• Pan Crust, 1 slice	290	10	38
• Skinny Crust, 1 slice	180	8	18
Large Chicken & Garlic Gourmet™			
Original Crust, 1 slice	230	9	25
• Pan Crust, 1 slice	320	11	39
• Skinny Crust, 1 slice	200	9	19
Large Chicken Smokehouse			
Original Crust, 1 slice	250	10	26
• Pan Crust, 1 slice	360	15	40
• Skinny Crust, 1 slice	220	10	20
Large Gourmet Veggie™			
Original Crust, 1 slice	220	9	26
• Pan Crust, 1 slice	310	10	40
• Skinny Crust, 1 slice	190	8	20
Large Guinevere's Garden Delight®			
Original Crust, 1 slice	210	7	26
• Pan Crust, 1 slice	290	9	39
• Skinny Crust, 1 slice	170	7	20
Large Hawaiian			
Original Crust, 1 slice	210	7	26
• Pan Crust, 1 slice	290	9	39
• Skinny Crust, 1 slice	180	7	20
Large Italian Garlic Supreme™			
Original Crust, 1 slice	270	14	25
• Pan Crust, 1 slice	360	16	39
• Skinny Crust, 1 slice	240	14	18
Large King Arthur's Supreme®			
Original Crust, 1 slice	270	14	26
• Pan Crust, 1 slice	340	14	39
• Skinny Crust, 1 slice	240	14	19
Large Maui Zaui™ (Polynesian Sauce)			
Original Crust, 1 slice	250	9	28
• Pan Crust, 1 slice	330	11	42
• Skinny Crust, 1 slice	210	9	21
Large Maui Zaui™ (Zesty Red Sauce)			
Original Crust, 1 slice	240	9	27
• Pan Crust, 1 slice	320	11	40

Round Table Pizza (cont.)

	Cal	Fat	Cbs
Large Maui Zaui™ (Zesty Red Sauce) (cont.)			
• Skinny Crust, 1 slice	210	9	20
Large Montague's All Meat Marvel®			
Original Crust, 1 slice	300	17	25
• Pan Crust, 1 slice	350	16	38
• Skinny Crust, 1 slice	260	16	18
Large Pepperoni			
Original Crust, 1 slice	240	11	24
• Pan Crust, 1 slice	320	12	38
• Skinny Crust, 1 slice	210	11	18
Large Smokehouse Combo			
Original Crust, 1 slice	270	13	26
• Pan Crust, 1 slice	360	15	40
• Skinny Crust, 1 slice	240	13	20
Large Ulti-Meat			
Original Crust, 1 slice	290	15	24
• Pan Crust, 1 slice	370	17	37
• Skinny Crust, 1 slice	260	15	18
Large Wombo Combo			
Original Crust, 1 slice	270	12	26
• Pan Crust, 1 slice	350	14	39
• Skinny Crust, 1 slice	230	12	19
Salads			
• Caesar Salad Small, 128 g	140	7	11
Garden Salad Small, 177 g	100	4	14
• Side of Chicken, 57 g	70	1	1

Rubio's

	Cal	Fat	Cbs
Burritos			
Baja Grill Burrito Carnitas, 379 g	660	32	57
• Baja Grill Burrito Chicken, 379 g	650	28	58
Baja Grill Burrito Steak, 379 g	650	29	57
Bean & Cheese Burrito, 371 g	810	37	87
• Big Burrito Especial Carnitas, 522 g	940	42	107
Big Burrito Especial Chicken, 522 g	940	38	107
Big Burrito Especial Steak, 522 g	940	39	106
Fish Burrito, 379 g	770	45	76
Grilled Mesquite Shrimp Burrito, 368 g	780	40	72
Mahi Mahi Burrito, 369 g	720	39	55
Make it a Wet Burrito, 132 g	120	8	9
Classic Taco Plates			
Original #1 (2 Fish Tacos), 429 g	900	42	110
• Pesky (2 Especial Fish Tacos), 485 g	1040	53	113
Two Carnitas Tacos, 429 g	780	29	100
Two Chicken Tacos, 457 g	930	42	101
• Two Steak Tacos, 429 g	780	27	100
Enchilada & Fish Taco			
• Carnitas Enchilada & Fish Taco, 594 g	1170	53	128
• Cheese Enchilada & Fish Taco, 559 g	1120	51	127
Chicken Enchilada & Fish Taco, 594 g	1170	51	128
Enchilada Plates			
• Carnitas, 626 g	1240	58	124
• Cheese, 555 g	1140	53	122
Chicken, 626 g	1240	54	124
HealthMex®			
Chicken Burrito, 359 g	550	16	70
Chicken Salad, 471 g	270	3	36
Chicken Taco, 132 g	150	2	21
• Mahi Mahi Burrito, 374 g	560	16	69
Mahi Mahi Salad, 484 g	270	3	35
• Mahi Mahi Taco, 139 g	150	2	21
Kid's Meals			
Add Black Beans, 103 g	100	2	14
Add Chips, 43 g	210	11	28
• Add Mini Churro, 23 g	80	4	11
Add Pinto Beans, 103 g	110	3	19

Rubio's (cont.)

	Cal	Fat	Cbs
Kid's Meals (cont.)			
Add Rice, 57 g	80	0	17
• Bean & Cheese Burrito, 258 g	570	21	71
Cheese Quesadilla, 116 g	360	18	32
Chicken Bites, 5 pcs.	230	8	19
• Chicken Taquitos, 2 pcs.	210	9	18
World Famous Fish Taco, 115 g	300	16	26
Quesadillas, Etc.			
Cheese Quesadilla, 338 g	890	59	55
Chicken Quesadilla, 423 g	1000	61	57
• Chicken Taquitos (3), 186 g	380	21	35
Nachos Grande Chicken, 536 g	1450	83	117
• Nachos Grande Steak, 536 g	1450	84	116
Nachos Grande, 451 g	1330	81	115
Shrimp Quesadilla, 446 g	1000	63	56
Steak Quesadilla, 423 g	1000	62	56
Salads & Bowls			
Baja Caesar Salad, 439 g	520	40	15
Chipotle Ranch Salad Chicken, 489 g	530	35	27
Chopped Salad Chicken, 512 g	600	35	37
• Fiesta Salad Chicken, 431 g	500	35	14
• Grande Bowl Chicken, 520 g	780	43	56
Sides			
Black Beans, large, 347 g	400	3	68
Black Beans, small, 96 g	110	1	19
Brownie, 85 g	430	22	57
Chips, large, 113 g	580	29	74
Chips, small, 43 g	220	11	28
Churro, 45 g	170	8	22
• Guacamole & Chips, 265 g	790	49	85
Make It A Combo (small beans & chips), 139 g	350	13	53
Pinto Beans, large, 347 g	460	4	90
Pinto Beans, small, 96 g	130	2	25
Rice, large, 227 g	390	21	48
• Rice, small, 57 g	100	5	12
Street Tacos			
Carnitas, 69 g	110	4	9
Chicken, 69 g	110	3	9
Steak, 69 g	110	3	9
Tacos			
Carnitas Taco, 136 g	210	9	21
Chicken Taco, 151 g	280	15	22
• Especial Fish Taco, 170 g	350	22	28
Mahi Mahi Taco, 158 g	280	15	22
Shrimp Taco, 149 g	290	16	23
• Steak Taco, 136 g	210	8	21
World Famous Fish Taco, 142 g	290	16	27

Ruby Tuesday

	Cal	Fat	Cbs
Appetizers			
• Asian Dumplings, 1/4 portion	110	5	11
Chicken Quesadilla, 1/4 portion	228	14	12
• Classic Sampler, 1/4 portion	338	19	25
Fire Wings, 1/4 portion	219	16	2
Fresh Avocado Quesadilla, 1/4 portion	172	13	12
Fresh Guacamole Dip, 1/4 portion	288	18	24
Grand Sampler, 1/4 portion	324	19	17
Jumbo Lump Crab Cake, 1/4 portion	111	8	3
Queso Dip & Chips, 1/4 portion	308	19	25
Southwestern Spring Rolls, 1/4 portion	176	10	14
Spinach Artichoke Dip, 1/4 portion	332	20	27
Thai Phoon Shrimp, 1/4 portion	194	13	11
Wisconsin Cheddar Fries, 1/4 portion	302	17	25
Chicken			
Bistro Barbecue Chicken	618	29	13
• Chicken & Broccoli Pasta	1713	95	105

Ruby Tuesday (cont.)

	Cal	Fat	Cbs
Appetizers (cont.)			
Chicken Bella	626	36	11
• Chicken Fresco	464	23	6
Chicken Oscar	469	22	3
Gourmet Chicken Pot Pie	1411	111	37
Parmesan Chicken Pasta	1654	96	115
Desserts			
Blondie	677	31	91
• Chocolate Chip Cookie	320	15	40
Chocolate Tall cake	605	21	93
• Double Chocolate Cake	979	48	118
Gourmet Cookie & Ice Cream	800	37	103
Strawberry Cream Puff	840	40	100
White Chocolate Macadamia Nut Cookie	340	20	38
Fresh Combinations			
Broccoli & Cheese Soup	443	34	20
Chicken & Broccoli Quiche	735	58	23
• Gourmet Chicken Pot Pie	985	80	29
Ruby Minis, 2 pcs.	655	45	36
Turkey Minis, 2 pcs.	517	33	32
• White Bean Chicken Chili	223	7	18
Handcrafted Burgers			
Alpine Swiss Burger	1374	98	60
Avocado Chicken Burger	864	51	47
Avocado Turkey Burger	1034	63	49
Bacon Cheeseburger	1193	85	48
Bella Turkey Burger	1145	71	56
Bison Bacon Cheeseburger	1072	71	48
Bison Burger	892	57	48
Blue Cheese Burger	1280	93	48
Buffalo Chicken Burger	1041	71	62
Chicken BLT Burger	981	63	59
Classic Cheeseburger	1103	78	48
Hickory Chicken Burger	863	47	59
Ruby's Classic Burger	1013	71	48
• Smokehouse Burger	1392	96	71
• Turkey Burger	812	45	49
Veggie Burger	953	52	60
Kids' Meals			
• Chicken Breast & broccoli	276	12	5
Chicken Tenders & fries	714	31	74
Chop Steak & mashed potatoes	517	37	21
Fried Shrimp & fries	571	21	71
• Grilled Cheese & fries	929	50	88
Macaroni & Cheese	595	33	54
Mini Cheeseburgers & fries	907	49	82
Pasta with Marinara	314	4	53
Turkey Minis & fries	893	47	82
Premium Burgers			
• Jumbo Lump Crab Burger	755	45	57
Triple Prime Burger	883	56	50
• Triple Prime Cheddar Burger	1063	70	50
Ribs: Premium Baby Back Ribs			
Classic BBQ , Full Rack	986	65	29
• Classic BBQ , Half Rack	493	32	14
• Memphis Dry Rub , Full Rack	1070	79	7
Memphis Dry Rub , Half Rack	535	40	3
Ruby Minis			
Ruby Minis, 4 pcs.	1310	90	72
Salads			
Carolina Chicken Salad	1022	72	38
Club House Salad	896	60	30
Seafood			
Asian Glazed Salmon	424	27	7
• Creole Catch	312	16	0

RESTAURANTS & FAST-FOOD CHAINS

Ruby Tuesday (cont.)

	Cal	Fat	Cbs
Seafood (cont.)			
Lemon Grilled Salmon	458	32	1
Louisiana Fried Shrimp	423	17	38
New Orleans Seafood	495	31	2
• Parmesan Shrimp Pasta	1221	64	98
Side Items			
Baked Potato (w/ butter & sour cream)	459	19	51
• Baked Potato (w/ cheese & bacon)	614	32	52
Brown Rice Pilaf (w/ cheese & tomatoes)	221	6	33
Creamy Mashed Cauliflower	153	10	9
Fresh Hot Fries	359	13	52
Fresh Steamed Broccoli	129	8	5
• Premium Baby Green Beans	85	5	5
Sautéed Baby Portabella Mushrooms	173	14	7
Toast	160	9	16
Tomato & Mozzarella Salad	112	7	6
Tossed Caesar Salad	174	15	5
White Cheddar Mashed Potatoes	274	16	21
Steaks			
• Peppercorn Mushroom Sirloin, 9 oz.	604	36	14
• Petite Sirloin, 7 oz.	206	5	2
Premium Aged Prime Sirloin, 12 oz.	544	30	0
Rib Eye, 9 oz.	591	35	5
Top Sirloin, 9 oz	256	6	2

Runza

	Cal	Fat	Cbs
Chicken Sandwiches			
• BBQ Chicken - Crispy, 196 g	517	19	56
BBQ Chicken - Grilled, 192 g	392	9	46
Smothered Chicken - Crispy, 213 g	497	19	52
• Smothered Chicken - Grilled, 207 g	381	10	41
Special Deluxe Chicken - Crispy, 201 g	483	19	51
Special Deluxe Chicken - Grilled, 207 g	382	12	40
Desserts			
Blue Raspberry Runza® Slushie™ - medium, 519 g	302	0	76
Cake Cone w/ Choco Ice Cream, 146 g	250	7	38
Cake Cone w/ Swirl Ice Cream, 146 g	250	7	38
Cake Cone w/ Vanilla Ice Cream, 146 g	250	7	38
Cherry Runza® Slushie™ - medium, 519 g	302	0	76
Choco Ice Cream Dish - medium, 140 g	230	7	33
Chocolate Shake - regular, 341 g	511	16	80
Chocolate Sundae, 168 g	300	7	51
Cookie Dough Sundae, 176 g	360	11	57
Crushed Butterfinger® Topping - regular, 41 g	179	7	29
Crushed Oreo® Topping - regular, 29 g	140	6	20
Grape Runza® Slushie™ - medium, 519 g	313	0	78
• Kid-size Cake Cone w/ Vanilla Ice Cream, 59 g	110	3	16
Mini M&M's® Topping - regular, 61 g	301	14	42
• Oreo® Cappuccino Shake - regular, 343 g	606	24	85
Pepsi® Runza® Slushie™ - medium, 519 g	224	0	60
Reeses® Mini Topping - regular, 58 g	297	15	34
Snickers® Topping - regular, 38 g	181	9	22
Strawberry Shake - regular, 314 g	471	16	72
Strawberry Sundae, 210 g	340	7	60
Swirl Ice Cream Dish - medium, 140 g	230	7	33
Turtle Sundae, 170 g	330	12	48
Vanilla Ice Cream Dish - medium, 140 g	230	7	33
Vanilla Shake - regular, 327 g	465	16	69
Waffle Cone w/ Choco Ice Cream, 146 g	270	7	42
Waffle Cone w/ Swirl Ice Cream, 146 g	270	7	42
Waffle Cone w/ Vanilla Ice Cream, 146 g	270	7	42
Dressings & Sauces			
Asian Sesame Ginger, 68 g	300	26	14
BBQ Sauce, 73 g	113	1	28
• Caesar, 71 g	408	45	3
Dorothy Lynch, 70 g	264	14	29

Runza (cont.)

	Cal	Fat	Cbs
Dressings & Sauces (cont.)			
Honey Mustard, 49 g	238	22	10
Jalapeño Ranch, 65 g	276	28	2
Lite Italian, 70 g	84	5	10
Poppyseed, 74 g	390	36	18
Ranch, 67 g	299	32	5
• Raspberry Vinaigrette, 58 g	25	0	6
• Reduced Calorie Ranch, 70 g	168	11	17
Fries & Onion Rings			
• French Fries - large, 196 g	625	35	70
French Fries - medium, 129 g	412	23	46
French Fries - small, 87 g	278	15	31
Frings®, 180 g	538	28	64
• Onion Ring Dip, 59 g	89	6	4
Onion Rings - large, 184 g	591	32	66
Onion Rings- medium, 115 g	369	20	41
Kids Meals (includes small fry, no drink)			
Kids Runza® Sandwich, 195 g	527	24	64
• Mini Corn Dogs (5), 79 g	276	17	25
• Mini Corn Dogs (10), 166 g	554	32	56
Polish Dog, 138 g	424	26	30
Legendary Hamburgers			
• 1/2 lb. Double Chzburger (The Runza® Way), 295 g	639	32	37
1/4 lb. Bacon Cheeseburger, 193 g	514	29	36
• 1/4 lb. Chzburger (The Runza® Way), 207 g	429	21	32
1/4 lb. French Onion Burger, 236 g	550	34	28
1/4 lb. Legend Supreme, 203 g	767	37	62
1/4 lb. Swiss Chz Mushroom, 174 g	448	25	36
Other Sandwiches/Variety			
Chicken Strips, 167 g	464	25	42
• Chicken Strips, 2 pcs.	186	10	11
Fish Sandwich, 178 g	492	24	50
Junior Cheeseburger, 133 g	327	17	28
Junior Chzburger (The Runza® Way), 149 g	306	14	30
Junior Swiss Mushroom Burger, 149 g	381	21	26
• Small Hamburger (plain), 168 g	497	24	55
Other			
American Cheese, 19 g	58	4	1
• Bacon, 20 g	122	11	0
Mayo, 9 g	35	3	1
• Mushrooms, 38 g	7	0	1
Swiss Cheese, 19 g	70	5	0
The Runza® Way, 68 g	25	0	5
OvenStuff'd® Sandwiches			
Cheese, 234 g	555	21	66
• Original, 215 g	497	17	65
• Swiss Cheese Mushroom, 275 g	589	25	68
Salads (w/o Dressing)			
Chicken Caesar w/ Croutons, 350 g	300	13	14
Shanghai Chicken, 370 g	300	7	32
• Side Salad, 129 g	28	1	4
Southwest Chicken w/ Salsa, 317 g	440	23	35
• Sweet Berry Chicken, 422 g	630	31	50
Tossed Salad w/ Crispy Chicken, 360 g	437	27	29
Tossed Salad w/ Croutons, 302 g	290	15	25
Tossed Salad w/ Grilled Chicken, 336 g	276	13	13
Soups			
Boston Clam Chowder - Bowl, 276 g	321	23	33
Boston Clam Chowder - Cup, 180 g	209	15	22
Broccoli Cheese - Bowl, 310 g	361	27	35
Broccoli Cheese - Cup, 209 g	243	18	23
Cauliflower Cheese - Bowl, 287 g	334	26	32
Cauliflower Cheese - Cup, 162 g	189	15	18
Chicken Noodle - Bowl, 305 g	171	5	21
Chicken Noodle - Cup, 191 g	107	3	13

Runza (cont.)

Soups (cont.)

	Cal	Fat	Cbs
Homemade Chili - Bowl, 334 g	309	10	26
Homemade Chili - Cup, 218 g	202	6	17
Potato w/ Bacon - Bowl, 296 g	306	20	40
Potato w/ Bacon - Cup, 180 g	186	12	24
Vegetable Beef - Bowl, 270 g	105	3	13
• Vegetable Beef - Cup, 191 g	74	2	9
Vegetable Cheese - Bowl, 296 g	332	22	28
Vegetable Cheese - Cup, 209 g	234	15	20
• Wisconsin Cheese - Bowl, 299 g	425	35	36
Wisconsin Cheese - Cup, 194 g	276	23	23

Sammy's Woodfired Pizza

	Cal	Fat	Cbs
Chinese Chicken Salad	450	12	47
Chopped Chicken Salad	425	11	30
• Fresh Tomato Basil Soup	110	5	10
Oak Roasted Salmon on Ponzu Salad	470	19	21
Roast Chicken Pesto Wrap	480	20	22
• Tomato Angel Hair Pasta	700	18	115

Samurai Sam's Teriyaki Grill

	Cal	Fat	Cbs
Other Bowls - Regular			
• Low Carb Bowl, 326 g	230	4	16
Spicy Beef 'n Broccoli Bowl - Brown Rice, 475 g	580	14	85
Spicy Beef 'n Broccoli Bowl, 475 g	620	13	97
Sumo Bowl - Brown Rice, 808 g	1022	23	111
• Sumo Bowl - White Rice, 808 g	1083	21	128
Sides, Salads & Kids Meals			
Asian Noodle Soup, 208 g	89	2	14
Chinese Ginger Dressing, 28 g	85	5	9
Chinese Salad Dressing, 100 g	230	7	44
Crab Rangoon, 3 pcs.	210	12	20
Grilled Chicken Egg Roll, 85 g	150	7	17
Kid's Bowl, White Chicken - Brown Rice, 198 g	262	3	37
Kid's Bowl, White Chicken - White Rice, 198 g	282	2	43
Oriental Chicken Salad, 283 g	220	4	9
Oriental Dressing, 28 g	70	2	12
• Sesame Garden Toss Salad, 475 g	490	13	57
• Side Salad, 57 g	10	0	2
Teriyaki Sauce (on the side), 28 g	40	0	9
Sweet & Sour Bowls - Regular			
Dark Chicken - Brown Rice, 665 g	570	12	84
• Dark Chicken, 665 g	610	10	96
White Chicken - Brown Rice, 665 g	540	6	85
White Chicken, 665 g	580	5	96
Teriyaki Bowls - Regular			
Dark Chicken - Brown Rice, 411 g	500	11	68
Dark Chicken - Reg, 411 g	540	10	79
Dark Chicken & Shrimp - Brown Rice, 404 g	451	7	67
Dark Chicken & Shrimp, 404 g	492	6	78
Dark Chicken & Steak , 411 g	540	9	83
Dark Chkn & Steak - Brown Rice, 411 g	490	10	71
Salmon - Brown Rice, 588 g	582	5	104
Salmon, 588 g	643	3	121
Shrimp - Brown Rice, 411 g	407	3	65
Steak - Brown Rice, 411 g	490	9	74
Steak & Shrimp Bowl - Brown Rice, 404 g	442	6	66
Steak & Shrimp Bowl, 404 g	483	5	77
Steak , 411 g	530	8	86
• Teriyaki Bowl White Chicken - Lrg, 581 g	740	6	114
• Veggie - Brown Rice, 369 g	323	2	69
Veggie, 369 g	363	1	81
White Chicken - Brown Rice, 411 g	470	5	68
White Chicken - Reg, 411 g	520	4	79
White Chicken & Shrimp - Brown, 404 g	437	4	67
White Chicken & Shrimp, 404 g	478	3	78

Samurai Sam's Teriyaki Grill (cont.)

	Cal	Fat	Cbs
Teriyaki Bowls - Regular (cont.)			
White Chicken & Steak, 411 g	520	6	83
White Chkn & Steak - Brown Rice, 411 g	480	7	71
Wraps			
Dark Chicken - Brown Rice, 391 g	650	17	90
Dark Chicken & Steak - Brown Rice, 391 g	630	14	93
Dark Chicken & Steak, 391 g	650	13	98
• Dark Chicken, 391 g	670	16	95
Steak - Brown Rice, 391 g	630	15	95
Steak, 391 g	650	14	101
• Veggie - Brown Rice, 320 g	490	9	89
Veggie, 320 g	510	8	94
White Chicken - Brown Rice, 391 g	620	12	90
White Chicken & Steak - Brn Rice, 391 g	628	13	89
White Chicken & Steak, 391 g	649	13	95
White Chicken, 391 g	640	11	96
Yakisoba Bowls			
Dark Chicken & Steak, 570 g	825	22	113
• Dark Chicken, 570 g	842	24	114
Steak, 570 g	809	20	112
• Veggie, 400 g	509	8	110
White Chicken & Steak, 570 g	801	17	113
White Chicken, 570 g	794	14	114
Yakisoba Bowl - Shrimp, 570 g	677	10	110

Schlotzsky's

	Cal	Fat	Cbs
Buns / Tortilla			
Dark Rye, Medium	330	2	68
• Dark Rye, Small	230	1	47
Flour Tortilla	300	9	47
• Jalapeño Cheese, Medium	340	4	63
Jalapeño Cheese, Small	230	3	44
Sourdough, Medium	330	2	67
Sourdough, Small	230	2	46
Wheat, Medium	340	3	67
Wheat, Small	230	2	46
Chips			
Barbecue, 2 oz. bag	220	12	25
Cracked Pepper, 2 oz. bag	220	12	25
Jalapeño, 2 oz. bag	220	12	25
Regular (Plain), 2 oz. bag	220	12	25
Salt & Vinegar, 2 oz. bag	220	12	25
Sour Cream & Onion, 2 oz. bag	220	12	25
Desserts			
Brownie	415	24	47
• Carrot Cake	717	42	80
Cheesecake	350	23	30
Cookie, Chocolate Chip	162	7	24
Cookie, Fudge Chocolate Chip	164	8	22
• Cookie, Oatmeal Raisin	148	5	24
Cookie, Sugar	154	7	22
Cookie, White Chocolate Macadamia	170	8	22
Drinks			
Lemonade Medium, 20 oz.	243	0	45
Raspberry Lemonade Medium, 20 oz.	243	0	45
Gourmet Pizzas			
• Baby Spinach Salad	471	8	83
Bacon Tomato & Portobello	614	22	76
BBQ Chicken & Jalapeño	684	16	98
Combination Special	639	25	76
Double Cheese	597	21	74
Fresh Tomato & Pesto	556	19	73
Grilled Chicken & Pesto	652	22	74
Mediterranean	560	20	74
Pepperoni & Double Cheese	686	30	74
Smoked Turkey & Jalapeño	642	19	78

RESTAURANTS & FAST-FOOD CHAINS

Schlotzsky's (cont.)	Cal	Fat	Cbs
Gourmet Pizzas (cont.)			
• Thai Chicken	693	22	85
Vegetarian Special	540	17	74
Kid's Meals			
Cheese Pizza	479	13	73
Cheese Sandwich	397	15	48
Ham & Cheese Sandwich	427	16	49
• Pepperoni Pizza	523	17	73
• Turkey Sandwich	298	5	49
Oven-Toasted Sandwiches			
• Albuquerque Turkey, Medium	964	40	80
Albuquerque Turkey, Small	687	36	56
Angus Beef & Provolone, Medium	757	29	80
Angus Beef & Provolone, Small	503	19	56
Angus Corned Beef Reuben, Medium	918	41	78
• Angus Corned Beef Reuben, Small	331	28	54
Angus Corned Beef, Medium	582	13	77
Angus Corned Beef, Small	395	9	53
Angus Pastrami & Swiss, Medium	905	36	82
Angus Pastrami & Swiss, Small	611	24	56
Angus Pastrami Reuben, Medium	918	40	78
Angus Pastrami Reuben, Small	629	27	54
Angus Roast Beef & Cheese, Medium	783	33	73
Angus Roast Beef & Cheese, Small	538	22	50
BLT, Medium	543	18	74
BLT, Small	364	12	50
Cheese The Original®-Style, Medium	790	38	74
Cheese The Original®-Style, Small	566	28	51
Chicken & Pesto, Medium	564	14	72
Chicken & Pesto, Small	387	9	50
Chicken Breast, Medium	509	6	77
Chicken Breast, Small	345	4	52
Chipotle Chicken, Medium	540	12	72
Chipotle Chicken, Small	379	10	47
Chipotle Grilled Chicken, Medium	578	13	76
Chipotle Grilled Chicken, Small	405	10	50
Deluxe The Original®-Style, Medium	954	46	78
Deluxe The Original®-Style, Small	742	38	55
Dijon Chicken, Medium	576	11	79
Dijon Chicken, Small	391	7	54
Dijon Grilled Chicken, Medium	614	12	83
Dijon Grilled Chicken, Small	417	8	57
Fresh Veggie, Medium	483	12	77
Fresh Veggie, Small	355	10	52
Grilled Chicken & Pesto, Medium	603	15	76
Grilled Chicken & Pesto, Small	413	10	52
Grilled Chicken Breast, Medium	545	7	80
Grilled Chicken Breast, Small	372	5	55
Ham & Cheese The Original®-Style, Med.	731	27	76
Ham & Cheese The Original®-Style, Small	512	19	54
Homestyle Tuna, Medium	596	20	73
Homestyle Tuna, Small	410	14	51
Mediterranean Tuna, Medium	536	11	76
Mediterranean Tuna, Small	363	8	52
Santa Fe Chicken, Medium	619	15	76
Santa Fe Chicken, Small	425	10	53
Santa Fe Grilled Chicken, Medium	657	16	80
Santa Fe Grilled Chicken, Small	452	11	55
Smoked Turkey Breast, Medium	500	7	76
Smoked Turkey Breast, Small	345	5	53
Smoked Turkey Reuben, Medium	889	37	83
Smoked Turkey Reuben, Small	609	25	58
Texas Schlotzsky's™, Medium	756	31	73
Texas Schlotzsky's™, Small	540	23	51
The Original®, Medium	770	34	76

Schlotzsky's (cont.)	Cal	Fat	Cbs
Oven-Toasted Sandwiches (cont.)			
The Original®, Small	563	27	52
Turkey & Guacamole, Medium	552	12	80
Turkey & Guacamole, Small	364	7	54
Turkey Bacon Club, Medium	770	29	76
Turkey Bacon Club, Small	562	23	53
Turkey The Original®-Style, Medium	815	33	78
Turkey The Original®-Style, Small	596	26	54
Panini			
Classic Swiss & Tomato	624	26	63
Grilled Chicken Romano	539	15	61
• Mozzarella & Portobello	485	15	63
• Panini Italiano	736	32	67
Smoked Ham Crostini	644	23	67
Smoked Turkey & Guacamole	579	21	67
Salads			
Baby Spinach & Feta	197	15	10
Caesar	103	5	10
Chicken Salad	292	15	12
Fruit	100	0	25
Garden	51	1	12
Greek	137	8	13
Grilled Chicken Caesar	221	8	12
Ham & Turkey Chef	249	13	14
Pasta Salad	68	3	12
Potato Salad	242	13	29
• Side Salad	26	1	7
• Turkey Chef	293	15	15
Soups			
Boston Clam Chowder, 1 bowl	323	17	34
Boston Clam Chowder, 1 cup	217	11	23
Broccoli Cheese Soup, 1 bowl	303	20	20
Broccoli Cheese Soup, 1 cup	187	12	13
Chicken Tortilla Soup, 1 bowl	225	9	20
Chicken Tortilla Soup, 1 cup	150	6	13
Hearty Vegetable Beef Soup, 1 bowl	165	8	18
Hearty Vegetable Beef Soup, 1 cup	109	5	12
Old Fshnd Chicken Noodle Soup, 1 bowl	135	2	17
Old Fshnd Chicken Noodle Soup, 1 cup	90	2	11
Potato w/ Bacon, 1 bowl	271	13	38
Potato w/ Bacon, 1 cup	182	9	26
Timberline Chili, 1 bowl	345	12	39
Timberline Chili, 1 cup	227	8	26
Vegetarian Vegetable Soup, 1 bowl	122	1	27
• Vegetarian Vegetable Soup, 1 cup	85	1	19
• Wisconsin Cheese Soup, 1 bowl	460	33	36
Wisconsin Cheese Soup, 1 cup	306	22	24
Wraps			
Asian Chicken	505	11	79
Parmesan Chicken Caesar	630	33	56
Wraps ~ Following Selections Vary by Restaurant			
Feta & Portobello	618	39	55
• Grilled Chicken & Guacamole	667	36	58
Homestyle Tuna	480	20	55
• Mediterranean Tuna	440	14	57

Sheetz	Cal	Fat	Cbs
Bakery Cookies			
Chocolate Chunk Cookie, 1 cookie	209	11	27
Chocolate No-Bake, 1 cookie	180	8	24
Oatmeal Raisin Cookie, 1 cookie	194	7	29
• Peanut Butter Cookie, 1 cookie	229	14	22
Peanut Butter No-Bake, 1 cookie	180	8	24
• Pink Iced Cookie, 1 cookie	180	7	29
Raisin Filled Cookie, 1 cookie	220	8	35

Sheetz (cont.)

	Cal	Fat	Cbs
Coffeez®			
Breakfast Blend, 16 g	10	0	2
Colombian, 16 g	10	0	2
House Blend, 16 g	10	0	2
Pumpkin Spice, 16 g	10	0	2
Serious Dark Roast, 16 g	10	0	2
Vanilla Nut Cream, 16 g	10	0	2
Winter Wonderland, 16 g	10	0	2
Coffeez® Creamer			
Amaretto Creamer, 1 g	40	2	7
Cinnamon Hazelnut Creamer, 1 g	40	2	7
• French Vanilla Creamer, 1 g	45	2	6
• Half & Half Creamer, 1 g	15	1	0
Mocha Creamer, 1 g	40	2	6
Cupo'ccino® / Hot Chocolate			
Almond Amaretto Cupo'ccino, 16 g	276	8	52
Blueberry Crumb Cupo'ccino, 16 g	280	8	52
Creme Burlee Cupo'ccino, 16 g	280	8	50
• Fat Free French Vanilla Cupo'ccino, 16 g	140	0	34
• French Vanilla Cupo'ccino, 16 g	284	10	50
Harvest Spice Cupo'ccino, 16 g	278	10	48
Hot Chocolate, 16 g	248	4	52
Mocha Canela, 16 g	240	4	52
PB Marshmallow Parfait, 16 g	260	7	52
Sugar Free Caramel Pecan, 16 g	224	7	40
Vanilla Chai Cupo'ccino, 16 g	277	8	51
Other Goodies			
Apple Turnover, 1 piece	340	6	33
Blueberry Muffin, 1 piece	377	2	53
Blueberry Pie, 1 piece	440	11	57
Carrot Muffin, 1 piece	415	3	58
Cherry Pie, 1 piece	460	11	61
Cherry Turnover, 1 piece	341	6	34
Chocolate Chunk Brownie, 1 piece	350	10	41
• Cinnamon Coffee Cake, 1 piece	550	6	68
Cinnamon Roll, 1 piece	240	3	32
• Double Dutch Brownie, 1 piece	180	2	28
Eclair Pie, 1 piece	550	16	63
Espresso Brownie, 1 piece	430	16	48
Glazed Honey Bun, 1 piece	246	2	35
Golden Honey Bun, 1 piece	334	3	41
Honey Pecan Bar, 1 piece	420	12	31
Peach Pie, 1 piece	430	11	54
Peanut Butter Gobbz, 1 piece	550	7	58
Rasp White Chocolate Scone, 1 piece	411	6	54
Sweet Dough Swirls, 1 piece	310	3	48

Shoney's

	Cal	Fat	Cbs
Blue Plate Specials			
Baked Whitefish	507	8	58
Bread Service - 2 sl. w/ Oleo	263	7	43
Cajun Whitefish	480	10	56
Corn	173	9	23
Cranberry Sauce, 2 oz.	64	0	17
Grandma's Meatloaf - w/ Glaze	1092	47	93
Grandma's Meatloaf - w/ Gravy	1089	49	87
Green Beans	124	6	14
Grilled Liver 'n' Onions	711	22	79
Ham Steak Dinner	667	26	60
Macaroni & Cheese	241	14	18
• Mashed Potatoes w/ Gravy	223	10	30
• Original Country Fried Steak	1151	62	103
Roast Beef Platter	880	30	96
Breakfast			
Apple Cinnamon Jelly, 1 packet	35	0	9
Bacon, 3 strips	120	11	0

Shoney's (cont.)

	Cal	Fat	Cbs
Breakfast (cont.)			
• Biscuits & Gravy	683	32	88
Biscuits, each	309	14	41
Creamer, Half & Half, 15 g	20	2	1
Grape Jelly, 1 packet	35	0	9
• Grits, 4 oz.	105	6	11
Hashbrowns, 4 oz.	238	15	25
Margarine, 1 packet	36	4	0
Sausage Patties, 1 pc.	209	18	1
Sourdough Toast w/ oleo, 2 slices	206	5	50
Strawberry Jam, 1 packet	35	0	9
Wheat Toast w/ oleo, 2 slices	188	9	24
White Toast w/ oleo, 2 slices	202	9	26
Breakfast Bar			
Bacon, 3 strips	120	11	0
Biscuits, each	309	14	41
Breakfast Bar Gravy, 2 oz.	54	4	5
Breakfast Potato Casserole, 4 oz.	43	4	1
Cake, Apple Spice, 1 piece	120	13	13
Cake, Banana Bash, 1 piece	130	9	13
Cake, Brunch Berry, 1 piece	120	13	41
Cake, Buttercreme, 1 piece	130	8	15
Cake, Double Chocolate, 1 piece	130	8	15
Cake, Luscious Lemon, 1 piece	130	7	15
Cake, Orange Cranberry, 1 piece	120	0	19
Cake, Shortcake, 1 piece	50	0	11
Cheese Sauce, 1 tbsp.	59	3	7
Cheese, Cheddar, Fancy, 1 tbsp.	27	2	1
Chicken Wings, Mild, 1 piece	64	3	3
• Cottage Cheese, 1 tbsp.	15	0	1
Donuts, Powdered, 1 piece	175	9	23
Eggs, Breakfast Bar, 1/2 cup	120	7	3
• French Toast Sticks, 4 pieces	380	16	53
Grits, 4 oz.	105	6	11
Ham, Diced, 1 tbsp.	16	1	0
Hashbrowns, 4 oz.	238	15	25
Honey, 1 packet	45	0	11
Jelly, Apple/Cinnamon, 1 packet	35	0	9
Jelly, Grape, 1 packet	35	0	9
Jelly, Strawberry Jam, 1 packet	35	0	9
Margarine, Parkay, 1 tbsp.	101	11	0
Milk, White, 1/2 cup	74	4	6
Oleo, Country Crock Individuals	36	4	0
Omelet Topping, 1 oz.	22	1	2
Pancakes, each	318	7	56
Peppers, Jalapeño, Sliced, 1 tbsp.	2	0	0
Sauce, Hot Louisiana, 1 tsp	0	0	0
Sauce, Salsa, 1 tbsp	5	0	1
Sausage Patty, 1 piece	209	18	1
Smoked Sausage, 1 piece	180	16	3
Strawberry Banana Topping, 4 oz.	84	0	20
Syrup, Pancake & Waffle, 2 tbsp	80	0	21
Topping, Apple Crisp, 1/4 cup	87	0	22
Topping, Apple, 1/4 cup	96	0	24
Topping, Peach, 1/4 cup	54	0	13
Topping, Strawberry, 1/4 cup	158	0	41
Tortillas, Flour, 1 piece	133	3	21
Whipped Topping, 1 scoop	9	1	1
Breakfast Menu Selections			
• All Star Breakfast (Add Options)	190	15	1
Big Eater Steak Breakfast (Add Options)	629	41	1
C/F Steak Breakfast	994	66	49
• Deluxe Pancake Platter	1609	32	299
Half Stack Pancake Platter	932	14	187
Sausage/Biscuit, 1 pc.	539	34	42

Shoney's (cont.)

Breakfast Menu Selections (cont.)	Cal	Fat	Cbs
Sunrise Breakfast	973	60	88
Burgers			
A-A Bacon Cheeseburger	891	49	44
• All-American Burger	688	32	44
Famous Patty Melt	946	60	40
• Half-O-Pound Burger	1351	53	130
Mushroom Swiss Burger	969	58	49
Chicken			
Charbroiled Blackened Chicken	831	26	100
• Charbroiled Chicken Breast	797	23	99
• Chicken Stir-Fry	1200	35	172
Fried Chicken Tenderloins	1157	61	121
Monterey Chicken	909	40	84
Smothered Chicken	891	34	90
Condiments/Add-Ons/Sides			
American Cheese, 1 slice	107	9	1
Bacon, 1 slice	40	4	0
BBQ Sauce, per 2 oz.	71	1	11
Catsup, 1 oz.	30	0	8
French Fries, 4 oz.	213	11	25
Grilled Onions, 2 oz.	67	6	4
Mayonnaise, 1 oz.	203	23	1
Monterey Jack Cheese, 1 slice	159	13	0
• Mustard, 1 oz.	21	1	2
• Onion Rings, 7 rings	500	15	83
Sauteed Mushrooms, 3 oz.	107	10	5
Secret Sauce, 1 2 oz.	168	16	4
Secret Sauce, per 2 oz.	168	16	4
Sweet & Sour Sauce, per, 2 oz.	67	0	17
Swiss Cheese, 1 slice	160	12	1
Desserts			
Apple Nutrasweet Pie	454	18	64
• Apple Pie a la Mode	1203	53	174
Caramel Sundae	621	27	83
Cheesecake, 1 slice	364	26	23
Cherry Nutrasweet Pie	467	18	66
Chocolate Milk Shake	1082	51	141
Hot Fudge Sundae	599	30	75
• Original Strawberry Pie	332	17	45
Peach Nutrasweet Pie	479	21	68
Strawberry Milk Shake	1115	50	151
Strawberry Sundae	609	27	85
Ultimate Hot Fudge Cake	875	37	126
Vanilla Milk Shake	1076	50	140
Walnut Brownie a la Mode	576	34	61

Silver Mine Subs

8" Cold Sub Sandwiches (on white bread)	Cal	Fat	Cbs
California Gulch, 363 g	736	36	66
Caribou - medium, 350 g	704	34	59
Comstock, 352 g	657	28	55
• Dodge City, 362 g	1011	69	57
Georgetown, 331 g	660	29	59
King Bullion, 352 g	636	26	55
Lawless Leadville, 352 g	629	26	56
Mother Lode, 500 g	999	56	58
Silver City, 380 g	870	53	58
• Tombstone, 362 g	617	24	55
Virginia City, 352 g	645	28	58
8" Hot Sub Sandwiches (on white bread)			
• Boomtown, 295 g	809	46	55
• Coeur D'Alene, 280 g	490	10	52
Cripple Creek, 337 g	708	31	58
Frontier, 321 g	679	23	67
Homestake, 344 g	547	15	61

Silver Mine Subs (cont.)

8" Hot Sub Sandwiches (on white bread) (cont.)	Cal	Fat	Cbs
Silver Plume, 358 g	710	30	58
Steam Engine, 387 g	804	43	61
8" Lowfat Sub Sandwiches (on white bread)			
Caribou, 276 g	380	4	58
Comstock, 308 g	440	7	54
Homestake, 314 g	440	7	60
King Bullion, 308 g	419	5	54
Lawless Leadville, 308 g	412	5	56
• Pikes Peak Or Bust, 216 g	327	4	58
• Silver Plume, 314 g	493	9	58
Tombstone, 318 g	400	3	55
Virginia City, 308 g	428	7	57
Bread and Tortilla Wraps			
• Wheat - 11", 149 g	373	5	69
• Wheat - 5", 75 g	187	3	35
Wheat- 8" 112 g	280	4	52
White - 11", 149 g	373	3	69
White bead - 5", 75 g	186	1	35
White bread - 8", 112 g	280	2	52
White Flour Tortilla Wrap - 10", 71 g	210	5	36
Cheeses (For 8" subs)			
Cheddar Cheese, 30 g	118	10	1
Provolone Cheese, 30 g	107	9	1
Desserts			
Chocolate Chunk Cookie, 85 g	387	15	59
Deluxe Fudge Brownie, 85 g	409	21	54
Kid's Subs (on white bread) & Kids Related Items			
Fruit Snacks, 25 g	80	0	19
Goldfish Crackers, 21 g	100	4	14
• Ham & Cheddar Cheese, 50 g	113	8	1
Ham & Provolone Cheese, 45 g	88	6	1
Turkey & Cheddar Cheese, 50 g	105	7	1
• Turkey & Provolone Cheese, 45 g	80	5	1
Meats (For 8" subs)			
Bacon - 3 strips, 21 g	101	8	0
Bacon - 9 strips (boomtown), 63 g	302	23	0
Grilled Chicken - Grilled Chkn Salad, 84 g	135	5	2
Grilled Chicken - Silver Plume, 126 g	203	7	3
Ham, 120 g	138	5	3
Meatballs, 140 g	383	32	2
Pepperoni, 84 g	420	39	0
Philly Cheesesteak, 126 g	150	5	6
Roast Beef - cold, 120 g	150	5	0
Roast Beef - hot, 168 g	210	8	0
• Salami, 120 g	493	45	0
Tuna Salad, 134 g	336	26	11
• Turkey, 120 g	107	1	0
Salads & Salad Related Items			
Blue Cheese Dressing - 1 packet, 43 g	180	19	2
Chef Salad, 208 g	82	2	6
Croutons - 1 package, 14 g	35	0	4
Fat Free Ranch Dressing - 1 packet, 43 g	60	0	14
Garden Salad, 148 g	21	0	5
Golden Italian Dressing - 1 packet, 43 g	110	10	3
Grilled Chicken Salad, 232 g	156	5	7
Honey Mustard, 42 g	182	15	10
• Ranch Dressing - 1 packet, 43 g	250	26	2
Romaine Lettuce Mix - Side Salad, 56 g	6	0	1
Romaine Lettuce Mix , 98 g	10	0	2
Side Salad, 81 g	11	0	3
Sandwich Dressings			
Avocado, 18 g	34	2	3
Dijon Mustard, 15 g	15	0	1
Honey Mustard, 15 g	65	6	4

Silver Mine Subs (cont.)

	Cal	Fat	Cbs
Sandwich Dressings (cont.)			
• Mayonnaise, 14 g	110	12	0
Oil, 5 g	40	5	0
Oregano, 0 g	0	0	0
Ranch Dressing, 14 g	75	8	1
• Vinegar, 5 g	0	0	0
Yellow Mustard, 15 g	0	0	0
Sides			
Fruit Cup, 113 g	80	0	19
• Potato Salad, 156 g	270	15	33
• Whole Dill Pickle, 168 g	5	0	0
Soup & Chili & Related Items			
Broccoli Cheese, 8 oz. cup	160	8	17
• Chili, 8 oz. cup	280	13	26
Oyster crackers, 1 package	60	2	10
Side of Wheat Bread, 75 g	187	3	35
Side of White Bread, 75 g	186	1	35
Veggie Sub Sandwiches (on white bread)			
• Pikes Peak Or Bust - large (11"), 398 g	906	47	78
Pikes Peak Or Bust - medium (8"), 290 g	651	33	59
• Pikes Peak Or Bust - small (5"), 188 g	396	19	39
Veggies (For 8" subs)			
• Black Olives, 44 g	69	7	3
Cucumbers, 28 g	4	0	1
Green Peppers, 22 g	5	0	1
Hot Banana Peppers, 18 g	3	0	1
Jalapeños, 20 g	3	0	1
Lettuce, 42 g	4	0	1
Mushrooms, 22 g	5	0	1
Onions, 18 g	8	0	2
• Pickle Slices, 44 g	0	0	0
Sprouts, 10 g	3	0	0
Tomato, 34 g	6	0	1

Skyline Chili

	Cal	Fat	Cbs
Bowls			
• Chili Bean Bowl	270	12	17
Chili Bowl	270	16	6
Chili Cheese Bowl	440	30	6
• Coney Bowl	870	69	9
Loaded Chili Bowl	580	40	18
Vegetarian Black Beans and Rice Bowl	320	9	46
Burritos			
All Chili Burrito	560	30	37
All Chili Burrito Deluxe	650	35	45
Black Bean Burrito	600	25	67
• Black Bean Burrito Deluxe	690	30	75
Chili Bean Mix Burrito	610	30	54
Chili Bean Mix Burrito Deluxe	700	36	62
• Chili Cheese Melt	350	16	33
Chili Spaghetti Dishes (Regular Size)			
3-Way	760	44	43
4-Way Bean	850	45	59
4-Way Onion	770	44	46
5-Way	840	45	58
Black Bean & Rice 3-Way	800	40	74
Black Bean & Rice 4-Way	810	40	77
• Black Bean & Rice 5-Way	880	40	89
Black Bean & Rice Spaghetti	490	12	79
• Chili Spaghetti	450	18	43
Chili Spaghetti Bean	520	17	61
Chili Spaghetti Bean & Onion	530	17	64
• Chili Spaghetti Onion	470	17	51
Coneys			
• Cheese Coney	340	22	17
Chili Cheese Sandwich	290	17	17

Skyline Chili (cont.)

	Cal	Fat	Cbs
Coneys (cont.)			
• Regular Chili Sandwich (w/o cheese)	180	7	17
Regular Coney (w/o cheese)	220	12	17
Dressings			
Buttermilk Ranch Dressing	230	24	2
Chili Ranch Dressing	275	29	0
Dijon Honey Mustard Dressing	180	17	8
• Greek Salad Dressing	250	28	1
Honey French Dressing	210	18	14
• Light Italian Dressing	20	1	2
Light Ranch Dressing	70	4	8
Fresh Selects Salads (No Dressing)			
Buffalo Chicken Salad	150	7	7
Classic Chicken Salad	150	7	8
Garden Salad	80	5	6
Greek Chicken Salad	170	8	9
• Greek Salad	60	4	5
• SW Chicken Salad w/ Tortilla Chips	760	44	66
SW Chicken Salad w/o Tortilla Chips	460	16	18
Fresh Selects Wraps (No Dressing)			
Buffalo Chicken Wrap	520	21	55
Classic Chicken Wrap	510	21	55
• Greek Chicken Wrap	510	21	54
• Southwest Chicken Wrap	670	30	65
Fries			
French Fries	630	33	79
Kids Meals			
• 3-Way Special	380	22	22
Coney Special w/ Chz	330	22	16
Coney Special w/o Chz	210	12	15
Double Wiener Hot Doggy w/ Chz	360	26	16
Double Wiener Hot Doggy w/o Chz	250	17	15
P'sghetti Special	280	16	19
Single Wiener Hot Doggy w/ Chz	270	18	15
• Single Wiener Hot Doggy w/o Chz	160	9	14
Sides			
Bowl of Crackers	100	3	20
• Cheddar Bread Full	520	39	32
Cheddar Bread Half	260	20	16
Garlic Bread Full	410	30	31
Garlic Bread Half	200	15	16
Side of Cheese	230	19	1
Side of Chili	130	8	3
Steamed Potatoes			
3-Way Potato	870	49	75
4-Way Potato	890	49	78
• 5-Way Potato	950	50	90
Cheddar Potato	740	41	72
Chili Potato	440	8	74
• Plain Potato	310	0	72
Sour Cream Potato	570	27	72

Smoothie King

	Cal	Fat	Cbs
Smoothies: Classic			
Açaí Adventure®, 20 oz.	437	5	93
Angel Food™, 20 oz.	370	0	89
Blackberry Dream™, 20 oz.	371	1	91
Blueberry Heaven®, 20 oz.	325	1	73
Celestial Cherry High™, 20 oz.	344	0	85
Coffee Smoothie Amaretto, 20 oz.	164	0	31
Coffee Smoothie French Roast, 20 oz.	187	0	39
• Coffee Smoothie French Vanilla, 20 oz.	164	0	31
Coffee Smoothie Hazelnut, 20 oz.	164	0	31
Coffee Smoothie Irish Creme, 20 oz.	164	0	31
Coffee Smoothie Mocha, 20 oz.	219	3	38
Cranberry Cooler™, 20 oz.	503	0	124

Smoothie King (cont.)

Smoothies: Classic (cont.)	Cal	Fat	Cbs
Cranberry Supreme®, 20 oz.	560	1	134
Gladiator®, 20 oz.	300	0	31
Go Goji™, 20 oz.	347	0	82
Green Tea Tango®, 20 oz.	368	4	72
Hearty Apple®, 20 oz.	405	1	86
High Protein Almond Mocha, 20 oz.	382	9	48
High Protein Banana, 20 oz.	322	9	32
High Protein Chocolate, 20 oz.	382	9	48
High Protein Lemon, 20 oz.	372	9	44
High Protein Pineapple, 20 oz.	315	9	29
Immune Builder®, 20 oz.	384	1	92
Instant Vigor™, 20 oz.	368	0	88
Island Impact®, 20 oz.	312	0	73
Island Treat®, 20 oz.	337	0	84
Kiwi Island Treat®, 20 oz.	504	1	119
Low-Carb Banana, 20 oz.	268	9	7
Low-Carb Chocolate, 20 oz.	268	9	7
Low-Carb Strawberry, 20 oz.	268	9	7
Low-Carb Vanilla, 20 oz.	268	9	7
MangoFest™, 20 oz.	285	0	72
Mangosteen Madness™, 20 oz.	343	0	84
Muscle Punch Plus™, 20 oz.	379	1	90
Muscle Punch®, 20 oz.	380	1	90
Orange Ka-BAM®, 20 oz.	469	0	120
Passion Passport®, 20 oz.	399	0	99
Peach Slice™, 20 oz.	333	0	78
Pep Upper®, 20 oz.	413	0	98
Pineapple Pleasure®, 20 oz.	284	0	69
Pomegranate Punch™, 20 oz.	425	0	100
Power Punch Plus®, 20 oz.	518	1	119
Power Punch®, 20 oz.	446	1	107
Raspberry Collider™, 20 oz.	344	0	88
Raspberry Sunrise™, 20 oz.	399	0	99
Slim-N-Trim Chocolate™, 20 oz.	224	1	49
Slim-N-Trim Orange-Vanilla™, 20 oz.	215	1	46
Slim-N-Trim Strawberry™, 20 oz.	379	1	87
Slim-N-Trim Vanilla™, 20 oz.	256	1	56
Strawberry Kiwi Breeze®, 20 oz.	376	0	90
Super Punch Plus®, 20 oz.	461	0	117
Super Punch™, 20 oz.	395	0	100
The Activator Chocolate®, 20 oz.	422	1	89
The Activator Strawberry®, 20 oz.	575	1	127
The Activator Vanilla®, 20 oz.	425	1	89
The Hulk Chocolate™, 20 oz.	919	35	128
• The Hulk Strawberry™, 20 oz.	1065	35	163
The Hulk Vanilla™, 20 oz.	915	35	125
The Shredder - Chocolate™, 20 oz.	311	3	36
The Shredder - Strawberry™, 20 oz.	356	1	57
The Shredder - Vanilla™, 20 oz.	283	2	30
Youth Fountain™, 20 oz.	252	0	64
Smoothies: Power Meal™			
Banana Berry Treat®, 20 oz.	372	0	90
Banana Boat®, 20 oz.	554	14	98
Berry Punch™, 20 oz.	367	0	93
Caribbean Way®, 20 oz.	399	0	100
Cherry Picker®, 20 oz.	441	0	105
Coconut Surprise®, 20 oz.	493	7	100
Fruit Fusion™, 20 oz.	360	0	84
Grape Expectations II™, 20 oz.	551	0	136
Grape Expectations®, 20 oz.	401	0	98
Kids' Kups Berry Interesting™, 20 oz.	277	0	69
• Kids' Kups Choc-A-Laka™, 20 oz.	191	3	30
Kids' Kups CW, Jr.™, 20 oz.	270	0	68
Kids' Kups Gimme-Grape™, 20 oz.	265	0	64

Smoothie King (cont.)

Smoothies: Power Meal™ (cont.)	Cal	Fat	Cbs
Kids' Kups Lil' Angel™, 20 oz.	223	0	56
Kids' Kups Smarti Tarti™, 20 oz.	200	0	49
Lemon Twist Banana®, 20 oz.	361	0	90
Lemon Twist Strawberry®, 20 oz.	442	0	110
Light & Fluffy®, 20 oz.	399	0	102
Malts, 20 oz.	771	39	87
Mo'cuccino™, 20 oz.	477	14	78
Peach Slice Plus®, 20 oz.	483	0	116
• Peanut Power Plus Grape™, 20 oz.	782	25	130
Peanut Power Plus Strawberry™, 20 oz.	732	25	120
Peanut Power®, 20 oz.	582	25	82
Piña Colada Island®, 20 oz.	632	10	120
Pineapple Surf®, 20 oz.	465	1	107
Shakes, 20 oz.	761	39	85
Strawberry X-Treme®, 20 oz.	369	0	93
Yogurt D-Lite®, 20 oz.	432	4	81

Sonic Drive-In

Add Ins (Medium)	Cal	Fat	Cbs
Blue Coconut, 18 g	35	0	9
Cherry, 23 g	50	0	14
• Chocolate Topping Add-In , 38 g	100	0	23
Diet Cherry, 19 g	10	0	2
Fresh Lemon Add-In, 18 g	5	0	2
• Fresh Lime Add-In, 14 g	5	0	1
Grape, 19 g	40	0	9
Orange, 18 g	40	0	10
Pineapple Topping, 35 g	60	0	14
Strawberry Topping, 35 g	70	0	17
Vanilla, 19 g	40	0	11
Watermelon, 19 g	45	0	12
Add Ons			
• Bacon, 13 g	70	5	0
Cheese, 18 g	60	5	2
• Chili, 33 g	50	4	2
Burgers			
Bacon Cheeseburger, 273 g	770	47	55
Burger w/ Ketchup, 235 g	540	25	54
Burger w/ Mayo, 242 g	630	37	53
Burger w/ Mustard, 235 g	540	25	52
Cheeseburger w/ Ketchup, 260 g	610	31	57
Cheeseburger w/ Mayo, 260 g	700	42	55
Cheeseburger w/ Mustard, 253 g	600	31	54
• Jr. Burger, 117 g	320	16	29
Jr. Cheeseburger, 135 g	380	21	30
SuperSONIC® Chzbrgr w/ Ketchup, 337 g	880	52	59
SuperSONIC® Chzbrgr w/ Mustard, 330 g	870	52	55
• SuperSONIC® Chzburger w/ Mayo, 337 g	970	63	56
Chicken			
• BBQ Sauce, 28 g	45	0	11
Breaded Chicken Sandwich, 255 g	670	33	66
• Chicken Strip Dinner, 4 pcs.	920	43	97
Grilled Chicken Sandwich, 204 g	340	12	32
Honey Mustard Sauce, 28 g	90	7	7
Jumbo Popcorn Chicken™ (Snack), 113 g	370	21	27
Ranch Sauce, 28 g	150	16	1
Coneys			
Corn Dog, 73 g	250	15	23
Extra-Long Cheese Coney, 237 g	600	33	54
Famous Slushes (Medium)			
Blue Coconut Slush, 20 oz.	290	0	76
Cherry Slush, 20 oz.	290	0	78
Grape Slush, 20 oz.	290	0	76
Lemon Fresh Fruit Slush, 20 oz.	290	0	78
• Lemon-Berry Fresh Fruit Slush, 20 oz.	310	0	83

Sonic Drive-In (cont.)

	Cal	Fat	Cbs
Famous Slushes (Medium) (cont.)			
Lime Fresh Fruit Slush, 20 oz.	290	0	78
Minute Maid® Apple Juice Slush, 20 oz.	280	0	76
Minute Maid® Cran Juice Slush, 20 oz.	290	0	77
• Mt. Blast® POWERADE® Slush, 20 oz.	280	0	76
Orange Slush, 20 oz.	290	0	77
Strawberry Fresh Fruit Slush, 20 oz.	310	0	82
Watermelon Slush, 20 oz.	290	0	78
Fresh Tastes® Salads			
Grilled Chicken Salad, 358 g	310	14	19
• Hidden Valley® Fat Free Golden Italian, 57 g	50	0	13
Hidden Valley® Honey Mustard, 57 g	240	21	14
Hidden Valley® Original Light Ranch, 57 g	120	7	14
Hidden Valley® Ranch Dressing, 57 g	260	28	0
• Jumbo Popcorn Chicken® Salad, 354 g	490	28	39
Santa Fe Grilled Chicken Salad, 406 g	380	15	29
Frozen Drinks & Desserts (Regular Size)			
Banana Cream Pie Shake, 14 oz.	690	23	113
Banana Malt, 14 oz.	560	20	89
Banana Shake, 14 oz.	550	19	87
Banana Split, 319 g	450	12	82
Barq's® Root Beer Float/Blended Float , 14 oz.	300	8	56
Blue Coconut CreamSlush® Treat, 14 oz.	430	13	76
Butterfinger® Sonic Blast®, 14 oz.	670	31	89
Cherry CreamSlush® Treat, 14 oz.	440	13	77
• Chocolate Cream Pie Shake, 14 oz.	750	23	127
Chocolate Malt, 14 oz.	630	20	102
Chocolate Shake, 14 oz.	610	19	101
Chocolate Sundae, 255 g	410	13	67
Coca-Cola® Float/Blended Float, 14 oz.	290	8	54
Coconut Cream Pie Shake, 14 oz.	680	24	108
Diet Coke® Float/Blended Float, 14 oz.	220	8	33
Diet Dr. Pepper® Float/Blended Float, 14 oz.	220	8	33
Dr. Pepper® Float/Blended Float, 14 oz.	310	8	58
Grape CreamSlush® Treat, 14 oz.	430	13	76
Hot Fudge Sundae, 253 g	440	18	63
Lemon CreamSlush® Treat, 14 oz.	430	13	77
Lemon-Berry CreamSlush® Treat, 14 oz.	460	12	85
Lime CreamSlush® Treat, 14 oz.	430	13	77
M&M's® Sonic Blast®, 14 oz.	660	28	95
Nuts Add-On, 4 g	20	2	1
Orange CreamSlush® Treat, 14 oz.	430	13	77
Oreo® Sonic Blast®, 14 oz.	660	28	94
Pineapple Malt, 14 oz.	590	20	93
Pineapple Shake, 14 oz.	570	19	92
Pineapple Sundae, 252 g	370	13	58
Reese's PB Cups® Sonic Blast®, 14 oz.	620	22	96
Strawberry Cream Pie Shake, 14 oz.	720	23	120
Strawberry CreamSlush® Treat, 14 oz.	450	12	84
Strawberry Malt, 14 oz.	590	20	96
Strawberry Shake, 14 oz.	580	19	94
Strawberry Sundae, 252 g	380	13	61
• Vanilla Cone, 133 g	180	6	30
Vanilla Dish, 184 g	240	9	36
Vanilla Malt, 14 oz.	550	21	84
Vanilla Shake, 14 oz.	540	20	82
Watermelon CreamSlush® Treat, 14 oz.	440	13	77
Kids' Meals			
• Chicken Strips - 2 strips, 72 g	210	11	13
Corn Dog, 73 g	250	15	23
• Grilled Cheese, 118 g	390	17	45
Jr. Burger, 117 g	320	16	29
Jr. Cheeseburger, 135 g	380	21	30
Sides (Regular)			
• French Fries, 75 g	210	10	28

Sonic Drive-In (cont.)

	Cal	Fat	Cbs
Sides (Regular) (cont.)			
w/ cheese, 93 g	280	15	29
w/ chili & cheese, 122 g	300	18	31
Mozzarella Sticks, 135 g	410	21	35
• Onion Rings, 156 g	500	28	55
Tater Tots, 84 g	220	14	23
w/ cheese, 102 g	290	19	25
w/ chili & cheese, 131 g	310	21	26
Toaster® Sandwiches			
Bacon Cheeseburger Toaster®, 251 g	690	37	58
Chicken Club Toaster®, 265 g	690	35	64
Wraps			
Chicken Strip Wrap, 234 g	480	20	56
• FRITOS® Chili Cheese Wrap, 239 g	670	38	66
• Grilled Chicken Wrap, 253 g	380	11	44
Your Ultimate Drink Stop! (Medium)			
Apple Juice Limeade , 20 oz.	200	0	54
Cherry Limeade, 20 oz.	220	0	59
Cranberry Limeade , 20 oz.	200	0	53
• Ice Tea, 20 oz.	5	0	1
Limeade, 20 oz.	170	0	47
Lo-Cal Diet Cherry Limeade, 20 oz.	15	0	3
Lo-Cal Diet Limeade, 20 oz.	10	0	1
Ocean Water®, 20 oz.	200	0	53
Peach Ice Tea, 20 oz.	5	0	1
Raspberry Ice Tea, 20 oz.	5	0	2
• Strawberry Limeade, 20 oz.	230	0	60

Souper Salad

	Cal	Fat	Cbs
Beverages			
Lemonade, Mango Premium, 24 oz.	220	0	58
• Lemonade, Premium, 24 oz.	190	0	49
Lemonade, Raspberry Premium, 24 oz.	220	0	58
Lemonade, Strawberry Premium, 24 oz.	220	0	57
• Smoothie, Mango, Grande, 20 oz.	350	0	89
Smoothie, Peach, Grande, 20 oz.	320	0	87
Smoothie, Raspberry, Grande, 20 oz.	320	0	87
Smoothie, Strawberry, Grande, 20 oz.	320	0	84
Bread			
Blueberry Bread, 1 piece	150	3	29
• Bread, Cheese Drop Biscuit, 1 piece	70	3	8
Breadstick, Garlic, 1 piece	130	5	18
Cornbread, 1 piece	170	5	30
• Gingerbread, 1 piece	180	6	30
Dessert			
Banana Pudding, 1/2 cup	160	6	26
Brownies, Prepared, 2 pcs.	120	5	21
Caramel Dessert Topping, 1 tbsp.	50	1	11
• Chocolate Pudding, 1/2 cup	170	5	30
Chocolate Syrup, 1 tbsp.	50	0	12
Cottage Cheese, Lowfat, 1/2 cup	90	2	5
Oreo Crumbles, 1 tbsp.	30	1	4
• Peaches, 1/2 cup	70	0	17
Pineapple Tidbits, 1/4 cup	60	0	15
Pineapple Topping, 1 tbsp.	35	0	9
Rainbow Sprinkles, 1 tbsp.	25	1	4
Sponge Cake, Yellow, 4 pcs.	80	2	14
Strawberries, Sliced, 1/2 cup	150	0	38
Strawberry Parfait, 1/2 cup	100	2	19
Vanilla Wafers, 4 pcs.	70	2	13
Whipped Topping, 1/2 cup	100	8	8
Dressing			
Balsamic Vinegar Dressing, 1 oz.	60	0	15
Bleu Cheese Dressing, 2 oz.	220	23	1
Caesar Dressing, 2 oz.	280	30	4
Chipotle Ranch Dressing, 2 oz.	280	28	8

Souper Salad (cont.)

	Cal	Fat	Cbs
Dressing			
Cranberry Vinaigrette, 2 oz.	100	0	24
French Dressing, Fat Free, 2 oz.	60	0	18
Green Goddess, 2 oz.	260	24	4
Honey Mustard, 2 oz.	240	26	2
House Vinaigrette, 2 oz.	220	22	4
• Italian Dressing w/ Chz, Fat Free, 2 oz.	30	0	6
Mayonnaise, 2 tbsp.	200	22	0
Olive Oil, 1 oz.	240	28	0
Peppercorn Ranch Dressing, 2 oz.	220	23	2
Ranch Dressing, 2 oz.	220	23	2
Ranch Dressing, Reduced Calorie, 2 oz.	120	11	3
Tangy Oriental, 2 oz.	160	12	10
• Thousand Island Dressing, 2 oz.	300	30	6
Featured Salad			
• Apple Walnut Salad for Bar, 1 cup	130	11	7
Asian Chicken Salad, 1 cup	80	3	10
Asian Shrimp Salad, 1 cup	100	4	13
Buffalo Chicken Salad, 1 cup	70	6	3
Capri Salad, 1 cup	50	2	8
Chicago Chopped Salad, 1 cup	120	10	3
Chicken Caesar Salad, 1 cup	90	7	4
Chicken Salsa Caesar Salad, 1 cup	80	5	4
Cobb Salad, 1 cup	100	8	2
Green Goddess Crab Salad, 1 cup	70	5	4
Italian Antipasto Salad, 1 cup	70	5	3
Mango Berry Salad, 1 cup	110	6	13
• Marinated Tomato Salad, 1 cup	60	2	11
Salmon Medley Salad, 1 cup	70	2	10
Shrimp and Crab Louie, 1 cup	130	10	5
Shrimp Caesar Salad, 1 cup	90	7	3
Southwest Chicken Chipotle, 1 cup	90	7	4
Hot Bar			
Bacon Bits, Real, 2 tbsp.	80	7	0
Chicken Fajita, 1/3 cup	45	3	3
Chili Potato Topping, 2 oz.	70	3	5
Chipotle Pepper Sauce, 1/4 tsp.	0	0	0
Cholula Hot Sauce, 1/4 tsp.	0	0	0
Colby, Shredded, 2 oz.	110	9	1
Crackers, 1 package	30	1	4
Flour Tortilla, 1 piece	90	3	16
Jalapeño Cheese Sauce, 2 oz.	35	2	5
Melba Toast, 1 slice	45	1	8
• Parmesan, 1 tbsp.	20	1	2
• Potato, Baked, Plain, 1 piece	200	0	46
Red Pepper, Crushed, 1/4 tsp.	0	0	0
Rice, White, Prepared, 1/3 cup	70	0	15
Romano, 1 tbsp.	30	2	0
Saltine Crackers, 1 package	40	1	7
Sour Cream, Light, 2 tbsp.	40	3	3
Southwestern Quesadilla, 1 slice	90	5	9
Spanish Rice, prepared, 1/3 cup	80	2	17
Sriracha Hot Sauce, 1/4 tsp.	0	0	0
SW Beans w/ Roasted Corn, 1/3 cup	60	1	10
Whipped Margarine for Hot Bar, 1 tbsp.	40	5	0
Hot Pasta			
Alfredo Sauce for Pasta Bar, 1 1/2 tbsp.	45	4	2
Basil Pesto for Pasta Bar, 1 tbsp.	45	5	0
Bowtie for Pasta Bar, 1 cup	240	5	42
Chicken Alfredo, 1 cup	320	9	40
• Macaroni & Cheese, 1 cup	380	18	38
• Marinara for Pasta Bar, 1 1/2 tbsp.	10	0	2
Meaty Marinara for Pasta Bar, 1 1/2 tbsp.	20	1	2
Penne for Hot Pasta Bar, 1 cup	230	5	42
Spaghetti & Meatballs, 1 cup	280	9	38

Souper Salad (cont.)

	Cal	Fat	Cbs
Hot Pasta (cont.)			
Spaghetti for Pasta Bar, 1 cup	240	5	41
Tortellini for Pasta Bar, 1 cup	290	11	38
Pizza			
• Cheese Pizza, 1 slice	70	3	8
Garden Pizza, 1 slice	80	3	9
• Pepperoni Pizza, 1 slice	90	4	8
Sausage Pizza, 1 slice	80	4	9
Signature Salad			
Broccoli Coleslaw, 1/3 cup	80	6	6
California Chicken Salad, 1/3 cup	80	6	4
Chickpea Salad, 1/3 cup	110	6	11
Edamame Salad, 1/3 cup	70	5	4
Fettuccine Pasta Salad, 1/3 cup	100	5	11
• Fisherman's Kettle Shrimp & Crab Salad, 1/3 cup	120	8	9
Gazpacho Salad, 1/3 cup	30	3	3
Marinated Mushrooms, 1/3 cup	60	7	1
• Marinated Oriental Cucumber, 1/3 cup	10	0	2
Melon Couscous Salad, 1/3 cup	50	1	10
Mustard Potato Salad, 1/3 cup	80	5	7
Paco's Taco Salad, 1/3 cup	100	5	12
Pasta de Garden, 1/3 cup	80	5	8
Pasta Primavera Salad, 1/3 cup	45	3	4
Red Potato Salad, 1/3 cup	50	4	5
Rice Florentine Salad, 1/3 cup	90	5	11
Roasted Vegetables, 1/3 cup	20	2	2
Rsted Mshrms & Artichokes w/ Feta Chz, 1/3 cup	40	3	3
Salad of the Sea, 1/3 cup	50	2	6
Santa Fe Corn Salad, 1/3 cup	100	4	13
Sweet Garden Slaw, 1/3 cup	35	2	4
Thai Chicken Pasta Salad, 1/3 cup	100	5	11
Tropical Tuxedo Salad, 1/3 cup	60	3	7
Tuna Fish Salad, 1/3 cup	70	5	1
Soup			
Adobe Rice and Chkn Soup, 5 oz. bowl	100	5	10
Alaskan Salmon Chowder, 5 oz. bowl	70	2	9
Beef Mushroom Barley, 5 oz. bowl	80	2	11
Beef Noodle Soup, 5 oz. bowl	80	3	10
Beef Shellini Soup, 5 oz. bowl	90	3	11
Beef Stroganoff, 5 oz. bowl	120	5	13
Black Bean Soup, 5 oz. bowl	80	2	20
Broccoli Cheese Soup, 5 oz. bowl	70	2	10
Cajun Gumbo Soup, 5 oz. bowl	110	4	13
Cauliflower Cheese Soup, 5 oz. bowl	70	2	11
Cheddar Chkn Broccoli Stew, 5 oz. bowl	140	6	15
Cherokee Joe's Cornbread Soup, 5 oz. bowl	70	2	13
Chicken Creole Soup, 5 oz. bowl	100	4	12
• Chicken Enchilada Soup, 5 oz. bowl	180	12	13
Chicken Gumbo Soup, 5 oz. bowl	90	4	10
Chicken Mshrm Barley Soup, 5 oz. bowl	80	3	9
Chicken Noodle Soup, 5 oz. bowl	80	3	9
Chicken Tetrazini Soup, 5 oz. bowl	120	5	13
• Chicken Tortilla Soup, 5 oz. bowl	60	2	7
Cream of Asparagus, 5 oz. bowl	140	10	7
Cream of Broccoli Soup, 5 oz. bowl	60	2	9
Cream of Cauliflower Soup, 5 oz. bowl	60	2	10
Cream of Chicken Soup, 5 oz. bowl	100	5	9
Cream of Mushroom Soup, 5 oz. bowl	80	4	10

Souplantation

	Cal	Fat	Cbs
Bakery			
Apple Cinnamon Bran Muffin, 1 piece	130	1	30
Apple Raisin Muffin, 1 piece	150	7	22
• Banana Crunch Muffin Top, 1 piece	120	5	19
Banana Nut Muffin, 1 piece	150	7	22
BBQ Chicken Focaccia, Honey Wheat Crust, 1 pc	200	8	23

Souplantation (cont.)

Bakery (cont.)	Cal	Fat	Cbs
Black Forest Muffin, 1 piece	230	9	36
Bruschetta Focaccia, 1 piece	140	7	15
Buffalo Chicken Focaccia, Honey Wht Crust, 1 pc	170	7	20
Buttermilk Biscuits, 1 biscuit	190	8	25
Buttermilk Cornbread, 1 piece	140	2	27
Cappuccino Chip Muffin, 1 piece	190	6	31
Caribbean Key Lime Muffin, 1 piece	170	6	28
Carrot Pineapple Muffin w/ Oat Bran, 1 piece	150	6	23
Cherry Nut Muffin, 1 piece	150	7	22
Chile Corn Muffin, 1 piece	140	3	27
Chipotle Lime Butter, 1 tbsp.	90	10	0
Chocolate Brownie Muffin, 1 piece	180	8	26
Chocolate Chip Muffin, 1 piece	170	8	22
Chocolate Peanut Butter Chip Muffin, 1 piece	220	10	31
Country Blackberry Muffin, 1 piece	170	6	27
Cranberry Orange Bran Muffin, 1 piece	130	1	30
Date N' Honey Bran, 1 piece	150	6	24
• French Quarter Praline Muffin, 1 piece	250	10	35
Fruit Medley Bran Muffin, 1 piece	130	1	29
Garlic Asiago Focaccia, 1 piece	160	8	19
Georgia Peach Poppyseed Muffin, 1 piece	150	6	20
Grilled Cheese Focaccia, 1 piece	190	10	18
Indian Grain Bread (Low-Fat), 1 piece	200	2	35
Irish Soda Bread, 1 piece	180	5	29
Lemon Vanilla Butter, 1 tbsp.	90	7	3
Mango Tropics Muffin w/ Coconut, 1 piece	180	7	28
Maple Walnut Muffin, 1 piece	230	10	32
Old World Greek Focaccia, 1 piece	190	9	24
Pauline's Apple Walnut Cake, 1 piece	220	12	24
Pepperoni Focaccia, 1 piece	190	9	21
Pesto & Sun-Dried Tomato Focaccia, 1 piece	170	8	20
Pumpkin Raisin Muffin, 1 piece	150	6	25
Quattro Formaggio Focaccia, 1 piece	140	5	19
Roasted Potato Focaccia, 1 piece	150	6	17
Roasted Red Pepper, Honey Wht Focaccia, 1 piece	170	8	20
Sauteed Vegetable Focaccia, 1 piece	180	9	19
Sourdough Bread, 1 piece	150	1	27
Southwest Chipotle Focaccia, 1 piece	160	8	19
Spiced Pumpkin Muffin w/ Cranberries, 1 piece	180	7	29
Strawberry Buttermilk Muffin, 1 piece	140	6	21
Sweet Cherry Butter, 1 tbsp.	80	7	4
Sweet Orange & Cranberry Muffin, 1 pc	200	7	33
Sweet Strawberry Butter, 1 tbsp.	80	7	4
Taffy Apple Muffin, 1 piece	160	6	25
Tangy Lemon Muffin, 1 piece	140	4	24
Thai Chicken Focaccia w/ Peanuts, 1 piece	170	7	20
Wildly Blue Blueberry Muffin, 1 piece	140	5	22
Wowie Maui Focaccia w/ Ham, 1 piece	170	7	21
Zucchini Nut Muffin, 1 piece	150	7	22
Desserts			
Apple Cobbler, 1/2 cup	360	10	67
Apple Medley (Fat- Free), 1/2 cup	70	0	18
Banana Pudding, 1/2 cup	160	4	27
Banana Royale (Fat- Free), 1/2 cup	80	0	20
Butterscotch Pudding (Low-Fat), 1/2 cup	140	3	24
Candy Sprinkles (Low-Fat), 1 tbsp.	70	3	11
• Caramel Apple Cobbler, 1/2 cup	390	12	68
Cherry Apple Cobbler, 1/2 cup	330	10	57
Chocolate Chip Cookie - 1 Small, 1 cookie	75	3	10
Chocolate Chip Cookie Bars, 1 piece	90	4	13
Chocolate Frozen Yogurt (Fat-Free), 1/2 cup	95	0	21
Chocolate Lava Cake, 1/2 cup	330	8	62
Chocolate PBCookie Cups, 1 piece	140	6	18
Chocolate Pudding (Low-Fat), 1/2 cup	150	3	25

Souplantation (cont.)

Desserts (cont.)	Cal	Fat	Cbs
Choco Pudding (No Sugar Added), 1/2 cup	90	2	21
Chocolate Syrup (Fat- Free), 2 tbsp.	70	0	18
Cranberry Apple Cobbler, 1/2 cup	370	10	58
Cran-Raspberry Gelatin (Fat-Free), 1/2 cup	100	0	26
Deep Chocolate Winter Mint Lava Cake, 1/2 cup	330	8	58
Gelatin (Fat-Free), 1/2 cup	80	0	20
• Gelatin (Sugar Free, Fat-Free), 1/2 cup	10	0	0
Granola Topping, 2 tbsp.	110	4	16
Green Tea Mousse, 1/2 cup	190	8	29
Holiday Cookies w/ Sprinkles, 1 cookie	80	4	12
Hot Lemon Lava Cake, 1/2 cup	320	11	51
Nutty Waldorf Salad (Low-Fat), 1/2 cup	90	3	14
Oatmeal Raisin Cookie - 1 small, 1 cookie	120	5	16
Pineapple Gelatin (Fat-Free), 1/2 cup	120	0	29
Pineapple Upside- Down Cake, 1/2 cup	270	10	42
Raspberry Apple Cobbler, 1/2 cup	380	11	67
Rice Pudding (Low- Fat), 1/2 cup	110	2	20
Shortcake, 1 piece	220	7	36
Strawberry Apple Cobbler, 1/2 cup	340	10	67
Sugar-free Chocolate Mousse, 1/2 cup	40	3	3
Sugar-free Lemon Mousse, 1/2 cup	40	3	4
Sugar-free Strawberry Mousse, 1/2 cup	40	3	4
Tapioca Pudding (Low-Fat), 1/2 cup	140	3	24
Vanilla Pudding, 1/2 cup	150	4	27
Vanilla Soft Serve (Reduced Fat), 1/2 cup	140	5	22
Warm Carrot Cake w/ Cream Chz Lava, 1/2 cup	320	15	40
Dressings			
Avocado Ranch Dressing, 2 tbsp.	150	14	4
Bacon Dressing, 2 tbsp.	110	11	7
• Balsamic Vinaigrette, 2 tbsp.	180	19	1
Basil Vinaigrette, 2 tbsp.	160	17	1
Blue Cheese Dressing, 2 tbsp.	130	13	3
Chow Mein Noodles, 1/4 cup	70	1	15
Cranberry Orange Vinaigrette (Low-Fat), 2 tbsp.	80	2	15
Creamy Italian Dressing, 2 tbsp.	120	13	0
Cucumber Dressing (Reduced Calorie), 2 tbsp.	70	7	3
Garlic Parmesan Seasoned Croutons, 5 pieces	80	5	6
Green Chili Ranch Dressing, 2 tbsp.	150	14	4
Honey Lime Cilantro Vinaigrette, 2 tbsp.	100	6	15
Honey Mint Lemonade, 2 tbsp.	130	7	19
Honey Mustard Dressing (Fat-Free), 2 tbsp.	45	0	10
Honey Mustard Dressing, 2 tbsp.	150	13	8
• Italian Dressing (Fat- Free), 2 tbsp.	25	0	7
Kahlena French Dressing, 2 tbsp.	120	9	10
Monterey Blue Salad Dressing, 2 tbsp.	120	11	5
Parmesan Pepper Cream Dressing, 2 tbsp.	140	16	1
Pineapple Vinaigrette, 2 tbsp.	120	11	5
Plain Croutons, 5 pieces	50	2	7
Ranch Dressing (Fat- Free), 2 tbsp.	50	0	2
Ranch Dressing, 2 tbsp.	150	15	4
Roasted Garlic Dressing, 2 tbsp.	100	10	3
Smoky BBQ Vinaigrette, 2 tbsp.	110	10	5
Spicy Buffalo Ranch Dressing, 2 tbsp.	130	14	2
Sweet Maple Dressing, 2 tbsp.	180	17	6
Thousand Island Dressing, 2 tbsp.	90	9	3
Tomato Basil Croutons, 5 pieces	70	5	5
Warm Bacon Dressing, 2 tbsp.	110	10	5
Hot Pastas & Kitchen Favorites			
4 Cheese Alfredo (Vegetarian), 1 cup	390	13	50
Arizona Marinara (Vegetarian), 1 cup	360	11	47
Beefy Meatball Stroganoff, 1 cup	340	21	28
Broccoli Alfredo w/ Basil, 1 cup	380	17	45
Bruschetta, 1 cup	260	4	41
Carbonara Pasta w/ Bacon, 1 cup	290	10	43

Souplantation (cont.)

Hot Pastas & Kitchen Favorites (cont.)	Cal	Fat	Cbs
Chicken Tetrazzini, 1 cup	480	23	47
Cilantro Lime Pesto (Vegetarian), 1 cup	370	21	36
Creamy Bruschetta (Vegetarian), 1 cup	360	16	43
Creamy Herb Chicken, 1 cup	310	17	32
Curried Pineapple & Ginger, 1 cup	200	2	40
Fettuccine Alfredo (Vegetarian), 1 cup	390	18	41
Fire-Roasted Tomato Basil Alfredo, 1 cup	370	14	44
Garden Vegetable w/ Italian Sausage, 1 cup	300	10	42
Garden Vegetable w/ Meatballs, 1 cup	310	10	44
Greek Mediterranean (Vegetarian), 1 cup	290	8	45
Hand-Crafted Mexican Beans, 1 cup	260	2	47
Italian Sausage w/ Red Pepper Puree, 1 cup	250	10	35
Italian Vegetable Beef, 1 cup	290	9	43
Lemon Cream w/ Capers, 1 cup	390	21	44
Linguini w/ Clam Sauce, 1 cup	380	10	56
Macaroni & Cheese (Vegetarian), 1 cup	290	10	40
Nutty Mushroom (Vegetarian), 1 cup	390	20	42
Oriental Noodle & Green Bean, 1 cup	240	3	45
Pasta Florentine (Vegetarian), 1 cup	360	10	54
Penne Arrabbiatta (Vegetarian), 1 cup	340	10	43
Roasted Eggplant Marinara, 1 cup	340	10	43
Roasted Garlic & Asiago Alfredo, 1 cup	330	11	45
Roasted Mushroom Alfredo w/ Rosemary, 1 cup	380	14	44
Salsa de Lupe (Fat- Free, Vegan), 1/4 cup	30	0	6
Sautéed Balsamic Vegetables, 1/2 cup	100	6	11
Smoked Salmon & Dill, 1 cup	360	16	41
Smoky BBQ Baked Beans, 1 cup	320	3	61
Spicy Italian Sausage & Peppers, 1 cup	360	11	43
Steamed Veggies w/ Lemon Herb Butter, 1/2 cup	130	9	10
Stuffing, 1 cup	211	12	20
Tomato Spinach Whole Wheat, 1 cup	290	10	38
Tuscany Sausage w/Capers & Olives, 1 cup	240	10	29
Vegetable Ragu (Vegetarian), 1 cup	250	6	41
Vegetarian Marinara w/ Basil, 1 cup	260	4	44
Walnut Pesto (Vegetarian), 1 cup	310	9	42
Morning Menu			
Belgian Waffles, 1 piece	90	0	16
Blueberry Sauce / Blueberry Stir-In, 2 tbsp.	60	0	15
Country Ham & Egg Breakfast Burrito	210	10	21
Egg Scramble Focaccia w/ Bacon , 1 piece	180	8	20
French Toast (Plain), 1 piece	150	4	25
Homemade Oatmeal (Plain), 3/4 cup	110	2	19
Mediterranean Sunrise Pasta, 1 piece	210	12	19
Potatoes O'Brien, 1/2 cup	140	6	19
Scrambled Eggs, 1/2 cup	135	8	2
Strawberry Sauce/ Strawberry Stir-In, 2 tbsp.	60	0	14
Sweet Cinnamon Biscuits w/ Frosting, 1 piece	270	13	37
Sweet Maple Buttermilk Biscuit, 1 piece	240	9	39
Sweet Pepper & Sausage Egg Breakfast Burrito	210	11	20
Sweet Strawberry Buttermilk Biscuit, 1 piece	250	9	40
Tom's Country Gravy, 2 tbsp.	90	5	8
Zucchini Fritatta, 1 piece	160	6	22
Salads			
Ambrosia w/ Coconut (Vegetarian), 1/2 cup	190	9	30
Artichoke Rice (Vegetarian), 1/2 cup	190	12	19
Aunt Doris' Red Pepper Slaw, 1/2 cup	70	0	18
Baja Bean & Cilantro, 1/2 cup	180	3	29
BBQ Potato (Vegetarian), 1/2 cup	170	9	21
Carrot Raisin, 1/2 cup	90	3	17
Chinese Krab, 1/2 cup	160	8	19
Citrus Noodles w/ Snow Peas, 1/2 cup	140	6	19
Confetti Avocado Slaw, 1/2 cup	140	9	12
Dijon Potato w/ Garlic Dill Vinaigrette, 1/2 cup	150	12	9
Field Corn & Very Wild Rice, 1/2 cup	170	9	19

Souplantation (cont.)

Salads (cont.)	Cal	Fat	Cbs
German Potato, 1/2 cup	150	6	23
Italian White Bean, 1/2 cup	140	5	19
Jalapeño Potato, 1/2 cup	170	9	21
Joan's Broccoli Madness, 1/2 cup	180	14	11
Lemon Rice w/ Cashews, 1/2 cup	160	7	23
Mandarin Noodles w/ Broccoli, 1/2 cup	170	3	31
Mandarin Shells w/ Almonds, 1/2 cup	120	3	19
Old Fashioned Macaroni w/ Ham, 1/2 cup	200	13	18
Oriental Ginger Slaw w/ Krab, 1/2 cup	70	3	8
Pesto Pasta, 1/2 cup	180	9	21
Picnic Potato, 1/2 cup	190	14	17
Pineapple Coconut Slaw, 1/2 cup	150	10	14
Poppyseed Coleslaw, 1/2 cup	120	9	9
Red Potato & Tomato, 1/2 cup	170	11	17
Rstd Potato w/ Chipotle-Chile Vinaigrette, 1/2 cup	140	6	18
San Francisco Herb Rice, 1/2 cup	180	6	27
Shrimp & Seafood Shells, 1/2 cup	210	13	20
Smoky Ham & Cheddar Broccoli Slaw, 1/2 cup	260	18	21
Southern Black-Eyed Pea, 1/2 cup	130	6	18
Southern Dill Potato, 1/2 cup	120	3	20
Southwestern Rice & Beans, 1/2 cup	90	3	15
Spicy Cajun Shells (Vegetarian), 1/2 cup	300	13	40
Spicy Southwestern Pasta, 1/2 cup	130	3	21
Summer Barley w/ Black Beans, 1/2 cup	110	3	19
Sweet & Sour Broccoli Slaw, 1/2 cup	150	3	28
Sweet Marinated Vegetables, 1/2 cup	80	0	19
Tabouli (Vegan), 1/2 cup	200	10	24
Thai Citrus & Brown Rice, 1/2 cup	220	12	26
Thai Noodle w/ Chicken & Peanut Sauce, 1/2 cup	190	10	19
Three Bean Marinade, 1/2 cup	170	6	27
Tomato Cucumber Marinade, 1/2 cup	80	5	8
Tuna Tarragon, 1/2 cup	250	15	21
Turkey Chutney Pasta, 1/2 cup	240	12	20
Wheat Berry & Curry, 1/2 cup	210	5	36
Whole Grain Fiesta Couscous, 1/2 cup	280	11	39
Wild Rice & Chicken, 1/2 cup	300	21	21
Zesty Tortellini, 1/2 cup	230	15	20
Soups			
8 Vegetable Chicken Stew, 1 cup	160	7	17
Albondigas Locas, 1 cup	210	11	19
Asian Ginger Broth, 1 cup	50	2	6
Beef & Barley Stew, 1 cup	240	10	19
Better Than Mom's Beef Stew, 1 cup	270	17	19
Big Chunk Chicken Noodle, 1 cup	170	3	19
Border Black Bean & Chorizo Soup, 1 cup	240	10	27
Broccoli Cheese, 1 cup	280	20	16
Canadian Cheese w/ Smoked Ham, 1 cup	370	27	20
Cheese Stuffed Cappelletti, 1 cup	250	11	31
Chesapeake Corn Chowder, 1 cup	290	17	30
Chicken & Rice, 1 cup	160	5	18
Chicken Fajitas & Black Bean, 1 cup	280	7	37
Chicken Pot Pie Stew, 1 cup	310	21	21
Chili Cheeseburger, 1 cup	290	12	29
Chunky Potato Cheese w/ Thyme, 1 cup	240	11	25
Classic Creamy Tomato Soup, 1 cup	200	13	19
Classical French Onion, 1 cup	150	6	21
Classical Minestrone, 1 cup	120	2	20
Classical Shrimp Bisque, 1 cup	240	16	15
Continental Lentil & Spinach, 1 cup	160	2	28
Corned Beef & Cabbage, 1 cup	150	6	17
Country Corn & Red Potato Chowder, 1 cup	220	8	35
Cream of Broccoli (Vegetarian), 1 cup	260	19	19
Cream of Chicken, 1 cup	290	21	16
Cream of Mushroom, 1 cup	290	24	15

Souplantation (cont.)

Soups (cont.)	Cal	Fat	Cbs
Cream of Rosemary Potato, 1 cup	320	22	26
Creamy Herbed Turkey, 1 cup	320	22	18
Creamy Vegetable Chowder, 1 cup	270	14	26
Curried Yellow Split Pea, 1 cup	230	2	40
Deep Kettle House Chili, 1 cup	230	3	26
Deep Kettle House Chili, 33% more meat!, 1 cup	250	8	26
Deep Kettle House Chili, 50% more meat!, 1 cup	290	11	29
El Paso Lime & Chicken, 1 cup	160	4	24
Field of Creams - Sweet Tomato Basil, 1 cup	220	15	20
Fire-Roasted Green Chile & Corn Chowder, 1 cup	240	15	21
Garden Fresh Vegetable, 1 cup	150	2	27
Garden of Eatin', 1 cup	150	3	25
Golden Yam Bisque, 1 cup	220	8	28
Green Chile Stew w/ Pork, 1 cup	170	6	18
Indian Lentil, 1 cup	160	3	25
Irish Potato Leek, 1 cup	260	16	23
Lemon Chicken Orzo, 1 cup	220	9	21
Loaded Baked Potato & Cheese w/ Bacon, 1 cup	290	18	24
Longhorn Beef Chili, 1 cup	190	6	25
Marvelous Minestrone w/ Bacon, 1 cup	220	8	31
Minestrone w/ Italian Sausage, 1 cup	220	12	17
Mulligatawny, 1 cup	240	14	17
Neighbor Joe's Gumbo, 1 cup	210	10	20
New Mexican Corn Tortilla w/ Chicken, 1 cup	200	10	19
New Orleans Jambalaya, 1 cup	210	11	18
Old Fashion Vegetable, 1 cup	100	2	18
Pinto Bean & Basil Barley, 1 cup	160	2	29
Posole w/ Pork, 1 cup	150	6	8
Potato Tomato & Spinach, 1 cup	150	2	28
Ratatouille Provencale, 1 cup	110	0	25
Roasted Mushroom w/ Sage, 1 cup	320	26	19
Rustic Tuscan Stew, 1 cup	140	2	25
Santa Fe Black Bean Chili, 1 cup	190	3	26
Savory Turkey Harvest, 1 cup	220	12	18
Smoky Pinto & Brown Rice, 1 cup	150	2	28
Southwest Tomato Cream, 1 cup	130	7	14
Southwest Turkey Chowder w/ Bacon, 1 cup	240	15	21
Spicy Sausage & Pasta, 1 cup	300	12	34
Spicy Vegetable Chili w/ Energy Boost, 1 cup	100	1	17
Split Pea & Potato Barley, 1 cup	200	2	37
Split Pea w/ Ham, 1 cup	290	10	36
Sweet Tomato Onion, 1 cup	90	3	13
Texas Red Chili, 1 cup	190	7	24
Three-Bean Turkey Chili, 1 cup	170	3	24
Tomato Chipotle Bisque, 1 cup	250	17	20
Tomato Parmesan & Vegetables, 1 cup	120	3	18
Turkey Cassoulet w/ Bacon, 1 cup	240	12	17
Turkey Vegetable, 1 cup	210	12	15
U.S. Senate Bean w/ Smoked Ham, 1 cup	150	4	20
Vegetable Bean & Barley Stew, 1 cup	150	2	0
Vegetable Medley, 1 cup	90	1	14
Vegetarian Harvest, 1 cup	200	10	23
White Bean & Lime Chicken Chili, 1 cup	220	5	29
Yankee Clipper Clam Chowder w/ Bacon, 1 cup	340	20	21
Sweet Tomatoes Extras			
Azteca Taco w/ Turkey, 1 cup	130	9	7
Bartlett Pear & Caramelized Walnut, 1 cup	180	12	13
BBQ Julienne Chopped w/ Chicken, 1 cup	210	11	23
BBQ Smokehouse Bacon & Peanuts, 1 cup	290	17	25
Buffalo Chicken, 1 cup	180	14	10
Caesar Salad Asiago, 1 cup	270	22	10
California Cobb w/ Bacon, 1 cup	190	15	7
Cambay Curry w/ Almonds & Coconut, 1 cup	220	17	17
Cape Cod Spinach Walnuts & Bacon, 1 cup	170	14	6

Souplantation (cont.)

Sweet Tomatoes Extras (cont.)	Cal	Fat	Cbs
Cherry Chipotle Spinach, 1 cup	160	8	20
Chicken Tortilla, 1 cup	180	10	16
• Classic Greek, 1 cup	120	9	4
Club Blue BLT w/ Bacon, 1 cup	270	17	20
Country French w/ Bacon, 1 cup	210	18	7
Crunchy Island Pineapple, 1 cup	160	8	20
Field of Greens: Citrus Vinaigrette, 1 cup	150	12	10
Field of Greens: Sweet Maple, 1 cup	180	15	10
• Green Chile Ranch Cornbread Bites, 1 cup	330	21	26
Honey Minted Fruit Toss, 1 cup	140	6	20
Mandarin Spinach w/ Caramelized Walnuts, 1 cup	170	11	14
Monterey Blue w/ Peanuts, 1 cup	270	17	25
Outrageous Orange w/ Cashews, 1 cup	210	15	16
Ragin' Cajun w/ Chicken, 1 cup	220	14	15
Ranch House BLT w/ Turkey & Bacon, 1 cup	190	13	11
Roasted Vegetables w/ Feta & Olives, 1 cup	190	15	12
Sedona Green Chile & Chipotle, 1 cup	220	16	15
Smoked Turkey & Spinach w/ Almonds, 1 cup	190	10	20
Sonoma Spinach w/ Dijon Vinaigrette, 1 cup	210	14	16
Spiced Pecan & Roasted Veggies w/ Bacon, 1 cup	200	13	15
Spinach Gorgonzola w/ Pecans & Bacon, 1 cup	230	19	9
Spinach w/ Pumpkin Seeds & Cranberries, 1 cup	200	15	11
Strawberry Fields w/ Caramelized Walnuts, 1 cup	130	8	15
Summer Lemon w/ Spiced Pecans, 1 cup	220	17	16
Sweet Tomato, Basil & Mozzarella, 1 cup	120	9	7
Thai Peanut & Red Pepper, 1 cup	220	11	23
Thai Udon & Peanut, 1 cup	220	13	19
Traditional Spinach w/ Bacon, 1 cup	190	13	11
Won Ton Chicken Happiness, 1 cup	170	9	15

Southern Tsunami

	Cal	Fat	Cbs
Blue Crab Roll, 251 g	674	14	112
California Roll, 270 g	628	5	129
Classic Miso Roll, 306 g	758	9	13
Cream Cheese Roll, 280 g	794	19	123
Crunchy Shrimp Roll, 294 g	773	18	129
Dragon Roll (FW Eel), 288 g	785	18	130
Dragon Roll (Sea Eel), 288 g	736	14	131
Eel Roll (FW Eel), 281 g	770	16	128
Eel Roll (Sea Eel), 281 g	713	11	130
Fullmoon Combo, 281 g	698	12	128
M&M Roll (Shrimp, Avocado), 214 g	609	4	125
M&M Roll (Tuna, Cucumber), 223 g	611	1	124
Marina Plate, 218 g	633	7	111
Meteor Special, 263 g	700	3	141
Nigiri (Egg Cake), 54 g	141	1	29
Nigiri (Fish Roe), 38 g	102	0	19
Nigiri (FW Eel), 45 g	149	5	20
• Nigiri (Octopus), 29 g	98	1	18
Nigiri (Salmon), 38 g	109	1	18
Nigiri (Sea Eel), 60 g	159	3	27
Nigiri (Shrimp), 45 g	112	0	25
Nigiri (Smoked Salmon), 53 g	136	1	25
Nigiri (Tilapia), 47 g	118	0	25
Nigiri (Tuna), 53 g	129	0	25
Nigiri (Yellowtail), 50 g	123	1	25
Ocean Crab Roll, 283 g	678	8	125
Orange Roll, 299 g	672	6	131
Rainbow Roll, 353 g	764	8	129
Red Chili Roll, 255 g	600	13	89
Seaside Combo (Tuna, Salmon), 238 g	684	4	124
Seaside Combo (Tuna, Salmon, Shrimp, Eel), 217 g	639	4	125
Sheroline Combo, 319 g	811	7	156
Snack Pack (Cucumber), 214 g	593	0	133
Snack Pack (Krab, Cucumber), 266 g	645	1	140

RESTAURANTS & FAST-FOOD CHAINS

▶ Southern Tsunami (cont.)

	Cal	Fat	Cbs
Spicy Roll (Baby Shrimp), 286 g	710	8	133
Spicy Roll (Salmon), 279 g	745	14	121
Spicy Roll (Tuna), 285 g	731	9	125
• Stardust Combo, 352 g	981	9	200
Tempura Roll, 315 g	806	11	146
Tsunami Roll, 260 g	734	12	133
Vegetable Combo (12 pcs.), 267 g	618	6	128
Vegetable Combo (24 pcs.), 331 g	877	3	191
Condiments			
• Green Horseradish, 4 g	7	0	1
Pickled Ginger, 13 g	9	0	24
• Soy Sauce, 7 g	16	0	2
Salads			
Edamame (Soybean), 75 g	90	5	3
• Edamame Salad, 113 g	124	7	9
• Seabreeze Salad, 113 g	13	3	23

▶ Starbucks

	Cal	Fat	Cbs
Brewed Coffees - Grande			
• Caffe Misto/Café Au Lait, 16 fl.oz.	110	4	10
• Coffee of the Week, 16 fl.oz.	5	0	0
Decaf Coffee Of the Week, 16 fl.oz.	16	0	0
Iced Brewed Coffee, 16 fl.oz.	90	0	21
Brownies, Cookies & Bars			
Blueberry Oat Bar w/ Organic Blueberries, 103 g	390	15	59
Chocolate Chip Cookie, 85 g	350	15	54
Crispy Marshmallow Square, 92 g	360	9	68
• Mini Chocolate Chip Cookie, 28 g	120	5	18
Oatmeal Raisin Cookie, 85 g	350	12	56
Seasonal Cookie, 102 g	410	16	64
• Snickerdoodle Cookie, 99 g	410	17	62
Classic Favorites			
Apple Juice, 16 fl.oz.	250	0	64
Caramel Apple Spice - no whip, 16 fl.oz.	310	0	74
Caramel Apple Spice - whip, 16 fl.oz.	380	8	76
Chocolate Milk, 16 fl.oz.	350	11	52
Cinnamon Dolce Crème - no whip, 16 fl.oz.	280	7	40
Cinnamon Dolce Crème - whip, 16 fl.oz.	350	14	42
Hot Chocolate - no whip, 16 fl.oz.	300	9	47
Hot Chocolate - whip, 16 fl.oz.	370	16	49
Milk, 16 fl.oz.	260	10	25
Steamed Apple Juice, 16 fl.oz.	230	0	56
Vanilla Crème - no whip, 16 fl.oz.	260	7	36
• Vanilla Crème - whip, 16 fl.oz.	33	14	38
White Hot Chocolate - no whip, 16 fl.oz.	40	12	61
• White Hot Chocolate - whip, 16 fl.oz.	490	19	63
Croissants, Bagels & Breads			
Butter Croissant, 102 g	370	21	37
• Chocolate Croissant, 120 g	470	26	54
• Lowfat Eight Grain Roll, 112 g	270	2	56
Plain Bagel, 113 g	310	1	62
Pretzel, 113 g	290	5	52
Strawberry Jam Buttermilk Biscuit, 113	340	13	50
Doughnuts, Sweet Rolls & Danishes			
Cheese Danish, 111 g	390	24	36
• Cinnamon Roll, 167 g	500	15	83
Doughnuts, Sweet Rolls & Danishes, 113 g	480	25	60
Top Pot Apple Fritter, 123 g	490	22	65
Top Pot Glazed Old Fashioned Doughnut, 113 g	480	23	64
• Top Pot Glazed Old Fashioned Mini Doughnut, 34 g	150	7	19
Drink Extras			
Flavored Syrup, 1 pump 10 g	20	0	5
Mocha Syrup, 1 Pump 17 fl.oz.	25	1	6
Plus Energy, 15 fl.oz.	5	0	1
• Sugar Free Flavored Syrup, 1 pump 10 g	0	0	0
Toppings - Caramel, 15 g	15	1	2

▶ Starbucks (cont.)

	Cal	Fat	Cbs
Drink Extras (cont.)			
Toppings - Chocolate, 4 g	5	0	1
• Whip Cream Grande & Venti Cold, 35 g	110	11	3
Whip Cream Grande & Venti Hot, 22 g	70	7	2
Espresso - Cold - Grande 2% Milk			
• Iced Caffe Americano, 16 fl.oz.	15	0	3
Iced Caffe Latte, 16 fl.oz.	130	5	13
Iced Caffe Mocha - no whip, 16 fl.oz.	200	6	35
Iced Caffe Mocha - whip, 16 fl.oz.	320	17	38
Iced Caramel Macchiato, 16 fl.oz.	230	6	33
Iced Doubleshot on Ice +Energy Bev, 16 fl.oz.	100	1	20
Iced Doubleshot on Ice Beverage, 16 fl.oz.	90	1	20
Iced Ppprmnt Wht Choc. Mocha no whip, 16 fl.oz.	400	9	72
• Iced Ppprmnt Wht Choc. Mocha - whip, 16 fl.oz.	510	20	75
Iced Sugar-Free Syrup Flavored Latte, 16 fl.oz.	110	4	12
Iced Syrup Flavored Latte, 16 fl.oz.	190	4	30
Iced Vanilla Latte, 16 fl.oz.	190	4	30
Iced White Chocolate Mocha - no whip, 16 fl.oz.	340	9	55
Iced White Chocolate Mocha - whip, 16 fl.oz.	450	20	58
Espresso - Hot - Grande			
• Caffe Americano, 16 fl.oz.	15	0	3
• Caffe Latte, 16 fl.oz.	190	7	18
Caffe Mocha - no whip, 16 fl.oz.	260	8	41
Caffe Mocha - whip, 16 fl.oz.	330	15	43
Cappuccino, 16 fl.oz.	120	4	12
Caramel Macchiato, 16 fl.oz.	240	7	34
Cinnamon Dolce Latte - no whip, 16 fl.oz.	260	6	40
Cinnamon Dolce Latte - whip, 16 fl.oz.	330	13	42
Cinnamon Dolce Latte, Sugar-Free Syrup, 16 fl.oz.	180	6	18
Peppermnt White Choc. Mocha - no whip, 16 fl.oz.	460	11	78
• Peppermnt White Choc. Mocha - whip, 16 fl.oz.	530	18	80
Syrup Flavored Latte, 16 fl.oz.	250	6	36
Vanilla Latte, 16 fl.oz.	250	6	36
White Choc. Mocha - no whip, 16 fl.oz.	400	11	61
White Choc. Mocha - whip, 16 fl.oz.	470	18	63
Frappuccino Blended Coffee - Grande 2% Milk			
Caffè Vanilla - no whip, 16 fl.oz.	310	3	67
Caffè Vanilla - whip, 16 fl.oz.	430	14	70
Caramel - no whip, 16 fl.oz.	270	4	53
Caramel - whip, 16 fl.oz.	380	15	57
Cinnamon Dolce - no whip, 16 fl.oz.	260	3	52
Cinnamon Dolce - whip, 16 fl.oz.	370	14	55
Coffee, 16 fl.oz.	240	3	48
• Espresso, 16 fl.oz.	190	3	38
Java Chip - no whip, 16 fl.oz.	340	8	64
• Java Chip - whip, 16 fl.oz.	460	19	67
Mocha - no whip, 16 fl.oz.	260	4	54
Mocha - whip, 16 fl.oz.	380	15	57
White Chocolate Mocha - no whip, 16 fl.oz.	300	5	59
White Chocolate Mocha - whip, 16 fl.oz.	410	16	62
Frappuccino Blended Crème - Grande 2% Milk			
• Chai - no whip, 16 fl.oz.	330	2	67
Chai - whip, 16 fl.oz.	440	13	71
Green Tea - no whip, 16 fl.oz.	380	3	78
Green Tea - whip, 16 fl.oz.	490	14	82
Double Chocolaty Chip - no whip, 16 fl.oz.	400	8	75
Double Chocolaty Chip - whip, 16 fl.oz.	510	19	78
Strawberries & Crème - no whip, 16 fl.oz.	440	3	92
• Strawberries & Crème - whip, 16 fl.oz.	570	15	95
Vanilla Bean - no whip, 16 fl.oz.	350	3	72
Vanilla Bean - whip, 16 fl.oz.	470	14	75
Frappuccino Light Blended Coffee - Grande			
Caffé Vanilla Light, 16 fl.oz.	190	1	42
Caramel Light, 16 fl.oz.	160	2	30
Cinnamon Dolce Light, 16 fl.oz.	140	1	29

Starbucks (cont.)

	Cal	Fat	Cbs
Frappuccino Light Blended Coffee - Grande (cont.)			
Coffee Light, 16 fl.oz.	130	1	25
• Espresso Light, 16 fl.oz.	110	1	20
Java Chip Light, 16 fl.oz.	200	5	36
• Mint Mocha Chip Light no whip, 16 fl.oz.	210	4	40
Mocha Light, 16 fl.oz.	140	1	29
White Chocolate Mocha Light, 16 fl.oz.	180	2	34
Loaves & Coffee Cakes			
Banana Walnut Loaf, 128 g	410	17	60
Classic Coffee Cake, 113 g	420	18	61
• Crumble Coffee Cake, 122 g	500	25	65
Lemon Loaf, 128 g	430	19	62
No Sugar Added Banana Nut Cake, 124 g	480	28	63
Rdcd.-Fat Strwbrries & Crème Cake, 124 g	330	9	57
Reduced-Fat Blueberry Cake, 122 g	320	6	54
• Reduced-Fat Cinnamon Swirl Cake, 105 g	300	6	53
Reduced-Fat Lemon Blueberry Loaf, 136 g	360	10	63
Muffins & Scones			
Banana Bran Muffin, 149 g	410	14	69
• Blueberry Muffin, 170 g	500	19	75
Blueberry Scone, 120 g	400	17	54
Cranberry Orange Scone, 135 g	450	16	72
Lowfat Apricot Blueberry Muffin, 159 g	380	5	77
Maple Oat Nut Scone, 113 g	440	22	56
• Mini Blueberry Muffin, 68 g	200	8	30
Triple Berry Cobbler Muffin, 150 g	480	25	61
Zucchini Walnut Mini Muffin, 105 g	390	24	42
Oven-Toasted Breakfast Items			
Bcn, Avocado, Aged Cheddar & Egg Wrap, 153 g	380	24	26
Bacon, Egg & Cheddar Bkfst. Sandwich, 156 g	370	17	37
Forest Ham, Egg & Cheddar Bkfst. Sand, 173 g	360	15	37
Sausage, Egg & Cheddar Bkfst. Sandwich, 184 g	440	23	37
• Spinach, Rsted Tomato, Feta & Egg Wrap, 144 g	240	10	29
Special Treats			
Triple Chocolate Cupcake, 90 g	360	20	46
Vanilla Cupcake, 86 g	330	16	43
Tazo Tea - Grande			
Black Shaken Iced Tea Lemonade, 16 fl.oz.	130	0	33
Black Shaken Iced Tea, 16 fl.oz.	80	0	21
Chai Iced Tea Latte, 16 fl.oz.	240	4	44
Chai Tea Latte, 16 fl.oz.	240	4	44
Green Shaken Iced Tea Lemonade, 16 fl.oz.	130	0	33
Green Shaken Iced Tea, 16 fl.oz.	80	0	21
Green Tea Latte, 16 fl.oz.	240	5	44
• Iced Green Tea Latte, 16 fl.oz.	270	5	44
Lemonade Blended with Zen™ Green Tea, 16 fl.oz.	190	0	47
Passion™ Shaken Iced Tea Lemonade, 16 fl.oz.	130	0	33
Passion™ Shaken Iced Tea, 16 fl.oz.	80	0	21
• Tea, 16 fl.oz.	0	0	0
Vivanno Nourishing Blends - Grande			
Banana Choc. Blend w/ Espresso Shot, 16 fl.oz.	260	5	42
Banana Chocolate Blend, 16 fl.oz.	270	5	44
• Orange Mango Banana Blend w/ Matcha, 16 fl.oz.	290	2	57
• Orange Mango Banana Blend, 16 fl.oz.	250	2	47

Steak Escape

7" Sandwiches	Cal	Fat	Cbs
Cajun Chicken, 245 g	408	5	58
• Capicola Portion, 28 g	31	1	0
Chicken Portion, 112 g	120	4	0
• Classic Italian, 238 g	471	11	60
Grand Chicken, 266 g	410	6	60
Ham Portion, 84 g	75	1	3
Salami Portion, 28 g	105	9	0
Steak Portion, 112 g	130	5	0
The Grand Escape, 266 g	420	6	60

Steak Escape (cont.)

	Cal	Fat	Cbs
7" Sandwiches (cont.)			
Turkey Club, 224 g	380	2	62
Turkey Portion, 84 g	75	1	3
Vegetarian, 252 g	311	1	65
Wild West BBQ, 273 g	455	6	60
Fries			
Fresh Cut Fries - 16 oz. cup, 224 g	651	34	87
Fresh Cut Fries - 32 oz. cup, 448 g	996	52	134
• Kids Meal Fresh Cut Fries, 84 g	249	13	34
Loaded Fries - Bacon & Cheddar, 308 g	905	44	88
• Loaded Fries - Ranch & Bacon, 308 g	1044	71	84
Kids Sandwiches			
Chicken, 110 g	205	7	29
Ham, 106 g	183	1	31
• Steak, 110 g	210	3	29
Turkey, 106 g	183	1	31
Loaded Smashed Potatoes			
Bacon & Cheddar, 476 g	636	26	91
Ranch & Bacon, 476 g	692	34	87
Salad			
• Side Salad, 168 g	40	1	8
with Chicken, 316 g	177	5	11
with Ham, 302 g	132	2	8
• with Meatball, 546 g	561	24	58
with Portabello, 532 g	290	1	63
with Steak, 316 g	187	6	11
with Turkey, 302 g	132	2	8
Smashed Potatoes			
• Plain, 392 g	246	0	53
with Chicken, 568 g	383	4	56
with Ham, 554 g	338	2	59
• with Meatball, 546 g	561	24	58
with Portabello, 532 g	290	1	63
with Steak, 568 g	393	5	56
with Turkey, 554 g	338	2	59
Toppings			
Bacon, 28 g	32	3	2
Balsamic Vinaigrette, 42 g	90	9	3
BBQ Sauce, 28 g	40	0	9
Black Olives, 42 g	11	0	2
Bleu Cheese Dressing, 42 g	184	18	3
• Brown Mustard, 28 g	0	0	0
Cheddar, 28 g	116	8	1
Italian Dressing, 14 g	51	5	1
Jalapeño Peppers, 42 g	11	N/A	N/A
Lettuce, 28 g	2	0	0
• Margarine, 28 g	203	23	0
Mayonnaise, 28 g	101	11	0
Mild Peppers, 42 g	11	0	4
Parmesan, 7 g	30	2	0
Provolone, 21 g	80	6	0
Ranch Dressing, 14 g	83	9	0
Sour Cream, 28 g	61	6	1
Tomatoes, 56 g	24	0	2
White American, 28 g	101	9	3

Sub Station II

	Cal	Fat	Cbs
Bologna & Cheese, 6"	658	47	44
Corned Beef & Cheese, 6"	613	39	40
• Genoa Salami, Pepperoni & Cheese, 6"	791	58	43
Ham & Cheese, 6"	582	36	48
Ham, Bologna & Cheese, 6"	645	44	42
Ham, Bologna, Cappicola & Cheese, 6"	624	42	41
• Ham, Cappicola & Cheese, 6"	580	36	42
Ham, Genoa Salami & Cheese, 6"	679	45	45
Ham, Genoa Salami, Pepperoni & Chz, 6"	789	55	48

Sub Station II (cont.)

	Cal	Fat	Cbs
Ham, Pepperoni & Cheese, 6"	720	49	48
Ham, Turkey & Cheese, 6"	606	37	49
Provolone, Swiss & American Cheese, 6"	700	49	40
Roast Beef & Cheese, 6"	631	40	44
Roast Beef, Ham & Cheese, 6"	608	38	42
Roast Beef, Ham, Turkey & Cheese, 6"	628	39	39
Roast Beef, Turkey & Cheese, 6"	603	38	41
Turkey & Cheese, 6"	601	37	48

Submarina

	Cal	Fat	Cbs
Salads			
Coleslaw, 1 side	170	12	14
Green Salad - large	31	0	6
• Green Salad - small	16	0	3
• Macaroni Salad, 1 side	230	13	23
Pasta Salad, 1 side	174	11	17
Potato Salad, 1 side	143	8	18
Specialities			
• Albacore Tuna, 6"	816	50	59
ATC, 6"	521	17	58
Avocado, Roast Beef & Cheese, 6"	542	18	61
California Sub, 6"	761	38	58
Chicken Caesar, 6"	611	26	60
Club Sub, 6"	712	32	57
East Coast Sub, 6"	632	26	57
Grilled Chicken, 6"	512	16	53
Italian Sub, 6"	666	31	59
Meatball & Cheese, 6"	648	29	67
NY Style Hot Pastrami, 6"	795	48	54
Santa Fe Chicken, 6"	716	36	58
• Triple Play, 6"	501	12	57
Veggie, 6"	544	24	58

Subway

	Cal	Fat	Cbs
4" Subway® Minis			
• Ham, 137 g	180	3	30
Roast Beef, 147 g	190	4	30
• Tuna (with cheese), 156 g	320	18	30
Turkey Breast, 147 g	190	3	30
6" Breads , Rolls & Wraps			
• Deli Style Roll, 71 g	170	3	32
Flatbread, 94 g	250	5	43
Hearty Italian Bread, 75 g	220	2	41
Honey Oat, 88 g	250	4	48
Italian Herbs & Cheese, 82 g	251	5	41
Italian (White) Bread, 71 g	200	2	38
Parmesan Oregano Bread, 75 g	220	3	41
Wheat Bread, 78 g	200	3	40
Monterey Cheddar, 82 g	240	5	39
• Wrap, 103 g	310	8	51
6" Breakfast Sandwiches			
• Cheese, 189 g	420	18	44
• Chipotle Steak & Cheese, 281 g	600	32	49
Double Bacon & Cheese, 207 g	510	25	45
Honey Mustard Ham & Cheese, 238 g	470	19	52
Western with Cheese, 229 g	450	19	46
6" Double Meat Subs			
Double Chicken & Bacon Ranch (w/ chz), 377 g	710	35	48
Double Cold Cut Combo (w/ cheese), 320 g	550	28	49
Double Ham, 281 g	350	7	49
Double Italian BMT (w/ cheese), 306 g	630	35	49
• Double Meatball Marinara (w/ cheese), 575 g	860	42	82
Double Oven Roasted Chicken, 309 g	400	8	51
Double Roast Beef, 281 g	360	7	46
Double Steak & Cheese, 632 g	540	18	52
Double Subway Club®, 347 g	420	8	50

Subway (cont.)

	Cal	Fat	Cbs
6" Double Meat Subs (cont.)			
Double Subway Melt® (w/ cheese), 330 g	490	17	51
Double Sweet Onion Chkn. Teriyaki, 373 g	480	7	65
Double Turkey Breast & Ham, 300 g	360	7	50
• Double Turkey Breast, 281 g	330	5	48
6" Jared Sandwiches			
Ham, 224 g	290	5	47
Oven Roasted Chicken Breast, 238 g	310	5	48
Roast Beef, 224 g	290	5	45
Subway Club®, 257 g	320	6	47
• Sweet Onion Chicken Teriyaki, 281 g	370	5	59
Turkey Breast & Ham, 234 g	290	5	47
Turkey Breast, 224 g	280	5	46
• Veggie Delite®, 167 g	230	3	44
6" Limited Time Subs			
• Barbecue Chicken, 238 g	310	6	52
Barbecue Rib Patty, 245 g	420	19	47
Buffalo Chicken, 274 g	380	18	46
Subway® Seafood Sensation (w/ cheese), 250 g	450	22	51
• The Feast (w/ cheese), 372 g	590	25	52
Veggie Patty, 252 g	390	8	56
6" Sandwiches			
• Chicken & Bacon Ranch, 297 g	580	30	47
Cold Cut Combo, 249 g	410	17	47
Italian BMT®, 243 g	450	21	47
Meatball Marinara, 377 g	560	24	63
Spicy Italian, 227 g	480	25	45
Steak & Cheese, 278 g	400	12	48
• Subway Melt®, 254 g	380	12	48
Tuna, 250 g	530	31	44
8" Pizza			
Cheese & Veggies, 381 g	740	25	100
• Cheese, 293 g	680	22	96
Pepperoni, 323 g	790	32	96
• Sausage, 339 g	830	35	97
Cheese (amount on 6" sub, wrap or salad)			
• American, Processed, 11 g	40	4	1
Monterey Cheddar, Shredded, 14 g	50	5	1
• Natural Cheddar, 15 g	60	5	0
Pepperjack, 14 g	50	4	0
Provolone, 14 g	50	4	0
Swiss, 14 g	50	5	0
Cookies & Desserts			
• Apple Pie, 71 g	250	10	37
• Apple Slices - 1 package, 71 g	35	0	9
Chocolate Chip, 45 g	210	10	30
Chocolate Chunk, 45 g	220	10	30
Double Chocolate Chip, 45 g	210	10	30
M & M®, 45 g	210	10	32
Oatmeal Raisin, 45 g	200	8	30
Peanut Butter, 45 g	220	12	26
Raisins - 1 package, 43 g	140	0	33
White Chip Macadamia Nut, 45 g	220	11	29
Yogurt - Dannon® All-Natural Strawberry, 113 g	110	1	20
Fruizle Express (Small)			
Berry Lishus (w/ banana), 396 g	140	0	35
Berry Lishus, 369 g	110	0	28
• Peach Pizzazz, 341 g	100	0	26
• Pineapple Delight (w/ banana), 396 g	160	0	40
Pineapple Delight, 369 g	130	0	33
Sunrise Refresher, 341 g	120	0	29
Individual Meats (amount on 6" sub or salad)			
Chicken Patty, Roasted, 71 g	90	3	4
Chicken Strips, 71 g	80	2	0
Cold Cut Combo Meats, 71 g	140	11	2

Subway (cont.)

	Cal	Fat	Cbs
Individual Meats (amount on 6″ sub or salad) (cont.)			
Egg Patty, 85 g	110	8	3
Ham, 57 g	60	2	3
Italian BMT® Meats, 64 g	180	14	2
• Meatballs, 198 g	300	18	19
Roast Beef, 57 g	70	2	1
Seafood Sensation, 71 g	190	16	7
Subway Club® Meats, 90 g	100	3	3
Tuna, 71 g	260	24	0
• Turkey Breast, 57 g	50	1	2
Veggie Patty, 85 g	160	5	12
Jared Salads			
Ham, 371 g	120	3	14
Oven Roasted Chicken Breast, 385 g	140	3	11
Roast Beef, 371 g	120	3	12
Subway Club®, 404 g	150	4	14
• Sweet Onion Chicken Teriyaki, 427 g	210	3	26
Turkey Breast & Ham, 380 g	120	3	14
Turkey Breast, 371 g	110	3	13
• Veggie Delite®, 314 g	60	1	11
Salad Dressing			
Fat Free Italian, 57 g	35	0	7
Ranch, 57 g	320	35	3
Sandwich Condiments (amount on 6″ sub)			
Bacon (2 strips), 9 g	45	4	0
Chipotle Southwest Sauce, 21 g	96	10	1
Honey Mustard Sauce, Fat Free, 21 g	30	0	7
Light Mayonnaise (1 tbsp.), 15 g	50	5	1
Mayonnaise (1 tbsp.), 15 g	110	12	0
Mustard yellow or deli brown (2 tsp.), 10 g	5	0	1
Olive Oil Blend (1 tsp.), 7 g	45	5	0
• Ranch Dressing, 21 g	120	13	1
Red Wine Vinaigrette, Fat Free, 21 g	29	0	6
Sweet Onion Sauce, Fat Free, 21 g	40	0	9
• Vinegar (1 tsp.), 8 g	0	0	0
Soup			
Chicken and Dumpling, 10 oz.	170	5	23
• Chili Con Carne, 10 oz.	290	8	35
Cream of Broccoli, 10 oz.	160	7	18
Cream of Potato with Bacon, 10 oz.	240	13	26
Golden Broccoli & Cheese, 10 oz.	200	12	17
• Minestrone, 10 oz.	80	1	15
New England Style Clam Chowder, 10 oz.	150	5	20
Roasted Chicken Noodle, 10 oz.	80	2	11
Spanish Style Chicken with Rice, 10 oz.	110	2	17
Tomato Garden Vegetable w/ Rotini, 10 oz.	90	0	20
Vegetable Beef, 10 oz.	100	2	15
Wild Rice with Chicken, 10 oz.	210	11	21
Vegetables (amount on 6″ sub)			
• Banana Peppers (3 rings), 4 g	0	0	0
Cucumbers (3 slices), 17 g	5	0	1
Green Peppers (3 strips), 7 g	0	0	0
Jalapeño Peppers (3 rings), 4 g	5	0	0
Lettuce, 21 g	5	0	0
Olives (3 rings), 3 g	5	0	0
Onions, 14 g	5	0	1
Pickles (3 chips), 9 g	0	0	0
• Tomatoes (3 wheels), 34 g	5	0	2

Sweet Tomatoes

	Cal	Fat	Cbs
Bakery			
Apple Cinnamon Bran Muffin, 1 piece	130	1	30
Apple Raisin Muffin, 1 piece	150	7	22
• Banana Crunch Muffin Top, 1 piece	120	5	19
Banana Nut Muffin, 1 piece	150	7	22
BBQ Chkn Focaccia, Honey Wheat Crust, 1 pc	200	8	23

Sweet Tomatoes (cont.)

	Cal	Fat	Cbs
Bakery (cont.)			
Black Forest Muffin, 1 piece	230	9	36
Bruschetta Focaccia, 1 piece	140	7	15
Buffalo Chkn Focaccia, Honey Wht. Crust, 1 pc	170	7	20
Buttermilk Biscuits, 1 biscuit	190	8	25
Buttermilk Cornbread, 1 piece	140	2	27
Cappuccino Chip Muffin, 1 piece	190	6	31
Caribbean Key Lime Muffin, 1 piece	170	6	28
Carrot Pineapple Muffin w/ Oat Bran, 1 pc	150	6	23
Cherry Nut Muffin, 1 piece	150	7	22
Chile Corn Muffin, 1 piece	140	3	27
Chipotle Lime Butter, 1 tbsp.	90	10	0
Chocolate Brownie Muffin, 1 piece	180	8	26
Chocolate Chip Muffin, 1 piece	170	8	22
Chocolate Peanut Butter Chip Muffin, 1 piece	220	10	31
Country Blackberry Muffin, 1 piece	170	6	27
Cranberry Orange Bran Muffin, 1 piece	130	1	30
Date N' Honey Bran, 1 piece	150	6	24
• French Quarter Praline Muffin, 1 piece	250	10	35
Fruit Medley Bran Muffin, 1 piece	130	1	29
Garlic Asiago Focaccia, 1 piece	160	8	19
Georgia Peach Poppyseed Muffin, 1 piece	150	6	20
Grilled Cheese Focaccia, 1 piece	190	10	18
Indian Grain Bread, 1 piece	200	2	35
Irish Soda Bread, 1 piece	180	5	29
Lemon Vanilla Butter, 1 tbsp.	90	8	3
Mango Tropics Muffin w/ Coconut, 1 piece	180	7	28
Maple Walnut Muffin, 1 piece	230	10	32
Old World Greek Focaccia, 1 piece	190	9	24
Pauline's Apple Walnut Cake, 1 piece	220	12	24
Pepperoni Focaccia, 1 piece	190	9	21
Pesto & Sun-Dried Tomato Focaccia, 1 piece	170	8	20
Pumpkin Raisin Muffin, 1 piece	150	6	25
Quattro Formaggio Focaccia, 1 piece	140	5	19
Roasted Potato Focaccia, 1 piece	150	6	17
Roasted Red Pepper, Honey Wht. Focaccia, 1 piece	170	8	20
Sautéed Vegetable Focaccia, 1 piece	180	9	19
Sourdough Bread, 1 piece	150	1	27
Southwest Chipotle Focaccia, 1 piece	160	8	19
Spiced Pumpkin Muffin w/ Cranberries, 1 piece	180	7	29
Strawberry Buttermilk Muffin, 1 piece	140	6	21
Sweet Cherry Butter, 1 tbsp.	80	7	4
Sweet Orange & Cranberry Muffin, 1 piece	200	7	33
Sweet Strawberry Butter, 1 tbsp.	80	7	4
Taffy Apple Muffin, 1 piece	160	6	25
Tangy Lemon Muffin, 1 piece	140	4	24
Thai Chicken Focaccia w/ Peanuts, 1 piece	170	7	20
Wildly Blue Blueberry Muffin, 1 piece	140	5	22
Wowie Maui Focaccia w/ Ham, 1 piece	170	7	21
Zucchini Nut Muffin, 1 piece	150	7	22
Desserts			
Apple Cobbler, 1/2 cup	360	10	67
Apple Medley, 1/2 cup	70	0	18
Banana Pudding, 1/2 cup	160	4	27
Banana Royale, 1/2 cup	80	0	20
Butterscotch Pudding, 1/2 cup	140	3	24
Candy Sprinkles, 1 tbsp.	70	3	11
• Caramel Apple Cobbler, 1/2 cup	390	12	68
Cherry Apple Cobbler, 1/2 cup	330	10	57
Chocolate Chip Cookie Bars, 1 piece	90	4	13
Chocolate Chip Cookie, 1 cookie	75	3	10
Chocolate Frozen Yogurt , 1/2 cup	95	0	21
Chocolate Lava Cake, 1/2 cup	330	8	62
Chocolate Peanut Butter Cookie Cups, 1 piece	140	6	18
Chocolate Pudding, 1/2 cup	150	3	25

Sweet Tomatoes (cont.)

Desserts (cont.)

	Cal	Fat	Cbs
Choco Pudding, Lowfat, No Added Sugar 1/2 cup	90	2	21
Chocolate Syrup, 2 tbsp.	70	0	18
Cranberry Apple Cobbler, 1/2 cup	370	10	58
Cran-Raspberry Gelatin , 1/2 cup	100	0	26
Deep Chocolate Winter Mint Lava Cake, 1/2 cup	330	8	58
Green Tea Mousse, 1/2 cup	190	8	29
Holiday Cookies w/ Sprinkles, 1 cookie	80	4	12
Hot Lemon Lava Cake, 1/2 cup	320	11	51
Nutty Waldorf Salad, 1/2 cup	90	3	14
Oatmeal Raisin Cookie, 1 cookie	120	5	16
Pineapple Gelatin, 1/2 cup	120	0	29
Pineapple Upside- Down Cake, 1/2 cup	270	10	42
Raspberry Apple Cobbler, 1/2 cup	380	11	67
Rice Pudding, 1/2 cup	110	2	20
Shortcake, 1 piece	220	7	36
Strawberry Apple Cobbler, 1/2 cup	340	10	67
Sugar-free Chocolate Mousse, 1/2 cup	40	3	3
Sugar-free Lemon Mousse, 1/2 cup	40	3	4
Sugar-free Strawberry Mousse, 1/2 cup	40	3	4
Tapioca Pudding, 1/2 cup	140	3	24
Vanilla Pudding, 1/2 cup	150	4	27
Vanilla Soft Serve, 1/2 cup	140	5	22
Warm Carrot Cake w/ Cream Chz Lava, 1/2 cup	320	15	40

Dressings

	Cal	Fat	Cbs
Avocado Ranch Dressing, 2 tbsp.	150	14	4
Bacon Dressing, 2 tbsp.	110	11	7
Balsamic Vinaigrette, 2 tbsp.	180	19	1
Basil Vinaigrette, 2 tbsp.	160	17	1
Blue Cheese Dressing, 2 tbsp.	130	13	3
Chow Mein Noodles, 1/4 Cup	70	1	15
Cranberry Orange Vinaigrette, 2 tbsp.	80	2	15
Creamy Italian Dressing, 2 tbsp.	120	13	0
Cucumber Dressing, 2 tbsp.	70	7	3
Garlic Parmesan Seasoned Croutons, 5 pieces	80	5	6
Green Chili Ranch Dressing, 2 tbsp.	150	14	4
Honey Lime Cilantro Vinaigrette, 2 tbsp.	100	6	15
Honey Mint Lemonade, 2 tbsp.	130	7	19
Honey Mustard Dressing, 2 tbsp.	150	13	8
Honey Mustard Dressing, 2 tbsp.	45	0	10
Italian Dressing, 2 tbsp.	25	0	7
Kahlena French Dressing, 2 tbsp.	120	9	10
Monterey Blue Salad Dressing, 2 tbsp.	120	11	5
Parmesan Pepper Cream Dressing, 2 tbsp.	140	16	1
Pineapple Vinaigrette, 2 tbsp.	120	11	5
Plain Croutons, 5 pieces	50	2	7
Ranch Dressing, 2 tbsp.	150	15	4
Ranch Dressing Fat Free, 2 tbsp.	50	0	2
Roasted Garlic Dressing, 2 tbsp.	100	10	3
Smoky BBQ Vinaigrette, 2 tbsp.	110	10	5
Spicy Buffalo Ranch Dressing, 2 tbsp.	130	14	2
Sweet Maple Dressing, 2 tbsp.	180	17	6
Thousand Island Dressing, 2 tbsp.	90	9	3
Tomato Basil Croutons, 5 pieces	70	5	5
Warm Bacon Dressing, 2 tbsp.	110	10	5

Hot Pastas & Kitchen Favorites

	Cal	Fat	Cbs
4 Cheese Alfredo, 1 cup	390	13	50
Arizona Marinara, 1 cup	360	11	47
Beefy Meatball Stroganoff, 1 cup	340	21	28
Broccoli Alfredo w/ Basil, 1 cup	380	17	45
Bruschetta, 1 cup	260	4	41
Carbonara Pasta w/ Bacon, 1 cup	290	10	43
Chicken Tetrazzini, 1 cup	480	23	47
Cilantro Lime Pesto, 1 cup	370	21	36
Creamy Bruschetta, 1 cup	360	16	43

Sweet Tomatoes (cont.)

Hot Pastas & Kitchen Favorites (cont.)

	Cal	Fat	Cbs
Creamy Herb Chicken, 1 cup	310	17	32
Curried Pineapple & Ginger, 1 cup	200	2	40
Fettuccine Alfredo, 1 cup	390	18	41
Fire-Roasted Tomato Basil Alfredo, 1 cup	370	14	44
Garden Vegetable w/ Italian Sausage, 1 cup	300	10	42
Garden Vegetable w/ Meatballs, 1 cup	310	10	44
Greek Mediterranean, 1 cup	290	8	45
Hand-Crafted Mexican Beans, 1 cup	260	2	47
Italian Sausage w/ Red Pepper Puree, 1 cup	250	10	35
Italian Vegetable Beef, 1 cup	290	9	43
Lemon Cream w/ Capers, 1 cup	390	21	44
Linguini w/ Clam Sauce, 1 cup	380	10	56
Macaroni & Cheese, 1 cup	290	10	40
Nutty Mushroom, 1 cup	390	20	42
Oriental Noodle & Green Bean, 1 cup	240	3	45
Pasta Florentine, 1 cup	360	10	54
Penne Arrabbiatta, 1 cup	340	10	43
Roasted Eggplant Marinara, 1 cup	340	10	43
Roasted Garlic & Asiago Alfredo, 1 cup	330	11	45
Roasted Mushroom Alfredo w/ Rosemary, 1 cup	380	14	44
Salsa de Lupe, 1/4 cup	30	0	6
Sautéed Balsamic Vegetables, 1/2 cup	100	6	11
Smoked Salmon & Dill, 1 cup	360	16	41
Smoky BBQ Baked Beans, 1 cup	320	3	61
Spicy Italian Sausage & Peppers, 1 cup	360	11	43
Steamed Veggies w/ Lemon Herb Butter, 1/2 cup	130	9	10
Stuffing, 1/2 cup	210	12	20
Tomato Spinach Whole Wheat, 1 cup	290	10	38
Tuscany Sausage w/ Capers & Olives, 1 cup	240	10	29
Vegetable Ragu, 1 cup	250	6	41
Vegetarian Marinara w/ Basil, 1 cup	260	4	44
Walnut Pesto, 1 cup	310	9	42

Morning Menu

	Cal	Fat	Cbs
Belgian Waffles, 1 piece	90	0	16
Blueberry Sauce, 2 tbsp.	60	0	15
Country Ham & Egg Breakfast Burrito, 1 burrito	210	10	21
Egg Scramble Focaccia w/ Bacon, 1 piece	180	8	20
French Toast (Plain), 1 piece	150	4	25
Homemade Oatmeal (Plain), 3/4 cup	110	2	19
Mediterranean Sunrise Pasta, 1 cup	210	12	19
Potatoes O'Brien, 1/2 cup	140	6	19
Scrambled Eggs, 1/2 cup	135	8	2
Strawberry Sauce, 2 tbsp.	60	0	14
Sweet Cinnamon Biscuits w/ Frosting, 1 piece	270	13	37
Sweet Maple Buttermilk Biscuit, 1 piece	240	9	39
Sweet Strawberry Buttermilk Biscuit, 1 piece	250	9	40
Swt. Pepper & Sausage Egg Bkfst. Burrito	210	11	20
Tom's Country Gravy, 2 tbsp.	90	5	8
Zucchini Fritatta, 1 piece	160	6	22

Salads

	Cal	Fat	Cbs
Ambrosia w/ Coconut, 1/2 cup	190	9	30
Artichoke Rice, 1/2 cup	190	12	19
Aunt Doris' Red Pepper Slaw, 1/2 cup	70	0	18
Baja Bean & Cilantro, 1/2 cup	180	3	29
BBQ Potato, 1/2 cup	170	9	21
Carrot Raisin, 1/2 cup	90	3	17
Chinese Krab, 1/2 cup	160	8	19
Citrus Noodles w/ Snow Peas, 1/2 cup	140	6	19
Confetti Avocado Slaw, 1/2 cup	140	9	12
Dijon Potato w/ Garlic Dill Vinaigrette, 1/2 cup	150	12	9
Field Corn & Very Wild Rice, 1/2 cup	170	9	19
German Potato, 1/2 cup	150	6	23
Greek Couscous w/ Feta & Pinenuts, 1/2 cup	210	10	25
Italian White Bean, 1/2 cup	140	5	19

Sweet Tomatoes (cont.)

	Cal	Fat	Cbs
Salads (cont.)			
Jalapeño Potato, 1/2 cup	170	9	21
Joan's Broccoli Madness, 1/2 cup	180	14	11
Lemon Rice w/ Cashews, 1/2 cup	160	7	23
Mandarin Noodles w/ Broccoli, 1/2 cup	170	3	31
Mandarin Shells w/ Almonds, 1/2 cup	120	3	19
Old Fashioned Macaroni w/ Ham, 1/2 cup	200	13	18
Oriental Ginger Slaw w/ Krab, 1/2 cup	70	3	8
Penne Pasta w/ Chkn & Citrus Vinaigrette, 1/2 cup	130	3	20
Pesto Pasta, 1/2 cup	180	9	21
Picnic Potato, 1/2 cup	190	14	17
Pineapple Coconut Slaw, 1/2 cup	150	10	14
Poppyseed Coleslaw, 1/2 cup	120	9	9
Red Potato & Tomato, 1/2 cup	170	11	17
Rstd Potato w/ Chipotle-Chile Vinaigrette, 1/2 cup	140	6	18
San Francisco Herb Rice, 1/2 cup	180	6	27
Shrimp & Seafood Shells, 1/2 cup	210	13	20
Smoky Ham & Cheddar Broccoli Slaw, 1/2 cup	260	18	21
Southern Black-Eyed Pea, 1/2 cup	130	6	18
Southern Dill Potato, 1/2 cup	120	3	20
Southwestern Rice & Beans, 1/2 cup	90	3	15
Spicy Cajun Shells, 1/2 cup	300	13	40
Spicy Southwestern Pasta, 1/2 cup	130	3	21
Summer Barley w/ Black Beans, 1/2 cup	110	3	19
Sweet & Sour Broccoli Slaw, 1/2 cup	150	3	28
Sweet Marinated Vegetables, 1/2 cup	80	0	19
Tabouli, 1/2 cup	200	10	24
Thai Citrus & Brown Rice, 1/2 cup	220	12	26
Thai Noodle w/ Chicken & Peanut Sauce, 1/2 cup	190	10	19
Three Bean Marinade, 1/2 cup	170	6	27
Tomato Cucumber Marinade, 1/2 cup	80	5	8
Tuna Tarragon, 1/2 cup	250	15	21
Turkey Chutney Pasta, 1/2 cup	240	12	20
Wheat Berry & Curry, 1/2 cup	210	5	36
Whole Grain Fiesta Couscous, 1/2 cup	280	11	39
• Wild Rice & Chicken, 1/2 cup	300	21	21
Zesty Tortellini, 1/2 cup	230	15	20
Soups			
8 Vegetable Chicken Stew, 1 cup	160	7	17
Albondigas Locas, 1 cup	210	11	19
• Asian Ginger Broth, 1 cup	50	2	6
Beef & Barley Stew, 1 cup	240	10	19
Better Than Mom's Beef Stew, 1 cup	270	17	19
Big Chunk Chicken Noodle, 1 cup	170	3	19
Border Black Bean & Chorizo Soup, 1 cup	240	10	27
Broccoli Cheese, 1 cup	280	20	16
• Canadian Cheese w/ Smoked Ham, 1 cup	370	27	20
Cheese Stuffed Cappelletti, 1 cup	250	11	31
Chesapeake Corn Chowder, 1 cup	290	17	30
Chicken & Rice, 1 cup	160	5	18
Chicken Fajitas & Black Bean, 1 cup	280	7	37
Chicken Pot Pie Stew, 1 cup	310	21	21
Chicken Tortilla w/ Jalapeño & Tomatoes, 1 cup	100	3	11
Chili Cheeseburger, 1 cup	290	12	29
Chunky Potato Cheese w/ Thyme, 1 cup	240	11	25
Classic Creamy Tomato Soup, 1 cup	200	13	19
Classical French Onion, 1 cup	150	6	21
Classical Minestrone, 1 cup	120	2	20
Classical Shrimp Bisque, 1 cup	240	16	15
Continental Lentil & Spinach, 1 cup	160	2	28
Corned Beef & Cabbage, 1 cup	150	6	17
Country Corn & Red Potato Chowder, 1 cup	220	8	35
Cream of Broccoli, 1 cup	260	19	19
Cream of Chicken, 1 cup	290	21	16
Cream of Mushroom, 1 cup	290	24	15

Sweet Tomatoes (cont.)

	Cal	Fat	Cbs
Soups (cont.)			
Cream of Rosemary Potato, 1 cup	320	22	26
Creamy Herbed Turkey, 1 cup	320	22	18
Creamy Vegetable Chowder, 1 cup	270	14	26
Curried Yellow Split Pea, 1 cup	230	2	40
Deep Kettle House Chili, 1 cup	230	3	26
Deep Kettle House Chili, 33% more meat!, 1 cup	250	8	26
Deep Kettle House Chili, 50% more meat!, 1 cup	290	11	29
El Paso Lime & Chicken, 1 cup	160	4	24
Field of Creams - Cauliflower w/ Cheese, 1 cup	280	21	17
Field of Creams - Sweet Tomato Basil, 1 cup	220	15	20
Fire-Roasted Green Chile & Corn Chowder, 1 cup	240	15	21
Garden Fresh Vegetable, 1 cup	150	2	27
Garden of Eatin', 1 cup	150	3	25
Golden Yam Bisque, 1 cup	220	8	28
Green Chile Stew w/ Pork, 1 cup	170	6	18
Indian Lentil, 1 cup	160	3	25
Irish Potato Leek, 1 cup	260	16	23
Lemon Chicken Orzo, 1 cup	220	9	21
Loaded Baked Potato & Cheese w/ Bacon, 1 cup	290	18	24
Longhorn Beef Chili, 1 cup	190	6	25
Marvelous Minestrone w/ Bacon, 1 cup	220	8	31
Minestrone w/ Italian Sausage, 1 cup	220	12	11
Moroccan Garbanzo & Lentil Bean, 1 cup	230	2	40
Mulligatawny, 1 cup	240	14	17
Neighbor Joe's Gumbo, 1 cup	210	10	20
New Mexican Corn Tortilla w/ Chicken, 1 cup	200	10	19
New Orleans Jambalaya, 1 cup	210	11	18
Old Fashion Vegetable, 1 cup	100	2	18
Pinto Bean & Basil Barley, 1 cup	160	2	29
Posole w/ Pork, 1 cup	150	6	8
Potato Tomato & Spinach, 1 cup	150	2	28
Ratatouille Provencale, 1 cup	110	0	25
Roasted Mushroom w/ Sage, 1 cup	320	26	19
Rustic Tuscan Stew, 1 cup	140	2	25
Santa Fe Black Bean Chili, 1 cup	190	3	26
Savory Turkey Harvest, 1 cup	220	12	18
Smoky Pinto & Brown Rice, 1 cup	150	2	28
Southwest Tomato Cream, 1 cup	130	7	14
Southwest Turkey Chowder w/ Bacon, 1 cup	240	15	21
Spicy Sausage & Pasta, 1 cup	300	12	34
Spicy Vegetable Chili w/ Energy Boost, 1 cup	100	1	17
Split Pea & Potato Barley, 1 cup	200	2	37
Split Pea w/ Ham, 1 cup	290	10	36
Sweet Tomato Onion, 1 cup	90	3	13
Texas Red Chili, 1 cup	190	7	24
Three-Bean Turkey Chili, 1 cup	170	3	24
Tomato Chipotle Bisque, 1 cup	250	17	20
Tomato Parmesan & Vegetables, 1 cup	120	3	18
Turkey Cassoulet w/ Bacon, 1 cup	240	12	17
Turkey Vegetable, 1 cup	210	12	15
U.S. Senate Bean w/ Smoked Ham, 1 cup	150	4	20
Vegetable Bean & Barley Stew, 1 cup	150	2	0
Vegetable Medley, 1 cup	90	1	14
Vegetarian Harvest, 1 cup	200	10	23
White Bean & Lime Chicken Chili, 1 cup	220	5	29
Yankee Clipper Clam Chowder w/ Bacon, 1 cup	340	20	21
Tossed Salads			
Azteca Taco w/ Turkey, 1 cup	130	9	7
Bartlett Pear & Caramelized Walnut, 1 cup	180	12	13
BBQ Julienne Chopped w/ Chicken, 1 cup	210	11	23
BBQ Smokehouse Bacon & Peanuts, 1 cup	290	17	25
Buffalo Chicken, 1 cup	180	14	10
Caesar Salad Asiago, 1 cup	270	22	10
California Cobb w/ Bacon, 1 cup	190	15	7

RESTAURANTS & FAST-FOOD CHAINS

Sweet Tomatoes (cont.)

	Cal	Fat	Cbs
Tossed Salads (cont.)			
Cambay Curry w/ Almonds & Coconut, 1 cup	220	17	17
Cape Cod Spinach Walnuts & Bacon, 1 cup	170	14	6
Cherry Chipotle Spinach, 1 cup	160	8	20
Chicken Tortilla, 1 cup	180	10	16
• Classic Greek, 1 cup	120	9	4
Club Blue BLT w/ Bacon, 1 cup	270	17	20
Country French w/ Bacon, 1 cup	210	18	7
Crunchy Island Pineapple, 1 cup	160	8	20
Field of Greens: Citrus Vinaigrette, 1 cup	150	12	10
Field of Greens: Sweet Maple, 1 cup	180	15	10
• Green Chile Ranch Cornbread Bites, 1 cup	330	21	26
Honey Minted Fruit Toss, 1 cup	140	6	20
Mandarin Spinach w/ Caramelized Walnuts, 1 cup	170	11	14
Monterey Blue w/ Peanuts, 1 cup	270	17	25
Outrageous Orange w/ Cashews, 1 cup	210	15	16
Ragin' Cajun w/ Chicken, 1 cup	220	14	15
Ranch House BLT w/ Turkey, 1 cup	190	13	11
Roasted Veggies w/ Feta & Olives, 1 cup	190	15	12
Sedona Green Chile & Chipotle, 1 cup	220	16	15
Smoked Turkey & Spinach w/ Almonds, 1 cup	190	10	20
Sonoma Spinach w/ Dijon Vinaigrette, 1 cup	210	14	16
Spiced Pecan & Rsted Veggies w/ Bacon, 1 cup	200	13	15
Spinach Gorgonzola w/ Pecans & Bacon, 1 cup	230	19	9
Spinach w/ Pumpkin Seeds & Cranberries, 1 cup	200	15	11
Strawberry Fields w/ Caramelized Walnuts, 1 cup	130	8	15
Summer Lemon w/ Spiced Pecans, 1 cup	220	17	16
Sweet Tomato, Basil & Mozzarella, 1 cup	120	9	7
Thai Peanut & Red Pepper, 1 cup	220	11	23
Thai Udon & Peanut, 1 cup	220	13	19
Traditional Spinach w/ Bacon, 1 cup	190	13	11
Won Ton Chicken Happiness, 1 cup	170	9	15

Swiss Chalet

	Cal	Fat	Cbs
Desserts			
Baked Apple Blossom, 160 g	470	28	52
Carrot Cake, 156 g	740	48	70
• Chocolate Eruption Cheesecake, 200 g	820	55	72
Classic Apple Pie, 136 g	330	14	49
Coconut Cream Pie, 106 g	310	20	23
Colossal Caramel Fudge Cheesecake, 200 g	700	39	78
• Lemon Meringue Pie, 113 g	295	9	65
Perfect Pecan Pie, 120 g	530	28	66
Sauce - Butterscotch, 34 g	100	0	24
Sauce - Chocolate, 34 g	80	0	20
Sauce - Strawberry, 34 g	40	0	10
Swiss Alps Chocolate Layer Cake, 125 g	590	39	55
From The Grill			
Feature Cut BBQ Ribs, 150 g	420	26	3
Grilled Chkn Breast (w/ rice and flatbread), 330 g	500	8	70
• Grilled Chkn Breast (w/o rice & flatbread), 115 g	130	2	1
Grilled Chicken Caesar (w/out flatbread), 285 g	490	34	16
• Large Cut BBQ Ribs, 452 g	1270	77	9
Regular Cut BBQ Ribs, 226 g	630	38	4
Kids' Meals (not including sides)			
Cheesy Pizza, 150 g	370	13	45
Chicken Strips, 3 strips	310	16	24
Chkn Thigh & Drumstick (w/ Skin), 139 g	310	19	2
• Grilled Cheese, 138 g	510	33	42
Mini Burgers (2), 138 g	360	18	32
• Mini Chicken Sandwiches (2), 151 g	281	8	30
Rotisserie Chicken			
Chicken Pot Pie, 428 g	580	33	42
• Double Leg (w/ skin), 278 g	630	38	4
Half Chicken (w/ skin), 298 g	610	31	5
• Quarter Chicken Breast (skinless), 124 g	210	7	0

Swiss Chalet (cont.)

	Cal	Fat	Cbs
Rotisserie Chicken (cont.)			
Quarter Chicken Breast (w/ skin), 149 g	300	11	3
Quarter Chicken Leg (skinless), 116 g	230	11	1
Quarter Chicken Leg (w/ skin), 139 g	310	19	2
Salad Dressings & Dips			
Famous Chalet Sauce, 100 ml	30	1	5
Asian Sesame Dressing, 15 ml	30	1	5
Balsamic Vinaigrette, 15 ml	40	4	2
Blue Cheese Dip, 15 ml	70	7	1
Caesar Dressing, 15 ml	90	9	1
• Cajun Sauce Dip, 57 ml	100	9	3
Chalet Dressing, 15 ml	80	7	3
• Fat-Free Raspberry Vinaigrette, 15 ml	15	0	3
Greek Dressing, 15 ml	70	7	1
Light Italian Dressing, 15 ml	35	4	1
Light Mayonnaise, 15 ml	45	5	1
Ranch Dressing, 15 ml	50	6	1
Salsa, 50 g	20	0	4
Tangy Plum Sauce, 28 g	50	0	24
Sides			
Baked Potato, 284 g	220	0	48
Butter, 10 g	70	8	0
Chinese Noodles, 160 g	230	2	44
Corn, 170 g	140	2	24
Flatbread, 46 g	140	4	22
Fresh Corn Chips, 28 g	140	7	19
• Fresh Cut Fries (Fried in Trans Fat-Free Oil), 168 g	470	25	56
Fresh Vegetables, 170 g	80	1	15
Gravy, 113 g	45	2	7
Mashed Potatoes, 140 g	100	4	17
Oven-baked Roll (Homestyle White), 51 g	130	1	27
Oven-baked Roll (Multigrain), 56 g	150	2	28
Ramekin of Coleslaw, 64 g	70	5	5
Rice Pilaf, 170 g	240	3	48
Sautéed Mushrooms, 170 g	220	16	11
Side Caesar Salad, 100 g	210	19	9
• Side Garden Salad (w/out dressing), 122 g	15	0	4
Side Greek Salad, 107 g	130	11	5
Sour Cream & Chives, 43 ml	70	5	3
Traditional Coleslaw, 180 g	200	14	15
Starters			
Caesar Salad, 170 g	360	32	15
Chalet Chicken Soup, 355 ml	160	4	17
Chalet Chicken Wings, 8 Mild Wings	640	44	16
Chicken Spring Rolls, 2 pieces	460	13	53
Dry Ribs, 400 g	920	64	4
• Garden Salad (no dressing), 162 g	30	0	6
Greek Salad, 183 g	220	18	9
Perogies (7 pieces), 196 g	420	10	69
Sundried Garlic Cheese Loaf, 276 g	910	57	78
Sundried Garlic Loaf (no cheese), 219 g	700	39	75
Wholesome Choices			
Garden Fresh Quarter Chkn Breast Dinner, 368 g	360	11	14
Oriental Chkn Salad, no dressing or noodles, 460 g	300	11	14
• Oriental Noodles, 28 g	130	6	16
Santa Fe Grilled Chkn Salad (no dressing), 354 g	300	4	35
• Spinach Chkn Salad, no dressing or tortillas, 428 g	370	10	19
Tortillas, 26 g	150	10	13
Vegetable Stir Fry (no rice or noodles), 432 g	270	3	54
with Grilled Chicken (no rice or noodles), 547 g	400	4	55
Wraps, Sandwiches & Burgers			
Bacon Cheese Burger (w/out bun), 200 g	630	42	2
• Bacon Cheese Burger (with bun), 285 g	870	46	45
Chicken Club Wrap, 364 g	840	40	61
Chicken on a Kaiser (dark meat), 241 g	570	15	44

RESTAURANTS & FAST-FOOD CHAINS

Swiss Chalet (cont.)

	Cal	Fat	Cbs
Wraps, Sandwiches & Burgers (cont.)			
Chicken on a Kaiser (white meat), 222 g	440	8	31
Chicken Quesadilla, 290 g	590	18	73
Grilled Santa Fe Chicken Sandwich, 240 g	380	4	49
Hamburger (w/out bun), 165 g	490	38	1
Hamburger (with bun), 250 g	730	49	44
Messy Chicken Sandwich (dark meat), 344 g	540	18	41
Messy Chicken Sandwich (white meat), 344 g	490	12	40
• Veggie Burger (w/out bun), 90 g	190	9	8
Veggie Burger (with bun), 175 g	430	13	51

T.J. Cinnamons

	Cal	Fat	Cbs
Original Gourmet Cinnamon Roll			
Cinnamon Roll, 149 g	507	10	73
Pecan Sticky Bun			
Cinnamon Roll, 1 piece, 149 g	507	10	73
Sticky Bun Smear w/ pecans, 1 piece, 35 g	181	12	18
T.J. Cinnamons Mocha Chill			
Mocha Chill, 340 g	264	4	46
Whipped Cream, 14 g	43	3	1
T.J. Icing			
Cream Cheese Icing, 28 g	117	5	18
Twists			
Chocolate Twist, 71 g	250	12	34
Cinnamon Twist, 71 g	260	14	33

Taco Time

	Cal	Fat	Cbs
Burrito			
Big Juan, Chicken, 13 oz.	594	19	68
Big Juan, Seasoned Ground Beef, 13 oz.	651	26	71
Big Juan, Shredded Beef, 13 oz.	633	25	67
Casita, Chicken, 12 oz.	494	18	43
Casita, Seasoned Ground Beef, 12 oz.	552	25	46
Casita, Shredded Beef, 12 oz.	533	25	42
• Cheddar Melt, 3 oz.	250	12	25
Chicken & Black Bean, 10 oz.	476	16	51
• Chicken B.L.T., 10 oz.	721	41	44
Chicken Ranchero, 11 oz.	654	32	52
Crisp Chicken, 6 oz.	336	10	32
Crisp Meat (Seasoned Ground Beef), 6 oz.	450	22	36
Crisp Pinto Bean, 6 oz.	394	16	50
Soft Meat (Seasoned Ground Beef), 7 oz.	426	16	43
Soft Pinto Bean, 7 oz.	377	11	54
Veggie, 11 oz.	534	18	74
Desserts			
Churro w/ cinn & sugar, 2 oz.	245	15	26
• Crustos, 4 oz.	294	6	58
Empanada, Apple, 4 oz.	234	7	40
Empanada, Cherry, 4 oz.	240	7	41
Empanada, Pumpkin, 4 oz.	256	8	42
• Plain Churro, 2 oz.	205	15	16
Extras			
Chicken Filling, 3 oz.	102	0	1
Chipotle Ranch, 1 oz.	165	18	1
Guacamole, 1 oz.	50	5	2
Mild Cheddar, 2 oz.	223	18	1
Ranch, 1 oz.	181	20	1
Salsa Nuevo, 1 oz.	8	0	2
• Salsa Verde, 1 oz.	6	0	2
Seasoned Ground Beef Filling, 3 oz.	143	7	4
Shredded Ground Beef Filling, 3 oz.	124	7	0
Sour Cream, 2 oz.	85	7	1
Taco Shells, 1 oz.	103	7	8
Thousand Island, 1 oz.	132	12	5
• Tortilla Salad Bowl, 10", 2 oz.	259	13	31
Tortilla Salad Bowl, 8", 3 oz.	155	9	17

Taco Time (cont.)

	Cal	Fat	Cbs
Salad			
• Taco, Regular - Chicken, 9 oz.	351	15	24
Taco, Regular - Seasoned Ground Beef, 8 oz.	396	23	24
Taco, Regular - Shredded Beef, 8 oz.	377	22	21
Tostada Delight, Chicken, 11 oz.	565	29	36
• Tostada Delight, Seasoned Ground Beef, 11 oz.	623	36	39
Tostada Delight, Shredded Beef, 11 oz.	604	36	35
Sides			
Chips, Taco, 2 oz.	150	3	27
Fries, Cheddar - Medium, 8 oz.	529	36	43
Fries, Mexi - Medium, 7 oz.	418	27	42
Fries, Stuffed - Medium, 7 oz.	463	9	42
• Mexi-Rice, 4 oz.	87	1	19
• Nachos, Grande, 17 oz.	1132	57	114
Refritos w/ chips, 7 oz.	304	11	35
Refritos w/o chips, 7 oz.	285	11	32
Taco			
1/2 lb. Soft, Chicken, 9 oz.	401	11	43
1/2 lb. Soft, Seasoned Ground Beef, 9 oz.	459	18	46
1/2 lb. Soft, Shredded Beef, 9 oz.	440	18	42
Crisp, Seasoned Ground Beef w/ Sour Cream, 5 oz.	254	14	13
• Crisp, Seasoned Ground Beef, 4 oz.	225	12	12
Super Soft, Chicken - Wheat Tortilla, 12 oz.	586	19	27
Super Soft, Chicken, 11 oz.	540	18	56
• Super Soft, Snd. Ground Beef - Wht. Tortilla, 12 oz.	644	26	30
Super Soft, Seasoned Ground Beef, 11 oz.	598	25	59
Super Soft, Shredded Beef - Wheat Tortilla, 12 oz.	626	26	26
Super Soft, Shredded Beef, 11 oz.	579	25	55
Value Soft, 5 oz.	314	13	28

Taco Bell

	Cal	Fat	Cbs
Big Bell Value Menu®			
• 1/2 lb. Beef & Potato Burrito, 252 g	530	23	66
1/2 lb. Beef Combo Burrito, 241 g	440	18	51
1/2 lb. Cheesy Bean & Rice Burrito, 227 g	470	20	58
Caramel Apple Empanada, 85 g	290	14	37
Cheesy Fiesta Potatoes, 135 g	290	17	29
Double Decker® Taco, 156 g	320	13	38
Grande Soft Taco, 206 g	430	20	43
Spicy Chicken Burrito, 191 g	400	17	48
• Spicy Chicken Soft Taco, 113 g	170	6	20
Burritos			
7-Layer Burrito, 283 g	490	18	65
Bean Burrito, 198 g	350	9	54
Burrito Supreme® - Beef, 248 g	420	17	51
Burrito Supreme® - Chicken, 248 g	400	13	49
Burrito Supreme® - Steak, 248 g	390	14	49
Fiesta Burrito - Beef, 184 g	370	13	49
Fiesta Burrito - Chicken, 184 g	350	10	47
• Fiesta Burrito - Steak, 184 g	340	11	47
• Grilled Stuft Burrito - Beef, 325 g	680	30	76
Grilled Stuft Burrito - Chicken, 325 g	640	23	73
Grilled Stuft Burrito - Steak, 325 g	630	25	72
Chalupas			
• Baja - Beef, 153 g	410	27	30
Baja - Chicken, 153 g	390	23	29
Baja - Steak, 153 g	390	24	28
Nacho Cheese - Beef, 153 g	370	22	32
Nacho Cheese - Chicken, 153 g	350	18	30
• Nacho Cheese - Steak, 153 g	340	19	30
Supreme - Beef, 153 g	380	23	30
Supreme - Chicken, 153 g	360	20	29
Supreme - Steak, 153 g	360	21	28
Gordita			
• Gordita Baja® - Beef, 153 g	340	19	29
Gordita Baja® - Chicken, 153 g	320	16	28

Taco Bell (Cont.)

	Cal	Fat	Cbs
Gordita (cont.)			
Gordita Baja® - Steak, 153 g	320	17	27
Gordita Nacho Cheese - Beef, 153 g	300	14	31
Gordita Nacho Cheese - Chicken, 153 g	280	11	29
• Gordita Nacho Cheese - Steak, 153 g	270	12	29
Gordita Supreme® - Beef, 153 g	310	16	29
Gordita Supreme® - Chicken, 153 g	290	12	28
Gordita Supreme® - Steak, 153 g	290	13	28
Nachos and Sides			
Cinnamon Twists, 35 g	170	7	26
Mexican Rice, 128 g	180	7	23
• Nachos BellGrande®, 305 g	770	44	77
Nachos Supreme, 191 g	440	26	41
Nachos, 99 g	330	21	32
• Pintos 'n Cheese, 128 g	160	6	19
New Fresco Menu			
Fresco Bean Burrito, 213 g	330	7	54
Fresco Burrito Supreme® - Chicken, 241 g	330	8	49
Fresco Burrito Supreme® - Steak, 241 g	330	8	48
• Fresco Crunchy Taco, 92 g	150	8	13
Fresco Fiesta Burrito - Chicken, 198 g	330	8	48
Fresco Grilled Steak Soft Taco, 128 g	160	5	20
Fresco Ranchero Chicken Soft Taco, 135 g	170	4	21
Fresco Soft Taco - Beef, 113 g	180	7	21
• Fresco Zesty Chkn. Border Bowl no drssing, 397 g	350	8	51
Regional Menu Items			
• Cheese Quesadilla, 142 g	470	26	39
Chili Cheese Burrito, 156 g	370	16	40
• Tostada, 170 g	240	10	27
Specialties			
Chicken Fiesta Taco Salad without Shell, 479 g	430	18	38
Chicken Fiesta Taco Salad, 544 g	790	38	77
Chicken Grilled Taquitos, 128 g	310	11	37
Chicken Quesadilla, 184 g	520	28	40
Crunchwrap Supreme®, 254 g	560	24	68
Enchirito® - Beef, 213 g	360	17	34
Enchirito® - Chicken, 213 g	340	13	33
Enchirito® - Steak, 213 g	330	14	33
Express Taco Salad, 475 g	610	32	56
Fiesta Taco Salad without Shell, 479 g	470	24	41
• Fiesta Taco Salad, 544 g	840	45	80
Guacamole Side, 43 g	70	5	5
Mexican Pizza, 213 g	530	30	46
Meximelt®, 128 g	280	14	22
Salsa Side, 43 g	15	0	3
Sour Cream Side, 43 g	80	7	3
Southwest Steak BORDER BOWL®, 443 g	600	24	68
Spicy Chicken Crunchwrap Supreme®, 254 g	540	23	67
• Steak Grilled Taquitos, 128 g	310	11	36
Steak Quesadilla, 184 g	520	28	39
Zesty Chicken Border Bowl no dressing, 376 g	440	15	57
Zesty Chicken Border Bowl, 418 g	640	35	60
Tacos			
Crunchy Taco Supreme®, 113 g	210	13	15
• Crunchy Taco, 78 g	170	10	13
• Double Decker® Taco Supreme®, 191 g	370	17	40
Grilled Steak Soft Taco, 128 g	270	16	20
Ranchero Chicken Soft Taco, 135 g	270	14	21
Soft Taco - Beef, 99 g	200	9	21
Soft Taco Supreme® - Beef, 135 g	250	13	23

Taco Cabana

	Cal	Fat	Cbs
Breakfast Tacos			
• Barbacoa, 1 ea.	307	15	2
Bacon & Egg, 1 ea.	246	12	22
Chorizon & Egg, 1 ea.	248	12	22

Taco Cabana (Cont.)

	Cal	Fat	Cbs
Breakfast Tacos (cont.)			
• Potato & Egg, 1 ea.	234	10	27
Burritos			
• Bean & Cheese, 1 ea.	710	27	85
• Beef, 1 ea.	353	24	76
Black Bean, 1 ea.	559	11	95
Chicken, 1 ea.	665	26	74
Fajitas			
• Beef, 4 oz.	245	12	3
Chicken Clark, 4 oz.	236	11	2
• Chicken White, 4 oz.	191	6	3
Grilled Chicken			
1/4 Chicken Dark, 5 oz.	298	18	1
• 1/4 Chicken no Skin, 4 oz.	167	3	0
1/4 Chicken White, 5 oz.	295	14	1
1/4 Dark no Skin, 3 oz.	170	7	1
Sides			
6" flour tortilla, 1 ea.	129	3	22
6" corn tortilla, 1 ea.	70	1	11
Black Beans, 4 oz.	111	1	21
Borracho Beans, 4 oz.	108	3	17
Calabacita, 4 oz.	78	5	6
Chips, 2 oz.	285	14	36
Elotes, 1 ea.	220	11	26
• Guacamole, 1 oz.	48	4	2
Queso, 3 oz.	184	12	7
Refried Beans, 4 oz.	171	6	21
Sour Cream, 1 oz.	57	5	1
Spanish Rice, 4 oz.	181	5	30
• Tortilla Soup Large, 19 oz.	371	13	32
Tortilla Soup Small, 9 oz.	249	8	26
Tacos			
• Bean & Cheese, 1 ea.	292	12	35
Black bean, 1 ea.	216	5	37
Carne gulsada, 1 ea.	202	8	20
• Crispy beef, 1 ea.	148	7	13
Soft Chicken, 1 ea.	217	9	21

Taco Del Mar

	Cal	Fat	Cbs
Almost Jumbo Burritos			
• Beef, Refried, 1 burrito	500	14	70
Cheese, Refried, 1 burrito	460	13	69
Chicken, Refried, 1 burrito	490	12	69
• Fish, Refried, 1 burrito	450	16	60
Pork, Refried, 1 burrito	490	13	70
Almost Super Burritos			
• Beef, Refried, 1 burrito	610	23	73
Chicken, Refried, 1 burrito	590	21	72
Fish, Refried, 1 burrito	520	24	57
Pork, Refried, 1 burrito	590	21	73
• Veggie, Refried, 1 burrito	510	17	72
Baja Bowls			
Beef, Refried, 1 bowl	830	35	81
• Chicken, Refried, 1 bowl	790	31	79
Fish, Refried, 1 bowl	880	41	95
Pork, Refried, 1 bowl	790	33	81
Breakfast Menu			
Almost Jumbo Brkfst Burrito, Refried, 1 burrito	590	27	60
Almost Super Brkfst Burrito, Refried, 1 burrito	640	31	62
Breakfast Taco, Flour, Refried, 1 taco	260	15	18
Egg & Cheese Brkfst Burrito, Refried, 1 burrito	490	19	59
Egg & Cheese Taco, Flour, Refried, 1 taco	200	10	17
Eggs, 2 oz. scoop	90	7	1
Hash Browns, 1 triangle	110	6	13
Jumbo Breakfast Burrito, Refried, 1 burrito	1080	50	105
• Potatoes Diced, 2 oz. scoop	60	1	11

RESTAURANTS & FAST-FOOD CHAINS

Taco Del Mar (Cont.)

	Cal	Fat	Cbs
Breakfast Menu (cont.)			
Sausage, 1 oz. scoop	100	8	1
• Super Breakfast Burrito, Refried, 1 burrito	1190	59	110
Carbohydrate Modified Items			
Carb Modified Almost Burrito, Beef, 1 burrito	340	17	26
• Carb Modified Almost Burrito, Chicken, 1 burrito	320	15	25
Carb Modified Almost Burrito, Pork, 1 burrito	320	16	26
Carb Modified Baja Bowl, Beef, 1 bowl	450	28	15
Carb Modified Baja Bowl, Chicken, 1 bowl	410	25	13
Carb Modified Baja Bowl, Pork, 1 bowl	410	26	14
• Carb Modified Quesadilla, Beef, 1 quesadilla	510	31	25
Carb Modified Quesadilla, Chicken, 1 quesadilla	490	29	24
Carb Modified Quesadilla, Pork, 1 quesadilla	490	30	25
Desserts			
• Butter Cookie, 1 cookie	220	10	31
Chocolate Chip Cookie, 1 cookie	240	12	34
Chocolate Chip/nut Cookie, 1 cookie	240	13	30
Milk Chocolate Cookie, 1 cookie	240	12	31
Oatmeal/Raisin/Walnut Cookie, 1 cookie	240	11	35
• Oreo Brownie, 1 brownie	400	17	59
Peanut Butter Cookie, 1 cookie	240	13	27
Triple Chocolate Cookie, 1 cookie	230	12	31
White Chocolate Cookie, 1 cookie	270	16	30
Enchiladas			
• Beef, 1 enchilada	1030	37	115
• Cheese, 1 enchilada	820	27	112
Chicken, 1 enchilada	990	33	113
Pork, 1 enchilada	990	35	114
Jumbo Burritos			
• Beef, Refried, 1 burrito	960	27	133
Cheese, Refried, 1 burrito	870	24	130
Chicken, Refried, 1 burrito	920	23	130
• Fish, Refried, 1 burrito	840	30	110
Pork, Refried, 1 burrito	920	24	132
Kids Menu			
• Kids Bean & Cheese Burrito & Chips, 1 meal	760	31	95
Kids Bean & Cheese Burrito, 1 burrito	480	17	58
Kids Chips & Cheese, 1 tray	400	22	38
Kids Quesadilla & Chips, 1 meal	600	27	71
Kids Quesadilla, 1 quesadilla	320	14	34
Kids Taco, Beef, 1 taco	270	15	16
• Kids Taco, Chicken, 1 taco	250	13	15
Kids Taco, Pork, 1 taco	250	14	16
Nachos & Chips			
Chips & Salsa, 1 tray	590	27	78
Super Nachos, Refried, 1 tray	1190	65	110
Quesadillas			
• Beef, 1 quesadilla	800	37	66
• Cheese, 1 quesadilla	710	35	63
Chicken, 1 quesadilla	770	33	64
Pork, 1 quesadilla	770	35	65
Sauces			
Enchilada Sauce, 3 oz.	35	0	7
• Green Sauce, 2 tbsp.	5	0	1
Guacamole, 1 oz scoop	40	4	2
Habanero Sauce, 2 tbsp.	10	0	1
Red Sauce, 2 tbsp.	5	0	1
Salsa, 3 oz. scoop	15	0	4
Sour Cream, 1 oz scoop	70	6	2
• White Sauce, 2 tbsp.	120	13	1
Sides			
Beans, Black, 4 oz. spoon	140	2	24
Beans, Refried, 4 oz. spoon	160	4	24
• Beans, Whole Pinto, 4 oz. spoon	90	0	20
Beef, 4 oz. scoop	200	11	4

Taco Del Mar (Cont.)

	Cal	Fat	Cbs
Sides (cont.)			
Cheese, 1 scoop	110	9	1
Chicken, 4 oz. scoop	170	7	1
Cod, 2 pieces	120	4	13
Pork, 4 oz. scoop	170	8	3
Rice & Black Beans, 1 tray	370	5	69
• Rice & Refried Beans, 1 tray	390	7	69
Rice & Whole Pinto Beans, 1 tray	320	3	66
Rice, 1 scoop	230	3	45
Super Burritos			
• Beef, Refried, 1 burrito	1180	44	138
Chicken, Refried, 1 burrito	1140	40	136
Fish, Refried, 1 burrito	1060	48	116
Pork, Refried, 1 burrito	1150	42	138
• Veggie, Refried, 1 burrito	980	33	136
Taco Salads			
Beef, Refried	930	49	75
• Chicken, Refried	900	45	73
• Fish, Refried	1040	61	89
Pork, Refried	900	46	74
Tacos			
Hard, Beef, 1 taco	270	15	17
Hard, Chicken, 1 taco	260	13	16
Hard, Fish, 1 taco	270	15	23
Hard, Pork, 1 taco	260	14	17
Soft, Beef, 1 taco	280	11	28
• Soft, Chicken, 1 taco	260	9	27
Soft, Fish, 1 taco	270	11	34
Soft, Pork, 1 taco	260	10	28
• Soft, Veggie, 1 taco	310	8	49
Tortillas			
Carb Modified Tortilla, 1 tortilla	110	3	19
Corn Tortillas, 2 each	120	2	24
Flour Tortilla 10", 1 each	210	5	33
Flour Tortilla 13", 1 each	350	9	57
• Flour Tortilla 6", 1 each	100	3	15
Spinach Tortilla 13", 1 each	350	10	56
Taco Salad Shell, 1 each	280	16	29
Taco Shell, 1 each	110	5	14
• Tomato Tortilla 13", 1 each	350	10	56
Whole Wheat Tortilla 13", 1 each	300	5	54
Vegan Burritos			
Almost Vegan, Refried, 1 burrito	430	11	70
Vegan Burrito, Refried, 1 burrito	800	19	133

Taco John's

	Cal	Fat	Cbs
10 g or less of Fat			
Bean Burrito, 7 oz.	320	7	53
Chicken Softshell Taco, 4 oz.	190	6	19
• Crispy Taco, 7 oz.	180	10	13
Mexican Rice, 6 oz.	240	3	36
• Refried Beans, 9 oz.	340	9	49
Softshell Taco, 4 oz.	230	10	20
Taco Burger, 5 oz.	250	9	30
Texas Style Chili, 8 oz.	210	8	26
Breakfast Menu			
Bravo Scrambler® (Bacon), 9 oz.	520	25	53
Bravo Scrambler® (Sausage), 10 oz.	675	44	48
Breakfast Burrito (Bacon), 8 oz.	515	25	52
Breakfast Burrito (Sausage), 9 oz.	620	32	55
Breakfast Egg Burrito, 7 oz.	400	19	39
Breakfast Quesadilla (Bacon), 9 oz.	665	41	41
Breakfast Quesadilla (Sausage), 9 oz.	735	45	42
Breakfast Quesadilla, 8 oz.	570	34	41
• Breakfast Taco (Bacon), 4 oz.	270	13	25
Breakfast Taco (Sausage), 4 oz.	320	17	26

RESTAURANTS & FAST-FOOD CHAINS

Taco John's (cont.)

	Cal	Fat	Cbs
Breakfast Menu (cont.)			
Scrambler Burrito (Bacon), 9 oz.	520	25	53
Scrambler Burrito (Sausage), 9 oz.	620	32	52
Super Olés Scrambler (Bacon), 14 oz.	960	62	75
• Super Olés Scrambler (Sausage), 16 oz.	1120	72	76
Burritos			
• Bean Burrito, 7 oz.	380	10	53
Beef Grilled Burrito, 8 oz.	590	30	49
Beefy Burrito, 7 oz.	430	20	41
Chicken & Potato Burrito, 8 oz.	460	20	54
Chicken & Rice Burrito, 10 oz.	520	20	68
Chicken Grilled Burrito, 8 oz.	590	30	47
Combination Burrito, 7 oz.	400	15	47
Crunchy Chicken and Potato Burrito, 9 oz.	590	30	62
Meat & Potato Burrito, 8 oz.	490	20	55
Steak & Potato Burrito, 8 oz.	460	20	53
Steak & Rice Burrito, 10 oz.	520	20	67
• Steak Grilled Burrito, 8 oz.	600	35	46
Super Burrito, 9 oz.	450	20	49
Desserts			
Apple Grande, 3 oz.	240	10	41
• Choco Taco, 4 oz.	385	20	48
Churro, 2 oz.	235	10	31
• Giant Goldfish® Grahams, 1 bag	120	5	19
Local Favorites			
• Chili Cheese Potato Olés®, 11 oz.	610	36	59
Chili Enchilada, 8 oz.	315	16	24
Mexi Rolls® - 2 Piece w/o Nacho Cheese, 2 oz.	155	7	16
• Nacho Cheese, 2 oz.	60	5	2
Ranch Burrito (Beef), 7 oz.	420	22	41
Ranch Burrito (Chicken), 7 oz.	390	18	40
Smothered Burrito, 11 oz.	505	21	55
Sides			
Chili, 8 oz.	270	10	26
Mexican Rice, 6 oz.	250	5	45
Nachos, 5 oz.	380	20	38
• Potato Olés® (Medium), 7 oz.	620	35	67
Potato Olés® with Nacho Cheese, 8 oz.	550	35	52
Refried Beans, 10 oz.	395	15	50
• Side Salad w/o dressing, 4 oz.	80	5	6
Specialties			
Cheese Quesadilla, 6 oz.	480	30	39
• Chicken Festiva Salad w/o dressing, 11 oz.	400	25	24
Chicken Quesadilla, 7 oz.	540	30	41
Chicken Super Nachos, 12 oz.	780	45	62
Chicken Taco Salad w/o dressing, 13 oz.	540	30	44
Crunchy Chkn Festiva Salad w/o dressing, 11 oz.	580	35	35
Crunchy Chicken Taco Salad w/o dressing, 14 oz.	710	40	56
Crunchy Chicken w/ Ketchipotle, 5 oz.	485	30	30
Crunchy Chicken, 5 oz.	455	30	24
Steak Festiva Salad w/o dressing, 11 oz.	410	25	23
Steak Quesadilla, 7 oz.	545	30	40
Steak Taco Salad w/o dressing, 13 oz.	545	30	43
Super Nachos, 13 oz.	830	50	73
• Super Potato Olés®, 17 oz.	1060	70	91
Taco Salad w/o dressing, 13 oz.	580	30	46
Tacos			
Chicken Softshell Taco, 4 oz.	190	5	19
• Crispy Taco, 3 oz.	180	10	13
Softshell Taco, 4 oz.	220	10	21
Steak Softshell Taco, 4 oz.	190	10	19
• Taco Bravo®, 7 oz.	340	15	39
Taco Burger, 5 oz.	280	10	28

Taco Mayo

	Cal	Fat	Cbs
Burritos			
Bean Burrito, 238 g	496	16	71
• Beef Burrito, 238 g	492	23	41
Beef N Bean Burrito, 238 g	494	19	56
• Super Burrito, 285 g	539	23	57
Drinks			
Piña Colada Chill, 560 g	479	25	59
Strawberry Chiller, 560 g	378	7	79
Favorites			
Beef Soft Taco, 119 g	229	11	17
Chicken Soft Taco, 105 g	184	6	16
• Taco Burger, 161 g	303	13	28
• Taco, 77 g	161	9	10
Tostada, 147 g	295	13	37
Fresh Grilled			
Cheese Quesadilla, 257 g	592	35	45
• Chicken Burrito Supreme, 194 g	407	16	39
Chicken Quesadilla, 313 g	672	37	46
Fajita Chicken Quesadilla, 327 g	698	39	47
• Fajita Steak Quesadilla, 327 g	725	40	47
Mexicali-Chicken Grill Burrito, 238 g	607	30	54
Mexicali-Steak Grill Burrito, 238 g	633	32	54
Steak Burrito Supreme, 194 g	434	18	39
Steak Quesadilla, 313 g	698	38	46
Fresh Grilled			
Chicken Mexicali Bowl, 572 g	1152	59	115
DoSmoChili-Beef, 547 g	955	40	100
DoSmoChili-Chicken, 519 g	879	32	99
DoSmoChili-Steak, 519 g	905	34	99
DoSmoQueso-Chicken, 519 g	883	32	101
DoSmoQueso-Steak, 519 g	910	34	101
DoSmoVerde-Chicken, 519 g	856	31	101
DoSmoVerde-Steak, 519 g	883	32	101
• Fajita-Chicken Grill Burrito, 224 g	492	23	42
Fajita-Steak Grill Burrito, 224 g	519	25	42
• Steak Mexicali Bowl, 557 g	1158	60	115
Tamale Grande Platter, 439 g	714	31	78
Nachos			
• Classic-Cheese Nachos, 135 g	377	19	45
Classic-Chicken Nacho Supreme, 313 g	510	26	48
Classic-Nacho Supreme, 342 g	719	37	70
Classic-Steak Nacho Supreme, 313 g	537	27	48
FB-Cheese Nachos, 123 g	505	31	40
FB-Chicken Nacho Supreme, 306 g	638	37	43
FB-Nacho Supreme, 335 g	846	49	65
FB-Steak Nacho Supreme, 306 g	664	39	43
Queso-Cheese Nacho, 142 g	407	21	45
Queso-Chicken Nacho Supreme, 320 g	539	27	47
Queso-Nacho Supreme, 345 g	748	38	70
Queso-Steak Nacho Supreme, 320 g	566	28	47
• Ultimate Nacho, 523 g	968	49	102
Salads			
Chicken Acapulco Salad, 350 g	678	50	35
• Chicken Taco Salad, 334 g	438	23	30
• Steak Acapulco Salad, 350 g	705	51	35
Steak Taco Salad, 320 g	444	25	30
Taco Salad, 460 g	705	38	57
Sides			
Guac N' Chips, 163 g	386	21	45
• Mexicali Rice, 140 g	160	1	36
• Potato Loco-Lg, 196 g	586	37	55
Potato Loco-Sm, 133 g	379	24	36
Queso N' Chips, 170 g	449	22	49
Refried Beans, 168 g	294	9	43

Tacone

	Cal	Fat	Cbs
Breakfast			
El Grande Wrap, 149 g	280	16	20
Venice Beach Wrap, 354 g	630	31	46
Desserts			
Fresh Fruit Salad, 227 g	80	0	21
Farm Fresh Salads			
• Caesar, 307 g	500	46	18
• Fiesta, 310 g	340	19	18
T.J. Cobb, 272 g	430	30	6
Flavor Sides			
• Grilled Veggies + Feta, 4 oz.	170	14	6
Spa Salad, 225 g	190	9	22
• Sweet Potato Fries, 109 g	190	9	23
Global Grill Platter			
Empire Steak, 468 g	380	21	14
Napa Valley Chicken, 355 g	320	15	10
• Rotisserie Chicken, 595 g	830	37	37
• Tradewind Shrimp, 457 g	250	12	14
Gourmet Wraps			
Baja Wrap with Chicken, 238 g	420	13	47
Baja, 215 g	370	11	54
• Buffalo Kickin' Chicken Wrap, 1/2 wrap	460	12	43
Campfire, 213 g	340	2	41
Kickin' Fried Chicken, 151 g	280	11	22
Kingston, 1/2 wrap	320	10	41
Malibu Melt, 173 g	360	17	25
Mambo, 146 g	220	7	26
Perfect Ten Wrap, 1/2 wrap	360	17	43
Pilgrim, 158 g	260	14	21
Spa, 136 g	200	9	26
Thai Cone, 177 g	300	9	35
• Try Our Lo-Carb Whole Wheat Tortilla, 90 g	180	6	33
Grilled Sandwiches			
• Angus Khan Burger, 411 g	1150	69	56
Chick-a-Boom, 256 g	570	38	25
Great Gobbler, 237 g	470	24	40
United Steak of America, 196 g	560	40	23
• Veggie Caprese, 115 g	310	18	29
Kids			
• Grilled Cheese + Tortilla Chips, 68 g	220	11	20
Kickin' Fried Chicken Jr., 142 g	250	24	7
• Quesadilla Jr., 122 g	420	22	35
Quesadillas			
• 4 Cheese, 85 g	210	11	18
• Apollonia, 225 g	640	39	39
BBQ Chicken, 136 g	300	13	28
Smoothies & Desserts			
Bikini Blast, 617 g	410	2	94
Blue Voodoo, 583 g	400	1	93
• Orangabang, 539 g	360	1	84
Palm Peach, 834 g	500	2	116
• Pink Flamingo, 658 g	520	1	125
Tacone® Sides			
Black Beans + Jack Cheese, 4 oz.	210	5	27
Down-Home Coleslaw, 4 oz.	35	1	7
• Homemade Tortilla Chips + Salsa, 142 g	300	12	42
Seasoned French Fries, 108 g	200	9	29
Seasoned Potato Chips, 86 g	160	8	21
Tacone® Rice, 170 g	240	1	51
Tacone® Side Salad, 100 g	140	11	9
• Thai Cucumber Salad, 122 g	20	0	5

Tastee-Freez

	Cal	Fat	Cbs

For Tastee-Freez nutritional information, please see Wienerschnitzel on pg. 384

TCBY

	Cal	Fat	Cbs
Hand-Scooped Frozen Yogurt & Sorbet			
Butter Pecan Perfection, 4 fl.oz.	110	5	14
Chocolate Chocolate Swirl, 4 fl.oz.	120	4	19
Chocolate Chunk Cookie Dough, 4 fl.oz.	160	6	24
Cookies & Cream, 4 fl.oz.	140	4	22
Cotton Candy, 4 fl.oz.	120	4	20
Mint Chocolate Chunk, 4 fl.oz.	140	5	22
Mocha Almond, 4 fl.oz.	150	5	22
No Sugar Added Choco Choco Swirl, 4 fl.oz.	90	1	23
No Sugar Added Vanilla Fudge Brownie, 4 fl.oz.	100	2	22
• No Sugar Added (NSA) Vanilla, 4 fl.oz.	80	1	19
Pralines & Cream, 4 fl.oz.	140	5	23
• Psychedelic Sorbet, 4 fl.oz.	290	0	75
Rainbow Cream, 4 fl.oz.	120	4	20
Rocky Road, 4 fl.oz.	220	7	36
Strawberries & Cream, 4 fl.oz.	120	3	21
Vanilla Bean, 4 fl.oz.	120	4	19
Vanilla Chocolate Chunk, 4 fl.oz.	140	5	22
Smoothies			
Berrylicious, 16 fl.oz.	290	3	65
• Black 'n Blueberry, 16 fl.oz.	280	3	63
Mango Tango, 16 fl.oz.	330	3	76
Mangolada, 16 fl.oz.	340	6	70
Mondo Mango, 16 fl.oz.	310	3	70
• Pina Paradise, 16 fl.oz.	350	12	58
Pink Pineapple, 16 fl.oz.	340	9	63
Straight-Up Strawberry, 16 fl.oz.	280	4	64
Strawberry Bananza, 16 fl.oz.	320	4	74
Strawberry Fling, 16 fl.oz.	340	3	78
Soft Serve Creamy Frozen Yogurt & Fruity Sorbet			
• 96% Fat Free Frozen Yogurt, 97 g	140	3	23
Low Carb Frozen Yogurt, 92 g	110	7	16
• No Sugar Added Nonfat Frozen Yogurt, 96 g	90	0	20
NonFat & NonDairy Sorbet, 97 g	100	0	24
NonFat Frozen Yogurt, 98 g	110	0	23

The Coffee Bean & Tea Leaf

	Cal	Fat	Cbs
Coffee Ice Blended® Drinks			
Blk Forest No Sgr Added Pwder & Soy Mlk, 16 oz.	270	5	46
Black Forest No Sugar Added Powder, 16 oz.	270	5	47
Black Forest Soy Milk, 16 oz.	490	11	90
• Black Forest, 16 oz.	500	10	91
Caramel NSA Powder & Soy Milk, 16 oz.	290	4	57
Caramel NSA Powder, 16 oz.	300	3	57
Caramel Soy Milk, 16 oz.	530	11	98
Caramel, 16 oz.	540	11	99
Extreme Caramel NSA Powder, 16 oz.	270	3	54
Extreme Caramel, 16 oz.	510	11	95
• Extreme Mocha NSA Powder, 16 oz.	110	1	21
Extreme Mocha, 16 oz.	340	7	65
Extreme Ultimate Mocha NSA Powder, 16 oz.	160	5	27
Extreme Ultimate Mocha, 16 oz.	390	10	71
Extreme Ultimate Vanilla NSA Powder, 16 oz.	170	4	28
Extreme Ultimate Vanilla, 16 oz.	410	12	70
Extreme Vanilla NSA Powder, 16 oz.	120	1	22
Extreme Vanilla, 16 oz.	360	9	63
Mocha NSA Powder & Soy Milk, 16 oz.	130	2	23
Mocha NSA Powder, 16 oz.	140	1	24
Mocha Soy Milk, 16 oz.	360	8	67
Mocha, 16 oz.	370	7	68
Ultimate Mocha NSA Powder & Soy Milk, 16 oz.	190	5	30
Ultimate Mocha NSA Powder, 16 oz.	190	5	31
Ultimate Mocha Soy Milk, 16 oz.	410	11	74
Ultimate Mocha, 16 oz.	420	10	75
Ultimate Vanilla NSA Powder & Soy Milk, 16 oz.	200	5	31
Ultimate Vanilla NSA Powder, 16 oz.	200	4	32

The Coffee Bean & Tea Leaf (cont.)

	Cal	Fat	Cbs
Coffee Ice Blended® Drinks (cont.)			
Ultimate Vanilla Soy Milk, 16 oz.	440	13	72
Ultimate Vanilla Ice, 16 oz.	440	12	73
Vanilla Ice NSA Powder & Soy Milk, 16 oz.	140	2	25
Vanilla Ice NSA Powder, 16 oz.	150	1	25
Vanilla Ice Soy Milk, 16 oz.	380	10	66
Vanilla Ice, 16 oz.	390	9	67
White Chocolate Dream® Soy Milk, 16 oz.	440	19	66
White Chocolate Dream®, 16 oz.	450	18	67
Espresso & Coffee Hot Drinks			
Americano, 16 oz.	10	0	1
Brewed Coffee, 16 oz.	5	0	0
Café Caramel NSA Powder & Soy Milk, 16 oz.	220	3	43
Café Caramel NSA Powder, 16 oz.	220	2	44
Café Caramel Soy Milk, 16 oz.	300	6	57
Café Caramel, 16 oz.	300	5	58
Café Latté Nonfat Milk, 16 oz.	160	0	24
Café Latté Soy Milk, 16 oz.	150	5	20
Café Latté Whole Milk, 16 oz.	270	14	24
Café Mocha NSA Powder & Soy Milk, 16 oz.	110	2	18
Café Mocha NSA Powder, 16 oz.	110	1	19
Café Mocha Soy Milk, 16 oz.	270	6	49
Café Mocha, 16 oz.	270	5	50
Café Vanilla NSA Powder & Soy Milk, 16 oz.	120	2	19
Café Vanilla NSA Powder, 16 oz.	120	1	20
Café Vanilla Soy Milk, 16 oz.	280	7	48
Café Vanilla, 16 oz.	290	7	48
Café White Chocolate Soy Milk, 16 oz.	330	14	49
Café White Chocolate, 16 oz.	330	14	49
Cappuccino Double Nonfat Milk, 12 oz.	70	0	10
Cappuccino Double Soy Milk, 12 oz.	60	2	9
Cappuccino Double Whole Milk, 12 oz.	110	6	10
Cappuccino Single Nonfat Milk, 12 oz.	80	0	11
Cappuccino Single Soy Milk, 12 oz.	70	2	10
Cappuccino Single Whole Milk, 12 oz.	130	7	11
Caramel Latté NSA Powder & Soy Milk, 16 oz.	320	6	57
Caramel Latté NSA Powder, 16 oz.	330	2	60
Caramel Latté Soy Milk, 16 oz.	400	9	72
Caramel Latté, 16 oz.	420	5	75
Double Espresso Macchiato Nonfat Milk, 4 oz.	10	0	2
Double Espresso Macchiato Soy Milk, 4 oz.	10	0	2
Double Espresso Macchiato Whole Milk, 4 oz.	15	1	2
Mocha Latté NSA Powder & Soy Milk, 16 oz.	210	5	32
Mocha Latté NSA Powder, 16 oz.	230	1	36
Mocha Latté Soy Milk, 16 oz.	370	9	64
Mocha Latté, 16 oz.	380	5	67
Single Espresso Macchiato Nonfat Milk, 4 oz.	10	0	1
Single Espresso Macchiato Soy Milk, 4 oz.	10	0	1
Single Espresso Macchiato Whole Milk, 4 oz.	10	1	1
• Single Espresso, 4 oz.	5	0	0
Vanilla Latté NSA Powder & Soy Milk, 16 oz.	220	5	33
Vanilla Latté NSA Powder, 16 oz.	230	1	37
Vanilla Latté Soy Milk, 16 oz.	390	10	63
Vanilla Latté, 16 oz.	400	7	66
White Chocolate Dream® Latté Soy Milk, 16 oz.	430	17	64
• White Chocolate Dream® Latté, 16 oz.	450	14	67
Fru Tea™ Ice Blended® Drinks			
• Lemon Zest FruTea™, 16 oz.	320	0	83
Mucho Mango FruTea™, 16 oz.	240	0	60
• Pomegranate FruTea™, 16 oz.	210	0	58
Hot Tea & Tea Lattés			
• Hot Tea, 16 oz.	5	0	1
Tea Latté w/ Choco & NSA Pwdr & Soy Milk, 16 oz.	110	2	19
Tea Latté w/ Choco Powder NSA Powder, 16 oz.	110	1	20
Tea Latté w/ Choco Powder Soy Milk, 16 oz.	270	6	50

The Coffee Bean & Tea Leaf (cont.)

	Cal	Fat	Cbs
Hot Tea & Tea Lattés (cont.)			
Tea Latté w/ Chocolate Powder, 16 oz.	270	5	51
Tea Latté w/ Vanilla NSA Powder, Soy Milk, 16 oz.	120	2	20
Tea Latté w/ Vanilla Powder NSA Powder, 16 oz.	120	1	21
Tea Latté w/ Vanilla Powder Soy Milk, 16 oz.	280	7	49
• Tea Latté w/ Vanilla Powder, 16 oz.	290	7	50
Iced Espresso & Coffee Drinks			
Iced Cappuccino Nonfat Milk, 16 oz.	60	0	9
Iced Cappuccino Soy Milk, 16 oz.	50	2	7
Iced Cappuccino, 16 oz.	90	5	9
Iced Caramel Latté NSA & Soy Milk, 16 oz.	270	5	51
Iced Caramel Latté NSA Powder, 16 oz.	280	2	53
Iced Caramel Latté Soy Milk, 16 oz.	350	7	65
• Iced Caramel Latté, 16 oz.	360	5	67
Iced Coffee, 16 oz.	10	0	1
Iced Latte Nonfat Milk, 16 oz.	100	0	14
Iced Latte Soy Milk, 16 oz.	90	3	12
Iced Latte, 16 oz.	160	8	14
Iced Mocha Latte NSA Powder & Soy Milk, 16 oz.	150	3	24
Iced Mocha Latte NSA Powder, 16 oz.	160	1	26
Iced Mocha Latte Soy Milk, 16 oz.	310	7	55
Iced Mocha Latte, 16 oz.	320	5	57
• Iced Tea, 16 oz.	0	0	1
Iced Vanilla Latte NSA Powder & Soy Milk, 16 oz.	160	3	25
Iced Vanilla Latte NSA Powder, 16 oz.	170	1	27
Iced Vanilla Latte Soy Milk, 16 oz.	320	8	54
Iced Vanilla Latte, 16 oz.	330	7	56
Kid Friendly! Non Coffee & Non Tea			
Hot Chocolate NSA Powder & Soy Milk, 16 oz.	230	6	34
Hot Chocolate NSA Powder, 16 oz.	250	1	39
Hot Chocolate Soy Milk, 16 oz.	380	10	66
Hot Chocolate, 16 oz.	400	5	69
• Hot Vanilla NSA Powder & Soy Milk, 16 oz.	230	5	35
Hot Vanilla NSA Powder, 16 oz.	250	1	40
Hot Vanilla Soy Milk, 16 oz.	400	11	64
• Hot Vanilla, 16 oz.	420	7	68
Non Coffee Ice Blended® Drinks			
Banana Caramel NSA Powder, 16 oz.	330	3	69
• Banana Caramel, 16 oz.	570	11	110
• Chai Ice NSA Powder, 16 oz.	110	1	20
Chai, 16 oz.	350	9	62
Green Tea Soy Milk, 16 oz.	480	11	81
Green Tea, 16 oz.	480	10	82
Malibu Dream™ NSA Powder, 16 oz.	200	1	41
Malibu Dream™, 16 oz.	440	9	82
Pomegranate Blueberry NSA Powder, 16 oz.	220	1	46
Pomegranate Blueberry, 16 oz.	460	9	87
Pure Chocolate NSA Powder & Soy Milk, 16 oz.	160	3	26
Pure Chocolate NSA Powder, 16 oz.	160	1	28
Pure Chocolate Soy Milk, 16 oz.	390	9	70
Pure Chocolate, 16 oz.	390	7	72
Pure Vanilla NSA Powder & Soy Milk, 16 oz.	170	3	27
Pure Vanilla NSA Powder, 16 oz.	170	1	29
Pure Vanilla Soy Milk, 16 oz.	410	11	69
Pure Vanilla, 16 oz.	410	9	70

The Great American Bagel

	Cal	Fat	Cbs
Bagels			
4-Grain Honey, 5 oz., 1 bagel	390	4	80
Apple Cinnamon Oat Bran, 5 oz., 1 bagel	370	4	73
Apple Cinnamon Sugar, 5 oz., 1 bagel	390	4	78
Apple Crumb, 9 oz., 1 bagel	620	11	118
Asiago w/ Bl & Gr Olives, 7 oz., 1 bagel	540	20	70
Asiago, 7 oz., 1 bagel	520	16	72
Banana Nut, 5 oz., 1 bagel	410	9	69
Blueberry Crumb, 9 oz., 1 bagel	630	10	122

The Great American Bagel (cont.)

	Cal	Fat	Cbs
Bagels (cont.)			
Blueberry, 5 oz., 1 bagel	370	4	75
Cheddar Bacon, 7 oz., 1 bagel	600	23	71
Cheddar Herb, 5 oz., 1 bagel	390	8	66
Cheddar Onion, 6 oz., 1 bagel	500	13	75
Cheddar Salsa, 7 oz., 1 bagel	500	17	68
• Cheddar Twist, 9 oz., 1 bagel	800	27	107
Chocolate Chip, 5 oz., 1 bagel	420	8	78
Cinnamon Delight, 7 oz., 1 bagel	640	18	108
Cinnamon Raisin, 5 oz., 1 bagel	380	4	76
Egg, 5 oz., 1 bagel	370	5	70
Everything, 5 oz., 1 bagel	380	5	73
French Toast, 5 oz., 1 bagel	430	8	77
Garlic, 5 oz., 1 bagel	390	4	75
Harvest 10-grain, 5 oz., 1 bagel	410	8	73
Hot Tomazzor, 8 oz., 1 bagel	520	13	77
Jalapeño Cheddar, 5 oz., 1 bagel	370	7	63
Onion, 5 oz., 1 bagel	380	4	74
PB Chocolate Chip, 5 oz., 1 bagel	420	8	76
Pesto, 5 oz., 1 bagel	360	5	67
Plain, 5 oz., 1 bagel	360	4	71
Poppy, 5 oz., 1 bagel	390	6	72
Provolone, 6 oz., 1 bagel	460	11	72
Pumpernickel, 5 oz., 1 bagel	360	4	71
Salt, 5 oz., 1 bagel	360	4	71
Sesame, 5 oz., 1 bagel	390	6	72
Sourdough Baguette, 4 oz.	300	4	56
Spinach Herb, 5 oz., 1 bagel	350	4	70
Strawberry Crumb, 9 oz., 1 bagel	630	10	123
Strawberry, 5 oz., 1 bagel	380	4	76
Stuffed Pepperoni, 9 oz., 1 bagel	570	17	78
Stuffed Spinach, 9 oz., 1 bagel	640	20	86
Sun-dried Tomato Basil, 5 oz., 1 bagel	390	4	74
Swiss Cheese, 6 oz., 1 bagel	470	12	72
Tomazzor, 8 oz., 1 bagel	520	13	77
Veggie, 5 oz., 1 bagel	310	4	61
• Whole Wheat Baguette, 4 oz.	290	4	56
Whole Wheat, 5 oz., 1 bagel	370	4	74
Cream Cheese Flavors			
Apple Cinnamon, 1 oz.	60	5	4
Blue Berry, 1 oz.	60	4	4
Chocolate Chip, 1 oz.	70	4	8
Cream Apple, 1 oz.	70	4	7
Cucumber, 1 oz.	60	5	1
Garlic Herb, 1 oz.	60	5	1
Lox, 1 oz.	60	5	1
Pineapple Walnut, 1 oz.	70	6	2
Plain, 1 oz.	60	5	1
Salsa, 1 oz.	50	5	1
Scallion, 1 oz.	50	5	1
Spinach, 1 oz.	50	4	1
Strawberry, 1 oz.	55	5	1
Vegetable, 1 oz.	62	5	1
• Walnut Raisin, 1 oz.	80	6	6

Tim Horton's

	Cal	Fat	Cbs
Bagels			
Blueberry, 1 bagel	270	1	55
Cinnamon Raisin, 1 bagel	270	1	55
Cream Cheese - Garden Vegetable, 1.5 oz.	120	11	3
Cream Cheese - Light Plain, 1.5 oz.	85	6	3
Cream Cheese - Plain, 1.5 oz.	130	12	2
Cream Cheese - Strawberry, 1.5 oz.	120	10	6
Everything, 1 bagel	280	2	53
Flax Seed, 1 bagel	290	5	53
Onion, 1 bagel	260	2	53

Tim Horton's (cont.)

	Cal	Fat	Cbs
Bagels (cont.)			
• Plain, 1 bagel	260	2	52
Poppy Seed, 1 bagel	270	2	53
Sesame Seed, 1 bagel	270	3	53
Sun Dried Tomato, 1 bagel	310	4	59
• Twelve Grain, 1 bagel	330	9	52
Breakfast			
Bacon, Egg, Cheese	410	25	31
Bagel B.E.L.T.	450	14	58
Egg, Cheese	360	21	30
• Hash Brown	100	5	12
Sausage, Egg, Cheese	520	37	30
Cookies			
Caramel Chocolate Pecan, 1 cookie	230	11	32
Chocolate Chip, 1 cookie	230	9	34
• Oatmeal Raisin Spice, 1 cookie	220	8	35
• Peanut Butter Chocolate Chunk, 1 cookie	260	15	28
Triple Chocolate, 1 cookie	250	13	31
White Chocolate Macadamia Nut, 1 cookie	240	12	31
Donuts			
Angel Cream, 1 donut	310	13	46
Apple Fritter, 1 donut	300	11	49
Blueberry Fritter, 1 donut	330	10	55
Blueberry, 1 donut	230	8	36
Boston Cream, 1 donut	250	9	38
Canadian Maple, 1 donut	260	9	41
Chocolate Dip, 1 donut	210	9	30
Chocolate Glazed, 1 donut	260	10	39
Honey Cruller, 1 donut	320	19	37
Honey Dip, 1 donut	210	8	33
• Maple Dip, 1 donut	210	8	31
Old Fashion Glazed, 1 donut	320	19	35
Old Fashion Plain, 1 donut	260	19	20
Sour Cream Plain, 1 donut	270	17	27
Strawberry, 1 donut	230	8	36
• Walnut Crunch, 1 donut	360	23	35
Muffins			
Blueberry Bran, 1 muffin	300	10	53
Blueberry, 1 muffin	330	11	55
• Chocolate Chip Plain, 1 muffin	430	16	69
Cranberry Blueberry Bran, 1 muffin	290	10	51
Cranberry Fruit, 1 muffin	350	12	59
Fruit Explosion, 1 muffin	360	11	61
• Lowfat Blueberry, 1 muffin	290	3	62
Lowfat Cranberry, 1 muffin	290	3	62
Raisin Bran, 1 muffin	360	10	65
Strawberry Sensation, 1 muffin	350	11	61
Wheat Carrot, 1 muffin	400	19	55
Sandwiches			
B.L.T. (w/ mayonnaise), 1 piece	450	18	53
Chicken Salad (with lettuce & tomato)	380	9	55
Country Bun – white	240	1	49
• Country Bun – whole wheat	230	1	46
Egg Salad (with lettuce)	390	13	52
Ham & Swiss (w/ Tim's Own dressing), 1 piece	440	12	56
• Toasted Chicken Club (w/ bacon), 1 piece	460	7	70
Turkey Bacon Club (w/ honey mustard), 1 piece	440	8	63
Turkey Breast (w/ Tim's Own dressing), 1 piece	390	5	59
Soups & Chili			
Beef Stew, 10 oz.	236	8	25
Chicken Noodle, 10 oz.	120	2	18
• Chili, 10 oz.	300	16	18
Cream of Broccoli, 10 oz.	160	9	16
Creamy Field Mushroom, 10 oz.	150	3	28
• Hearty Vegetable, 10 oz.	70	0	14

Tim Horton's (cont.)

	Cal	Fat	Cbs
Soups & Chili (cont.)			
Minestrone, 10 oz.	120	3	24
Potato Bacon, 10 oz.	180	6	30
Split Pea with Ham, 10 oz.	150	3	27
Turkey Rice, 10 oz.	120	2	21
Vegetable Beef Barley, 10 oz.	110	2	21
Specialty Baked Goods			
Butter Croissant, 1 croissant	340	18	38
Cheese Croissant, 1 croissant	370	20	37
Cherry Cheese Danish, 1 danish	330	13	46
Chocolate Danish, 1 danish	430	24	51
• Cinnamon Roll – Frosted, 1 roll	470	25	57
Cinnamon Roll – Glazed, 1 roll	420	23	50
Maple Pecan Danish, 1 danish	380	20	46
• Plain Tea Biscuit, 1 biscuit	250	9	35
Raisin Tea Biscuit, 1 biscuit	290	10	45
Timbits®			
• Apple Fritter, 1 timbit	50	2	9
Banana Cream, 1 timbit	60	2	9
Blueberry, 1 timbit	60	2	10
Chocolate Glazed, 1 timbit	70	3	10
Honey Dip, 1 timbit	60	2	9
Lemon, 1 timbit	60	2	9
Old Fashion Plain, 1 timbit	70	5	5
• Sour Cream Glazed, 1 timbit	90	5	12
Strawberry, 1 timbit	60	2	10
Yogurt & Berries			
Lowfat Creamy Vanilla Yogurt w/ Berries, 6 oz.	160	3	32
Lowfat Strawberry Yogurt w/ Berries, 6 oz.	150	3	32

Topz

	Cal	Fat	Cbs
Aero Fries, Rings & Nuggets			
Aero Fries, 158 g	380	14	58
• Aero Onion Rings, 166 g	298	11	46
• Chili Cheese Fries, 301 g	589	27	66
Dessertz			
Brownie, 105 g	350	5	67
• Chocolate Chip Cookie, 105 g	385	9	67
• Lowfat Ice Cream w/ Choc. Syrup, 162 g	255	7	43
Oatmeal Raisin Cookie, 105 g	385	9	67
Fresh Gourmet Salads			
• Chinese Chicken Salad, 392 g	322	14	17
Dijon Deli Chopped Salad, 382 g	229	13	9
Ginger Grilled Ahi Salad, 392 g	312	15	10
• Small Dijon Deli Salad, 21 g	101	6	3
Fruit Shakez			
• Chocolate Banana Shake, 472 g	460	8	80
Chocolate Shake, 372 g	360	9	55
Raspberry Shake, 427 g	404	9	64
• Strawberry Shake, 427 g	356	9	54
Gourmet Hot Dogs			
• Beef Chili Dog, 269 g	485	24	49
Double Turkey Dog, 242 g	390	8	60
Hebrew National Beef Dog, 230 g	450	21	52
• Turkey Chili Dog, 255 g	355	9	53
Gourmet Lean Burgers			
1/2 lb. Black Angus Burger w/o Sauce, 392 g	672	34	37
• 1/2 lb. Black Angus Burger, 415 g	735	40	40
1/4 lb. Black Angus Burger, w/o sauce, 278 g	444	19	37
1/4 lb. Black Angus Burger, 301 g	507	25	40
1/4 lb. Black Angus Chili Burger, 318 g	489	21	42
• Garden Burger, 228 g	355	12	46
Turkey Burger, 301 g	449	19	40
Kidz Mealz			
• Kidz Grilled Cheese, 62 g	207	9	24
• Kidz Beef Dog, 145 g	405	21	40

Topz (cont.)

	Cal	Fat	Cbs
Kidz Mealz (cont.)			
Kidz Burger, 184 g	408	19	33
Kidz Turkey Dog, 131 g	275	7	44
Signature Chili			
Signature Chili, 291 g	329	17	17
Signature Lean Sandwiches			
Classic Grilled Cheese Sandwich, 123 g	414	18	47
• Ginger Grilled Ahi Sandwich, 268 g	384	11	37
• Grilled Cheese & Tomato Sandwich, 144 g	418	18	40
Grilled Chicken Breast Sandwich, 290 g	396	10	39

Tropical Smoothie

	Cal	Fat	Cbs
Cheeses			
American, 2/3 oz.	53	4	0
Lowfat Mozzarella, 3 oz.	80	5	1
Pepper Jack, 2/3 oz.	50	5	0
Provolone	50	4	1
• Shredded Cheddar, 1/3 cup	177	15	1
• Shredded Parmesan, 1 oz.	50	3	0
Swiss, 2/3 oz.	55	4	0
Dessert Smoothies: w/ Splenda			
Beach Bum (Chocolate)	366	5	75
Beach Bum (Vanilla)	370	6	66
Chocolate Chiller	356	7	68
Coconut Royale	531	11	105
Mocha Madness	447	12	77
• Peanut Butter Cup	638	24	92
• Tropi-colada	299	6	61
Kid's Menu			
Cheese Quesadilla	559	26	53
• Cheese Quesadilla w/Chicken	611	27	54
Ham and American Sandwich	257	7	32
Ham and American Wrap	422	14	53
• Turkey and American Sandwich	268	6	32
Turkey and American Wrap	433	13	53
Kids Smoothies: w/ Splenda			
• Chocolate Chimp	160	3	32
• Jetty Jr.	85	0	20
Orange Delight	100	3	17
Lowfat Smoothies: w/ Splenda			
Blimey Limey	210	0	52
• Blue Lagoon	130	1	30
Cool Breeze	209	0	49
Hawaiian Breeze	160	0	38
Island Fever	253	1	61
Jetty Punch	169	1	39
Kiwi Quencher	217	0	52
Mango Magic	203	0	47
Orange Passion	250	0	59
Paradise Point	263	1	62
Peaches n' Silk	182	1	43
• Raspberry Rush	384	1	90
Rockin' Raspberry	213	1	50
Strawberry Beach	151	0	34
Sunny Day	301	1	72
Sunrise Sunset	191	0	46
Toucan Delight	232	1	54
Power Smoothies: w/ Splenda			
Fat Buster	173	1	41
Health Nut	418	11	54
• Lean Machine	173	1	40
Morning After	241	1	57
Muscle Blaster	397	3	69
• Peanut Paradise	610	22	69
Salads			
Caesar Salad, 1 salad	116	1	8

Tropical Smoothie (cont.)

	Cal	Fat	Cbs
Salads (cont.)			
Chef Salad, 1 salad	172	2	11
• Garden Classic Salad, 1 salad	59	1	10
• Sesame Chicken Salad, 1 salad	417	10	53
Thai Chicken Salad, 1 salad	353	4	54
Sauces			
Balsamic Vinaigrette Dressing, 1 oz.	61	5	4
Caesar Dressing, 1 oz.	160	17	1
• Chipotle Dressing, 1 oz.	180	20	2
• Fat Free Italian, 1 oz.	8	0	2
Franks Red Hot Sauce, 1 oz.	10	0	1
Jamaican Jerk Sauce, 1 oz.	40	0	9
Light Ranch, 1 oz.	100	10	1
Light Ranch, 1/2 oz.	50	5	1
Mango Habanero Sauce, 1 oz.	30	0	7
Mayonnaise, Lowfat 1 oz.	50	5	1
Mayonnaise, Reduced Calorie, 1 oz.	80	7	4
Salsa, 1 oz.	10	0	3
Sesame Dressing, 1 oz.	90	5	11
Texas Petal Sauce, 1 oz.	160	17	1
Texas Petal Sauce, 1/2 oz.	80	9	1
Thai Peanut Dressing, 1 oz.	74	3	10
Specialty Breads			
Focaccia, 1 pc.	295	3	60
Specialty Sandwiches			
American Albacore	725	29	85
Cheese BLT Sandwich	717	37	72
Chicken Caesar Sandwich	624	25	66
Chipolte Chicken Sandwich	660	27	71
Club	703	26	77
Ham and Cheese	604	19	78
Roast Beef	681	30	63
• The Italian	748	39	71
Turkey Bacon Ranch	669	23	69
• Tuscan Turkey	439	13	67
Splendid Dessert Smoothies: w/ Splenda			
Chocolate Banana	410	7	81
Orange Dream	377	5	79
Splendid Smoothies: w/ Splenda			
• Citrus Split	196	1	47
Cranberry Crush	184	0	45
Pineapple Delight	181	0	44
• Strawberry Light	139	0	31
Supercharged Smoothies: w/ Splenda			
Banana Berry Boost	197	2	45
Get Up and Goji	225	0	53
Island Intensity	202	2	45
Mango Moxie	253	0	60
• Pomegranate Plunge	275	0	67
• Strawberry Stamina	197	1	45
Tortillas			
Garlic Herb Tortilla, 1 pc.	299	8	49
White Tortilla, 1 pc.	312	8	51
Wraps			
Breakfast Wrap (Bacon)	537	23	55
• Breakfast Wrap (Ham)	524	18	57
Buffalo Chicken	566	21	61
Chicken Cordon Bleu	610	26	56
Chicken Mango Habanero	654	14	95
Cool Tuna Wrap	646	27	71
Early Bird	672	34	56
Jamaican Jerk	579	13	79
King Caesar	557	26	55
Popeyes Favorite	578	20	60
Salsa Sunrise	594	24	57

Tropical Smoothie (cont.)

	Cal	Fat	Cbs
Wraps (cont.)			
• Sesame Chicken	754	24	103
Thai Chicken Wrap	744	15	116
Totally Turkey	653	27	58
Veggie Veggie	615	26	72
Western Wrap	537	18	59

Tubby's

	Cal	Fat	Cbs
Regular: Burger Subs			
American Cheeseburger	810	48	56
• Big Tub	671	56	55
Burger Special	898	59	59
Cheeseburger	911	60	59
Mushroom Burger	868	59	53
• Pizza Burger	929	60	62
Taco	827	47	67
Regular: Burger Wraps			
American Cheeseburger	660	48	19
Burger Special	748	58	22
Cheeseburger	969	61	67
Mushroom Burger	776	59	24
• Pizza Burger	988	61	70
Taco	734	48	38
• Tub	579	57	26
Regular: Chicken Subs			
Chicken & Broccoli	552	23	56
Chicken & Cheddar	543	23	54
• Chicken Club	705	41	53
Chicken Fajita	445	12	57
• Chicken Parmesan	426	14	51
Grilled Chicken	346	5	52
Regular: Chicken Wraps			
Chicken & Broccoli	552	23	56
Chicken & Cheddar	451	24	25
• Chicken Club	613	42	24
Chicken Fajita	353	12	28
Chicken Parmesan	334	15	22
• Grilled Chicken	254	5	23
Regular: Deli Subs			
• Club Sub	701	41	53
Famous	664	39	55
• Ham & Cheese	568	30	54
Turkey & Cheese	598	32	51
Turkey Club	678	38	52
Regular: Deli Wraps			
Club Sub	591	41	23
Famous	570	40	26
• Ham & Cheese	476	31	25
Turkey & Cheese	534	32	22
• Turkey Club	614	38	23
Regular: Specialty Subs			
BLT	636	42	50
Cold Veggie	462	14	66
• Italian Sausage	729	45	56
• Tuna	417	18	47
Veggie Stir Fry	652	27	89
Regular: Steak Subs			
Mushroom Steak	833	26	52
Pepper Steak	709	46	56
• Philly Cheesesteak	685	40	49
• Pizza Steak	986	57	85
Portabella Mushroom	801	48	54
Steak & Cheddar	833	56	52
Steak & Cheese	823	56	51
Steak Special	746	46	58

RESTAURANTS & FAST-FOOD CHAINS

Tubby's (cont.)

Regular: Steak Wraps	Cal	Fat	Cbs
Mushroom Steak	738	56	23
Pepper Steak	617	46	23
• Philly Cheesesteak	593	40	20
• Pizza Steak	750	56	25
Portabella Mushroom	709	48	25
Steak & Cheddar	741	57	23
Steak & Cheese	731	56	22
Steak Special	654	46	29

Una Mas

Burritos	Cal	Fat	Cbs
Bean & Cheese (The Works), 527 g	1063	57	91
Bean & Cheese Burrito, 442 g	923	44	85
Butternut Squash Burrito (The Works), 641 g	842	44	97
Butternut Squash Burrito, 556 g	701	31	91
• Carnitas Burrito (The Works), 626 g	1560	100	84
Carnitas Burrito, 525 g	1367	83	78
Foghead Burrito, 584 g	876	36	102
Fresca Burrito (The Works), 598 g	774	29	105
Fresca Burrito, 499 g	581	12	99
Gallito Griller (The Works), 527 g	1085	63	63
Gallito Griller, 499 g	1024	57	62
Grilled Fajita Burrito-Chicken, 587 g	766	31	87
Grilled Fajita Burrito-Steak, 587 g	851	36	88
Grilled Fajita Burrito-Veggie, 502 g	666	28	86
Lobster Burrito (The Works), 570 g	1029	50	93
Lobster Burrito, 527 g	915	40	92
Mahi-Mahi Burrito (The Works), 587 g	937	53	81
Mahi-Mahi Burrito, 487 g	744	35	75
• Nino Burrito, 255 g	403	12	58
Pineapple Thai Burrito, 390 g	660	19	87
Roasted Pasilla Veggie (The Works), 556 g	710	32	89
Roasted Pasilla Veggie Burrito, 528 g	649	26	88
San Lucas Fish Baja Style (The Works), 550 g	948	53	84
San Lucas Fish Burrito-Baja Style, 451 g	755	36	78
San Lucas Fish Burrito Cabo Style (The Works), 514 g	841	46	75
San Lucas Fish Burrito-Cabo Style, 415 g	648	29	69
Una Mas Burrito- Chicken (The Works), 570 g	779	32	89
Una Mas Burrito-Chicken, 471 g	587	15	84
Una Mas Burrito- Steak (The Works), 570 g	864	36	90
Una Mas Burrito-Steak, 471 g	671	19	84
Vera Cruz Shrimp Baja Style (The Works), 520 g	1149	74	82
Vera Cruz Shrimp Burrito-Baja Style, 491 g	1082	67	81
Vera Cruz Shrimp Cabo Style (The Works), 558 g	940	50	88
Vera Cruz Shrimp Burrito-Cabo Style, 516 g	826	40	86
Wet Style Burrito, 669 g	960	45	95
Dinner Plates			
• Fajitas Plato Combo, 723 g	846	35	81
• Mahi-Mahi Dinner Plate, 707 g	874	45	77
Pescado Ranchero Dinner Plate, 707 g	859	46	75
Enchiladas			
Enchiladas Rojas, 435 g	532	24	50
Nachos			
Mas Nachos with Chicken, 765 g	1949	106	189
• Mas Nachos with Steak, 765 g	2033	110	189
Mas Nachos, 680 g	1850	102	188
• Nachos Ninos, 227 g	564	31	52
Quesadillas			
Monterey Butternut Squash Quesadilla, 458 g	925	57	67
Monterey Quesadilla- Chicken, 429 g	958	57	61
Monterey Quesadilla- Steak, 429 g	1042	61	61
• Monterey Shrimp Quesadilla, 446 g	1073	67	63
• Nino Quesadilla, 242 g	524	26	50
• Quesadilla Chica, 157 g	447	24	38

Una Mas (cont.)

Salad Dressings	Cal	Fat	Cbs
Lime-Jalapeño Vinaigrette, 1 oz.	133	15	1
Tangy Lime Vinaigrette, 1 oz.	153	17	1
Sides			
• Bottomless Bskt of Chips/Salsa Fresca, 340 g	1104	48	158
Chipotle Sauce, 1 tbsp	82	9	0
Corn Salsa, 1/4 cup	22	0	5
Frijoles Negros, 1/2 cup	138	2	24
Frijoles Picantes, 1/2 cup	132	1	24
Guacamole, 1/4 cup	133	12	8
Mexican Fried Rice, 1/2 cup	70	2	12
Nacho Style Fried Tortilla Chips, 1 oz.	135	6	19
Pinto Beans, 1/2 cup	152	2	26
Roasted Pineapple Salsa, 1/4 cup	32	1	6
Salsa Barrio, 1/4 cup	26	1	5
Salsa Blanca, 1/4 cup	376	40	2
• Salsa Fresca, 1/4 cup	12	0	3
Salsa Picante, 1/4 cup	62	5	5
Salsa Ranchera, 1/4 cup	20	1	3
Salsa Roja, 1/4 cup	13	0	3
Salsa Verde, 1/4 cup	21	0	4
Soups & Salads			
Caesar Salad with Chicken, 511 g	886	58	53
Crispy Taco Salad, 426 g	500	26	48
w/ Chicken, 511 g	600	30	49
w/ Steak, 511 g	684	34	50
Crispy Taco & Soup, 1 Taco/8 oz. Soup	728	39	64
Margarita Salad, 554 g	892	70	55
w/ Chicken, 724 g	1078	73	57
• w/ Steak, 724 g	1260	86	58
Spicy Chipotle Chicken Breast Salad, 511 g	571	36	18
• Tortilla Soup (Small), 8 oz.	194	11	10
Verde Salad, 284 g	434	37	22
Tacos			
Crispy Chicken Taco Plate, 224 g	327	17	30
Flautas Puebla (Chicken) Plate, 619 g	784	38	86
Flautas Puebla (Chicken) Side Order, 256 g	362	20	35
• Flautas Puebla (Steak) Plate, 619 g	915	52	86
Flautas Puebla (Steak) Side Order, 256 g	405	25	32
Mahi-Mahi Taco (The Works), 259 g	494	33	32
Mahi-Mahi Taco, 188 g	341	20	28
San Lucas Fish Taco-Baja Style (The Works), 259 g	579	40	38
San Lucas Fish Taco-Baja Style, 188 g	426	26	34
San Lucas Fish Cabo Style (The Works), 223 g	472	33	29
San Lucas Fish Taco-Cabo Style, 153 g	319	19	26
Taco-Butternut Squash, 137 g	218	11	27
Taco-Carnitas, 180 g	460	27	28
• Taqueria Taco (per taco), 86 g	136	7	9
Taqueria Taco Combo Basket (/w Beans), 229 g	320	15	27
Taqueria Taco Combo Basket (/w Rice), 229 g	308	16	24
Una Mas Taco - Steak, 180 g	278	9	33
Una Mas Taco- Chicken (The Works), 222 g	320	14	36
Una Mas Taco- Chicken, 180 g	250	8	33
Una Mas Taco- Steak (The Works), 222 g	348	16	36
Una Mas Taco- Veggie (The Works), 279 g	304	13	40
Una Mas Taco- Veggie, 236 g	234	6	37
Vera Cruz Shrimp Baja Style (The Works), 222 g	549	39	33
Vera Cruz Shrimp Taco-Baja Style, 151 g	396	26	29
Vera Cruz Shrimp Cabo Style (The Works), 239 g	493	34	32
Vera Cruz Shrimp Taco-Cabo Style, 168 g	339	20	28

Village Inn

Breakfast	Cal	Fat	Cbs
• Cinnamon Raisin French Toast	370	11	57
Fruit & Nut Multigrain Pancakes	490	10	91
• Veggie Omelette	490	16	69

Village Inn (cont.)	Cal	Fat	Cbs
Entrees			
3-Course Sirloin Steak	640	22	70
• Chicken Stir-Fry Dinner Skillet	710	24	83
• Grilled Tilapia	630	20	64
Sandwiches			
• Grilled Chicken Sandwich	460	16	46
• Half Sandwich & Soup	290	9	27
Soup & Salads			
• Chicken Caesar Salad	380	16	25
• Chicken Noodle Soup	80	2	10
Garden Grand Salad	350	20	25
Minestrone Soup	100	2	17
Side Salad	80	4	8
Vegetable Beef Soup	140	7	12

Wahoo's Fish Taco	Cal	Fat	Cbs
Appetizers			
Baja Rolls	475	20	49
Banzai Burrito			
Blackened Chicken	680	14	89
Blackened Fish	590	11	89
Carne Asada	675	18	87
• Carnitas	735	23	87
Charbroiled Chicken	675	14	87
Charbroiled Fish	585	11	87
Shrimp	600	11	87
• Vegetarian	520	9	96
Classic Burrito			
Blackened Chicken	545	17	51
Blackened Fish	460	14	53
Carne Asada	515	20	49
Carnitas	595	26	49
Charbroiled Chicken	540	17	49
Charbroiled Fish	455	14	51
• Mushroom	415	17	57
Shrimp	470	14	51
• Veggie	600	14	98
Combo Platters: #1 w/1 Taco			
• Blackened Chicken	750	11	121
Blackened Fish	715	9	122
Carne Asada	735	12	121
Carnitas	770	14	121
Charbroiled Chicken	745	10	121
Charbroiled Fish	710	9	121
• Mushroom	690	10	124
Shrimp	725	9	122
Veggie	740	9	136
Combo Platters: #2 w/2 Tacos			
2 Blackened Chicken	960	16	140
Blackened Chicken, Carne Asada	945	17	139
Blackened Chicken, Carnitas	980	20	139
Blackened Chicken, Mushroom	900	16	143
Blackened Chicken, Shrimp	935	15	140
Blackened Chicken, Veggie	950	15	154
Blackened Fish, Blackened Chicken	920	15	141
2 Blackened Fish	885	14	142
Blackened Fish, Carne Asada	905	16	140
Blackened Fish, Carnitas	945	19	140
Blackened Fish, Mushroom	865	15	143
Blackened Fish, Shrimp	895	14	141
Blackened Fish, Veggie	910	13	155
2 Carne Asada	930	18	138
Carne Asada, Carnitas	965	21	138
Carne Asada, Mushroom	885	17	142
Carne Asada, Shrimp	920	16	140
Carne Asada, Veggie	935	16	154

Wahoo's Fish Taco (cont.)	Cal	Fat	Cbs
Combo Platters: #2 w/2 Tacos (cont.)			
• 2 Carnitas	1005	24	138
Carnitas, Mushroom	925	20	142
Carnitas, Shrimp	955	19	139
Carnitas, Veggie	970	19	154
Chicken, Blackened Chicken	955	16	139
Chicken, Blackened Fish	920	15	140
Chicken, Carne Asada	940	17	138
Chicken, Carnitas	975	20	138
Chicken, Chicken	950	16	138
Chicken, Mushroom	900	16	142
Chicken, Shrimp	930	15	139
Chicken, Veggie	945	15	154
Fish, Blackened Chicken	920	15	140
Fish, Blackened Fish	885	14	141
Fish, Carne Asada	905	16	139
Fish, Carnitas	940	19	139
Fish, Chicken	915	15	139
Fish, Fish	880	13	140
Fish, Mushroom	860	15	143
Fish, Shrimp	895	14	140
Fish, Veggie	910	13	155
• 2 Mushroom	845	16	145
Shrimp, Mushroom	875	15	143
Shrimp, Shrimp	905	14	141
Shrimp, Veggie	925	13	140
Veggie, Mushroom	890	14	157
2 Veggie	940	13	169
Combo Platters: #3 Classic Burrito			
Blackened Chicken	1085	22	154
Blackened Fish	1000	19	155
Carne Asada	1055	25	152
Carnitas	1135	31	152
Charbroiled Chicken	1080	22	152
Charbroiled Fish	995	19	154
• Mushroom	955	21	160
Shrimp	1010	19	154
• Veggie	1140	19	201
Combo Platters: #3 Banzaiai Burrito			
Blackened Chicken	1220	19	192
Blackened Fish	1130	15	192
Carne Asada	1215	22	190
• Carnitas	1275	27	190
Charbroiled Chicken	1215	19	190
Charbroiled Fish	1125	15	190
Shrimp	1140	16	190
• Vegetarian	1060	14	199
Combo Platters: #4 Burrito, Taco			
Blackened Chicken Banzaiai Burrito	680	14	89
Blackened Chicken Burrito	545	17	51
Blackened Chicken Taco	210	6	19
Blackened Fish Banzai Burrito	590	11	89
Blackened Fish Burrito	460	14	53
Blackened Fish Taco	175	4	19
Carne Asada Banzaiai Burrito	675	18	87
Carne Asada Burrito	515	20	49
Carne Asada Taco	195	7	16
• Carnitas Banzaiai Burrito	735	23	87
Carnitas Burrito	595	26	49
Carnitas Taco	230	10	18
Charbroiled Chicken Banzaiai Burrito	675	14	87
Charbroiled Chicken Burrito	540	17	49
Charbroiled Chicken Taco	205	6	18
Charbroiled Fish Banzai Burrito	585	11	87
Charbroiled Fish Burrito	455	14	51

Wahoo's Fish Taco (cont.)

	Cal	Fat	Cbs
Combo Platters: #4 Burrito, Taco (cont.)			
• Charbroiled Fish Taco	170	4	19
Mushroom Burrito	415	17	57
Mushroom Taco	150	5	21
Rice Beans	540	5	103
Shrimp Banzai Burrito	600	11	87
Shrimp Burrito	470	14	51
Shrimp Taco	180	5	19
Vegetable Banzai Burrito	520	9	96
Veggie Burrito	600	14	98
Veggie Taco	200	4	33
Combo Platters: #6 Maui Bowl			
Maui Bowl	1115	19	163
Combo Platters: #7 Chicken Bowl			
Blackened Chicken	1050	15	145
• Charbroiled Chicken	1035	15	143
• Teriyaki Chicken	1140	15	163
Combo Platters: #8 Wahoo Bowl			
Blackened Fish	913	10	145
• Charbroiled Fish	900	10	143
Shrimp	980	11	143
• Teriyaki Fish	1040	10	170
Combo Platters: #9 and #10			
#9 Veggie Bowl	995	8	195
#10 Kalua Pig Bowl	1230	28	163
Combo Platters: #11 Banzaiai Bowl			
Blackened Chicken	1080	13	172
Blackened Fish	990	9	172
Carne Asada	1049	15	171
• Carnitas	1130	21	171
Charbroiled Chicken	1075	13	171
• Charbroiled Fish	980	9	171
Shrimp	995	10	171
Kid's Bowl			
• Bean & Cheese Burrito	635	26	71
Blackened Chicken	435	5	66
Blackened Fish	395	4	66
Carne Asada	430	7	65
Carnitas	455	9	65
Charbroiled Chicken	430	5	65
• Charbroiled Fish	390	4	65
Shrimp	405	4	66
Kid's Sides			
Beans	445	2	80
Rice	475	6	94
Kid's Taco With Rice & Beans			
Carne Asada	570	10	89
• Carnitas	590	12	89
Charbroiled Chicken	570	9	89
• Charbroiled Fish	535	8	90
Shrimp	540	8	90
Soup			
Chicken Tortilla Soup	140	4	8
Taco			
Blackened Chicken	210	6	19
Blackened Fish	175	4	19
Carne Asada	195	7	18
• Carnitas	230	10	18
Charbroiled Chicken	205	6	18
Charbroiled Fish	170	4	19
• Mushroom	150	5	21
Shrimp	180	5	19
Veggie	200	4	33
Wahoo's Salad (-chips)			
Blackened Chicken	565	28	16

Wahoo's Fish Taco (cont.)

	Cal	Fat	Cbs
Wahoo's Salad (-chips) (cont.)			
Blackened Fish	430	23	16
Carne Asada	555	33	13
• Carnitas	640	41	13
Charbroiled Chicken	550	27	13
Charbroiled Fish	415	22	13
• Sautee'd Veggies	345	20	32
Shrimp	500	24	14
Veggie	490	22	56
Wahoo's Sandwich			
Blackened Chicken	650	25	58
Blackened Fish	570	22	58
Carne Asada	645	28	57
• Carnitas	695	33	57
Charbroiled Chicken	640	25	57
Charbroiled Fish	560	22	57
• Sautee'd Veggies	520	20	68
Shrimp	575	22	57

Wendy's

	Cal	Fat	Cbs
Chicken Temptations and Fish			
10-piece Chicken Nuggets, 150 g	460	22	24
Chicken Club, 246 g	540	7	48
Crispy Chicken Deluxe, 180 g	400	25	35
• Crispy Chicken Sandwich, 285 g	660	25	68
• Grilled Chicken Go Wrap, 122 g	260	16	23
Homestyle Chicken Fillet, 220 g	430	30	48
Homestyle Chicken Go Wrap, 252 g	630	11	57
Premium Fish Fillet Sandwich, 177 g	450	29	47
Spicy Chicken Go Wrap, 128 g	320	20	28
Spicy Chicken Sandwich, 223 g	440	16	46
Ultimate Chicken Grill, 211 g	320	16	36
Frosty			
• Frosty™ Float, 467 g	380	7	75
M&M® Twisted Frosty™, 269 g	560	19	86
Medium Original Choco Frosty™, 298 g	411	11	68
• Medium Vanilla Frosty™, 596 g	820	21	135
Nestle® Cookie Dough Twisted Frosty™, 257 g	480	16	77
Oreo® Twisted Frosty™, 247 g	450	14	72
Small Chocolate Fudge Frosty™ Shake, 329 g	410	11	69
Small Strawberry Frosty™ Shake, 325 g	390	11	67
Small Vanilla Bean Frosty™ Shake, 322 g	380	11	65
Garden Sensation Salads			
• Chicken BLT Salad w/ Homestyle Chkn, 417 g	780	53	42
• Chicken Caesar Salad w/ Grilled Chkn, 318 g	490	33	20
Mandarin Chicken® Salad w/ Grilled Chkn, 402 g	540	25	50
Southwest Taco Salad, 520 g	640	39	44
Hot Stuffed Baked Potatoes			
• Bacon and Cheese Potato, 366 g	450	13	67
• Broccoli and Cheese Potato, 397 g	320	2	69
Sour Cream and Chives Potato, 308 g	320	4	63
Side Dishes			
4-piece Nuggets, Kids' Meal, 60 g	190	12	10
5-piece Crispy Chicken Nuggets, 75 g	230	15	12
• Bacon and Cheese Potato, 366 g	450	13	67
Broccoli and Cheese Potato, 397 g	320	2	69
Caesar Side Salad, 142 g	260	19	14
Chili, Chips and Cheese, 0 g	305	10	29
Chocolate Chip Cookie, 57 g	270	12	37
• Mandarin Oranges, 142 g	80	0	19
Medium French Fries, 142 g	430	20	56
Side Salad, 225 g	130	8	11
Small Chili, 227 g	190	6	19
Sour Cream and Chives Potato, 308 g	320	4	63
Super Value Menu			
5-piece Crispy Chicken Nuggets, 75 g	230	15	12

Wendy's (cont.)

Super Value Menu (cont.)	Cal	Fat	Cbs
Caesar Side Salad, 142 g	260	19	14
Crispy Chicken Sandwich, 142 g	330	14	34
Jr. Bacon Cheeseburger, 136 g	310	16	25
• Side Salad, 225 g	130	8	11
Small Chili, 227 g	190	6	19
• Small French Fries, 113 g	340	16	45
Small Original Chocolate Frosty™, 227 g	320	8	52
Sour Cream and Chives Potato, 308 g	320	4	63
Wendy's Old Fashioned Hamburgers			
1/2 lb. Double with Cheese, 318 g	700	40	38
1/4 lb. Deluxe Double Stack, 184 g	400	22	28
1/4 lb. Double Stack, 143 g	360	18	26
1/4 lb. Single, 226 g	430	20	37
• 3/4 lb. Triple with Cheese, 410 g	960	60	39
Baconator™, 276 g	830	51	35
Double Jr. Cheeseburger Deluxe, 186 g	390	20	28
Jr. Bacon Cheeseburger, 136 g	310	16	25
Jr. Cheeseburger Deluxe, 152 g	300	14	28
Jr. Cheeseburger, 109 g	260	11	26
• Jr. Hamburger, 98 g	220	8	26
Stack Attack™ Double Cheeseburger, 135 g	380	20	26
Triple Stack, 178 g	490	28	26

We're Rolling Pretzel Company

Pretzel	Cal	Fat	Cbs
Cinnamon Sugar Pretzel, 1 pretzel	492	5	102
Garlic Pretzel, 1 pretzel	448	10	78
• Plain Pretzel, 1 pretzel	368	1	78
Pretzel Rod 10 packs, 1 pretzel	641	8	125
Pretzel Rod 15 packs, 1 pretzel	962	12	188
• Pretzel Rod 20 packs, 1 pretzel	1282	16	250
Pretzel w/Butter & Salt, 1 pretzel	401	5	78
Raisin Pretzel, 1 pretzel	473	5	97
Sandwiches			
• Chicken Salad	574	20	70
Classic Italian	573	17	69
Ham & Swiss	491	10	69
• Turkey & Swiss	439	6	71

Wetzel's Pretzels

Pretzels	Cal	Fat	Cbs
Wetzel's Original w/o Butter, 1 pretzel	336	1	N/A
Wetzel's Original w/ Butter, 1 pretzel	384	4	N/A

Whataburger

Breakfast	Cal	Fat	Cbs
• Biscuit	300	17	32
Biscuit and Gravy	530	36	52
Biscuit Sandwich w/ bacon, egg & cheese	500	32	33
Biscuit Sandwich w/ egg & cheese	450	28	33
Biscuit Sandwich w/ sausage, egg & cheese	690	49	33
Biscuit w/ bacon	350	20	32
Biscuit w/ sausage	540	37	32
Breakfast On A Bun® w/ bacon	380	22	29
Breakfast On A Bun® w/ sausage	570	39	29
Breakfast Platter w/ bacon	740	45	53
• Breakfast Platter w/ sausage	930	62	53
Egg Sandwich	330	18	29
Honey Butter Chicken Biscuit	610	38	51
Pancakes w/ bacon	630	12	112
Pancakes w/ sausage	820	29	112
Pancakes, plain	580	8	112
Taquito w/ bacon & egg	380	21	27
Taquito w/ bacon, egg, & cheese	420	24	27
Taquito w/ potato & egg	430	23	37

Whataburger (cont.)

Breakfast (cont.)	Cal	Fat	Cbs
Taquito w/ potato, egg & cheese	470	27	37
Taquito w/ sausage & egg	410	24	27
Taquito w/ sausage, egg, & cheese	450	28	27
Burgers			
• Justaburger®	320	16	30
Whataburger Jr.®	330	16	32
Whataburger®	640	32	61
Whataburger® with bacon & cheese	800	45	62
Whataburger®, Double Meat	890	51	61
• Whataburger®, Triple Meat	1140	70	61
Chicken and Fish			
• Chicken Strips, 2 pieces	380	24	22
Chicken Strips, 4 pieces (with gravy)	840	54	53
Grilled Chicken Sandwich	450	18	45
• Whatacatch® Dinner, 2 piece	1580	92	161
Whatacatch® Sandwich	480	30	42
Whatachick'n® Sandwich	530	20	61
Kid's Menu			
Kid's Meal Chicken Strips	770	51	53
Kid's Meal Justaburger®	570	29	60
Desserts			
• Cinnamon Roll	400	7	80
Cookie, Chocolate Chunk	230	11	33
Cookie, White Chocolate Chunk Macadamia Nut	250	14	30
• Hot Apple Pie	230	11	29
Hot Peach Pie	280	14	36
Drinks (Medium)			
• Chocolate Malt	1050	25	188
Chocolate Shake	1000	26	171
Strawberry Malt	1040	24	188
Strawberry Shake	990	26	171
Vanilla Malt	940	27	155
• Vanilla Shake	890	28	139
Salads			
Chicken Strips	570	38	34
• Garden	60	0	12
Grilled Chicken	230	7	19
Sides			
French Fries (Medium)	400	20	47
Hash Brown Sticks (4 each)	200	12	20
• Onion Rings (Medium)	420	28	36
• Texas Toast, 1 slice	180	8	25
White Peppered Gravy, 1 gravy	60	5	8

White Castle

Beverages - Medium	Cal	Fat	Cbs
Chocolate Shake - Chicago region, 32 g	600	7	125
Chocolate Shake - Cincinnati region, 32 g	830	24	134
Chocolate Shake - Columbus & Detroit regions, 32 g	650	18	103
Chocolate Shake - Indianapolis region, 32 g	620	16	100
• Chocolate Shake - New Jersey region, 32 g	890	23	148
Chocolate Shake - New York region, 32 g	740	20	128
Chocolate Shake - St. Louis region, 32 g	690	21	109
Chocolate Shake Louisville region, 32 g	810	23	134
Chocolate Shake Nashville region, 32 g	860	23	143
Strawberry Shake - Chicago region, 32 g	610	7	127
Strawberry Shake - Cincinnati region, 32 g	840	24	136
Strawberry Shake - Columbus/Detroit regions, 32 g	730	18	124
Strawberry Shake - Minneapolis region, 32 g	790	21	146
• Vanilla Shake - Chicago region, 32 g	490	7	99
Vanilla Shake - Cincinnati region, 32 g	840	24	134
Vanilla Shake - Columbus/Detroit regions, 32 g	620	18	97
Vanilla Shake - Minneapolis regions, 32 g	680	21	118
Vanilla Shake - New Jersey region, 32 g	860	23	140
Vanilla Shake - New York region, 32 g	720	21	121

White Castle (cont.)

	Cal	Fat	Cbs
Beverages - Medium (Cont.)			
Vanilla Shake Nashville region, 32 g	790	23	126
Cheeses			
• American Cheese Slice, 7 g	25	2	0
Cheddar Cheese Sauce - New York region, 43 g	70	5	6
Cheddar Cheese Sauce - St Louis region, 43 g	40	3	3
• Cheese Sauce, 43 g	130	10	6
Jalapeño Cheese Slice, 9 g	35	3	1
Nacho Cheese Sauce, 47 g	50	4	3
Sandwiches			
Bacon Cheeseburger, 71 g	200	11	15
Cheeseburger, 65 g	170	9	15
Chicken Breast Sandwich w/Cheese, 82 g	200	8	21
Chicken Ring Sandwich w/Cheese, 69 g	200	10	19
Chicken Ring Sandwich, 62 g	180	8	19
Chicken Supreme , 88 g	230	10	21
• Double Bacon Cheeseburger, 130 g	370	22	23
Double Cheeseburger, 118 g	300	17	23
Double Jalapeño Cheeseburger, 122 g	320	19	23
Double White Castle, 104 g	250	13	22
Fish w/Cheese, 77 g	180	8	19
Jalapeño Cheeseburger, 67 g	180	10	15
Surf & Turf, 157 g	390	22	28
• White Castle, 58 g	140	7	14
Sides			
Chicken Rings: 6 Rings, 110 g	340	23	15
Clam Strips: Regular, 113 g	250	22	5
Fish Nibblers: Regular, 117 g	280	16	24
French Fries: Regular, 108 g	310	15	39
Homestyle Onion Rings: Regular, 96 g	430	24	49
Mozzarella Cheese Sticks: 5 Sticks, 132 g	420	23	37
• Onion Chips: Regular, 112 g	480	23	62
• Onion Rings: Regular, 96 g	210	10	28

Wienerschnitzel

	Cal	Fat	Cbs
Breakfast			
• Biscuit, 81 g	260	11	35
with Bacon, 97 g	330	17	35
with Egg & Bacon, 154 g	390	21	36
with Egg & Sausage, 181 g	490	30	40
with Egg, 138 g	320	15	36
with Egg, Bacon & Cheese, 168 g	440	25	36
with Egg, Sausage & Cheese, 195 g	540	34	40
with Sausage, 124 g	430	26	39
Biscuit & Gravy, 138 g	350	17	42
Breakfast Platter with Bacon, 267 g	600	40	40
• with Sausage, 293 g	700	49	44
Burrito with Egg, Bacon & Cheese, 244 g	490	25	39
Burrito with Egg, Sausage & Chz, 271 g	590	34	43
Chili Cheese Burrito, 261 g	470	21	43
Country Breakfast, 294 g	640	40	47
Croissant with Egg, Bacon & Chz, 172 g	520	31	40
with Egg, Sausage & Cheese, 199 g	620	40	44
French Toast Sticks, 148 g	490	29	49
Hash Browns, 80 g	290	25	14
Sandwich with Egg, Bacon & Chz, 144 g	300	15	26
with Egg, Sausage & Cheese, 171 g	400	24	30
Burgers & Sandwiches			
Bacon Ranch Chicken Sandwich, 200 g	430	21	37
Chili Cheese Fries Burrito, 196 g	470	21	53
Chili Cheeseburger, 159 g	350	13	32
Chipotle Ranch Pupsters, 147 g	440	24	43
Deluxe Cheeseburger, 235 g	450	23	33
Deluxe Hamburger, 221 g	400	19	33
Double Chili Cheeseburger, 260 g	560	24	35
Italian Sausage Sandwich, 156 g	350	17	31

Wienerschnitzel (cont.)

	Cal	Fat	Cbs
Burgers & Sandwiches (cont.)			
• Original Burger, 150 g	290	9	29
Pastrami Burger, 202 g	510	26	30
• Pastrami Sandwich, 221 g	580	35	38
Polish Sausage Sandwich, 208 g	490	29	39
Ranch Dressing, 35 g	120	12	2
Desserts			
Apple Pie, 92 g	310	19	31
Fries & Sides			
• Chili Cheese Fries, 231 g	540	38	39
Jalapeño Poppers, 65 g	210	11	21
Large Fries, 181 g	470	34	39
Onion Straws, 98 g	430	35	25
• Ranch Dressing, 35 g	120	12	2
Regular Fries, 131 g	340	25	28
Hot Dogs			
All Beef Chili Cheese Dog Pretzel Bun, 214 g	570	28	59
All Beef Chili Cheese Dog, 175 g	430	25	33
All Beef Chili Dog Pretzel Bun, 200 g	520	24	59
All Beef Chili Dog, 161 g	380	21	33
All Beef Deluxe Dog Pretzel Bun, 238 g	510	23	58
All Beef Deluxe Dog, 200 g	370	20	32
All Beef Kraut Dog Pretzel Bun, 201 g	500	23	56
All Beef Kraut Dog, 162 g	360	20	30
All Beef Mustard Dog Pretzel Bun, 176 g	490	23	56
All Beef Mustard Dog, 137 g	350	20	30
All Beef Relish Dog Pretzel Bun, 192 g	500	23	58
All Beef Relish Dog, 154 g	360	20	32
Chicago Dog, 290 g	410	20	43
Chili Cheese Dog Pretzel Bun, 179 g	480	20	57
Chili Cheese Dog, 140 g	340	17	31
Chili Dog on a Pretzel Bun, 165 g	430	16	57
Chili Dog, 126 g	290	13	31
Deluxe Dog on a Pretzel Bun, 203 g	410	15	56
Deluxe Dog, 165 g	270	12	30
Kraut Dog on a Pretzel Bun, 166 g	400	15	54
Kraut Dog, 127 g	260	12	28
Mustard Dog on a Pretzel Bun, 141 g	400	15	54
Mustard Dog, 102 g	260	12	28
• Pastrami Dog, 245 g	640	34	57
Relish Dog on a Pretzel Bun, 157 g	410	15	56
Relish Dog, 119 g	270	12	30
Stadium Dog, 157 g	370	20	32
Turkey Chili Cheese Dog, 143 g	320	15	31
Turkey Chili Dog, 129 g	270	11	31
Turkey Deluxe Dog, 168 g	250	10	30
Turkey Kraut Dog, 130 g	250	10	28
• Turkey Mustard Dog, 106 g	240	10	28
Turkey Relish Dog, 122 g	250	10	30
Kids Bags			
• Corn Dog, 82 g	250	17	15
Hamburger, 199 g	290	8	31
• Mini Corn Dogs (6-pack), 99 g	320	22	22
Mustard Dog, 102 g	260	12	28
Tastee-Freez Desserts			
• Banana Split, 450 g	820	24	149
Cone, 4 oz. Kids Chocolate Dipped, 122 g	400	25	43
• Cone, 4 oz. Kids Plain, 94 g	210	7	34
Cone, 6 oz. Chocolate Dipped, 166 g	490	29	57
Cone, 6 oz. Plain, 138 g	300	11	49
Freezee, Butterfinger, 279 g	620	24	100
Freezee, M&M, 279 g	630	25	99
Freezee, Oreo, 279 g	630	25	99
Freezee, Reese's Peanut Butter Cup, 279 g	630	26	97
Old Fashion Sundae, Caramel, 181 g	400	14	66

RESTAURANTS & FAST-FOOD CHAINS

Wienerschnitzel (cont.)	Cal	Fat	Cbs
Tastee-Freez Desserts (cont.)			
Old Fashion Sundae, Chocolate, 181 g	390	14	64
Old Fashion Sundae, Hot Fudge, 181 g	400	16	63
Old Fashion Sundae, Pineapple, 181 g	370	14	59
Old Fashion Sundae, Strawberry, 181 g	370	14	59
Shake, Chocolate, 311 g	650	23	110
Shake, Strawberry, 312 g	650	23	111
Shake, Vanilla, 312 g	650	23	110

Winchell's	Cal	Fat	Cbs
Baked Products			
Croissant	260	17	28
Cake Products			
Chocolate Iced Cake	230	15	28
Traditional Cake	215	14	26
Yeast Raised Products			
Chocolate Bar	240	16	29
• Chocolate Round	240	16	29
Chocolate Twist	240	16	29
• Glazed Round	230	15	27
Glazed Twist	230	15	27

WingStreet	Cal	Fat	Cbs
Bone In Wings			
• All American (2 pieces), 48 g	170	13	7
Buffalo Burnin Hot (2 pieces), 65 g	210	13	14
Buffalo Medium (2 pieces), 65 g	210	13	14
Buffalo Mild (2 pieces), 65 g	210	13	14
Cajun (2 pieces), 65 g	210	13	15
Garlic Parmesan (2 pieces), 56 g	210	16	8
• Honey BBQ (2 pieces), 70 g	230	13	20
Spicy Asian (2 pieces), 70 g	220	13	19
Spicy BBQ (2 pieces), 70 g	220	13	18
Teriyaki (2 pieces), 74 g	230	13	20
Bone Out Wings			
• All American (2 pieces), 61 g	190	10	11
Buffalo Burnin Hot (2 pieces), 78 g	220	11	18
Buffalo Medium (2 pieces), 78 g	220	11	18
Buffalo Mild (2 pieces), 78 g	220	11	18
Cajun (2 pieces), 78 g	220	10	19
Garlic Parmesan (2 pieces), 69 g	220	14	12
• Honey BBQ (2 pieces), 84 g	240	10	24
Spicy Asian (2 pieces), 84 g	230	10	23
Spicy BBQ (2 pieces), 84 g	230	10	22
Teriyaki (2 pieces), 87 g	240	10	24
Sides			
Apple Pie (2 pies), 105 g	370	17	50
• Fried Cheese Sticks, 96 g	310	19	23
• Taters, 227 g	790	52	74
Traditional Wings			
• All American (2 pieces), 41 g	80	5	0
Buffalo Burnin Hot (2 pieces), 58 g	110	6	7
Buffalo Medium (2 pieces), 58 g	120	6	7
Buffalo Mild (2 pieces), 58 g	120	6	7
Cajun (2 pieces), 58 g	120	6	8
Garlic Parmesan (2 pieces), 49 g	120	9	1
• Honey BBQ (2 pieces), 63 g	140	6	13
Spicy Asian (2 pieces), 63 g	130	6	12
Spicy BBQ (2 pieces), 63 g	130	6	11
Teriyaki (2 pieces), 67 g	110	6	6

Yard House	Cal	Fat	Cbs
Appetizers			
Apple Plum Sauce, 1 tbsp.	20	1	2
Blue Crabs Cakes	540	46	18
Buffalo Chicken Wings w/o sauce	1050	66	20

Yard House (cont.)	Cal	Fat	Cbs
Appetizers (cont.)			
California Roll	545	28	48
• Chicken Nachos	1980	120	148
Chilled Edamame	300	9	27
Chinese Garlic Noodle	865	57	75
Coconut Shrimp	600	25	71
Firecrackers Chicken Wings	1370	83	55
Fried Calamari w/o sauce	665	39	31
Fried Chicken Strips - 4 strips	920	64	54
w/o sides and sauce	470	27	26
Grilled Artichoke w/ mayo	855	84	27
w/o chips & aioli mayonnaise	300	27	13
Grilled Korean BBQ Beef Ribs	870	42	55
Hawaiian Poke Stack	650	47	36
Jamaican Jerks Wings	1075	56	40
Lettuce Wraps with Chicken	1140	58	82
Lettuce Wraps with Mushrooms	1030	62	92
Lettuce Wraps with Shrimp	1060	53	82
Lobster Dip with Pita & Chips	1230	54	148
Moo Shu Egg Rolls	725	31	65
• w/o carrots and sauce	270	8	25
Onion Ring Tower w/o dressing	1380	70	170
Roasted Garlic Aioli, 1 tbsp.	70	7	2
Seared Ahi Sashimi	400	22	24
w/o dressing	195	4	13
Soy Vinaigrette, 1 tbsp.	50	5	3
Spicy Tuna Roll	625	38	38
Spinach Cheese Dip	945	53	88
Dressing			
• Balsamic Vinaigrette, 1 tbsp.	80	8	2
Bleu Cheese Dressing, 1 tbsp.	75	8	1
Caesar Dressing, 1 tbsp.	75	8	0
• Thai Peanut Vinaigrette, 1 tbsp.	45	2	5
Dressings			
Buttermilk Ranch Dressing, 1 tbsp.	55	6	1
• Caesar Dressing, 1 tbsp.	75	8	0
Chipotle Ranch Dressing, 1 tbsp.	50	5	1
Gorgonzola Dressing, 1 tbsp.	65	6	0
Soy Vinaigrette, 1 tbsp.	50	5	3
• Thai Peanut Vinaigrette, 1 tbsp.	45	2	5
Entrée Salads			
Ahi Crunchy Salad	815	51	58
w/o dressing	205	4	12
• BBQ Chicken Salad	1655	106	108
w/o fr. onions, tortilla strips & dressing	710	25	61
Caesar Salad with Ahi	525	39	9
w/o dressing	220	7	8
Caesar Salad with Chicken	755	52	11
w/o dressing	445	20	10
Caesar Salad with Shrimp	610	49	10
w/o dressing	305	17	8
Grilled Hearts of Romaine	600	52	22
w/o dressing	225	15	20
• w/o dressing & walnuts	60	2	8
Roasted Turkey Cobb Salad	1065	84	17
w/o dressing and bacon	420	25	14
Steak Salad w/o dressing & chips	760	51	23
Thai Chicken Salad	845	28	99
w/o dressing	490	8	56
Grilled Burgers (burger only)			
Avocado & Swiss Burger	1225	81	65
BBQ Bacon & Cheese Burger	1400	81	94
• Bearnaise Burger	1930	151	85
Chile Pepper Jack Burger	1285	85	63
Classic Cheese Burger	1160	75	62

RESTAURANTS & FAST-FOOD CHAINS

Yard House (cont.)

	Cal	Fat	Cbs
Grilled Burgers (burger only) (cont.)			
• Grilled Portabella Burger	875	53	77
Hawaiian Burger	1390	81	99
Turkey Burger	1255	78	80
Healthy Dining Menu			
Ahi Crunchy Salad (w/o dressing)	205	4	12
BBQ Chicken Pizza, 2 slices	325	13	34
Caesar Dressing, 1 tbsp.	75	8	0
Caesar Salad with Ahi (w/o dressing)	220	7	8
Caesar Salad with Chicken (w/o dressing)	445	20	10
Caesar Salad with Shrimp (w/o dressing)	305	17	8
• California Roll	545	28	48
Chopped Salad, no bacon, 1/4 avocado	255	16	27
• Edamame Appetizer, 1/2 order	150	5	14
Margherita Pizza, 2 slices	250	10	29
Soy Vinaigrette, 1 tbsp.	50	5	3
Spicy Tuna Dynamite Roll, 1/2 order	315	19	19
Thai Chicken Pizza, 2 slices	340	16	32
Thai Chicken Salad (w/o dressing)	490	8	56
Thai Peanut Vinaigrette, 1 tbsp.	45	2	5
House Favorites			
Angel Hair Pasta	1535	113	96
Chicken Enchilada Stack	1810	128	73
• Chicken Garlic Noodles	1410	93	84
Chicken Rice Bowl	1445	78	133
Jerk Chicken with Shrimp Stack	1520	96	67
Macaroni and Cheese	1780	120	95
Maui Chicken	1510	77	141
Orange Peel Chicken	1815	84	197
Parmesan Crusted Chicken	1415	71	106
Penne with Roasted Chicken w/o bread	1645	116	87
Southern Fried Chicken Breast	1485	110	78
• Turkey Pot Pie	2020	125	132
Kids Klub			
Cheese Burger only	840	49	56
Chicken Fingers w/o sides & sauce	470	27	26
Fish and Chips w/o sides & sauce	275	14	18
• Four Cheese Pizza, 2 slices	235	10	26
Fries	555	35	54
Grilled Cheese w/o sides	670	42	55
Hot Dog only	380	14	48
• Mac and Cheese	890	59	54
Pasta	720	49	59
Pepperoni Cheese Pizza, 2 slices	350	21	27
Ranch Dressing, 1 tbsp.	55	6	1
Sundae	325	15	48
Tartar Sauce, 1 tbsp.	75	8	1
Pizza			
BBQ Chicken Pizza, 2 slices	325	13	34
Four Cheese Pizza, 2 slices	280	14	26
Ham & Pineapple Pizza, 2 slices	275	12	29
• Margherita Pizza, 2 slices	250	10	31
• Pepperoni & Mushroom Pizza, 2 slices	350	21	27
Thai Chicken Pizza, 2 slices	340	16	32
Sandwiches (sandwiches only)			
Ahi Steak Sandwich	695	35	42
• w/o mayo	520	16	40
Blue Crab Cake Hoagie	1165	71	98
Cuban Roast Pork Dip Sandwich	1355	77	79
Grilled Chicken and Avocado Sandwich	1230	76	64
Grilled Pastrami Sandwich	980	56	71
• New York Steak Sandwich	1620	93	121
Portabello BLT Sandwich	870	62	61
Roast Beef Dip	1135	55	66
Roasted Turkey Club	1125	58	94

Yard House (cont.)

	Cal	Fat	Cbs
Sandwiches (sandwiches only) (cont.)			
w/o mayo & bacon	755	19	92
Roasted Turkey Melt Sandwich	1000	56	69
w/o mayo & butter	700	22	68
Spicy Chicken Breast Sandwich	1175	68	71
Seafood			
Crab Crusted Swordfish	1320	93	58
• Fried Fish w/o fries	550	28	36
Fries with Fish	1110	70	109
Ginger Crusted Salmon	1440	93	97
Grilled Jumbo Shrimp	1330	75	107
• Linguine and Clams	1500	113	79
Lobster Garlic Noodles	1065	56	80
Miso Chilean Sea Bass	1200	49	126
Orzo Scallops	1305	82	78
Pan Seared Ahi	980	40	89
Porcini Mushroom Crusted Halibut	1360	105	46
Shrimp Rice Bowl	1370	74	133
Vodka Shrimp Pasta	1200	72	73
Sides & Sauces			
Chipotle Ranch Dressing, 1 tbsp.	50	5	1
Cocktail Sauce, 1 tbsp.	15	0	4
Cole Slaw, 5 oz.	202	16	16
French Fries, 6 oz.	665	42	65
• Pickle, half	6	0	1
• Potato Chips, 3 cups	440	25	50
Ranch Dressing, 1 tbsp.	55	6	1
Sourdough Bread, 3 oz.	235	3	44
Sweet Potato Fries, 6 oz.	525	30	60
Tartar Sauce, 1 tbsp.	75	8	1
Starters			
Baby Leaf Spinach Salad	645	55	25
w/o dressing	330	24	16
Caesar Salad	395	36	9
w/o dressing	90	4	8
Chopped Salad	470	36	31
w/o bacon and only 1/4 avocado	255	16	27
Clam Chowder	340	20	39
French Onion Soup	485	36	23
House Salad	390	21	46
w/o dressing	220	12	25
• w/o dressing and wontons	65	2	10
Iceberg Wedge	550	51	20
w/o dressing	85	3	13
Mixed Fields Greens	395	34	22
w/o dressing	80	2	12
• Summer Salad	815	66	56
w/o dressing	580	43	50
w/o dressing and walnuts	235	16	25
Walnut Pear Salad	665	53	41
w/o dressing	345	22	31
w/o dressing and walnuts	186	9	20
Steaks, Ribs, Chops			
• BBQ Baby Back Ribs	2275	115	206
BBQ Pork Tenderloin	1445	86	98
Grilled Ribeye Steak	1195	77	47
New York Steak	1135	63	46
New Zealand Lamb Chops	1630	128	77
Ribeye Steak and Grilled Shrimp	1410	90	48
Three Peppercorn Beef Tenderloin	1450	108	58
• Top Sirloin Steak	960	43	58

Yoshinoya

	Cal	Fat	Cbs
Bowls			
Combo Bowl (Bf & Ckn) No Skin, 25 oz.	1043	28	171
Combo Bowl (Beef & Chicken)	1220	36	171

Yoshinoya (cont.)

Bowls (cont.)	Cal	Fat	Cbs
• Kids Meal Beef Bowl	340	11	48
Kids Meal Chicken Bowl	370	9	53
Regular Beef Bowl	840	30	109
Regular Beef Bowl With Vegetables	770	23	114
Regular Chicken Bowl (Teriyaki or Spicy)	760	15	125
Regular Chicken Bowl No Skin, 17 oz.	608	7	125
Regular Vegetable Bowl	530	4	116
• Shrimp & Beef Combo Bowl	1280	44	184
Shrimp & Chicken Combo Bowl	1260	35	191
Shrimp Bowl	910	29	143
Desserts			
Cheesecake	280	15	31
• Chocolate Cake	330	17	44
• Flan	230	7	35
Strawberry Shortcake	290	15	37
Side Orders			
Beef	370	28	6
Chicken and Vegetables only	300	12	21
Rice	460	3	104
Vegetables	60	1	12

Z'Tejas Southwestern Grill

	Cal	Fat	Cbs
Grilled Cilantro Pesto-Rubbed Ruby Trout	530	25	31
• Grilled Miso Salmon	645	27	48
• Jerk Chicken Salad	515	24	27
Voodoo Blackened Tuna	540	19	41

Zero's Subs

6 " Sandwiches	Cal	Fat	Cbs
BLT	411	19	48
BLT no Mayo	330	12	43
Cosmo Vegetarian	469	23	46
• no cheese, no oil and no vinegar	216	2	45
Cosmo Vegetarian Deluxe	488	25	48
no cheese, no oil and no vinegar	235	3	47
Grilled Veggie Sub	394	14	52
no cheese, no oil and vinegar	244	3	51
Grinder	557	31	48
Grinder multigrain	559	32	50
no cheese, no oil & vinegar	401	18	49
no cheese, no oil & vinegar	399	17	47
Ham & Cheese	439	19	44
no cheese, no oil & vinegar	286	5	43
• Hot Italian Sausage	663	37	45
Meatball & Cheese	565	30	50
no cheese	465	22	50
Pepperoni & Cheese	545	31	48
no Cheese	346	15	41
Philly Chicken & Cheese	402	10	48
no cheese	319	4	45
w/ M&GP	410	10	49
w/M&GP, no cheese	328	4	47
Philly Steak & Cheese	492	21	49
w/ M&GP	500	21	50
w/ M&GP, no cheese	418	15	48
no cheese	409	15	46
Roast Beef & Cheese	460	19	45
no cheese, no oil & vinegar	307	5	45
The Club	514	23	44
no cheese, no oil & vinegar	361	10	43
Tuna & Cheese	519	26	47
no cheese, no oil & vinegar	366	12	46
Turkey & Cheese	454	17	44
no cheese, no oil & vinegar	301	3	43

Other Food Items

Other Food Items	Cal	Fat	Cbs
Write down the calories, fat, and carbs of your favorite food items			

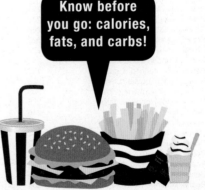

Know before you go: calories, fats, and carbs!

A	Cal	Fat	Cbs
Alcohol, 100 proof, 1 fl.oz.	82	0	0
Alcohol, 86 proof, 1 fl.oz.	70	0	0
Alcohol, 90 proof, 1 fl.oz.	73	0	0
Alcohol, 94 proof, 1 fl.oz.	76	0	0
Alcohol, dessert wine, dry, 1 glass	157	0	12
Alcohol, dessert wine, sweet, 1 glass	165	0	14
Alcohol, liquors, 1 fl.oz.	107	0	11
Alcohol, pina colada, 8 fl.oz.	440	5	57
Alfalfa seeds, 1 tbsp	1	0	0
Allspice, ground, 1 tsp	5	0	1
Almond butter, w/ salt, 1 tbsp	101	10	3
Almond butter, w/o salt, 1 tbsp	101	10	3
Almonds, roasted, 1 oz. (12 nuts)	169	15	6
Anchovies, 3 oz.	111	4	0
Apple cider, powdered, 1 packet	83	0	21
Apple juice, 8 fl.oz.	120	0	29
Apples, w/o skin, 1 medium	61	0	16
Apples, w/ skin, 1 medium	72	0	19
Applesauce, 1 cup	194	1	51
Apricots, 1 apricot	17	0	4
Arrowroot, 1 cup, sliced	78	0	16
Arrowroot flour, 1 cup	457	0	113
Artichokes, 1 artichoke	76	0	17
Arugula, 1 cup	4	0	1
Asparagus, 1 spear	2	0	1
Avocados, 1 cup, cubes	240	22	13

B	Cal	Fat	Cbs
Bacon bits, meatless, 1 tbsp	33	2	2
Bacon, canadian, cooked, 1 slice	43	2	0
Bacon, meatless, 1 slice	16	2	0
Bacon, pork, cooked, 1 slice	42	3	0
Bagels, cinnamon-raisin, 1 bagel, 4" dia	244	2	49
Bagels, egg, 1 bagel, 4" dia	292	2	56
Bagels, oat-bran, 1 bagel, 4" dia	227	1	47
Bagels, plain , 1 bagel, 4" dia	245	1	47
Bagels, deli gourmet style, 1 bagel	370	3	71
Balsam pear, 1 balsam pear	21	0	5
Bamboo shoots, 1 cup	41	1	8
Banana chips, 1 oz.	147	10	17
Bananas, 1 medium, 7"-8"	105	0	27
Barley, 1 cup	651	4	135
Barley flour, 1 cup	511	2	110
Barley, pearled, cooked, 1 cup	193	1	44
Basil, 5 leaves	1	0	0
Basil, dried, 1 tsp	2	0	1
Bay leaf, 1 tsp, crumbled	2	0	1
Beans, adzuki, cooked, 1 cup	294	0	57
Beans, baked, canned, plain, 1 cup	239	1	54
Beans, baked, canned, w/o salt, 1 cup	266	1	52
Beans, baked, canned, w/ beef, 1 cup	322	9	45
Beans, black, cooked, 1 cup	227	1	40
Beans, cranberry, cooked, 1 cup	241	1	43
Beans, fava, canned, 1 cup	182	1	31
Beans, french, cooked, 1 cup	228	1	43
Beans, great northern, cooked, 1 cup	209	1	37
Beans, kidney, cooked, 1 cup	225	1	40
Beans, lima, cooked, 1 cup	216	1	39
Beans, lima, canned, 1 can	190	0	36
Beans, mung, cooked, 1 cup	212	1	39
Beans, mungo, cooked, 1 cup	189	1	33
Beans, navy, cooked, 1 cup	255	1	47
Beans, pink, cooked, 1 cup	252	1	47
Beans, pinto, cooked, 1 cup	245	1	44
Beans, small white, cooked, 1 cup	254	1	46

B (cont.)	Cal	Fat	Cbs
Beans, snap, green, cooked, 1 cup	44	0	10
Beans, snap, yellow, cooked, 1 cup	44	0	10
Beans, white, cooked, 1 cup	249	1	45
Beans, yellow, 1 cup	255	2	48
Beechnuts, dried, 1 oz.	163	14	10
Beef, choice short rib, cooked, 3 oz.	400	36	0
Beef bologna, 1 slice	88	8	1
Beef jerky, chopped, 1 piece	81	5	2
Beef sausage, precooked, 1 link	134	12	1
Beef stew, canned, 1 serving	218	13	16
Beef, tri-tip roast, roasted, 3 oz.	174	9	0
Beef, brisket, lean and fat, roasted, 3 oz.	328	27	0
Beef, brisket, lean, roasted, 3 oz.	206	11	0
Beef, chuck, arm roast, lean, braised, 3 oz.	179	7	0
Beef, chuck, top blade, raw, 3 oz.	138	8	0
Beef, cured breakfast strips, 3 slices	276	26	1
Beef, cured, corned, canned, 3 oz.	213	13	0
Beef, cured, dried, 1 serving	43	1	1
Beef, cured, luncheon meat, 1 slice	31	1	0
Beef, flank, raw, 1 oz.	47	2	0
Beef, ground patties, frozen, 3 oz.	240	20	0
Beef, ground, 70% lean, raw, 1 oz.	94	9	0
Beef, ground, 80% lean, raw, 1 oz.	72	6	0
Beef, ground, 95% lean, raw, 1 oz.	39	1	0
Beef, rib, large end, boneless, raw, 1 oz.	94	8	0
Beef, rib, shortribs, boneless, raw, 1 oz.	110	10	0
Beef, rib, whole, boneless, raw, 1 oz.	91	8	0
Beef, rib-eye, small end, raw, 1 oz.	78	6	0
Beef, round, bottom, raw, 1 oz.	56	3	0
Beef, round, eye, raw, 1 oz.	49	3	0
Beef, round, full cut, raw, 1 oz.	55	3	0
Beef, round, tip, raw, 1 oz.	56	4	0
Beef, round, top, raw, 1 oz.	48	2	0
Beef, shank crosscuts, raw, 1 oz.	50	3	0
Beef, short loin, porterhouse, raw, 1 oz.	73	6	0
Beef, short loin, t-bone, raw, 1 oz.	66	5	0
Beef, short loin, top, raw, 1 oz.	66	5	0
Beef, sirloin, tri-tip, raw, 1 oz.	50	3	0
Beef, tenderloin, raw, 1 oz.	70	5	0
Beef, top sirloin, raw, 1 oz.	61	4	0
Beer, light, 12 fl.oz.	110	12	7
Beer, nonalcoholic, 12 fl.oz.	80	1	70
Beer, regular, 12 fl.oz.	140	12	10
Beets, 1 beet	35	0	8
Bratwurst, chicken, 1 serving	148	9	0
Bratwurst, pork, 1 serving	281	25	2
Bratwurst, veal, 1 serving	286	27	0
Bread stuffing, dry mix, prepared, 1/2 cup	178	9	22
Bread, banana, 1 slice	196	6	33
Bread, corn, 1 piece	188	6	29
Bread, cracked-wheat, 1 slice	65	1	12
Bread, french, 1 slice	70	1	15
Bread, garlic, 1 slice	160	10	14
Bread, Irish soda, 1 oz.	82	1	16
Bread, pita, 2 oz.	150	1	30
Bread, pumpernickel, 1 slice	75	1	15
Bread, raisin, 1 slice	80	2	15
Bread, rice bran, 1 oz.	69	1	12
Bread, sandwich slice, 1 slice	70	1	13
Bread, sourdough, 1 slice	100	1	20
Broad beans, cooked, 1 cup	187	1	33
Brownies, 1 brownie	220	13	27
Buckwheat, 1 cup	583	6	122
Buckwheat flour, 1 cup	402	4	85
Buckwheat groats, roasted, cooked, 1 cup	155	1	34

B (cont.)	Cal	Fat	Cbs
Buffalo, raw, 1 oz.	28	0	0
Burbot, raw, 3 oz.	77	1	0
Burdock root, 1 cup	85	0	21
Butter, whipped, w/ salt, 1 tbsp	67	8	0
Butternuts, dried,1 oz.	174	16	3

C	Cal	Fat	Cbs
Cabbage, common, 1 cup, shredded	17	1	4
Cabbage, pak choi, 1 cup, shredded	9	0	2
Cabbage, pe-tsai, 1 cup, shredded	12	0	3
Cake, angel food, 1 slice	180	4	36
Cake, boston cream pie, 1 slice	260	9	32
Cake, carrot, 1 slice	310	16	39
Cake, cheesecake, 1 slice	500	30	50
Cake, chocolate, 1 slice	270	13	36
Cake, chocolate mousse, 1 slice	250	10	35
Cake, devil's food, 1 slice	270	13	35
Cake, pineapple upside-down, 1 piece	367	14	58
Cake, pound, 1 slice	320	16	38
Cake, sponge w/ cream, berries, 1 slice	325	8	38
Cake, yellow, 1 slice	260	11	36
Candy, butterscotch, 5 pieces	120	3	20
Candy, caramels, 1 piece	30	1	6
Candy, carob, 1 bar	470	27	49
Candy, chocolate fudge, 1 oz.	125	5	18
Candy, chocolate mints, 1 mint	45	1	9
Candy, milk chocolate w/ almonds, 2 oz.	216	14	21
Candy, choco-coated peanuts, 12 peanuts	160	11	15
Candy, gumdrops, 4 pieces	130	0	31
Candy, hard candy, 1 piece	18	0	5
Candy, jelly beans, 12 beans	100	0	24
Candy, licorice, 1 piece	30	0	7
Candy, lollipop, 1 lollipop	20	0	5
Candy, milk chocolate bar, 2 oz.	235	13	26
Candy, mints, 1 mint	30	0	7
Cantaloupe, 1 cup, cubed	54	0	13
Cardoon, 1 cup, shredded	36	0	9
Carrots, 1 medium	65	0	15
Cashew butter, w/ salt, 1 tbsp	94	8	4
Cashew nuts, 1 oz.	157	12	9
Cassava, 1 cup	330	1	78
Celeriac, 1 cup	66	1	14
Chard, swiss, 1 cup	7	0	1
Cheese, american, 1 slice	110	9	1
Cheese, brick, 1 oz.	100	8	0
Cheese, brie, 1 oz.	95	8	1
Cheese, camembert, 1 oz.	90	7	1
Cheese, cheddar, 1 oz.	110	9	1
Cheese, colby jack, 1 oz.	110	9	1
Cheese, cottage, 2%, 1 cup	203	4	8
Cheese, edam, 1 oz.	100	8	1
Cheese, feta, 1 oz.	100	8	1
Cheese, goat, 1 oz.	128	10	1
Cheese, goat, semisoft, 1 oz.	103	9	1
Cheese, goat, soft, 1 oz.	76	6	0
Cheese, gouda, 1/2	100	8	1
Cheese, monterey jack, 1 oz.	110	9	0
Cheese, mozzarella, 1 oz.	90	7	1
Cheese, parmesan, hard, 1 oz.	110	7	1
Cheese, parmesan, shredded, 1 tbsp	22	2	0
Cheese, provolone, 1 oz.	100	8	1
Cheese, queso, 2 tbsp	110	9	2
Cheese, ricotta, 2 tbsp	50	4	1
Cheese, roquefort, 1 oz.	105	9	1
Cheese, swiss, 1 oz.	110	9	1

C (cont.)	Cal	Fat	Cbs
Cherries, sour, 8 pieces	30	0	7
Cherries, sweet, 8 pieces	30	0	7
Chewing gum, 1 piece	25	0	5
Chicken, breast, w/ skin, 1/2 breast	249	13	0
Chicken, breast, w/o skin, 1/2 breast	130	2	0
Chicken, capons, boneless, 1/2 capon	1459	74	0
Chicken, capons, giblets, cooked, 1 cup	238	8	1
Chicken, cornish game hen, rsted, 1/2 bird	336	24	0
Chicken, cornish game hen, meat, 1 bird	295	9	0
Chicken, dark meat, w/o skin, 1 cup diced	287	14	0
Chicken, drumstick, w/ skin, 1 drumstick	118	6	0
Chicken, drumstick, w/o skin, 1 drumstick	74	2	0
Chicken, leg, w/ skin, 1 leg	312	20	0
Chicken, leg, w/o skin, 1 leg	156	5	0
Chicken, light meat, w/o skin, 1 cup diced	214	6	0
Chicken, thigh, w/ skin, 1 thigh	198	14	0
Chicken, thigh, w/o skin, 1 thigh	82	3	0
Chicken, wing, w/ skin, 1 wing	109	8	0
Chicken, wing, w/o skin, 1 wing	37	1	0
Chickpeas, cooked, 1 cup	269	4	45
Chicory greens, 1 cup, chopped	41	1	9
Chicory roots, 1/2 cup	33	0	8
Chicory, witloof, 1/2 cup	8	0	2
Chili con carne w/ beans, 1 cup	298	13	28
Chili powder, 1 tsp	8	0	1
Chili w/ beans, canned, 1 cup	287	14	31
Chili w/o beans, canned, 1 cup	194	7	18
Chinese chestnuts, 1 oz.	64	0	14
Chives, 1 tbsp, chopped	1	0	0
Chocolate chip crisped rice bar, 1 bar	115	4	21
Chocolate chips, 1/4 cup	210	12	24
Chocolate milkshake, ready-to-drink, 8 fl.oz.	181	5	26
Chocolate, semi sweet bars, baking, 1 oz.	160	8	20
Chorizo, pork and beef, 1 link	273	23	1
Chow mein noodles, 1 cup	237	14	26
Cinnamon, ground, 1 tsp	6	0	2
Cisco, 3 oz.	83	2	0
Citrus fruit drink, from concentrate, 8 fl.oz.	124	0	30
Clam, mixed species, raw, 1 large	15	0	1
Cloves, ground, 1 tsp	7	0	1
Cocktail mix, nonalcoholic, 1 fl.oz.	103	0	26
Cocoa mix, powder, 1 serving	113	1	24
Cocoa mix, powder, unsweetened, 1 tbsp	12	1	3
Coconut meat, 1 cup, shredded	283	27	12
Coconut milk, 1 cup	552	57	13
Coffee, brewed, decaf, 1 cup	0	0	0
Coffee, brewed, regular, 1 cup	2	0	0
Coffee, café au lait, 8 fl.oz.	65	3	6
Coffee, cappuccino, 8 fl.oz.	70	4	6
Coffee, espresso, 1 shot	4	0	1
Coffee, instant, decaf, 1 tsp	0	0	0
Coffee, instant, regular, 1 tsp, dry	2	0	0
Coffee, latte, 8 fl.oz.	100	5	8
Coffee, mocha, 8 fl.oz.	180	12	16
Coffeecake, 3 oz.	230	7	38
Coleslaw, 1/2 cup	41	2	7
Collards, 1 cup, chopped	11	0	2
Conch, baked or broiled, 1 cup, sliced	165	2	2
Cookies, animal crackers, 1 cookie	22	1	4
Cookies, brownies, 4 oz.	430	25	52
Cookies, butter, 1 cookie	23	1	3
Cookies, choco chip, deli fresh baked, 1	275	15	38
Cookies, chocolate chip, commercial, 1	130	7	17
Cookies, chocolate wafers, 1 wafer	26	1	4
Cookies, fig bars, 1 cookie	150	3	31

NUTRITIONAL FACTS FOR POPULAR FOOD ITEMS

C (cont.)	Cal	Fat	Cbs
Cookies, fudge, 1 cookie	73	1	16
Cookies, gingersnap, 1 cookie	29	1	5
Cookies, graham, plain/honey, 2 1/2" square	30	1	5
Cookies, marshmallow w/ choco coating, 1	118	5	19
Cookies, molasses, 1 cookie	138	4	24
Cookies, oatmeal, 1 cookie	238	9	38
Cookies, oatmeal w/ raisins, 1 cookie	238	9	38
Cookies, oatmeal, commercial, iced, 1	123	5	18
Cookies, oatmeal, refrigerated dough,1	68	3	10
Cookies, peanut butter sandwich,1 cookie	67	3	9
Cookies, peanut butter, dough, 1	73	4	8
Cookies, sugar, 1 cookie	66	3	8
Cookies, sugar wafers w/ cream filling, 1	46	2	6
Cookies, sugar, refrigerated dough, 1	113	5	15
Cookies, vanilla wafers, 1 wafer	28	1	4
Coriander leaves, 9 sprigs	5	0	1
Corn flour, yellow, 1 cup	416	4	87
Corn, sweet, white, 1 ear	77	1	17
Corn, sweet, yellow, 1 ear	77	1	17
Corn, sweet, white, cream style, 1 cup	184	1	46
Corn, sweet, yellow, cream style, 1 cup	184	1	46
Cornnuts, 1 oz.	126	4	20
Cornstarch, 1 cup	488	0	117
Couscous, cooked, 1 cup	176	0	37
Cowpeas (black-eyed peas), cooked, 1 cup	160	1	34
Cowpeas, catjang, cooked, 1 cup	200	1	35
Cowpeas, leafy tips, 1 cup, chopped	10	0	2
Crab, alaska king, raw, 1 leg	144	1	0
Crab, blue, canned, 1 cup	134	2	0
Crab, dungeness, cooked, 1 crab	140	2	1
Crabapples, 1 cup, sliced	84	0	22
Crackers w/ cheese filling, 6 crackers	191	10	23
Crackers w/ peanut butter filling, 6 cracker	193	10	22
Crackers, cheese, regular, crackers	312	16	36
Crackers, graham, 1 cracker	30	1	5
Crackers, matzo, plain, 1 matzo	112	0	24
Crackers, matzo, whole-wheat, 1 matzo	100	0	22
Crackers, melba toast, 1 cup	129	1	25
Crackers, milk, 1 cracker	50	2	8
Crackers, regular, 1 cup, bite size	311	16	38
Crackers, rusk toast, 1 rusk	41	1	7
Crackers, rye, 1 cracker	37	0	9
Crackers, saltines, 1 cracker	20	0	4
Crackers, soda, 1 cracker	23	1	4
Crackers, wheat, 1 cracker	9	0	1
Crackers, whole-wheat, 1 cracker	18	1	3
Cranberries, 1 cup, whole	44	0	12
Cranberry juice cocktail, 1 cup	144	0	36
Cranberry-apple juice, 1 cup	174	0	44
Cranberry-grape juice, 1 cup	137	0	34
Crayfish, wild, raw, 8 crayfish	21	0	0
Cream cheese, 1 tbsp	51	0	0
Cream of tartar, 1 tsp	8	0	2
Cream, half & half, 1 tbsp	20	2	1
Cream, heavy whipping, 1 cup, fluid	821	88	7
Crepes, 1 crepe	120	6	14
Croissants, apple, 1 croissant	145	5	21
Croissants, butter, 1 croissant	115	6	13
Croissants, cheese, 1 croissant	174	9	20
Croutons, plain, 1 cup	122	2	22
Croutons, seasoned, 1 cup	186	7	25
Cucumber, 1 cucumber	45	0	11
Cucumber, peeled, 1 cup, sliced	14	0	3
Cumin seed, 1 tsp	8	1	1
Currants, black, 1 cup	71	1	17

C (cont.)	Cal	Fat	Cbs
Currants, red & white, 1 cup	63	0	16
Curry powder, 1 tsp	7	0	1

D	Cal	Fat	Cbs
Dandelion greens, 1 cup, chopped	25	0	5
Danish pastry, cheese, 4 1/4" diameter, 1	266	16	26
Danish pastry, cinnamon, 4 1/4" diameter, 1	262	15	29
Danish pastry, fruit, 4 1/4" diameter, 1	263	13	34
Danish pastry, nut, 4 1/4" diameter, 1	280	16	30
Danish pastry, raspberry, 4 1/4" diameter, 1	263	13	34
Deer, ground, raw, 1 oz.	45	2	0
Deer, raw, 1 oz.	34	1	0
Doughnuts, chocolate coated or frosted, 1	133	9	13
Doughnuts, choco, sugared or glazed, 1	250	12	34
Doughnuts, french crullers, 1 cruller	169	8	24
Doughnuts, plain, 1 doughnut, stick	219	12	26
Doughnuts, wheat, sugared or glazed, 1	101	5	12
Duck liver, raw, 1 liver	60	2	2
Duck, meat only, roasted, 1/2 duck	444	25	0
Duck, skinless, raw, 1/2 duck	400	18	0
Durian, 1 cup, chopped	357	13	66

E	Cal	Fat	Cbs
Eclairs w/ chocolate glaze, 1 éclair	293	18	27
Eel, mixed species, raw, 3 oz.	156	10	0
Egg noodles, cooked, 1 cup	213	2	40
Egg substitute, liquid, 1 tbsp	13	1	0
Egg white, fried, 1 large	92	7	0
Egg white, raw, 1 large	17	0	0
Egg yolk, raw, 1 large	53	4	1
Egg, hard-boiled, 1 cup, chopped	211	14	2
Egg, omelette, 1 large	93	7	0
Egg, poached, 1 large	74	5	0
Egg, raw, 1 large	85	6	0
Egg, scrambled, 1 cup	365	27	5
Eggnog, 8 fl.oz.	343	19	34
Eggplant, 1 eggplant	110	10	26
Elderberries, 1 cup	106	1	27
Elk, ground, raw, 1 oz.	49	3	0
Elk, raw, 1 oz.	31	0	0
Endive, 1 head	87	1	17
English muffins, plain, 1 muffin	134	1	26
English muffins, cinnamon-raisin, 1 muffin	139	2	49
English muffins, wheat, 1 muffin	127	1	26
English muffins, whole-wheat, 1 muffin	134	1	27
English muffins, whole-wheat/multigrain,1	155	1	31
European chestnuts, peeled, 1 oz.	56	0	13
European chestnuts, unpeeled, 1 oz.	60	1	13

F	Cal	Fat	Cbs
Farina, cooked, 1 cup.	471	0	24
Fast food, biscuit w/ egg, 1 biscuit	373	22	32
Fast food, biscuit w/ egg & bacon, 1 biscuit	458	31	29
Fast food, biscuit w/ sausage, 1 biscuit	485	32	40
Fast food, caramel sundae, 1 sundae	304	9	49
Fast food, chz, large, double patty, 1	704	44	40
Fast food, chz, large, single patty, 1	563	33	38
Fast food, corndog, 1 corndog	460	19	56
Fast food, croissant w/ egg, chz, 1	368	25	24
Fast food, croissant w/ egg, chz, bacon, 1	413	28	24
Fast food, croissant w/ egg, chz, sausage,1	523	38	25
Fast food, Danish pastry, cheese, 1 pastry	353	25	29
Fast food, Danish pastry, cinnamon, 1	349	17	47
Fast food, Danish pastry, fruit, 1 pastry	335	16	45
Fast food, fish sandwich w/ tartar sauce, 1	431	23	41
Fast food, french toast sticks, 5 pieces	513	29	58

NUTRITIONAL FACTS FOR POPULAR FOOD ITEMS

F (cont.)	Cal	Fat	Cbs
Fast food, fried chicken, boneless, 6 pieces	285	18	16
Fast food, hamburger, large, double patty, 1	540	27	40
Fast food, hamburger, large, single patty, 1	425	21	37
Fast food, hot fudge sundae, 1 sundae	284	9	48
Fast food, hot dog w/ chili, 1 hot dog	296	13	31
Fast food, hot dog, plain, 1 hot dog	242	15	18
Fast food, McDonald's Big Mac® w/ chz,1	560	30	46
Fast food, McDonald's Big Mac® w/o chz,1	495	25	43
Fast food, McDonald's cheeseburger, 1	310	12	35
Fast food, McDonald's Chicken McGrill®, 1	400	16	38
Fast food, McDonald's Crispy Chicken, 1	500	23	50
Fast food, McDonald's Filet-o-Fish®, 1	400	18	42
Fast food, McDonald's french fries, ,1 med	350	11	47
Fast food, McDonald's hamburger, 1	260	9	33
Fast food, McDonald's 1/4 Pounder®,chz,1	510	25	43
Fast food, McDonald's 1/4 Pounder®,1	420	18	40
Fast food, onion rings, 8-9 rings, 1 portion	276	16	31
Fast food, strawberry sundae, 1 sundae	268	8	45
Fast food, sub w/ cold cuts, 1 sub 6"	456	19	51
Fast food, sub w/ roast beef, 1 sub 6"	410	13	44
Fast food, sub w/ tuna,1 sub 6"	584	28	55
Fast food, vanilla soft-serve w/ cone, 1	164	6	24
Fennel bulb, 1 cup, sliced	27	0	6
Fennel seed, 1 tbsp	20	1	3
Fenugreek seed, 1 tbsp	36	1	7
Figs, 1 medium	37	0	10
Figs, dried, 1 fig	21	0	5
Fireweed leaves, 1 cup, chopped	24	1	4
Fish oil, cod liver, 1 tbsp	123	14	0
Fish oil, herring, 1 tbsp	123	14	0
Fish oil, menhaden, 1 tbsp	123	14	0
Fish oil, salmon, 1 tbsp	123	14	0
Fish oil, sardine, 1 tbsp	123	14	0
Fish, bluefin tuna, raw, 3 oz.	122	4	0
Fish, bluefish, raw, 3 oz.	105	4	0
Fish, butterfish, raw, 3 oz.	124	7	0
Fish, carp, raw, 3 oz.	108	5	0
Fish, catfish, raw, 3 oz.	81	2	0
Fish, cod, atlantic, raw, 3 oz.	70	1	0
Fish, croaker, atlantic, raw, 3 oz.	88	3	0
Fish, flatfish, raw, 3 oz.	77	1	0
Fish, gefilte fish, 1 piece	35	1	3
Fish, grouper, mixed species, raw, 3 oz.	78	1	0
Fish, haddock, raw, 3 oz.	74	1	0
Fish, halibut, raw, 3 oz.	94	2	0
Fish, herring, atlantic, raw, 3 oz.	134	8	0
Fish, herring, pacific, raw, 3 oz.	166	12	0
Fish, mackerel, atlantic, raw, 3 oz.	174	12	0
Fish, mackerel, king, raw, 3 oz.	89	2	0
Fish, mackerel, pacific, raw, 3 oz.	134	7	0
Fish, mackerel, spanish, raw, 3 oz.	118	5	0
Fish, milkfish, raw, 3 oz.	126	6	0
Fish, monkfish, raw, 3 oz.	65	1	0
Fish, ocean perch, atlantic, raw, 3 oz.	80	1	0
Fish, perch, mixed species, raw, 3 oz.	77	1	0
Fish, pike, northern, raw, 3 oz.	75	1	0
Fish, pollock, atlantic, raw, 3 oz.	78	1	0
Fish, pout, ocean, raw, 3 oz.	67	1	0
Fish, rainbow smelt, raw, 3 oz.	82	2	0
Fish, rockfish, pacific, raw, 3 oz.	80	1	0
Fish, roe, mixed species, raw, 1 tbsp	20	10	0
Fish, sablefish, raw, 3 oz.	166	13	0
Fish, salmon, atlantic, farmed, raw, 3 oz.	156	9	0
Fish, salmon, atlantic, wild, raw, 3 oz.	121	5	0
Fish, salmon, chinook, raw, 3 oz.	152	9	0

F (cont.)	Cal	Fat	Cbs
Fish, salmon, pink, raw, 3 oz.	99	3	0
Fish, sea bass, mixed species, raw, 3 oz.	82	2	0
Fish, seatrout, mixed species, raw, 3 oz.	88	3	0
Fish, shad, raw, 3 oz.	167	12	0
Fish, skipjack tuna, raw, 3 oz.	88	1	0
Fish, snapper, mixed species, raw, 3 oz.	85	1	0
Fish, striped bass, raw, 3 oz.	82	2	0
Fish, striped mullet, 3 oz.	99	3	0
Fish, sturgeon, mixed species, raw, 3 oz.	89	3	0
Fish, swordfish, raw, 3 oz.	103	3	0
Fish, trout, mixed species, raw, 3 oz.	126	6	0
Fish, white sucker, raw, 3 oz.	78	2	0
Fish, whitefish, raw, 3 oz.	114	5	0
Fish, wolffish, atlantic, raw, 3 oz.	82	2	0
Fish, yellowfin tuna, raw, 3 oz.	93	1	0
Fish, yellowtail, mixed species, raw, 3 oz.	124	5	0
Flan, caramel custard, 5 1/2 oz.	303	12	43
Flaxseed, 1 tbsp	59	4	4
Flaxseed oil, 1 tbsp	120	14	0
Frankfurter, 1 serving	151	13	2
Frankfurter, beef, 1 frankfurter	188	17	2
Frankfurter, beef & pork, 1 frankfurter	174	16	1
Frankfurter, chicken, 1 frankfurter	116	9	3
Frankfurter, meat, 1 frankfurter	151	13	2
Frankfurter, meatless, 1 frankfurter	163	10	5
Frankfurter, pork, 1 frankfurter	204	18	0
Frankfurter, turkey, 1 frankfurter	102	8	1
French fries, frozen, unprepared, 18 fries	170	7	28
French toast, frozen, ready-to-heat, 1 piece	126	4	19
Frosting, creamy chocolate, 2 tbsp	164	7	26
Frosting, creamy vanilla, 2 tbsp	160	6	26
Frozen yogurt, choco, soft-serve, 1/2 cup	115	4	18
Frozen yogurt, vanilla, soft-serve, 1/2 cup	117	4	17
Fruit cocktail, canned, 1 cup	229	0	60
Fruit punch, from concentrate, 8 fl.oz.	124	1	30
Fruit salad, canned in syrup, 1 cup	186	0	49
Fruit salad, canned in water, 1 cup	74	0	19

G (cont.)	Cal	Fat	Cbs
Garden cress, raw, 1 cup	16	0	3
Garlic, 1 clove	4	0	1
Garlic powder, 1 tsp	9	0	2
Gelatin dessert mix, w/ water, 1/2 cup	84	0	19
Gin, 80 Proof, 1 fl.oz.	73	0	0
Ginger root, 1 tsp	2	0	0
Ginger, ground, 1 tsp	6	0	1
Ginkgo nuts, 1 oz.	52	1	11
Ginkgo nuts, dried, 1 oz.	99	1	21
Goose liver, raw, 1 liver	125	4	6
Goose, meat only, roasted, cup chopped	340	18	0
Gourd, white-flowered, 1 gourd	108	0	26
Granola bars, hard, plain, 1 bar	134	6	18
Granola bars, soft, plain, 1 bar	126	5	19
Grape juice, 8 fl.oz.	160	0	40
Grapefruit, 1/2 fruit	50	0	12
Grapefruit juice, sweetened, 8 fl.oz.	125	0	33
Grapefruit juice, unsweetened, 8 fl.oz.	91	0	22
Grapes, canned, heavy syrup, 1 cup	187	0	50
Grapes, red or green, 1 cup	106	0	28
Gravy, mushroom, canned, 1 can	149	8	16
Gravy, au jus, canned, 1 can	48	1	8
Gravy, beef, canned, 1 can	154	7	14
Gravy, chicken, canned, 1 can	235	17	16
Gravy, turkey, canned, 1 can	152	6	15
Guacamole dip, 2 tbsp	50	4	4
Guavas, 1 fruit	37	1	8

NUTRITIONAL FACTS FOR POPULAR FOOD ITEMS

H	Cal	Fat	Cbs
Ham, chopped, 1 slice	50	3	1
Ham, minced, 1 slice	55	4	0
Ham, sliced, 1 slice	46	2	1
Hazlenuts, dry roasted, 1 oz.	183	18	5
Hazlenuts, blanched, 1 oz.	178	17	5
Hominy, canned, white, 1 cup	119	2	24
Hominy, canned, yellow, 1 cup	115	1	23
Honey, 1 tbsp	64	0	17
Honeydew melons, 1 cup, diced	61	0	16
Horseradish, 1 tsp	2	0	1
Hot chocolate, 8 fl.oz.	200	10	25
Hummus, 1 tbsp	23	1	2
Hush puppies, 1 hush puppy	74	3	10
Ice cream cone, rolled or sugar type, 1 cone	40	0	8
Ice cream cone, wafer or cake type, 1 cone	17	0	3
Ice cream, chocolate, 1/2 cup	143	7	19
Ice cream, strawberry, 1/2 cup	127	6	18
Ice cream, vanilla, 1/2 cup	144	8	17
Iced tea, presweetened, 8 fl.oz.	100	0	25
Iced tea, unsweetened, 8 fl.oz.	2	0	0
Italian seasoning, 1 tsp	4	0	1

J	Cal	Fat	Cbs
Jams and preserves, 1 tbsp	56	0	14
Japanese chestnuts, 1 oz.	44	0	10
Japanese soba noodles, cooked, 1 cup	113	0	24
Japanese ramen noodles, packaged, dry, 1	195	7	28
Jellies, 1 tbsp	55	0	14

K	Cal	Fat	Cbs
Kale, 1 cup, chopped	34	1	7
Kiwifruit, 1 medium	45	0	11
Kumquats, 1 fruit	13	0	3

L	Cal	Fat	Cbs
Lamb, cubed, raw, 1 oz.	38	2	0
Lamb, foreshank, raw, 1 oz.	57	4	0
Lamb, ground, raw, 1 oz.	80	7	0
Lamb, leg, shank half, raw, 1 oz.	52	3	0
Lamb, leg, sirloin half, raw, 1 oz.	74	6	0
Lamb, leg, whole, choice, raw, 1 oz.	65	5	0
Lamb, loin, choice, raw, 1 oz.	79	6	0
Lamb, rib, choice, raw, 1 oz.	97	9	0
Lamb, shoulder, arm, raw, 1 oz.	69	5	0
Lamb, shoulder, blade, raw, 1 oz.	69	5	0
Lamb, shoulder, whole, raw, 1 oz.	69	5	0
Lard, 1 tbsp	115	13	0
Leeks, 1 leek	54	0	13
Lemon juice, 1 cup	61	0	21
Lemon juice, canned or bottled, 1 tbsp	3	0	1
Lemon pepper seasoning, 1 tsp	7	0	1
Lemonade powder, 1 scoop	102	0	27
Lemonade, pink concentrate, 8 fl.oz.	99	0	26
Lemonade, white concentrate, 8 fl.oz.	131	0	34
Lemons w/ peel, 1 fruit	22	0	12
Lentils, cooked, 1 cup	230	1	40
Lentils, sprouted, raw, 1 cup	82	0	17
Lettuce, green leaf, 1 cup, shredded	5	0	1
Lettuce, iceberg, 1 cup, shredded	10	0	2
Lettuce, red leaf, 1 cup, shredded	3	0	0
Lettuce, romaine, 1 cup, shredded	8	0	2
Lime juice, 1 cup	62	0	21
Limes, 1 fruit	20	0	7
Liverwurst, pork, 1 slice	59	5	0
Lobster, northern, raw, 1 lobster	135	1	1
Luncheon meat, beef, loaved, 1 oz.	87	7	1

L (cont.)	Cal	Fat	Cbs
Luncheon meat, beef, thin sliced, 1 oz.	50	1	2
Luncheon meat, meatless slices, 1 slice	26	2	1
Luncheon meat, pork & chkn, minced, 1 oz.	56	4	0
Luncheon meat, pork & ham, minced, 1 oz.	88	75	1
Luncheon meat, pork or beef, 1 oz.	99	9	1
Luncheon meat, pork, canned, 1 oz.	95	9	1
Luncheon sausage, pork & beef, 1 oz.	74	6	0

M	Cal	Fat	Cbs
Macadamia nuts, 1 oz. (10-12 nuts)	203	22	4
Macaroni and cheese, commercial, 1 cup	259	3	48
Macaroni, cooked, 1 cup	197	1	40
Malt drink mix, dry, 3 heaping tsp	87	2	16
Malt beverage, 8 fl.oz.	144	0	32
Mangos, 1 fruit	135	1	35
Maraschino cherries, 1 cherry	8	0	2
Margarine, fat free spread, 1 tbsp	6	0	1
Margarine, stick, 1 tbsp	100	11	0
Margarine, stick, unsalted, 1 tbsp	102	11	0
Margarine, tub, 1 tbsp	102	11	0
Martini, 1 fl.oz.	69	0	1
Mayonnaise, 1 tbsp	100	11	0
Milk, 1% low fat, 1 cup	102	2	12
Milk, 2% low fat, 1 cup	138	5	14
Milk, buttermilk, cultured, reduced fat, 1 cup	137	5	13
Milk, chocolate, 1 cup	208	9	26
Milk, dry, nonfat, instant, 1/3 cup dry	82	0	12
Milk, evaporated, 1/2 cup	169	10	13
Milk, skim or nonfat, 1 cup	83	0	12
Milk, canned, sweetened condensed, 1 cup	982	27	167
Milk, whole, 1 cup	146	8	11
Milkshake, dry mix, vanilla, 1 packet	69	1	11
Millet, 1 cup	756	8	146
Miso soup, 1 cup	37	17	73
Mixed nuts, 1 cup	814	71	35
Molasses, 1 tablespoon	58	0	15
Muffins, apple bran, 1 muffin	300	3	61
Muffins, banana nut, 1 muffin	480	24	60
Muffins, blueberry, 1 muffin	313	7	54
Muffins, chocolate chip, 1 muffin	510	24	69
Muffins, corn, 1 muffin	345	10	58
Muffins, oat bran, 1 muffin	305	8	55
Muffins, plain, 1 muffin	242	9	36
Mushrooms, 1 cup, pieces	15	0	2
Mushrooms, enoki, 1 large	2	0	0
Mushrooms, oyster, 1 large	55	1	9
Mushrooms, portobello, 1 large	0	0	0
Mushrooms, shiitake, 1 mushroom	11	0	3
Mussels, blue, raw, 1 cup	129	3	6
Mustard greens, 1 cup, chopped	15	0	3
Mustard seed, yellow, 1 tbsp	53	3	4
Mustard spinach, 1 cup, chopped	33	1	6
Mustard, prepared, yellow, 1 tsp	3	0	0

N	Cal	Fat	Cbs
Natto (fermented soybeans), 1 cup	371	19	25
Nectarines, 1 fruit	60	0	14
New Zealand spinach, 1 cup, chopped	8	0	1
Nutmeg, ground, 1 tsp	12	1	1

O	Cal	Fat	Cbs
Oat bran, 1 cup	231	7	62
Oatmeal, instant, prepared w/ water, 1 cup	129	2	22
Oil, canola, 1 tbsp	124	14	0
Oil, canola & soybean, 1 tbsp	119	14	0
Oil, coconut, 1 tbsp	120	14	0

NUTRITIONAL FACTS FOR POPULAR FOOD ITEMS

O (cont.)	Cal	Fat	Cbs
Oil, corn, peanut & olive, 1 tbsp	120	14	0
Oil, olive, 1 tbsp	119	14	0
Oil, peanut, 1 tbsp	119	14	0
Oil, sesame, 1 tbsp	120	14	0
Oil, soy, 1 tbsp	120	14	0
Oil, vegetable, almond, 1 tbsp	120	14	0
Oil, vegetable, cocoa butter, 1 tbsp	120	14	0
Oil, vegetable, coconut, 1 tbsp	117	14	0
Oil, vegetable, grapeseed, 1 tbsp	120	14	0
Oil, vegetable, hazelnut, 1 tbsp	120	14	0
Oil, vegetable, nutmeg butter, 1 tbsp	120	14	0
Oil, vegetable, palm, 1 tbsp	120	14	0
Oil, vegetable, poppyseed, 1 tbsp	120	14	0
Oil, vegetable, rice bran, 1 tbsp	120	14	0
Oil, vegetable, sheanut, 1 tbsp	120	14	0
Oil, vegetable, tomatoseed, 1 tbsp	120	14	0
Oil, vegetable, walnut, 1 tbsp	1927	218	0
Okra, 1 cup	31	0	7
Onion powder, 1 tsp	8	0	2
Onions, 1 cup, chopped	67	0	16
Onions, sweet, 1 onion	106	0	25
Orange juice, 8 fl.oz.	109	1	25
Orange marmalade, 1 tbsp	49	0	13
Oranges, 1 large	86	0	22
Oregano, dried, 1 tsp, ground	6	0	1
Oyster, eastern, raw, 3 oz.	50	1	5
Oyster, pacific, raw, 3 oz.	69	2	4

P	Cal	Fat	Cbs
Pancakes, blueberry, 1 pancake	84	4	11
Pancakes, buttermilk, 1 pancake	86	4	11
Pancakes, plain, dry mix, 1 pancake	74	1	14
Papayas, 1 cup, cubed	55	0	14
Paprika, 1 tsp	6	0	1
Parsley, 1 cup	22	1	4
Parsley, dried, 1 tsp	1	0	0
Parsnips, 1 cup, sliced	100	0	24
Passion fruit, 1 fruit	17	0	4
Pasta, corn, cooked, 1 cup	176	1	39
Pasta, plain, cooked, 1 cup	197	1	40
Pasta, spinach, cooked, 1 cup	195	1	38
Pastrami, turkey, 1 oz.	40	2	1
Pate de foie gras, 1 tbsp	60	6	1
Pate, chicken liver, canned, 1 tbsp	26	2	1
Pate, goose liver, canned, 1 tbsp	60	6	1
Peaches, 1 large	61	0	15
Peaches, canned, 1 cup, halved	59	0	15
Peanut butter, chunky, 2 tbsp	188	16	7
Peanut butter, smooth, 2 tbsp	188	16	6
Peanuts, dry roasted w/ salt, 1 oz.	166	14	6
Peanuts, raw, 1 oz.	161	14	5
Pears, 1 pear	121	0	32
Pears, asian, 1 pear	116	1	29
Pears, canned, 1 cup	71	0	19
Peas, green, fresh, cooked, 1 cup	134	0	25
Peas, green, frozen, cooked, 1 cup	125	0	23
Peas, split, cooked, 1 cup	231	1	41
Pecans, 1 oz. (20 halves)	196	20	40
Pepper, black, 1 tsp	5	0	1
Pepper, red or cayenne, 1 tsp	6	0	1
Pepperoni, 15 slices	135	12	1
Peppers, chili, green, 1 cup	29	0	6
Peppers, chili, red, 1 pepper	18	0	4
Peppers, chili, sun-dried, 1 pepper	2	0	0
Peppers, jalapeno, 1 pepper	4	0	1
Peppers, sweet, green, 1 medium	24	0	6

P (cont.)	Cal	Fat	Cbs
Peppers, sweet, red, 1 medium	31	0	7
Peppers, sweet, yellow, 1 medium	32	0	8
Persimmons, 1 fruit	32	0	8
Pheasant, boneless, raw, 1/2 pheasant	724	37	0
Pheasant, leg, skinless, boneless, raw, 1 leg	143	5	0
Pheasant, skinless, raw, 1/2 pheasant	468	13	0
Pickle relish, sweet, 1 tbsp	20	0	5
Pickle, sour, 1 large 4"	15	0	3
Pickle, sweet, 1 large 4"	158	0	43
Pickles, dill, 1 large 4"	24	0	6
Pie crust, graham cracker, baked, 1	1037	52	137
Pie, apple, 1 piece	411	19	58
Pie, blueberry, 1 piece	290	13	44
Pie, cherry, 1 piece	325	14	50
Pie, lemon meringue, 1 piece	303	10	53
Pie, pecan, 1 piece	452	21	65
Pie, pumpkin, 1 piece	229	10	30
Pine nuts, 1 oz. (167 kernels)	191	19	4
Pineapple, 1 fruit	227	1	60
Pineapple, canned, 1 slice	15	0	4
Pita bread, whole wheat, 1 pita	170	2	35
Pistachio nuts, 1 oz. (49 kernels)	161	13	8
Pizza, cheese, 1 slice (3.7 oz.)	250	10	29
Pizza, pepperoni, 1 slice (3.7 oz.)	288	15	26
Plantains, 1 medium	218	1	57
Plums, 1 fruit	30	0	8
Plums, canned, 1 plum	19	0	5
Polenta, 1/2 cup	220	2	24
Pomegranates, 1 fruit	105	1	26
Popcorn cakes, 1 cake	38	0	8
Popcorn, air-popped, 1 cup	31	0	6
Popcorn, caramel-coated, 1 oz.	122	4	22
Popcorn, cheese, 1 cup	58	4	6
Popcorn, oil-popped, 1 cup	55	3	6
Popovers, dry mix, 1 oz.	105	1	20
Poppy seed, 1 tsp	15	1	1
Pork, cured, brkfst strips, cooked, 3 slices	156	12	0
Pork, cured, ham, extra lean, canned, 3 oz.	116	4	0
Pork, cured, ham, patties, 1 patty	205	18	1
Pork, cured, ham, extra lean, cooked, 3 oz.	140	7	0
Pork, cured, salt pork, raw, 1 oz.	212	23	0
Pork, fresh ground, cooked, 3 oz.	252	18	0
Pork, leg, rump half, cooked, 3 oz.	214	12	0
Pork, leg, shank half, cooked, 3 oz.	246	17	0
Pork, leg, whole, cooked, 3 oz.	232	15	0
Pork, loin, blade, cooked, 3 oz.	275	21	0
Pork, loin, center loin, cooked, 3 oz.	199	11	0
Pork, loin, center rib, cooked, 3 oz.	214	13	0
Pork, loin, sirloin, cooked, 3 oz.	176	8	0
Pork, loin, tenderloin, cooked, 3 oz.	147	5	0
Pork, loin, top loin, cooked, 3 oz.	192	10	0
Pork, loin, whole, cooked, 3 oz.	211	12	0
Pork, shoulder, arm, cooked, 3 oz.	238	18	0
Pork, shoulder, blade, cooked, 3 oz.	229	16	0
Pork, shoulder, whole, cooked, 3 oz.	248	18	0
Pork, spareribs, cooked, 3 oz.	337	26	0
Potato chips, barbecue, 1 oz.	139	5	15
Potato chips, cheese, 1 oz.	141	8	16
Potato chips, salted, 1 oz.	152	10	15
Potato chips, sour cream & onion, 1 oz.	151	10	15
Potato chips, reduced fat, 1 oz.	134	6	19
Potato chips, unsalted, 1 oz.	152	10	15
Potato flour, 1 cup	571	1	133
Potato salad, 1 cup	358	21	28
Potatoes, 1 medium	164	0	37

P (cont.)	Cal	Fat	Cbs
Potatoes, baked, w/ skin, 1 medium	160	0	37
Potatoes, baked, w/o skin, 1 medium	143	0	33
Potatoes, mashed, 1 cup	237	9	35
Potatoes, red, 1 medium	153	0	34
Potatoes, russet, 1 medium	168	0	39
Potatoes, scalloped, 1 cup	211	9	26
Potatoes, white, 1 medium	149	0	34
Pretzels, hard, plain, salted, 1 oz.	108	1	22
Prune juice, 8 fl.oz.	180	0	43
Pudding, banana1/2 cup	154	3	29
Pudding, chocolate, 1/2 cup	154	3	28
Pudding, coconut cream, 1/2 cup	157	3	28
Pudding, lemon, 1/2 cup	157	3	30
Pudding, rice, 1/2 cup	163	2	31
Pudding, tapioca, 1/2 cup	154	2	29
Pudding, vanilla, 1/2 cup	148	3	27
Pumpkin, 1 cup	30	0	8
Pumpkin pie mix, 1 cup	281	0	71
Pumpkin, canned, 1 cup	83	1	20

R	Cal	Fat	Cbs
Rabbit, cooked, 3 oz.	167	7	0
Radicchio, 1 cup, shredded	9	0	2
Radishes, 1 cup, sliced	19	0	4
Raisins, 1 1/2 oz.	129	0	34
Raisins, 1 1/2 oz.	130	0	34
Raspberries, 1 cup	64	1	15
Rhubarb, 1 cup, diced	26	0	6
Rice cakes, brown rice, corn, 1 cake	35	0	7
Rice cakes, brown rice, multigrain, 1 cake	35	0	7
Rice cakes, brown rice, plain, 1 cake	35	0	7
Rice, brown, cooked, 1 cup	218	2	46
Rice, white, cooked, 1 cup	242	0	53
Rice, wild, 1 cup	166	1	35
Rolls, dinner, 1 roll	136	3	23
Rolls, dinner, wheat, 1 roll	117	3	20
Rolls, dinner, whole-wheat, 1 roll	114	2	22
Rolls, french, 1 roll	119	2	22
Rolls, hamburger or hotdog, 1 roll	120	2	21
Rolls, hard (incl. kaiser), 1 roll	126	2	23
Rolls, pumpernickel, 1 roll	119	1	23
Rosemary, 1 tsp	1	0	0
Rosemary, dried, 1 tsp	4	0	1
Rum, 80 proof, 1 fl.oz.	64	0	0
Rutabagas, 1 cup, cubed	50	0	11
Rye, 1 cup	566	4	118
Rye flour, dark, 1 cup	415	3	88
Rye flour, light, 1 cup	374	1	82
Rye flour, medium, 1 cup	361	2	79

S	Cal	Fat	Cbs
Sage, ground, 1 tsp	2	0	0
Sake, 1 fl.oz.	39	0	2
Salad dressing, 1000 island, 1 tbsp	58	6	2
Salad dressing, bacon & tomato, 1 tbsp	49	5	0
Salad dressing, blue cheese, 1 tbsp	77	8	1
Salad dressing, caesar, 1 tbsp	78	9	1
Salad dressing, coleslaw, 1 tbsp	61	5	4
Salad dressing, french, 1 tbsp	71	7	2
Salad dressing, honey dijon, 1 tbsp	58	5	3
Salad dressing, italian, 1 tbsp	43	4	2
Salad dressing, mayo-based, 1 tbsp	57	5	4
Salad dressing, mayonnaise, 1 tbsp	103	12	0
Salad dressing, peppercorn, 1 tbsp	76	8	1
Salad dressing, ranch, 1 tbsp	73	8	1
Salad dressing, russian, 1 tbsp	53	4	5

S (cont.)	Cal	Fat	Cbs
Salad, chicken, 6 oz.	420	33	11
Salad, egg, 6 oz.	300	23	14
Salad, prima pasta, 6 oz.	360	30	18
Salad, seafood w/ crab & shrimp, 6 oz.	420	34	20
Salad, tuna, 6 oz.	450	36	14
Salami, cooked, turkey, 1 oz.	38	2	0
Salami, dry, pork or beef, 3 slices	104	8	1
Salami, italian pork, 1 oz.	119	10	0
Salsa, w/ oil, 2 tbsp	40	3	8
Salsa, w/o oil, 2 tbsp	15	0	4
Salt, 1 tbsp	0	0	0
Sauce, alfredo, 1/4 cup	120	11	3
Sauce, barbecue, 1 cup	188	5	32
Sauce, cheese, 1 cup	479	36	13
Sauce, cranberry, 1 cup	418	0	108
Sauce, hollandaise, 1 cup	62	2	10
Sauce, honey mustard, 1 tbsp	30	1	5
Sauce, marinara, 1 cup	185	6	28
Sauce, salsa, 1 cup	70	0	16
Sauce, soy, 1 tbsp	10	0	0
Sauce, steak, 1 tbsp	25	0	6
Sauce, teriyaki, 1 tbsp	15	0	2
Sauce, tomato chili, 1 cup	284	1	54
Sauce, worcestershire, 1 cup	184	0	54
Sauerkraut, 1/2 cup	25	0	5
Sausage, italian pork, raw, 1 link	391	35	1
Sausage, pork, 1 link	85	7	0
Sausage, smoked linked, pork, 1 link	265	22	1
Sausage, turkey, 1 link	65	5	0
Savory, ground, 1 tsp	4	0	1
Scallops, 1 scallop	26	0	1
Seaweed, dried, 1 oz.	50	0	13
Sesame seeds, dried, 1 tbsp	52	5	2
Shallots, 1 tbsp, chopped	7	0	2
Shortening, 1 tbsp	113	13	0
Shrimp, mixed species, raw, 1 medium	6	0	0
Snacks, cheese puffs or twists, 1 oz.	157	10	15
Soda, club, 12 fl.oz.	0	0	0
Soda, cream, 12 fl.oz.	252	0	66
Soda, diet cola, 12 fl.oz.	0	0	0
Soda, ginger ale, 12 fl.oz.	166	0	43
Soda, lemon-lime, 12 fl.oz.	196	0	51
Soda, regular, w/ caffeine, 12 fl.oz.	155	0	40
Soda, regular, w/o caffeine, 12 fl.oz.	207	0	53
Soda, root beer, 12 fl.oz.	202	0	52
Soda, tonic water, 12 fl.oz.	166	0	43
Soup, beef broth, 1 cup	29	0	2
Soup, beef stroganoff, 1 cup	235	11	22
Soup, beef vegetable, 1 cup	82	2	13
Soup, chicken broth, 1 cup	39	1	1
Soup, chicken noodle, 1 cup	75	2	9
Soup, chicken vegetable, 1 cup	75	3	9
Soup, chicken w/ dumplings, 1 cup	96	6	6
Soup, clam chowder, 1 cup	95	3	12
Soup, cream of chicken, 1 cup	117	7	9
Soup, cream of mushroom, 1 cup	129	9	9
Soup, cream of potato, 1 cup	149	6	17
Soup, minestrone, 1 cup	82	3	11
Soup, split-pea w/ham, 1 cup	190	4	28
Soup, tomato, 1 cup	161	6	22
Soup, vegetarian, 1 cup	72	2	12
Sour cream, 1 tbsp	26	3	1
Sour cream, fat free, 1 tbsp	9	0	2
Sour cream, reduced fat, 1 tbsp	22	2	1
Soy milk, 1 cup	127	5	12

NUTRITIONAL FACTS FOR POPULAR FOOD ITEMS

S (cont.)	Cal	Fat	Cbs
Soy protein isolate, 1 oz.	96	1	2
Soybeans, green, cooked, 1 cup	254	12	12
Soybeans, nuts, roasted, 1/4 cup	194	9	14
Soyburger, 1 patty	125	4	9
Spaghetti, cooked, 1 cup	197	1	40
Spaghetti, spinach, cooked, 1 cup	182	1	37
Spaghetti, whole-wheat, cooked, 1 cup	174	1	37
Spinach, 1 cup	7	0	1
Squab, boneless, raw, 1 squab	585	47	0
Squab, skinless, raw, 1 squab	239	13	0
Squash, summer, 1 cup, sliced	18	0	4
Squash, winter, 1 cup, cubed	39	0	10
Squid, mixed species, raw, 1 oz.	26	0	1
Stock, beef, 1 cup	31	0	3
Stock, chicken, 1 cup	86	3	9
Stock, fish, 1 cup	40	2	0
Strawberries, 1 cup	49	1	12
Succotash, 1 cup	145	1	31
Sugar, brown, 1 tsp	12	0	3
Sugar, granulated, 1 tsp	16	0	4
Sugar, maple, 1 tsp	11	0	3
Sugar, powdered, 1 tsp	10	0	3
Sunflower seeds, 1 tbsp	45	10	2
Sweet potato, 1 cup, cubed	114	0	27
Syrup, chocolate, 1 tbsp	67	2	12
Syrup, dark corn, 1 tbsp	57	0	16
Syrup, grenadine, 1 tbsp	53	0	13
Syrup, light corn, 1 tbsp	59	0	16
Syrup, maple, 1 tbsp	52	0	13
Syrup, pancake, 1 tbsp	47	0	12

T	Cal	Fat	Cbs
Taco shell, hard, 1 shell	55	3	6
Tangerines, 1 large	52	0	13
Tarragon, dried, 1 tsp	2	0	0
Tea, instant, 1 cup	2	0	0
Thyme, 1 tsp	1	0	0
Thyme, dried, 1 tsp	3	0	1
Tofu, firm, 1/2 cup	183	11	5
Tofu, fried, 1 piece	35	3	1
Tofu, soft, 1/2 cup	76	5	2
Tomato juice, canned, with salt, 6 fl.oz.	31	0	8
Tomato juice, canned, without salt, 6 fl.oz.	30	0	8
Tomato paste, canned, 1/2 cup	107	1	25
Tomato sauce, canned, 1 cup	78	1	18
Tomatoes, canned, crushed, 1 cup	82	1	19
Tomatoes, green, 1 cup, chopped	41	0	9
Tomatoes, orange, 1 cup, chopped	25	0	5
Tomatoes, red, 1 cup, chopped	32	0	7
Tomatoes, sun-dried, 1 cup, chopped	139	2	30
Toppings, butterscotch or caramel, 2 tbsp	103	0	27
Toppings, marshmallow cream, 2 tbsp	132	0	32
Toppings, nuts in syrup, 2 tbsp	184	9	24
Toppings, pineapple, 2 tbsp	106	0	28
Toppings, strawberry, 2 tbsp	107	0	28
Tortilla chips, plain, 1 oz.	142	7	18
Tortilla, corn, 1 tortilla	45	1	9
Tortilla, flour, 1 tortilla	160	3	28
Trail mix, 1/4 cup	173	11	17
Turkey, deli sliced, white meat, 1 oz.	30	1	1
Turkey, back, skinless, boneless, raw, 1/2	180	5	0
Turkey, breast, boneless, raw, 1/2	541	12	0
Turkey, breast, skinless, boneless, raw, 1/2	433	3	0
Turkey, dark meat, bnless, raw,1/2 turkey	686	26	0
Turkey, leg, boneless, raw, 1 leg	412	13	0
Turkey, leg, skinless, boneless, raw, 1 leg	355	8	0

T (cont.)	Cal	Fat	Cbs
Turkey, wing, boneless, raw, 1 wing	204	10	0
Turkey, wing, skinless, bnless, raw, 1 wing	95	1	0
Turkey, young hen, back, bnless, raw, 1/2	650	48	0
Turkey, yng hen, breast, bnless, raw, 1/2	1460	73	0
Turkey, young hen, leg, bnless, raw, 1 leg	991	49	0
Turkey, young hen, wing, bnless, raw, 1	470	31	0
Turkey, young tom, back, bnless, raw, 1/2	938	58	0
Turkey, yng tom, breast, bnless, raw, 1/2	2701	113	0
Turkey, yng tm, drk meat, bnless, raw, 1/2	1884	63	0
Turkey, young tom, leg, bnless, raw, 1 leg	1740	78	0
Turkey, young tom, wing, bnless, raw, 1	654	39	0
Turnip greens, 1 cup, chopped	18	0	4
Turnips, 1 cup, cubed	36	0	8

V	Cal	Fat	Cbs
Vanilla extract, 1 tbsp	37	0	2
Veal, breast, raw, 1 oz.	59	4	0
Veal, cubed, raw, 1 oz.	31	1	0
Veal, ground, raw, 1 oz.	41	2	0
Veal, leg, raw, 1 oz.	33	1	0
Veal, loin, raw, 1 oz.	46	3	0
Veal, rib, raw, 1 oz.	46	3	0
Veal, shank, raw, 1 oz.	32	1	0
Veal, shoulder, arm, raw, 1 oz.	37	2	0
Veal, shoulder, blade, raw, 1 oz.	37	2	0
Veal, shoulder, whole, raw, 1 oz.	37	2	0
Veal, sirloin, raw, 1 oz.	43	2	0
Vegetable juice, 8 fl.oz.	50	0	12
Vinegar, 1 tbsp	2	0	1

W	Cal	Fat	Cbs
Waffles, plain, 1 waffle	218	11	25
Walnuts, 1 oz. (14 halves)	185	19	4
Wasabi root, 1 cup, sliced	142	1	31
Water chestnuts, chinese, 1/2 cup, sliced	60	0	15
Watercress, 1 cup, chopped	4	0	0
Watermelon, 1 cup, diced	46	0	12
Wheat bran, 1 cup	125	3	37
Wheat flour, whole grain, 1 cup	407	2	87
Wheat germ, 1 cup	414	11	60
Whipped cream, 1 cup	154	13	8
Wine, cooking, 1 tsp	2	0	0
Wine, red, 3-1/2 oz. glass	74	0	2
Wine, rose, 3-1/2 oz. glass	73	0	1
Wine, white, 3-1/2 oz. glass	70	0	1
Yam, 1 cup, cubed	177	0	42
Yeast, active, dry, 1 tsp	12	0	2
Yogurt, fruit, low fat, 8 oz. container	118	0	24
Yogurt, fruit, whole milk, 8 oz. container	250	6	38
Yogurt, plain, lowfat, 8 oz. container	110	4	7
Yogurt, plain, whole milk, 8 oz. container	138	7	11

Z	Cal	Fat	Cbs
Zucchini, 1 medium	45	0	10

NUTRITIONAL FACTS FOR POPULAR FOOD ITEMS

Other Food Items	Cal	Fat	Cbs
Write down the calories, fat, and carbs of your favorite food items			

Other Food Items	Cal	Fat	Cbs
Write down the calories, fat, and carbs of your favorite food items			

JOURNAL PAGES

With this diet journal as your companion, you can make better, more informed choices that will help you lose weight, look better, and improve your health.

Use the five months of journal space to record the nutritional values of your meals. This allows you to monitor what you eat, plan ahead, and reach your weight-loss goal.

DAILY TARGETS

Based on the number of calories your diet allows, list the daily targets that you would like to meet. (Nutritional websites or your primary care physician can help you determine the appropriate amounts.)

DAILY CALORIES:	FAT gms:	CARBS gms:

RESULTS

Fill in the following information so that you can keep track of your results!

STATISTICS:	BEFORE:	DESIRED:	AFTER:
WEIGHT			
BODY FAT %			
BMI			
CHEST			
WAIST			
HIPS			
THIGH			
BICEP			

MONDAY

DATE: 07 / 01 / 10

······· Daily Tip ·······

Try not to eat while w [EXAMPLE] eading or any other
activity. It can mak ch you are eating.

WEIGHT:
147

WATER INTAKE:
# of 8oz. glasses

☑ ☑ ☑ ☑
☑ ☑ ☐ ☐

VITAMINS & SUPPLEMENTS:
Calcium
vitamin C

ENERGY LEVEL:
☐ low
☑ medium
☐ high

CALORIES BURNED:
250

DAILY NUTRITIONAL INTAKE:

FOOD/BEVERAGES	CALORIES	FAT	CARBS
Breakfast			
Blueberry scone	400	17	55
Orange juice	110	0	26
Lunch			
Pita w/turkey	290	4	36
American cheese	32	1	1
Baby carrots	60	0	12
Pepsi	180	0	45
Snack			
Apple slices and	245	17	21
peanut butter			
Dinner			
Salmon	175	11	0
Wild rice	83	1	17
Broccoli	54	1	12
Crystal Light	5	0	0
iced tea			
DAILY TOTALS:	1,634	52	225

NOTES/REMINDERS:

Buy fruit and yogurt for breakfast.
Do 30 minutes of cardio tomorrow.

MONDAY

.... **Daily Tip** ....

Try not to eat while watching television, driving, reading or any other activity. It can make you lose track of how much you are eating.

....

DAILY NUTRITIONAL INTAKE:

FOOD/BEVERAGES	CALORIES	FAT	CARBS
DAILY TOTALS:			

WEIGHT:

WATER INTAKE:
# of 8oz. glasses
☐ ☐ ☐ ☐
☐ ☐ ☐ ☐

VITAMINS & SUPPLEMENTS:

ENERGY LEVEL:
☐ low
☐ medium
☐ high

CALORIES BURNED:

NOTES/REMINDERS:

TUESDAY

DATE: ___ / ___ / ___

······································ **Daily Tip** ································

Celebrate your success every day. Be proud of what you have accomplished and continue to envision the future you.

··

WEIGHT:

WATER INTAKE:
# of 8oz. glasses

☐ ☐ ☐ ☐
☐ ☐ ☐ ☐

VITAMINS & SUPPLEMENTS:

_____
_____
_____
_____
_____
_____
_____
_____

ENERGY LEVEL:
☐ low
☐ medium
☐ high

CALORIES BURNED:

DAILY NUTRITIONAL INTAKE:

FOOD/BEVERAGES	CALORIES	FAT	CARBS
DAILY TOTALS:			

NOTES/REMINDERS:

WEDNESDAY

WEEK 1

· **Daily Tip** ·

Adding new food and variety to your plan will help keep
your diet interesting and keep you motivated.

· ·

DAILY NUTRITIONAL INTAKE:

FOOD/BEVERAGES	CALORIES	FAT	CARBS

DAILY TOTALS:

WEIGHT:

WATER INTAKE:
# of 8oz. glasses
☐ ☐ ☐ ☐
☐ ☐ ☐ ☐

**VITAMINS &
SUPPLEMENTS:**

ENERGY LEVEL:
☐ low
☐ medium
☐ high

CALORIES BURNED:

NOTES/REMINDERS:

WEEK 1

THURSDAY

DATE: ___/___/___

························ **Daily Tip** ·························

Balance out a high-calorie breakfast by
eating a moderate lunch and dinner.

··

WEIGHT:

WATER INTAKE:
# of 8oz. glasses

☐ ☐ ☐ ☐
☐ ☐ ☐ ☐

**VITAMINS &
SUPPLEMENTS:**

_____
_____
_____
_____
_____
_____
_____

ENERGY LEVEL:
☐ low
☐ medium
☐ high

CALORIES BURNED:

DAILY NUTRITIONAL INTAKE:

FOOD/BEVERAGES	CALORIES	FAT	CARBS
DAILY TOTALS:			

NOTES/REMINDERS:

DATE: ___ / ___ / ___

FRIDAY

· **Daily Tip** ·

Disassociate diets with restriction and deprivation.
Look at diets as eating the right foods in the right amounts.

· ·

DAILY NUTRITIONAL INTAKE:

FOOD/BEVERAGES	CALORIES	FAT	CARBS
DAILY TOTALS:			

WEIGHT:

WATER INTAKE:
# of 8oz. glasses
☐ ☐ ☐ ☐
☐ ☐ ☐ ☐

VITAMINS & SUPPLEMENTS:

ENERGY LEVEL:
☐ low
☐ medium
☐ high

CALORIES BURNED:

NOTES/REMINDERS:

SATURDAY

DATE: ___ / ___ / ___

······················· Daily Tip ·······················

Don't be too hard on yourself if you stumble along the way. Just remind yourself that tomorrow is another day, and you can get back on track.

WEIGHT:

WATER INTAKE:
# of 8oz. glasses

☐ ☐ ☐ ☐
☐ ☐ ☐ ☐

VITAMINS & SUPPLEMENTS:

ENERGY LEVEL:
☐ low
☐ medium
☐ high

CALORIES BURNED:

DAILY NUTRITIONAL INTAKE:

FOOD/BEVERAGES	CALORIES	FAT	CARBS
DAILY TOTALS:			

NOTES/REMINDERS:

DATE:
_____ / _____ / _____

SUNDAY

·· **Daily Tip** ··

The gratification of gradual weight loss will be much more
satisfying than the instant gratification of food.

··

DAILY NUTRITIONAL INTAKE:

FOOD/BEVERAGES	CALORIES	FAT	CARBS
DAILY TOTALS:			

WEIGHT:

WATER INTAKE:
# of 8oz. glasses

☐ ☐ ☐ ☐
☐ ☐ ☐ ☐

**VITAMINS &
SUPPLEMENTS:**

ENERGY LEVEL:
☐ low
☐ medium
☐ high

CALORIES BURNED:

NOTES/REMINDERS:

End-of-the-Week

WRAP-UP

START WEIGHT:

END WEIGHT:

WEEKLY ENERGY LEVEL:

☐ low ☐ med ☐ high

WEEKLY CALORIES BURNED:

DAYS I TRACKED MY DIET:

☐ Monday ☐ Tuesday ☐ Wednesday ☐ Thursday ☐ Friday ☐ Saturday ☐ Sunday

HOW I FELT THIS WEEK:

_____
_____
_____
_____
_____
_____
_____
_____

GOALS FOR NEXT WEEK:

_____
_____
_____
_____
_____
_____
_____
_____

NOTES/REMINDERS:

DATE: ___ / ___ / ___

MONDAY

· **Daily Tip** ·

Set temporary or short-term goals for yourself. Breaking the journey
down into smaller sections can make it easier to stay on track.

· ·

DAILY NUTRITIONAL INTAKE:

FOOD/BEVERAGES	CALORIES	FAT	CARBS
DAILY TOTALS:			

WEIGHT:

WATER INTAKE:
# of 8oz. glasses

☐ ☐ ☐ ☐
☐ ☐ ☐ ☐

VITAMINS & SUPPLEMENTS:

ENERGY LEVEL:
☐ low
☐ medium
☐ high

CALORIES BURNED:

NOTES/REMINDERS:

TUESDAY

DATE: ___ / ___ / ___

··· **Daily Tip** ·································

Find a friend to share in your weight-loss journey—
it can help you remain on track and stay motivated.

WEIGHT:

WATER INTAKE:
# of 8oz. glasses
☐ ☐ ☐ ☐
☐ ☐ ☐ ☐

**VITAMINS &
SUPPLEMENTS:**

ENERGY LEVEL:
☐ low
☐ medium
☐ high

CALORIES BURNED:

DAILY NUTRITIONAL INTAKE:

FOOD/BEVERAGES	CALORIES	FAT	CARBS
DAILY TOTALS:			

NOTES/REMINDERS:

WEDNESDAY

· **Daily Tip** ·

Stick to your dietary commitment for at least 30 days.
After the first 30 days, you will have practiced the
behavior long enough to consider it a habit.

· ·

DAILY NUTRITIONAL INTAKE:

FOOD/BEVERAGES	CALORIES	FAT	CARBS
DAILY TOTALS:			

WEIGHT:

WATER INTAKE:
# of 8oz. glasses
☐ ☐ ☐ ☐
☐ ☐ ☐ ☐

**VITAMINS &
SUPPLEMENTS:**

ENERGY LEVEL:
☐ low
☐ medium
☐ high

CALORIES BURNED:

NOTES/REMINDERS:

THURSDAY

DATE: ___ / ___ / ___

······················· **Daily Tip** ·······················

Moderation is the key to a healthy
lifestyle and to losing weight.

···

WEIGHT:

WATER INTAKE:
# of 8oz. glasses

☐ ☐ ☐ ☐
☐ ☐ ☐ ☐

**VITAMINS &
SUPPLEMENTS:**

ENERGY LEVEL:
☐ low
☐ medium
☐ high

CALORIES BURNED:

DAILY NUTRITIONAL INTAKE:

FOOD/BEVERAGES	CALORIES	FAT	CARBS
DAILY TOTALS:			

NOTES/REMINDERS:

DATE: ____ / ____ / ____

FRIDAY

Daily Tip

Order a sandwich with whole
grain bread instead of white.

DAILY NUTRITIONAL INTAKE:

FOOD/BEVERAGES	CALORIES	FAT	CARBS
DAILY TOTALS:			

WEIGHT:

WATER INTAKE:
# of 8oz. glasses
☐ ☐ ☐ ☐
☐ ☐ ☐ ☐

**VITAMINS &
SUPPLEMENTS:**

ENERGY LEVEL:
☐ low
☐ medium
☐ high

CALORIES BURNED:

NOTES/REMINDERS:

SATURDAY

DATE: ___ / ___ / ___

··· **Daily Tip** ·································

Incorporate foods from each of the 6 main
food groups into your diet plan.

··

WEIGHT:

WATER INTAKE:
# of 8oz. glasses

☐ ☐ ☐ ☐
☐ ☐ ☐ ☐

**VITAMINS &
SUPPLEMENTS:**

ENERGY LEVEL:
☐ low
☐ medium
☐ high

CALORIES BURNED:

DAILY NUTRITIONAL INTAKE:

FOOD/BEVERAGES	CALORIES	FAT	CARBS
DAILY TOTALS:			

NOTES/REMINDERS:

DATE: ___/___/___

SUNDAY

WEEK 2

······················ **Daily Tip** ······························

Drink plenty of water each day. Often we think we are hungry when our body is sending us signals that we are actually thirsty or dehydrated.

··

DAILY NUTRITIONAL INTAKE:

FOOD/BEVERAGES	CALORIES	FAT	CARBS
DAILY TOTALS:			

WEIGHT:

WATER INTAKE:
# of 8oz. glasses
☐ ☐ ☐ ☐
☐ ☐ ☐ ☐

VITAMINS & SUPPLEMENTS:

ENERGY LEVEL:
☐ low
☐ medium
☐ high

CALORIES BURNED:

NOTES/REMINDERS:

WEEK 2

End-of-the-Week

WRAP-UP

START WEIGHT:

END WEIGHT:

WEEKLY ENERGY LEVEL:
☐ low ☐ med ☐ high

WEEKLY CALORIES BURNED:

DAYS I TRACKED MY DIET:
☐ Monday ☐ Tuesday ☐ Wednesday ☐ Thursday ☐ Friday ☐ Saturday ☐ Sunday

HOW I FELT THIS WEEK:

_____
_____
_____
_____
_____
_____
_____
_____
_____

GOALS FOR NEXT WEEK:

_____
_____
_____
_____
_____
_____
_____
_____
_____

NOTES/REMINDERS:

DATE:
____ / ____ / ____

MONDAY

······························· **Daily Tip** ·······························

Get adequate vitamins and minerals by eating
a wide variety of fruits and vegetables.

··

DAILY NUTRITIONAL INTAKE:

FOOD/BEVERAGES	CALORIES	FAT	CARBS
DAILY TOTALS:			

WEIGHT:

WATER INTAKE:
# of 8oz. glasses
☐ ☐ ☐ ☐
☐ ☐ ☐ ☐

**VITAMINS &
SUPPLEMENTS:**

ENERGY LEVEL:
☐ low
☐ medium
☐ high

CALORIES BURNED:

NOTES/REMINDERS:

TUESDAY

DATE: _____ / _____ / _____

··· **Daily Tip** ·································

Complex carbohydrates are crucial for losing
weight as well as for maintaining energy.

··

WEIGHT:

WATER INTAKE:
# of 8oz. glasses
☐ ☐ ☐ ☐
☐ ☐ ☐ ☐

**VITAMINS &
SUPPLEMENTS:**

_____
_____
_____
_____
_____
_____
_____
_____

ENERGY LEVEL:
☐ low
☐ medium
☐ high

CALORIES BURNED:

DAILY NUTRITIONAL INTAKE:

FOOD/BEVERAGES	CALORIES	FAT	CARBS
DAILY TOTALS:			

NOTES/REMINDERS:

DATE: _____ / _____ / _____

WEDNESDAY

· **Daily Tip** ·

Diets that rely on "tricks" are difficult to maintain
and can damage your body. Learn how to
distinguish a fad diet from a sensible one.

· ·

DAILY NUTRITIONAL INTAKE:

FOOD/BEVERAGES	CALORIES	FAT	CARBS
DAILY TOTALS:			

WEIGHT:

WATER INTAKE:
# of 8oz. glasses

☐ ☐ ☐ ☐
☐ ☐ ☐ ☐

VITAMINS & SUPPLEMENTS:

_____
_____
_____
_____
_____
_____
_____
_____

ENERGY LEVEL:
☐ low
☐ medium
☐ high

CALORIES BURNED:

NOTES/REMINDERS:

THURSDAY

DATE: ___ / ___ / ___

································ **Daily Tip** ································

Give yourself a planned break from your diet every
once in a while. Figure out what you can enjoy
without undermining your weight loss.

··

WEIGHT:

WATER INTAKE:
# of 8oz. glasses

☐ ☐ ☐ ☐
☐ ☐ ☐ ☐

**VITAMINS &
SUPPLEMENTS:**

_____
_____
_____
_____
_____
_____
_____

ENERGY LEVEL:
☐ low
☐ medium
☐ high

CALORIES BURNED:

DAILY NUTRITIONAL INTAKE:

FOOD/BEVERAGES	CALORIES	FAT	CARBS
DAILY TOTALS:			

NOTES/REMINDERS:

FRIDAY

···························· **Daily Tip** ····························

Try to eat several hours before going to bed so your
body has a chance to burn off extra calories.

··

DAILY NUTRITIONAL INTAKE:

FOOD/BEVERAGES	CALORIES	FAT	CARBS
DAILY TOTALS:			

WEIGHT:

WATER INTAKE:
# of 8oz. glasses

☐ ☐ ☐ ☐
☐ ☐ ☐ ☐

VITAMINS & SUPPLEMENTS:

ENERGY LEVEL:
☐ low
☐ medium
☐ high

CALORIES BURNED:

NOTES/REMINDERS:

SATURDAY

DATE: ___ / ___ / ___

Eat fewer carbohydrates, such as white bread,
chips and cookies, at nighttime.

WEIGHT:

WATER INTAKE:
# of 8oz. glasses

☐ ☐ ☐ ☐
☐ ☐ ☐ ☐

**VITAMINS &
SUPPLEMENTS:**

ENERGY LEVEL:
☐ low
☐ medium
☐ high

CALORIES BURNED:

DAILY NUTRITIONAL INTAKE:

FOOD/BEVERAGES	CALORIES	FAT	CARBS
DAILY TOTALS:			

NOTES/REMINDERS:

DATE:
____ / ____ / ____

SUNDAY

WEEK 3

Make your weight-loss goals reasonable and reachable; that way you will be more likely to reach them and achieve your resolutions.

DAILY NUTRITIONAL INTAKE:

FOOD/BEVERAGES	CALORIES	FAT	CARBS
DAILY TOTALS:			

WEIGHT:

WATER INTAKE:
# of 8oz. glasses
☐ ☐ ☐ ☐
☐ ☐ ☐ ☐

VITAMINS & SUPPLEMENTS:

ENERGY LEVEL:
☐ low
☐ medium
☐ high

CALORIES BURNED:

NOTES/REMINDERS:

End-of-the-Week

WRAP-UP

START WEIGHT:

END WEIGHT:

WEEKLY ENERGY LEVEL:
☐ low ☐ med ☐ high

WEEKLY CALORIES BURNED:

DAYS I TRACKED MY DIET:
☐ Monday ☐ Tuesday ☐ Wednesday ☐ Thursday ☐ Friday ☐ Saturday ☐ Sunday

HOW I FELT THIS WEEK:

_____
_____
_____
_____
_____
_____
_____
_____
_____

GOALS FOR NEXT WEEK:

_____
_____
_____
_____
_____
_____
_____
_____

NOTES/REMINDERS:

MONDAY

DATE: ____ / ____ / ____

· **Daily Tip** ·

Take into account your age and health status. Understand what your body needs before coming up with an appropriate weight-loss program.

· ·

DAILY NUTRITIONAL INTAKE:

FOOD/BEVERAGES	CALORIES	FAT	CARBS
DAILY TOTALS:			

WEIGHT:

WATER INTAKE:
# of 8oz. glasses
☐ ☐ ☐ ☐
☐ ☐ ☐ ☐

VITAMINS & SUPPLEMENTS:

ENERGY LEVEL:
☐ low
☐ medium
☐ high

CALORIES BURNED:

NOTES/REMINDERS:

WEEK 4

TUESDAY

DATE: ___ / ___ / ___

· **Daily Tip** ·

Know the effects of every diet, and whether or not there are any downsides, will help you make the correct decision.

· ·

WEIGHT:

WATER INTAKE:
# of 8oz. glasses

☐ ☐ ☐ ☐
☐ ☐ ☐ ☐

VITAMINS & SUPPLEMENTS:

_____
_____
_____
_____
_____
_____
_____

ENERGY LEVEL:
☐ low
☐ medium
☐ high

CALORIES BURNED:

DAILY NUTRITIONAL INTAKE:

FOOD/BEVERAGES	CALORIES	FAT	CARBS
DAILY TOTALS:			

NOTES/REMINDERS:

WEDNESDAY

· Daily Tip ·

Get lots of sleep. Lack of sleep can lead to an increase
in appetite, and cravings for fatty and sugary foods.

· ·

DAILY NUTRITIONAL INTAKE:

FOOD/BEVERAGES	CALORIES	FAT	CARBS
DAILY TOTALS:			

WEIGHT:

WATER INTAKE:
# of 8oz. glasses
☐ ☐ ☐ ☐
☐ ☐ ☐ ☐

VITAMINS &
SUPPLEMENTS:

ENERGY LEVEL:
☐ low
☐ medium
☐ high

CALORIES BURNED:

NOTES/REMINDERS:

THURSDAY

DATE:
___ / ___ / ___

··· **Daily Tip** ·······································

Whole grains are very beneficial to your body. They can help
reduce the risk of high cholesterol or blood pressure,
diabetes, and certain heart diseases.

···

WEIGHT:

WATER INTAKE:
# of 8oz. glasses

☐ ☐ ☐ ☐
☐ ☐ ☐ ☐

**VITAMINS &
SUPPLEMENTS:**

_____
_____
_____
_____
_____
_____
_____
_____

ENERGY LEVEL:
☐ low
☐ medium
☐ high

CALORIES BURNED:

DAILY NUTRITIONAL INTAKE:

FOOD/BEVERAGES	CALORIES	FAT	CARBS
DAILY TOTALS:			

NOTES/REMINDERS:

FRIDAY

··· **Daily Tip** ·······································

Avoid foods with trans fats, such as candy, chips, packaged snacks, pastries, donuts, cookies, and fried foods.

··

DAILY NUTRITIONAL INTAKE:

FOOD/BEVERAGES	CALORIES	FAT	CARBS
DAILY TOTALS:			

WEIGHT:

WATER INTAKE:
# of 8oz. glasses
☐ ☐ ☐ ☐
☐ ☐ ☐ ☐

VITAMINS & SUPPLEMENTS:

ENERGY LEVEL:
☐ low
☐ medium
☐ high

CALORIES BURNED:

NOTES/REMINDERS:

SATURDAY

DATE: ___ / ___ / ___

· **Daily Tip** ·

Achieving a healthy lifestyle takes time
and practice, but you can do it.

· ·

WEIGHT:

WATER INTAKE:
# of 8oz. glasses
☐ ☐ ☐ ☐
☐ ☐ ☐ ☐

**VITAMINS &
SUPPLEMENTS:**

ENERGY LEVEL:
☐ low
☐ medium
☐ high

CALORIES BURNED:

DAILY NUTRITIONAL INTAKE:

FOOD/BEVERAGES	CALORIES	FAT	CARBS
DAILY TOTALS:			

NOTES/REMINDERS:

DATE:
_____ / _____ / _____

SUNDAY

· **Daily Tip** ·

Keep physical fitness a priority through exercise routines
that are realistic, maintainable, and fun.

· ·

DAILY NUTRITIONAL INTAKE:

FOOD/BEVERAGES	CALORIES	FAT	CARBS
DAILY TOTALS:			

WEIGHT:

WATER INTAKE:
\# of 8oz. glasses
☐ ☐ ☐ ☐
☐ ☐ ☐ ☐

VITAMINS & SUPPLEMENTS:

ENERGY LEVEL:
☐ low
☐ medium
☐ high

CALORIES BURNED:

NOTES/REMINDERS:

End-of-the-Week

WRAP-UP

START WEIGHT:

END WEIGHT:

WEEKLY ENERGY LEVEL:

☐ low ☐ med ☐ high

WEEKLY CALORIES BURNED:

DAYS I TRACKED MY DIET:

☐ Monday ☐ Tuesday ☐ Wednesday ☐ Thursday ☐ Friday ☐ Saturday ☐ Sunday

HOW I FELT THIS WEEK:

_____
_____
_____
_____
_____
_____
_____
_____
_____

GOALS FOR NEXT WEEK:

_____
_____
_____
_____
_____
_____
_____
_____
_____

NOTES/REMINDERS:

DATE:
___ / ___ / ___

MONDAY

························· **Daily Tip** ·································

Avoid high-fructose corn syrup, found in sweets and other processed foods like condiments, salad dressing, canned fruit, and soups.

···

DAILY NUTRITIONAL INTAKE:

FOOD/BEVERAGES	CALORIES	FAT	CARBS
DAILY TOTALS:			

WEIGHT:

WATER INTAKE:
# of 8oz. glasses
☐ ☐ ☐ ☐
☐ ☐ ☐ ☐

VITAMINS & SUPPLEMENTS:

ENERGY LEVEL:
☐ low
☐ medium
☐ high

CALORIES BURNED:

NOTES/REMINDERS:

TUESDAY

DATE: ___ / ___ / ___

·· **Daily Tip** ··

If you cannot make it to the gym every day,
try to incorporate other physical activities into your day,
such as gardening, vacuuming, or shopping.

···

WEIGHT:

WATER INTAKE:
# of 8oz. glasses

☐ ☐ ☐ ☐
☐ ☐ ☐ ☐

**VITAMINS &
SUPPLEMENTS:**

_____
_____
_____
_____
_____
_____
_____

ENERGY LEVEL:
☐ low
☐ medium
☐ high

CALORIES BURNED:

DAILY NUTRITIONAL INTAKE:

FOOD/BEVERAGES	CALORIES	FAT	CARBS
DAILY TOTALS:			

NOTES/REMINDERS:

WEDNESDAY

WEEK
5

························· **Daily Tip** ·························

Occasionally get up from your desk and stretch.
Take every opportunity to add movement to your day.

DAILY NUTRITIONAL INTAKE:

FOOD/BEVERAGES	CALORIES	FAT	CARBS
DAILY TOTALS:			

WEIGHT:

WATER INTAKE:
# of 8oz. glasses

☐ ☐ ☐ ☐
☐ ☐ ☐ ☐

VITAMINS & SUPPLEMENTS:

ENERGY LEVEL:
☐ low
☐ medium
☐ high

CALORIES BURNED:

NOTES/REMINDERS:

THURSDAY

DATE: ___/___/___

············· **Daily Tip** ·············

When dining out, be aware of hidden calories, sodium, and fats that could be included in sauces or the way the meals are prepared in the kitchen.

WEIGHT:

WATER INTAKE:
# of 8oz. glasses

☐ ☐ ☐ ☐
☐ ☐ ☐ ☐

VITAMINS & SUPPLEMENTS:

ENERGY LEVEL:
☐ low
☐ medium
☐ high

CALORIES BURNED:

DAILY NUTRITIONAL INTAKE:

FOOD/BEVERAGES	CALORIES	FAT	CARBS
DAILY TOTALS:			

NOTES/REMINDERS:

FRIDAY

WEEK 5

Don't be afraid to ask your server how the meal is prepared,
or to request that the food be prepared in a way that
is in keeping with your diet program.

DAILY NUTRITIONAL INTAKE:

FOOD/BEVERAGES	CALORIES	FAT	CARBS
DAILY TOTALS:			

WEIGHT:

WATER INTAKE:
# of 8oz. glasses
☐ ☐ ☐ ☐
☐ ☐ ☐ ☐

VITAMINS & SUPPLEMENTS:

ENERGY LEVEL:
☐ low
☐ medium
☐ high

CALORIES BURNED:

NOTES/REMINDERS:

SATURDAY

DATE: ___ / ___ / ___

.... Daily Tip ....

Try to eat only part of what is on your plate
and eat the rest as leftovers the next day.

....

WEIGHT:

WATER INTAKE:
# of 8oz. glasses

☐ ☐ ☐ ☐
☐ ☐ ☐ ☐

**VITAMINS &
SUPPLEMENTS:**

_____

_____

_____

_____

_____

_____

_____

ENERGY LEVEL:
☐ low
☐ medium
☐ high

CALORIES BURNED:

DAILY NUTRITIONAL INTAKE:

FOOD/BEVERAGES	CALORIES	FAT	CARBS
DAILY TOTALS:			

NOTES/REMINDERS:

SUNDAY

· **Daily Tip** ·

Read the Nutritional Facts Labels to help you measure
out correct serving sizes so you don't overeat.

· ·

DAILY NUTRITIONAL INTAKE:

FOOD/BEVERAGES	CALORIES	FAT	CARBS
DAILY TOTALS:			

WEIGHT:

WATER INTAKE:
# of 8oz. glasses
☐ ☐ ☐ ☐
☐ ☐ ☐ ☐

VITAMINS & SUPPLEMENTS:

ENERGY LEVEL:
☐ low
☐ medium
☐ high

CALORIES BURNED:

NOTES/REMINDERS:

WEEK
5

End-of-the-Week

WRAP-UP

START WEIGHT:

END WEIGHT:

WEEKLY ENERGY LEVEL:

☐ low ☐ med ☐ high

WEEKLY CALORIES BURNED:

DAYS I TRACKED MY DIET:

☐ Monday ☐ Tuesday ☐ Wednesday ☐ Thursday ☐ Friday ☐ Saturday ☐ Sunday

HOW I FELT THIS WEEK:

_____
_____
_____
_____
_____
_____
_____
_____
_____

GOALS FOR NEXT WEEK:

_____
_____
_____
_____
_____
_____
_____
_____

NOTES/REMINDERS:

DATE: ___/___/___

MONDAY

WEEK 6

································· **Daily Tip** ·································

If having a party, try to provide low-calorie, healthy snacks like
vegetables and dip, baked potato chips, fruit slices, and water.

··

DAILY NUTRITIONAL INTAKE:

FOOD/BEVERAGES	CALORIES	FAT	CARBS
DAILY TOTALS:			

WEIGHT:

WATER INTAKE:
# of 8oz. glasses
☐ ☐ ☐ ☐
☐ ☐ ☐ ☐

**VITAMINS &
SUPPLEMENTS:**

ENERGY LEVEL:
☐ low
☐ medium
☐ high

CALORIES BURNED:

NOTES/REMINDERS:

TUESDAY

DATE: ___/___/___

Consult a registered dietician, a highly trained
food and nutrition expert, who can help
you with your nutrition questions.

WEIGHT:

WATER INTAKE:
# of 8oz. glasses

☐ ☐ ☐ ☐
☐ ☐ ☐ ☐

**VITAMINS &
SUPPLEMENTS:**

ENERGY LEVEL:
☐ low
☐ medium
☐ high

CALORIES BURNED:

DAILY NUTRITIONAL INTAKE:

FOOD/BEVERAGES	CALORIES	FAT	CARBS
DAILY TOTALS:			

NOTES/REMINDERS:

DATE:
____ / ____ / ____

WEDNESDAY

····························· **Daily Tip** ·····························

Get moving: an active person burns approximately 30 percent
of their calories through daily non-exercise activity,
versus 15 percent for sedentary people.

··

DAILY NUTRITIONAL INTAKE:

FOOD/BEVERAGES	CALORIES	FAT	CARBS
DAILY TOTALS:			

WEIGHT:

WATER INTAKE:
# of 8oz. glasses
☐ ☐ ☐ ☐
☐ ☐ ☐ ☐

**VITAMINS &
SUPPLEMENTS:**

ENERGY LEVEL:
☐ low
☐ medium
☐ high

CALORIES BURNED:

NOTES/REMINDERS:

THURSDAY

DATE: ___/___/___

· **Daily Tip** ·

Weight loss will help lower your risk of certain diseases, improve your overall health, and build your self-confidence.

· ·

WEIGHT:

WATER INTAKE:
# of 8oz. glasses

☐ ☐ ☐ ☐
☐ ☐ ☐ ☐

VITAMINS & SUPPLEMENTS:

_____
_____
_____
_____
_____
_____
_____
_____

ENERGY LEVEL:
☐ low
☐ medium
☐ high

CALORIES BURNED:

DAILY NUTRITIONAL INTAKE:

FOOD/BEVERAGES	CALORIES	FAT	CARBS
DAILY TOTALS:			

NOTES/REMINDERS:

DATE:
___/___/___

FRIDAY

· **Daily Tip** ·

Stay hydrated: Water enables your body to work effectively at burning stored fat.

· ·

DAILY NUTRITIONAL INTAKE:

FOOD/BEVERAGES	CALORIES	FAT	CARBS
DAILY TOTALS:			

WEIGHT:

WATER INTAKE:
# of 8oz. glasses

☐ ☐ ☐ ☐
☐ ☐ ☐ ☐

VITAMINS & SUPPLEMENTS:

ENERGY LEVEL:
☐ low
☐ medium
☐ high

CALORIES BURNED:

NOTES/REMINDERS:

SATURDAY

DATE: _____ / _____ / _____

········· Daily Tip ·········

If having a cookout or barbecue, choose lean cuts of meat
that have less fat or trim off excess fat before cooking.

WEIGHT:

WATER INTAKE:
# of 8oz. glasses

☐ ☐ ☐ ☐
☐ ☐ ☐ ☐

**VITAMINS &
SUPPLEMENTS:**

ENERGY LEVEL:
☐ low
☐ medium
☐ high

CALORIES BURNED:

DAILY NUTRITIONAL INTAKE:

FOOD/BEVERAGES	CALORIES	FAT	CARBS
DAILY TOTALS:			

NOTES/REMINDERS:

SUNDAY

·········· **Daily Tip** ··········

Fill up on low-density, high-volume foods, such as fruits, vegetables, soups and stews, cooked grains, lean meats, fish, and lean poultry.

DAILY NUTRITIONAL INTAKE:

FOOD/BEVERAGES	CALORIES	FAT	CARBS
DAILY TOTALS:			

WEIGHT:

WATER INTAKE:
# of 8oz. glasses

☐ ☐ ☐ ☐
☐ ☐ ☐ ☐

VITAMINS & SUPPLEMENTS:

ENERGY LEVEL:
☐ low
☐ medium
☐ high

CALORIES BURNED:

NOTES/REMINDERS:

WEEK 6

End-of-the-Week

WRAP-UP

START WEIGHT:

END WEIGHT:

WEEKLY ENERGY LEVEL:
☐ low ☐ med ☐ high

WEEKLY CALORIES BURNED:

DAYS I TRACKED MY DIET:
☐ Monday ☐ Tuesday ☐ Wednesday ☐ Thursday ☐ Friday ☐ Saturday ☐ Sunday

HOW I FELT THIS WEEK:

_____
_____
_____
_____
_____
_____
_____
_____

GOALS FOR NEXT WEEK:

_____
_____
_____
_____
_____
_____
_____
_____

NOTES/REMINDERS:

DATE: ___ / ___ / ___

MONDAY

WEEK 7

·········· **Daily Tip** ··········

All oils are high in fat and calories,
so be sure to go easy on the portions.

·······························

DAILY NUTRITIONAL INTAKE:

FOOD/BEVERAGES	CALORIES	FAT	CARBS
DAILY TOTALS:			

WEIGHT:

WATER INTAKE:
# of 8oz. glasses
☐ ☐ ☐ ☐
☐ ☐ ☐ ☐

VITAMINS & SUPPLEMENTS:

ENERGY LEVEL:
☐ low
☐ medium
☐ high

CALORIES BURNED:

NOTES/REMINDERS:

TUESDAY

DATE: ___ / ___ / ___

Caffeine can give you that boost you need to wake up
in the morning, but it can trick your body into
thinking it is hungry when it is not.

WEIGHT:

WATER INTAKE:
# of 8oz. glasses

☐ ☐ ☐ ☐
☐ ☐ ☐ ☐

**VITAMINS &
SUPPLEMENTS:**

ENERGY LEVEL:
☐ low
☐ medium
☐ high

CALORIES BURNED:

DAILY NUTRITIONAL INTAKE:

FOOD/BEVERAGES	CALORIES	FAT	CARBS
DAILY TOTALS:			

NOTES/REMINDERS:

DATE:
____ / ____ / ____

WEDNESDAY

WEEK
7

·· **Daily Tip** ··

Make the switch from sodas and coffee to water by gradually
reducing the amount of caffeine you consume each day.

DAILY NUTRITIONAL INTAKE:

FOOD/BEVERAGES	CALORIES	FAT	CARBS
DAILY TOTALS:			

WEIGHT:

WATER INTAKE:
# of 8oz. glasses
☐ ☐ ☐ ☐
☐ ☐ ☐ ☐

**VITAMINS &
SUPPLEMENTS:**

ENERGY LEVEL:
☐ low
☐ medium
☐ high

CALORIES BURNED:

NOTES/REMINDERS:

THURSDAY

DATE: ___ / ___ / ___

····· Daily Tip ·····

If you have diabetes, food allergies, or are a vegetarian, consult a dietetics professional on how you can safely lose weight.

WEIGHT:

WATER INTAKE:
# of 8oz. glasses

☐ ☐ ☐ ☐
☐ ☐ ☐ ☐

VITAMINS & SUPPLEMENTS:

ENERGY LEVEL:
☐ low
☐ medium
☐ high

CALORIES BURNED:

DAILY NUTRITIONAL INTAKE:

FOOD/BEVERAGES	CALORIES	FAT	CARBS
DAILY TOTALS:			

NOTES/REMINDERS:

DATE:

___ / ___ / ___

FRIDAY

.... **Daily Tip** ....

Replacing full-sugar soda with water at mealtimes
can help you lose around a pound a week.

....

DAILY NUTRITIONAL INTAKE:

FOOD/BEVERAGES	CALORIES	FAT	CARBS
DAILY TOTALS:			

WEIGHT:

WATER INTAKE:
# of 8oz. glasses

☐ ☐ ☐ ☐
☐ ☐ ☐ ☐

VITAMINS & SUPPLEMENTS:

ENERGY LEVEL:
☐ low
☐ medium
☐ high

CALORIES BURNED:

NOTES/REMINDERS:

SATURDAY

DATE: ___ / ___ / ___

If you are always on the go, traveling, or on vacation, pack healthy snacks like trail mix, dried fruits, nuts, or healthy crackers.

WEIGHT:

WATER INTAKE:
# of 8oz. glasses

☐ ☐ ☐ ☐
☐ ☐ ☐ ☐

VITAMINS & SUPPLEMENTS:

ENERGY LEVEL:
☐ low
☐ medium
☐ high

CALORIES BURNED:

DAILY NUTRITIONAL INTAKE:

FOOD/BEVERAGES	CALORIES	FAT	CARBS
DAILY TOTALS:			

NOTES/REMINDERS:

DATE:

_____ / _____ / _____

SUNDAY

·············· **Daily Tip** ··············

Avoid processed foods, such as packaged snack foods and boxed meals, which contain high amounts of trans fats, artificial flavors, and preservatives.

···

DAILY NUTRITIONAL INTAKE:

FOOD/BEVERAGES	CALORIES	FAT	CARBS
DAILY TOTALS:			

WEIGHT:

WATER INTAKE:
# of 8oz. glasses

☐ ☐ ☐ ☐
☐ ☐ ☐ ☐

VITAMINS & SUPPLEMENTS:

ENERGY LEVEL:
☐ low
☐ medium
☐ high

CALORIES BURNED:

NOTES/REMINDERS:

WEEK 7

End-of-the-Week
WRAP-UP

START WEIGHT:

END WEIGHT:

WEEKLY ENERGY LEVEL:
☐ low ☐ med ☐ high

WEEKLY CALORIES BURNED:

DAYS I TRACKED MY DIET:
☐ Monday ☐ Tuesday ☐ Wednesday ☐ Thursday ☐ Friday ☐ Saturday ☐ Sunday

HOW I FELT THIS WEEK:

_____
_____
_____
_____
_____
_____
_____
_____
_____

GOALS FOR NEXT WEEK:

_____
_____
_____
_____
_____
_____
_____
_____

NOTES/REMINDERS:

DATE:

_____ / _____ / _____

MONDAY

Educate yourself on how to read a nutrition label. Understanding what is in the food you eat is an important step in your weight-loss program.

DAILY NUTRITIONAL INTAKE:

FOOD/BEVERAGES	CALORIES	FAT	CARBS
DAILY TOTALS:			

WEIGHT:

WATER INTAKE:
# of 8oz. glasses
☐ ☐ ☐ ☐
☐ ☐ ☐ ☐

VITAMINS & SUPPLEMENTS:

_____
_____
_____
_____
_____
_____
_____
_____

ENERGY LEVEL:
☐ low
☐ medium
☐ high

CALORIES BURNED:

NOTES/REMINDERS:

TUESDAY

DATE: ___ / ___ / ___

······· **Daily Tip** ·······

Skip sugary juice in favor of eating whole fruits, or else make sure the juice you are drinking is 100 percent fruit juice.

WEIGHT:

WATER INTAKE:
# of 8oz. glasses

☐ ☐ ☐ ☐
☐ ☐ ☐ ☐

VITAMINS & SUPPLEMENTS:

ENERGY LEVEL:
☐ low
☐ medium
☐ high

CALORIES BURNED:

DAILY NUTRITIONAL INTAKE:

FOOD/BEVERAGES	CALORIES	FAT	CARBS
DAILY TOTALS:			

NOTES/REMINDERS:

WEDNESDAY

.... **Daily Tip** ....

Adopt a relaxation technique, such as yoga or deep breathing,
to reduce your stress levels and lose weight.

....

DAILY NUTRITIONAL INTAKE:

FOOD/BEVERAGES	CALORIES	FAT	CARBS
DAILY TOTALS:			

WEIGHT:

WATER INTAKE:
# of 8oz. glasses

☐ ☐ ☐ ☐
☐ ☐ ☐ ☐

**VITAMINS &
SUPPLEMENTS:**

_____
_____
_____
_____
_____
_____
_____
_____
_____

ENERGY LEVEL:
☐ low
☐ medium
☐ high

CALORIES BURNED:

NOTES/REMINDERS:

THURSDAY

DATE: ___ / ___ / ___

·· Daily Tip ··

Eating fish is a good way to increase the healthy fats in your diet, which can help reduce the risk of heart attacks.

WEIGHT:

WATER INTAKE:
# of 8oz. glasses

☐ ☐ ☐ ☐
☐ ☐ ☐ ☐

VITAMINS & SUPPLEMENTS:

ENERGY LEVEL:
☐ low
☐ medium
☐ high

CALORIES BURNED:

DAILY NUTRITIONAL INTAKE:

FOOD/BEVERAGES	CALORIES	FAT	CARBS
DAILY TOTALS:			

NOTES/REMINDERS:

FRIDAY

· **Daily Tip** ·

Choose carbs wisely. Eat a 100-calorie apple
versus eating a 100-calorie serving of chips.

· ·

DAILY NUTRITIONAL INTAKE:

FOOD/BEVERAGES	CALORIES	FAT	CARBS
DAILY TOTALS:			

WEIGHT:

WATER INTAKE:
# of 8oz. glasses
☐ ☐ ☐ ☐
☐ ☐ ☐ ☐

VITAMINS & SUPPLEMENTS:

ENERGY LEVEL:
☐ low
☐ medium
☐ high

CALORIES BURNED:

NOTES/REMINDERS:

SATURDAY

DATE: ___ / ___ / ___

· **Daily Tip** ·

Be sure to get enough calcium in your diet, through
dairy, green leafy vegetables, or supplements.

· ·

WEIGHT:

WATER INTAKE:
# of 8oz. glasses

☐ ☐ ☐ ☐
☐ ☐ ☐ ☐

**VITAMINS &
SUPPLEMENTS:**

ENERGY LEVEL:
☐ low
☐ medium
☐ high

CALORIES BURNED:

DAILY NUTRITIONAL INTAKE:

FOOD/BEVERAGES	CALORIES	FAT	CARBS
DAILY TOTALS:			

NOTES/REMINDERS:

SUNDAY

WEEK
8

Having a small snack between meals can help you
control your appetite, provides you with energy,
and keeps your metabolism active.

DAILY NUTRITIONAL INTAKE:

FOOD/BEVERAGES	CALORIES	FAT	CARBS
DAILY TOTALS:			

WEIGHT:

WATER INTAKE:
# of 8oz. glasses
☐ ☐ ☐ ☐
☐ ☐ ☐ ☐

**VITAMINS &
SUPPLEMENTS:**

_____

_____

_____

_____

_____

_____

_____

ENERGY LEVEL:
☐ low
☐ medium
☐ high

CALORIES BURNED:

NOTES/REMINDERS:

End-of-the-Week
WRAP-UP

START WEIGHT:

END WEIGHT:

WEEKLY ENERGY LEVEL:

☐ low ☐ med ☐ high

WEEKLY CALORIES BURNED:

DAYS I TRACKED MY DIET:

☐ Monday ☐ Tuesday ☐ Wednesday ☐ Thursday ☐ Friday ☐ Saturday ☐ Sunday

HOW I FELT THIS WEEK:

_____

_____

_____

_____

_____

_____

_____

_____

_____

GOALS FOR NEXT WEEK:

_____

_____

_____

_____

_____

_____

_____

_____

_____

NOTES/REMINDERS:

DATE:

_____ / _____ / _____

MONDAY

· **Daily Tip** ·

Body mass index (BMI) is a good indicator of
whether or not you are at a healthy weight.

· ·

DAILY NUTRITIONAL INTAKE:

FOOD/BEVERAGES	CALORIES	FAT	CARBS
DAILY TOTALS:			

WEIGHT:

WATER INTAKE:
# of 8oz. glasses

☐ ☐ ☐ ☐
☐ ☐ ☐ ☐

VITAMINS & SUPPLEMENTS:

_____
_____
_____
_____
_____
_____
_____

ENERGY LEVEL:
☐ low
☐ medium
☐ high

CALORIES BURNED:

NOTES/REMINDERS:

TUESDAY

DATE: ___ / ___ / ___

························· **Daily Tip** ·························

Try to prepare meals in advance if you know you are going
to be busy and unable to cook a proper meal.

···

WEIGHT:

WATER INTAKE:
# of 8oz. glasses

☐ ☐ ☐ ☐
☐ ☐ ☐ ☐

**VITAMINS &
SUPPLEMENTS:**

_____

_____

_____

_____

_____

_____

_____

ENERGY LEVEL:
☐ low
☐ medium
☐ high

CALORIES BURNED:

DAILY NUTRITIONAL INTAKE:

FOOD/BEVERAGES	CALORIES	FAT	CARBS
DAILY TOTALS:			

NOTES/REMINDERS:

DATE: ___ / ___ / ___

WEDNESDAY

Maintain your weight loss by adopting a lifestyle that includes all foods in moderation, healthy alternatives to foods high in fat and calories, and daily activities.

DAILY NUTRITIONAL INTAKE:

FOOD/BEVERAGES	CALORIES	FAT	CARBS
DAILY TOTALS:			

WEIGHT:

WATER INTAKE:
# of 8oz. glasses
☐ ☐ ☐ ☐
☐ ☐ ☐ ☐

VITAMINS & SUPPLEMENTS:

ENERGY LEVEL:
☐ low
☐ medium
☐ high

CALORIES BURNED:

NOTES/REMINDERS:

THURSDAY

DATE:
___ / ___ / ___

· **Daily Tip** ·

Studies have shown that adding more plant foods to your diet is
a good way to lower your LDL or "bad" cholesterol levels.

WEIGHT:

WATER INTAKE:
# of 8oz. glasses

☐ ☐ ☐ ☐
☐ ☐ ☐ ☐

**VITAMINS &
SUPPLEMENTS:**

ENERGY LEVEL:
☐ low
☐ medium
☐ high

CALORIES BURNED:

DAILY NUTRITIONAL INTAKE:

FOOD/BEVERAGES	CALORIES	FAT	CARBS
DAILY TOTALS:			

NOTES/REMINDERS:

DATE:
____ / ____ / ____

FRIDAY

························ **Daily Tip** ························

Add more plant foods to your diet by including oats,
barley, dried beans, oranges, apples, and nuts.

DAILY NUTRITIONAL INTAKE:

FOOD/BEVERAGES	CALORIES	FAT	CARBS
DAILY TOTALS:			

WEIGHT:

WATER INTAKE:
# of 8oz. glasses
☐ ☐ ☐ ☐
☐ ☐ ☐ ☐

**VITAMINS &
SUPPLEMENTS:**

ENERGY LEVEL:
☐ low
☐ medium
☐ high

CALORIES BURNED:

NOTES/REMINDERS:

SATURDAY

DATE: ___ / ___ / ___

········· **Daily Tip** ·········

Enriched foods have nutrients added to them that were lost during food processing. Fortified foods have nutrients added that were not originally present.

WEIGHT:

WATER INTAKE:
# of 8oz. glasses

☐ ☐ ☐ ☐
☐ ☐ ☐ ☐

VITAMINS & SUPPLEMENTS:

_____
_____
_____
_____
_____
_____
_____

ENERGY LEVEL:
☐ low
☐ medium
☐ high

CALORIES BURNED:

DAILY NUTRITIONAL INTAKE:

FOOD/BEVERAGES	CALORIES	FAT	CARBS
DAILY TOTALS:			

NOTES/REMINDERS:

DATE:

_____ / _____ / _____

SUNDAY

WEEK
9

··· **Daily Tip** ·································

Fruits and vegetables have a high fiber and water content,
which means they fill you up and keep you full longer.

···

DAILY NUTRITIONAL INTAKE:

FOOD/BEVERAGES	CALORIES	FAT	CARBS
DAILY TOTALS:			

WEIGHT:

WATER INTAKE:
# of 8oz. glasses

☐ ☐ ☐ ☐
☐ ☐ ☐ ☐

**VITAMINS &
SUPPLEMENTS:**

ENERGY LEVEL:
☐ low
☐ medium
☐ high

CALORIES BURNED:

NOTES/REMINDERS:

End-of-the-Week
WRAP-UP

START WEIGHT: **END WEIGHT:**   **WEEKLY ENERGY LEVEL:**   **WEEKLY CALORIES BURNED:**

☐ low ☐ med ☐ high

DAYS I TRACKED MY DIET:
☐ Monday ☐ Tuesday ☐ Wednesday ☐ Thursday ☐ Friday ☐ Saturday ☐ Sunday

HOW I FELT THIS WEEK:

_____
_____
_____
_____
_____
_____
_____
_____

GOALS FOR NEXT WEEK:

_____
_____
_____
_____
_____
_____
_____
_____

NOTES/REMINDERS:

MONDAY

························· **Daily Tip** ·······························

Eating 5 small meals a day is a good way to
control your eating habits and portion sizes.

···

DAILY NUTRITIONAL INTAKE:

FOOD/BEVERAGES	CALORIES	FAT	CARBS
DAILY TOTALS:			

WEIGHT:

WATER INTAKE:
# of 8oz. glasses
☐ ☐ ☐ ☐
☐ ☐ ☐ ☐

VITAMINS & SUPPLEMENTS:

ENERGY LEVEL:
☐ low
☐ medium
☐ high

CALORIES BURNED:

NOTES/REMINDERS:

TUESDAY

DATE: ___ / ___ / ___

······················· **Daily Tip** ·······················

Ginger, cinnamon, nutmeg, and vanilla are all good
additions to food in order to curb a sweet tooth.

WEIGHT:

WATER INTAKE:
# of 8oz. glasses

☐ ☐ ☐ ☐
☐ ☐ ☐ ☐

**VITAMINS &
SUPPLEMENTS:**

ENERGY LEVEL:
☐ low
☐ medium
☐ high

CALORIES BURNED:

DAILY NUTRITIONAL INTAKE:

FOOD/BEVERAGES	CALORIES	FAT	CARBS
DAILY TOTALS:			

NOTES/REMINDERS:

DATE: ___ / ___ / ___

WEDNESDAY

······························ **Daily Tip** ······························

Just because a product claims that it's "low fat," "fat-free,"
"sugar-free," or "low carb" does not necessarily
mean it will help you lose weight.

··

DAILY NUTRITIONAL INTAKE:

FOOD/BEVERAGES	CALORIES	FAT	CARBS
DAILY TOTALS:			

WEIGHT:

WATER INTAKE:
# of 8oz. glasses
☐ ☐ ☐ ☐
☐ ☐ ☐ ☐

VITAMINS & SUPPLEMENTS:

ENERGY LEVEL:
☐ low
☐ medium
☐ high

CALORIES BURNED:

NOTES/REMINDERS:

THURSDAY

DATE: ___ / ___ / ___

····················· **Daily Tip** ·····················

If you're looking for a quick, healthy afternoon snack,
try munching on slices of fruit, low-fat popcorn,
mixed nuts, or trail mix.

··

WEIGHT:

WATER INTAKE:
# of 8oz. glasses

☐ ☐ ☐ ☐
☐ ☐ ☐ ☐

VITAMINS & SUPPLEMENTS:

_____
_____
_____
_____
_____
_____
_____

ENERGY LEVEL:
☐ low
☐ medium
☐ high

CALORIES BURNED:

DAILY NUTRITIONAL INTAKE:

FOOD/BEVERAGES	CALORIES	FAT	CARBS
DAILY TOTALS:			

NOTES/REMINDERS:

DATE:
_____ / _____ / _____

FRIDAY

································ **Daily Tip** ································

Make your meals seem like more food
by serving them on smaller plates.

···

DAILY NUTRITIONAL INTAKE:

FOOD/BEVERAGES	CALORIES	FAT	CARBS
DAILY TOTALS:			

WEIGHT:

WATER INTAKE:
# of 8oz. glasses
☐ ☐ ☐ ☐
☐ ☐ ☐ ☐

VITAMINS & SUPPLEMENTS:

ENERGY LEVEL:
☐ low
☐ medium
☐ high

CALORIES BURNED:

NOTES/REMINDERS:

SATURDAY

DATE: ___/___/___

······················· Daily Tip ·······················

Eat more slowly. When you eat at a slower pace, you give
yourself more time to recognize when you are full.

···

WEIGHT:

WATER INTAKE:
# of 8oz. glasses
☐ ☐ ☐ ☐
☐ ☐ ☐ ☐

**VITAMINS &
SUPPLEMENTS:**

_____
_____
_____
_____
_____
_____
_____

ENERGY LEVEL:
☐ low
☐ medium
☐ high

CALORIES BURNED:

DAILY NUTRITIONAL INTAKE:

FOOD/BEVERAGES	CALORIES	FAT	CARBS
DAILY TOTALS:			

NOTES/REMINDERS:

DATE: ____ / ____ / ____

SUNDAY

········· **Daily Tip** ·········

Heat up your food. Foods served hot can be
more satiating so you are likely to eat less.

DAILY NUTRITIONAL INTAKE:

FOOD/BEVERAGES	CALORIES	FAT	CARBS
DAILY TOTALS:			

WEIGHT:

WATER INTAKE:
# of 8oz. glasses

☐ ☐ ☐ ☐
☐ ☐ ☐ ☐

VITAMINS & SUPPLEMENTS:

ENERGY LEVEL:
☐ low
☐ medium
☐ high

CALORIES BURNED:

NOTES/REMINDERS:

WEEK 10

End-of-the-Week
WRAP-UP

START WEIGHT:

END WEIGHT:

WEEKLY ENERGY LEVEL:
☐ low ☐ med ☐ high

WEEKLY CALORIES BURNED:

DAYS I TRACKED MY DIET:
☐ Monday ☐ Tuesday ☐ Wednesday ☐ Thursday ☐ Friday ☐ Saturday ☐ Sunday

HOW I FELT THIS WEEK:

GOALS FOR NEXT WEEK:

NOTES/REMINDERS:

MONDAY

DATE:

_____ / _____ / _____

.... **Daily Tip** ....

When eating, try to savor each bite of food. Putting your
fork down between bites can help you control your
portion sizes so you don't overeat.

....

DAILY NUTRITIONAL INTAKE:

FOOD/BEVERAGES	CALORIES	FAT	CARBS
DAILY TOTALS:			

WEIGHT:

WATER INTAKE:
# of 8oz. glasses

☐ ☐ ☐ ☐
☐ ☐ ☐ ☐

**VITAMINS &
SUPPLEMENTS:**

_____
_____
_____
_____
_____
_____
_____
_____

ENERGY LEVEL:
☐ low
☐ medium
☐ high

CALORIES BURNED:

NOTES/REMINDERS:

TUESDAY

DATE:

____ / ____ / ____

· **Daily Tip** ·

Men and women who eat breakfast in the mornings are far
less likely to become obese than those who skip
the most important meal of the day.

· ·

WEIGHT:

WATER INTAKE:
# of 8oz. glasses

☐ ☐ ☐ ☐
☐ ☐ ☐ ☐

**VITAMINS &
SUPPLEMENTS:**

_____
_____
_____
_____
_____
_____
_____
_____

ENERGY LEVEL:
☐ low
☐ medium
☐ high

CALORIES BURNED:

DAILY NUTRITIONAL INTAKE:

FOOD/BEVERAGES	CALORIES	FAT	CARBS
DAILY TOTALS:			

NOTES/REMINDERS:

WEDNESDAY

DATE: ____ / ____ / ____

.... **Daily Tip** ....

Switch to taller, narrow glasses to keep from drinking
extra calories. People tend to think that a tall glass
contains more liquid than a short, wide tumbler.

....

DAILY NUTRITIONAL INTAKE:

FOOD/BEVERAGES	CALORIES	FAT	CARBS
DAILY TOTALS:			

WEIGHT:

WATER INTAKE:
# of 8oz. glasses

☐ ☐ ☐ ☐
☐ ☐ ☐ ☐

VITAMINS & SUPPLEMENTS:

_____
_____
_____
_____
_____
_____
_____

ENERGY LEVEL:
☐ low
☐ medium
☐ high

CALORIES BURNED:

NOTES/REMINDERS:

THURSDAY

DATE:

_____ / _____ / _____

························· Daily Tip ·······························

Try not to go to the grocery store when you are hungry.
It can lead to buying more food than you need.

···

WEIGHT:

WATER INTAKE:
# of 8oz. glasses

☐ ☐ ☐ ☐
☐ ☐ ☐ ☐

**VITAMINS &
SUPPLEMENTS:**

_____
_____
_____
_____
_____
_____
_____
_____

ENERGY LEVEL:
☐ low
☐ medium
☐ high

CALORIES BURNED:

DAILY NUTRITIONAL INTAKE:

FOOD/BEVERAGES	CALORIES	FAT	CARBS
DAILY TOTALS:			

NOTES/REMINDERS:

DATE:
___ / ___ / ___

FRIDAY

······························· **Daily Tip** ·······························

Instead of fixating on all the "bad stuff," write down all of
the physical qualities you like about yourself and the
good things you have done for your body.

···

DAILY NUTRITIONAL INTAKE:

FOOD/BEVERAGES	CALORIES	FAT	CARBS
DAILY TOTALS:			

WEIGHT:

WATER INTAKE:
# of 8oz. glasses
☐ ☐ ☐ ☐
☐ ☐ ☐ ☐

**VITAMINS &
SUPPLEMENTS:**

ENERGY LEVEL:
☐ low
☐ medium
☐ high

CALORIES BURNED:

NOTES/REMINDERS:

SATURDAY

DATE: ___/___/___

········· **Daily Tip** ·········

Nuts are a great snack item. They are high in monounsaturated fats, protein, and carbohydrates, as well as vitamins and minerals.

WEIGHT:

WATER INTAKE:
# of 8oz. glasses

☐ ☐ ☐ ☐
☐ ☐ ☐ ☐

VITAMINS & SUPPLEMENTS:

ENERGY LEVEL:
☐ low
☐ medium
☐ high

CALORIES BURNED:

DAILY NUTRITIONAL INTAKE:

FOOD/BEVERAGES	CALORIES	FAT	CARBS
DAILY TOTALS:			

NOTES/REMINDERS:

DATE:
_____ / _____ / _____

SUNDAY

· **Daily Tip** ·

Snacking on nuts can lead to eating less and losing weight.
However, because nuts are high in calories, just be
sure to eat only small servings at a time.

· ·

DAILY NUTRITIONAL INTAKE:

FOOD/BEVERAGES	CALORIES	FAT	CARBS
DAILY TOTALS:			

WEIGHT:

WATER INTAKE:
# of 8oz. glasses
☐ ☐ ☐ ☐
☐ ☐ ☐ ☐

**VITAMINS &
SUPPLEMENTS:**

ENERGY LEVEL:
☐ low
☐ medium
☐ high

CALORIES BURNED:

NOTES/REMINDERS:

End-of-the-Week
WRAP-UP

START WEIGHT:

END WEIGHT:

WEEKLY ENERGY LEVEL:

☐ low ☐ med ☐ high

WEEKLY CALORIES BURNED:

DAYS I TRACKED MY DIET:

☐ Monday ☐ Tuesday ☐ Wednesday ☐ Thursday ☐ Friday ☐ Saturday ☐ Sunday

HOW I FELT THIS WEEK:

_____

_____

_____

_____

_____

_____

_____

_____

_____

GOALS FOR NEXT WEEK:

_____

_____

_____

_____

_____

_____

_____

_____

_____

NOTES/REMINDERS:

MONDAY

Drinking 1 glass of red wine at night may help improve
your HDL, or "good" cholesterol levels while reducing
your LDL, or "bad" cholesterol levels.

DAILY NUTRITIONAL INTAKE:

FOOD/BEVERAGES	CALORIES	FAT	CARBS
DAILY TOTALS:			

WEIGHT:

WATER INTAKE:
# of 8oz. glasses
☐ ☐ ☐ ☐
☐ ☐ ☐ ☐

VITAMINS & SUPPLEMENTS:
_____
_____
_____
_____
_____
_____
_____

ENERGY LEVEL:
☐ low
☐ medium
☐ high

CALORIES BURNED:

NOTES/REMINDERS:

TUESDAY

DATE:

_____ / _____ / _____

Try grilling, sautéing, or baking your food instead of
frying it. The way you prepare your food has a
big influence on how good it is for you.

WEIGHT:

WATER INTAKE:
# of 8oz. glasses

☐ ☐ ☐ ☐
☐ ☐ ☐ ☐

**VITAMINS &
SUPPLEMENTS:**

_____
_____
_____
_____
_____
_____
_____

ENERGY LEVEL:
☐ low
☐ medium
☐ high

CALORIES BURNED:

DAILY NUTRITIONAL INTAKE:

FOOD/BEVERAGES	CALORIES	FAT	CARBS
DAILY TOTALS:			

NOTES/REMINDERS:

WEDNESDAY

· **Daily Tip** ·

Schedule an event that you would like to lose weight for, such as your birthday, a vacation, or high school reunion.

· ·

DAILY NUTRITIONAL INTAKE:

FOOD/BEVERAGES	CALORIES	FAT	CARBS
DAILY TOTALS:			

WEIGHT:

WATER INTAKE:
# of 8oz. glasses
☐ ☐ ☐ ☐
☐ ☐ ☐ ☐

VITAMINS & SUPPLEMENTS:

ENERGY LEVEL:
☐ low
☐ medium
☐ high

CALORIES BURNED:

NOTES/REMINDERS:

THURSDAY

DATE: ___ / ___ / ___

·· **Daily Tip** ··

Remember that small measurable steps toward
weight loss are often the most gratifying.

···

WEIGHT:

WATER INTAKE:
# of 8oz. glasses

☐ ☐ ☐ ☐
☐ ☐ ☐ ☐

**VITAMINS &
SUPPLEMENTS:**

_____
_____
_____
_____
_____
_____
_____

ENERGY LEVEL:
☐ low
☐ medium
☐ high

CALORIES BURNED:

DAILY NUTRITIONAL INTAKE:

FOOD/BEVERAGES	CALORIES	FAT	CARBS
DAILY TOTALS:			

NOTES/REMINDERS:

DATE:

____ / ____ / ____

FRIDAY

························· **Daily Tip** ·························

Stay motivated by documenting changes to your
weight, body size, energy and mood on a
weekly and monthly basis.

··

DAILY NUTRITIONAL INTAKE:

FOOD/BEVERAGES	CALORIES	FAT	CARBS
DAILY TOTALS:			

WEIGHT:

WATER INTAKE:
# of 8oz. glasses

☐ ☐ ☐ ☐
☐ ☐ ☐ ☐

VITAMINS & SUPPLEMENTS:

ENERGY LEVEL:
☐ low
☐ medium
☐ high

CALORIES BURNED:

NOTES/REMINDERS:

SATURDAY

DATE: ___ / ___ / ___

······························· **Daily Tip** ·······························

If you feel a craving coming on, try to distract
yourself by taking a walk or calling a friend.

···

WEIGHT:

WATER INTAKE:
# of 8oz. glasses

☐ ☐ ☐ ☐
☐ ☐ ☐ ☐

**VITAMINS &
SUPPLEMENTS:**

_____
_____
_____
_____
_____
_____
_____

ENERGY LEVEL:
☐ low
☐ medium
☐ high

CALORIES BURNED:

DAILY NUTRITIONAL INTAKE:

FOOD/BEVERAGES	CALORIES	FAT	CARBS
DAILY TOTALS:			

NOTES/REMINDERS:

SUNDAY

WEEK 12

··· **Daily Tip** ·································

Tracking your weight on a daily basis can help you keep a
close eye on what eating patterns help you lose weight.

··

DAILY NUTRITIONAL INTAKE:

FOOD/BEVERAGES	CALORIES	FAT	CARBS
DAILY TOTALS:			

WEIGHT:

WATER INTAKE:
# of 8oz. glasses

☐ ☐ ☐ ☐
☐ ☐ ☐ ☐

VITAMINS & SUPPLEMENTS:

_____

_____

_____

_____

_____

_____

_____

_____

ENERGY LEVEL:
☐ low
☐ medium
☐ high

CALORIES BURNED:

NOTES/REMINDERS:

End-of-the-Week

WRAP-UP

START WEIGHT:

END WEIGHT:

WEEKLY ENERGY LEVEL:
☐ low ☐ med ☐ high

WEEKLY CALORIES BURNED:

DAYS I TRACKED MY DIET:
☐ Monday ☐ Tuesday ☐ Wednesday ☐ Thursday ☐ Friday ☐ Saturday ☐ Sunday

HOW I FELT THIS WEEK:

_____
_____
_____
_____
_____
_____
_____
_____

GOALS FOR NEXT WEEK:

_____
_____
_____
_____
_____
_____
_____
_____

NOTES/REMINDERS:

MONDAY

WEEK
13

Keep healthy snacks in your kitchen. That way, when you have the urge to munch on something, you will have better choices on hand.

· ·

DAILY NUTRITIONAL INTAKE:

FOOD/BEVERAGES	CALORIES	FAT	CARBS
DAILY TOTALS:			

WEIGHT:

WATER INTAKE:
# of 8oz. glasses
☐ ☐ ☐ ☐
☐ ☐ ☐ ☐

VITAMINS & SUPPLEMENTS:

ENERGY LEVEL:
☐ low
☐ medium
☐ high

CALORIES BURNED:

NOTES/REMINDERS:

TUESDAY

DATE: ___ / ___ / ___

Fat is an important nutrient: Just make sure that the fat you consume is the healthy, unsaturated kind found in fish, nuts, and seeds.

WEIGHT:

WATER INTAKE:
# of 8oz. glasses

☐ ☐ ☐ ☐
☐ ☐ ☐ ☐

VITAMINS & SUPPLEMENTS:

ENERGY LEVEL:
☐ low
☐ medium
☐ high

CALORIES BURNED:

DAILY NUTRITIONAL INTAKE:

FOOD/BEVERAGES	CALORIES	FAT	CARBS
DAILY TOTALS:			

NOTES/REMINDERS:

WEDNESDAY

· **Daily Tip** ·

Consider your resolution to lose weight as a benefit to yourself, not a test of your willpower.

· ·

DAILY NUTRITIONAL INTAKE:

FOOD/BEVERAGES	CALORIES	FAT	CARBS
DAILY TOTALS:			

WEIGHT:

WATER INTAKE:
# of 8oz. glasses

☐ ☐ ☐ ☐
☐ ☐ ☐ ☐

VITAMINS & SUPPLEMENTS:

_____

_____

_____

_____

_____

_____

ENERGY LEVEL:
☐ low
☐ medium
☐ high

CALORIES BURNED:

NOTES/REMINDERS:

THURSDAY

DATE:

_____ / _____ / _____

························· **Daily Tip** ·························

If using butter or margarine in your meal, try to enjoy them
in small portions and from a tub, rather than a stick.

WEIGHT:

WATER INTAKE:
# of 8oz. glasses

☐ ☐ ☐ ☐
☐ ☐ ☐ ☐

**VITAMINS &
SUPPLEMENTS:**

ENERGY LEVEL:
☐ low
☐ medium
☐ high

CALORIES BURNED:

DAILY NUTRITIONAL INTAKE:

FOOD/BEVERAGES	CALORIES	FAT	CARBS
DAILY TOTALS:			

NOTES/REMINDERS:

DATE:
_____ / _____ / _____

FRIDAY

•••••••••••••••••••••••••••••• **Daily Tip** ••••••••••••••••••••••••••••••

Share your intentions to eat healthy with the people
around you to create a sense of accountability.

•••

DAILY NUTRITIONAL INTAKE:

FOOD/BEVERAGES	CALORIES	FAT	CARBS
DAILY TOTALS:			

WEIGHT:

WATER INTAKE:
# of 8oz. glasses
☐ ☐ ☐ ☐
☐ ☐ ☐ ☐

**VITAMINS &
SUPPLEMENTS:**

_____
_____
_____
_____
_____
_____
_____
_____

ENERGY LEVEL:
☐ low
☐ medium
☐ high

CALORIES BURNED:

NOTES/REMINDERS:

SATURDAY

DATE:
____ / ____ / ____

······································ **Daily Tip** ································

If you are headed to a party where hors d'oeuvres and bowls of
snacks will be served, try to eat a small meal beforehand.

WEIGHT:

WATER INTAKE:
# of 8oz. glasses

☐ ☐ ☐ ☐
☐ ☐ ☐ ☐

**VITAMINS &
SUPPLEMENTS:**

ENERGY LEVEL:
☐ low
☐ medium
☐ high

CALORIES BURNED:

DAILY NUTRITIONAL INTAKE:

FOOD/BEVERAGES	CALORIES	FAT	CARBS
DAILY TOTALS:			

NOTES/REMINDERS:

DATE:

_____ / _____ / _____

SUNDAY

WEEK
13

····································· **Daily Tip** ·····································

Look for local or online weight-loss support communities where
you can share your story, get tips, and ask for advice.

···

DAILY NUTRITIONAL INTAKE:

FOOD/BEVERAGES	CALORIES	FAT	CARBS
DAILY TOTALS:			

WEIGHT:

WATER INTAKE:
# of 8oz. glasses

☐ ☐ ☐ ☐
☐ ☐ ☐ ☐

**VITAMINS &
SUPPLEMENTS:**

_____

_____

_____

_____

_____

_____

_____

_____

ENERGY LEVEL:
☐ low
☐ medium
☐ high

CALORIES BURNED:

NOTES/REMINDERS:

WEEK
13

End-of-the-Week
WRAP-UP

START WEIGHT: **END WEIGHT:** **WEEKLY ENERGY LEVEL:** **WEEKLY CALORIES BURNED:**

☐ low ☐ med ☐ high

DAYS I TRACKED MY DIET:
☐ Monday ☐ Tuesday ☐ Wednesday ☐ Thursday ☐ Friday ☐ Saturday ☐ Sunday

HOW I FELT THIS WEEK:

_____
_____
_____
_____
_____
_____
_____
_____

GOALS FOR NEXT WEEK:

_____
_____
_____
_____
_____
_____
_____
_____

NOTES/REMINDERS:

DATE:

_____ / _____ / _____

MONDAY

········· **Daily Tip** ·········

Cereal is an excellent source of fiber. Check out the label for cereals that have at least 5 grams of fiber per serving.

DAILY NUTRITIONAL INTAKE:

FOOD/BEVERAGES	CALORIES	FAT	CARBS

DAILY TOTALS:

WEIGHT:

WATER INTAKE:
# of 8oz. glasses

☐ ☐ ☐ ☐
☐ ☐ ☐ ☐

VITAMINS & SUPPLEMENTS:

ENERGY LEVEL:
☐ low
☐ medium
☐ high

CALORIES BURNED:

NOTES/REMINDERS:

TUESDAY

DATE: ___ / ___ / ___

.... Daily Tip ....

Enjoy an occasional splurge, but mentally prepare
to go back to your routine the following day.

WEIGHT:

WATER INTAKE:
# of 8oz. glasses

☐ ☐ ☐ ☐
☐ ☐ ☐ ☐

VITAMINS &
SUPPLEMENTS:

ENERGY LEVEL:
☐ low
☐ medium
☐ high

CALORIES BURNED:

DAILY NUTRITIONAL INTAKE:

FOOD/BEVERAGES	CALORIES	FAT	CARBS
DAILY TOTALS:			

NOTES/REMINDERS:

DATE: ____ / ____ / ____

WEDNESDAY

WEEK
14

· **Daily Tip** ·

Schedule rewards into your program to congratulate yourself for every positive step you make.

· ·

DAILY NUTRITIONAL INTAKE:

FOOD/BEVERAGES	CALORIES	FAT	CARBS
DAILY TOTALS:			

WEIGHT:

WATER INTAKE:
# of 8oz. glasses
☐ ☐ ☐ ☐
☐ ☐ ☐ ☐

VITAMINS & SUPPLEMENTS:

ENERGY LEVEL:
☐ low
☐ medium
☐ high

CALORIES BURNED:

NOTES/REMINDERS:

THURSDAY

DATE: _____ / _____ / _____

······································· **Daily Tip** ·······································

Do not confuse water loss with fat loss.

WEIGHT:

WATER INTAKE:
# of 8oz. glasses

☐ ☐ ☐ ☐
☐ ☐ ☐ ☐

VITAMINS & SUPPLEMENTS:

ENERGY LEVEL:
☐ low
☐ medium
☐ high

CALORIES BURNED:

DAILY NUTRITIONAL INTAKE:

FOOD/BEVERAGES	CALORIES	FAT	CARBS
DAILY TOTALS:			

NOTES/REMINDERS:

FRIDAY

························ **Daily Tip** ·························

Eating a salad before the start of your meal can help curb your appetite, allowing you to eat smaller portions of your main course.

DAILY NUTRITIONAL INTAKE:

FOOD/BEVERAGES	CALORIES	FAT	CARBS
DAILY TOTALS:			

WEIGHT:

WATER INTAKE:
# of 8oz. glasses
☐ ☐ ☐ ☐
☐ ☐ ☐ ☐

VITAMINS & SUPPLEMENTS:

ENERGY LEVEL:
☐ low
☐ medium
☐ high

CALORIES BURNED:

NOTES/REMINDERS:

SATURDAY

DATE: ___/___/___

······· **Daily Tip** ·······

Start a moderate exercise routine by adding 10 to 15 minutes of aerobic activity to your daily schedule.

··

WEIGHT:

WATER INTAKE:
# of 8oz. glasses
☐ ☐ ☐ ☐
☐ ☐ ☐ ☐

VITAMINS & SUPPLEMENTS:

_____
_____
_____
_____
_____
_____
_____
_____

ENERGY LEVEL:
☐ low
☐ medium
☐ high

CALORIES BURNED:

DAILY NUTRITIONAL INTAKE:

FOOD/BEVERAGES	CALORIES	FAT	CARBS
DAILY TOTALS:			

NOTES/REMINDERS:

DATE:

____ / ____ / ____

SUNDAY

··· **Daily Tip** ·································

Realize that the last 5 pounds can be
the most challenging to lose.

···

DAILY NUTRITIONAL INTAKE:

FOOD/BEVERAGES	CALORIES	FAT	CARBS
DAILY TOTALS:			

WEIGHT:

WATER INTAKE:
# of 8oz. glasses

☐ ☐ ☐ ☐
☐ ☐ ☐ ☐

VITAMINS & SUPPLEMENTS:

_____

_____

_____

_____

_____

_____

_____

ENERGY LEVEL:
☐ low
☐ medium
☐ high

CALORIES BURNED:

NOTES/REMINDERS:

End-of-the-Week
WRAP-UP

START WEIGHT: **END WEIGHT:** **WEEKLY ENERGY LEVEL:** **WEEKLY CALORIES BURNED:**

☐ low ☐ med ☐ high

DAYS I TRACKED MY DIET:
☐ Monday ☐ Tuesday ☐ Wednesday ☐ Thursday ☐ Friday ☐ Saturday ☐ Sunday

HOW I FELT THIS WEEK:

_____

_____

_____

_____

_____

_____

_____

_____

GOALS FOR NEXT WEEK:

_____

_____

_____

_____

_____

_____

_____

_____

NOTES/REMINDERS:

MONDAY

······························ **Daily Tip** ······························

Instead of thinking of dieting as "giving up" foods, think of it as eating your favorite foods, but in moderation.

··

DAILY NUTRITIONAL INTAKE:

FOOD/BEVERAGES	CALORIES	FAT	CARBS
DAILY TOTALS:			

WEIGHT:

WATER INTAKE:
# of 8oz. glasses
☐ ☐ ☐ ☐
☐ ☐ ☐ ☐

VITAMINS & SUPPLEMENTS:

ENERGY LEVEL:
☐ low
☐ medium
☐ high

CALORIES BURNED:

NOTES/REMINDERS:

TUESDAY

DATE: ____ / ____ / ____

························· **Daily Tip** ·························

Smaller portion sizes and higher-calorie foods eaten in
small amounts can help you lose weight without
making you feel like you are depriving yourself.

WEIGHT:

WATER INTAKE:
# of 8oz. glasses

☐ ☐ ☐ ☐
☐ ☐ ☐ ☐

**VITAMINS &
SUPPLEMENTS:**

_____
_____
_____
_____
_____
_____
_____
_____

ENERGY LEVEL:
☐ low
☐ medium
☐ high

CALORIES BURNED:

DAILY NUTRITIONAL INTAKE:

FOOD/BEVERAGES	CALORIES	FAT	CARBS
DAILY TOTALS:			

NOTES/REMINDERS:

DATE:
____ / ____ / ____

WEDNESDAY

··· **Daily Tip** ·································

Make slow, small changes to your diet instead of
fast, big changes. This way, your healthy
lifestyle is easier to maintain.

···

DAILY NUTRITIONAL INTAKE:

FOOD/BEVERAGES	CALORIES	FAT	CARBS
DAILY TOTALS:			

WEIGHT:

WATER INTAKE:
# of 8oz. glasses
☐ ☐ ☐ ☐
☐ ☐ ☐ ☐

**VITAMINS &
SUPPLEMENTS:**

ENERGY LEVEL:
☐ low
☐ medium
☐ high

CALORIES BURNED:

NOTES/REMINDERS:

THURSDAY

DATE: ___ / ___ / ___

Plan your meals ahead of time. That way, you won't be caught off guard or forced to make unhealthy food choices.

WEIGHT:

WATER INTAKE:
# of 8oz. glasses

☐ ☐ ☐ ☐
☐ ☐ ☐ ☐

VITAMINS & SUPPLEMENTS:

ENERGY LEVEL:
☐ low
☐ medium
☐ high

CALORIES BURNED:

DAILY NUTRITIONAL INTAKE:

FOOD/BEVERAGES	CALORIES	FAT	CARBS
DAILY TOTALS:			

NOTES/REMINDERS:

FRIDAY

WEEK
15

Skipping breakfast will actually train your body to store more
fat when it senses you are not getting enough food.

DAILY NUTRITIONAL INTAKE:

FOOD/BEVERAGES	CALORIES	FAT	CARBS
DAILY TOTALS:			

WEIGHT:

WATER INTAKE:
# of 8oz. glasses
☐ ☐ ☐ ☐
☐ ☐ ☐ ☐

**VITAMINS &
SUPPLEMENTS:**

ENERGY LEVEL:
☐ low
☐ medium
☐ high

CALORIES BURNED:

NOTES/REMINDERS:

SATURDAY

DATE: ___ / ___ / ___

Drinking 5 cups of green tea may burn
70 to 80 extra calories a day.

WEIGHT:

WATER INTAKE:
# of 8oz. glasses

☐ ☐ ☐ ☐
☐ ☐ ☐ ☐

**VITAMINS &
SUPPLEMENTS:**

_____
_____
_____
_____
_____
_____
_____

ENERGY LEVEL:
☐ low
☐ medium
☐ high

CALORIES BURNED:

DAILY NUTRITIONAL INTAKE:

FOOD/BEVERAGES	CALORIES	FAT	CARBS
DAILY TOTALS:			

NOTES/REMINDERS:

DATE:
____ / ____ / ____

SUNDAY

Working out on an empty stomach, such as in the morning or before you eat dinner, will help you burn the maximum amount of fat and calories.

DAILY NUTRITIONAL INTAKE:

FOOD/BEVERAGES	CALORIES	FAT	CARBS

DAILY TOTALS:

WEIGHT:

WATER INTAKE:
# of 8oz. glasses
☐ ☐ ☐ ☐
☐ ☐ ☐ ☐

VITAMINS & SUPPLEMENTS:

ENERGY LEVEL:
☐ low
☐ medium
☐ high

CALORIES BURNED:

NOTES/REMINDERS:

WEEK 15

End-of-the-Week

WRAP-UP

START WEIGHT:

END WEIGHT:

WEEKLY ENERGY LEVEL:

☐ low ☐ med ☐ high

WEEKLY CALORIES BURNED:

DAYS I TRACKED MY DIET:

☐ Monday ☐ Tuesday ☐ Wednesday ☐ Thursday ☐ Friday ☐ Saturday ☐ Sunday

HOW I FELT THIS WEEK:

GOALS FOR NEXT WEEK:

NOTES/REMINDERS:

MONDAY

DATE:
___ / ___ / ___

······················· **Daily Tip** ·······························

If you need a burst of energy during your workout, have a
snack with complex carbohydrates and protein handy,
like a small piece of fruit and cheese.

··

DAILY NUTRITIONAL INTAKE:

FOOD/BEVERAGES	CALORIES	FAT	CARBS
DAILY TOTALS:			

WEIGHT:

WATER INTAKE:
# of 8oz. glasses
☐ ☐ ☐ ☐
☐ ☐ ☐ ☐

**VITAMINS &
SUPPLEMENTS:**

ENERGY LEVEL:
☐ low
☐ medium
☐ high

CALORIES BURNED:

NOTES/REMINDERS:

TUESDAY

DATE:

____ / ____ / ____

······················· **Daily Tip** ·······························

Strive for consistency with your weight-loss program, not perfection.

··

WEIGHT:

WATER INTAKE:
# of 8oz. glasses

☐ ☐ ☐ ☐
☐ ☐ ☐ ☐

VITAMINS & SUPPLEMENTS:

ENERGY LEVEL:
☐ low
☐ medium
☐ high

CALORIES BURNED:

DAILY NUTRITIONAL INTAKE:

FOOD/BEVERAGES	CALORIES	FAT	CARBS
DAILY TOTALS:			

NOTES/REMINDERS:

WEDNESDAY

WEEK
16

Don't eat snack foods directly out of the package. Measure the portion you want to eat on a plate, and put the rest away.

DAILY NUTRITIONAL INTAKE:

FOOD/BEVERAGES	CALORIES	FAT	CARBS

DAILY TOTALS:

WEIGHT:

WATER INTAKE:
# of 8oz. glasses
☐ ☐ ☐ ☐
☐ ☐ ☐ ☐

VITAMINS & SUPPLEMENTS:

ENERGY LEVEL:
☐ low
☐ medium
☐ high

CALORIES BURNED:

NOTES/REMINDERS:

THURSDAY

DATE:
___ / ___ / ___

······················· **Daily Tip** ·······························

It takes 20 minutes for your brain to register that your stomach is full. If you eat slower while enjoying every bite, you are less likely to overeat.

WEIGHT:

WATER INTAKE:
# of 8oz. glasses

☐ ☐ ☐ ☐
☐ ☐ ☐ ☐

VITAMINS & SUPPLEMENTS:

ENERGY LEVEL:
☐ low
☐ medium
☐ high

CALORIES BURNED:

DAILY NUTRITIONAL INTAKE:

FOOD/BEVERAGES	CALORIES	FAT	CARBS
DAILY TOTALS:			

NOTES/REMINDERS:

FRIDAY

· **Daily Tip** ·

Some research suggests that spicy foods, primarily red pepper, cayenne and chili pepper, may help raise your metabolism.

· ·

DAILY NUTRITIONAL INTAKE:

FOOD/BEVERAGES	CALORIES	FAT	CARBS
DAILY TOTALS:			

WEIGHT:

WATER INTAKE:
# of 8oz. glasses
☐ ☐ ☐ ☐
☐ ☐ ☐ ☐

VITAMINS & SUPPLEMENTS:

ENERGY LEVEL:
☐ low
☐ medium
☐ high

CALORIES BURNED:

NOTES/REMINDERS:

WEEK 16

SATURDAY

DATE:
___ / ___ / ___

········· **Daily Tip** ·········

Plan ahead before going to the grocery store. Make a list of exactly what you want to buy, and don't spend time in the cookie or snack aisles.

WEIGHT:

WATER INTAKE:
# of 8oz. glasses

☐ ☐ ☐ ☐
☐ ☐ ☐ ☐

VITAMINS & SUPPLEMENTS:

ENERGY LEVEL:
☐ low
☐ medium
☐ high

CALORIES BURNED:

DAILY NUTRITIONAL INTAKE:

FOOD/BEVERAGES	CALORIES	FAT	CARBS
DAILY TOTALS:			

NOTES/REMINDERS:

DATE:
____ / ____ / ____

SUNDAY

· **Daily Tip** ·

Create a healthy diet that focuses on unprocessed foods
such as fruit, vegetables, whole grains, legumes
(lentils, dry beans and peas), and lean protein.

· ·

DAILY NUTRITIONAL INTAKE:

FOOD/BEVERAGES	CALORIES	FAT	CARBS
DAILY TOTALS:			

WEIGHT:

WATER INTAKE:
# of 8oz. glasses

☐ ☐ ☐ ☐
☐ ☐ ☐ ☐

VITAMINS & SUPPLEMENTS:

_____

_____

_____

_____

_____

_____

_____

ENERGY LEVEL:
☐ low
☐ medium
☐ high

CALORIES BURNED:

NOTES/REMINDERS:

End-of-the-Week
WRAP-UP

START WEIGHT:

END WEIGHT:

WEEKLY ENERGY LEVEL:
☐ low ☐ med ☐ high

WEEKLY CALORIES BURNED:

DAYS I TRACKED MY DIET:
☐ Monday ☐ Tuesday ☐ Wednesday ☐ Thursday ☐ Friday ☐ Saturday ☐ Sunday

HOW I FELT THIS WEEK:

_____
_____
_____
_____
_____
_____
_____
_____

GOALS FOR NEXT WEEK:

_____
_____
_____
_____
_____
_____
_____
_____

NOTES/REMINDERS:

MONDAY

DATE:

_____ / _____ / _____

··· **Daily Tip** ·································

Tofu is a good substitute for many foods because it is rich in
high-quality protein and contains no cholesterol.
Try using it in place of cream in sauces.

···

DAILY NUTRITIONAL INTAKE:

FOOD/BEVERAGES	CALORIES	FAT	CARBS
DAILY TOTALS:			

WEIGHT:

WATER INTAKE:
# of 8oz. glasses
☐ ☐ ☐ ☐
☐ ☐ ☐ ☐

VITAMINS & SUPPLEMENTS:

ENERGY LEVEL:
☐ low
☐ medium
☐ high

CALORIES BURNED:

NOTES/REMINDERS:

TUESDAY

DATE: ___ / ___ / ___

· **Daily Tip** ·

Chicken broth and fresh herbs are an excellent and delicious substitute for butter and margarine when cooking.

· ·

WEIGHT:

WATER INTAKE:
# of 8oz. glasses

☐ ☐ ☐ ☐
☐ ☐ ☐ ☐

**VITAMINS &
SUPPLEMENTS:**

ENERGY LEVEL:
☐ low
☐ medium
☐ high

CALORIES BURNED:

DAILY NUTRITIONAL INTAKE:

FOOD/BEVERAGES	CALORIES	FAT	CARBS
DAILY TOTALS:			

NOTES/REMINDERS:

DATE: ___ / ___ / ___

WEDNESDAY

Add lean protein to your diet, such as ground turkey, skinless white-meat poultry, as well as egg whites, fish, and legumes.

DAILY NUTRITIONAL INTAKE:

FOOD/BEVERAGES	CALORIES	FAT	CARBS

DAILY TOTALS:

WEIGHT:

WATER INTAKE:
# of 8oz. glasses
☐ ☐ ☐ ☐
☐ ☐ ☐ ☐

VITAMINS & SUPPLEMENTS:

ENERGY LEVEL:
☐ low
☐ medium
☐ high

CALORIES BURNED:

NOTES/REMINDERS:

THURSDAY

DATE: ___ / ___ / ___

························· Daily Tip ·························

After dinner or other large meals, try going for a long walk with a friend.

···

WEIGHT:

WATER INTAKE:
# of 8oz. glasses

☐ ☐ ☐ ☐
☐ ☐ ☐ ☐

VITAMINS & SUPPLEMENTS:

_____
_____
_____
_____
_____
_____
_____

ENERGY LEVEL:
☐ low
☐ medium
☐ high

CALORIES BURNED:

DAILY NUTRITIONAL INTAKE:

FOOD/BEVERAGES	CALORIES	FAT	CARBS
DAILY TOTALS:			

NOTES/REMINDERS:

DATE:
___ / ___ / ___

FRIDAY

Try to have something small to eat every 2 to 3 hours. Avoid large gaps of time without food where your hunger completely takes over.

DAILY NUTRITIONAL INTAKE:

FOOD/BEVERAGES	CALORIES	FAT	CARBS
DAILY TOTALS:			

WEIGHT:

WATER INTAKE:
# of 8oz. glasses
☐ ☐ ☐ ☐
☐ ☐ ☐ ☐

VITAMINS & SUPPLEMENTS:

ENERGY LEVEL:
☐ low
☐ medium
☐ high

CALORIES BURNED:

NOTES/REMINDERS:

SATURDAY

DATE: ___ / ___ / ___

· **Daily Tip** ·

Each time you sit down to eat, think of it as a new opportunity to make healthy food choices!

· ·

WEIGHT:

WATER INTAKE:
# of 8oz. glasses

☐ ☐ ☐ ☐
☐ ☐ ☐ ☐

VITAMINS & SUPPLEMENTS:

_____
_____
_____
_____
_____
_____
_____

ENERGY LEVEL:
☐ low
☐ medium
☐ high

CALORIES BURNED:

DAILY NUTRITIONAL INTAKE:

FOOD/BEVERAGES	CALORIES	FAT	CARBS
DAILY TOTALS:			

NOTES/REMINDERS:

SUNDAY

DATE:

_____ / _____ / _____

··· **Daily Tip** ·································

Burn more calories than you eat with nutrient- and
fiber-dense foods like fruits and vegetables.

DAILY NUTRITIONAL INTAKE:

FOOD/BEVERAGES	CALORIES	FAT	CARBS
DAILY TOTALS:			

WEIGHT:

WATER INTAKE:
# of 8oz. glasses

☐ ☐ ☐ ☐
☐ ☐ ☐ ☐

**VITAMINS &
SUPPLEMENTS:**

ENERGY LEVEL:
☐ low
☐ medium
☐ high

CALORIES BURNED:

NOTES/REMINDERS:

End-of-the-Week
WRAP-UP

START WEIGHT:

END WEIGHT:

WEEKLY ENERGY LEVEL:
☐ low ☐ med ☐ high

WEEKLY CALORIES BURNED:

DAYS I TRACKED MY DIET:
☐ Monday ☐ Tuesday ☐ Wednesday ☐ Thursday ☐ Friday ☐ Saturday ☐ Sunday

HOW I FELT THIS WEEK:

GOALS FOR NEXT WEEK:

NOTES/REMINDERS:

MONDAY

································ **Daily Tip** ································

Try to choose snacks that are rich in vitamins and will give
you the proper nutrients your body needs. That way,
you won't just be consuming empty calories.

··

DAILY NUTRITIONAL INTAKE:

FOOD/BEVERAGES	CALORIES	FAT	CARBS
DAILY TOTALS:			

WEIGHT:

WATER INTAKE:
# of 8oz. glasses
☐ ☐ ☐ ☐
☐ ☐ ☐ ☐

**VITAMINS &
SUPPLEMENTS:**

ENERGY LEVEL:
☐ low
☐ medium
☐ high

CALORIES BURNED:

NOTES/REMINDERS:

TUESDAY

DATE:
_____ / _____ / _____

Buy a healthy cookbook or food magazine. It will be filled
with delicious recipes to help you cook healthier meals.

WEIGHT:

WATER INTAKE:
# of 8oz. glasses

☐ ☐ ☐ ☐
☐ ☐ ☐ ☐

**VITAMINS &
SUPPLEMENTS:**

ENERGY LEVEL:
☐ low
☐ medium
☐ high

CALORIES BURNED:

DAILY NUTRITIONAL INTAKE:

FOOD/BEVERAGES	CALORIES	FAT	CARBS
DAILY TOTALS:			

NOTES/REMINDERS:

WEDNESDAY

······························ **Daily Tip** ································

Eat soon after exercising to heal your body and restore energy.

··

DAILY NUTRITIONAL INTAKE:

FOOD/BEVERAGES	CALORIES	FAT	CARBS
DAILY TOTALS:			

WEIGHT:

WATER INTAKE:
# of 8oz. glasses

☐ ☐ ☐ ☐
☐ ☐ ☐ ☐

VITAMINS & SUPPLEMENTS:

ENERGY LEVEL:
☐ low
☐ medium
☐ high

CALORIES BURNED:

NOTES/REMINDERS:

THURSDAY

DATE:
___ / ___ / ___

······· **Daily Tip** ·······

When possible, take the stairs or park farther away
from the store. Extra steps in your day mean
extra calories burned over the long run.

WEIGHT:

WATER INTAKE:
# of 8oz. glasses

☐ ☐ ☐ ☐
☐ ☐ ☐ ☐

**VITAMINS &
SUPPLEMENTS:**

ENERGY LEVEL:
☐ low
☐ medium
☐ high

CALORIES BURNED:

DAILY NUTRITIONAL INTAKE:

FOOD/BEVERAGES	CALORIES	FAT	CARBS
DAILY TOTALS:			

NOTES/REMINDERS:

DATE:
_____ / _____ / _____

FRIDAY

································· **Daily Tip** ·································

Check-out aisles in grocery stores are laden with foods
that are high in fat, calories, sugar, and salt;
recognize this and resist temptation.

···

DAILY NUTRITIONAL INTAKE:

FOOD/BEVERAGES	CALORIES	FAT	CARBS
DAILY TOTALS:			

WEIGHT:

WATER INTAKE:
# of 8oz. glasses
☐ ☐ ☐ ☐
☐ ☐ ☐ ☐

**VITAMINS &
SUPPLEMENTS:**

_____
_____
_____
_____
_____
_____
_____

ENERGY LEVEL:
☐ low
☐ medium
☐ high

CALORIES BURNED:

NOTES/REMINDERS:

SATURDAY

DATE:
___/___/___

If joining a gym is not your thing, try organizing a game
of basketball or Frisbee. Take a jog outdoors or
walk your dog, if the weather is nice.

WEIGHT:

WATER INTAKE:
# of 8oz. glasses

☐ ☐ ☐ ☐
☐ ☐ ☐ ☐

**VITAMINS &
SUPPLEMENTS:**

_____
_____
_____
_____
_____
_____
_____
_____

ENERGY LEVEL:
☐ low
☐ medium
☐ high

CALORIES BURNED:

DAILY NUTRITIONAL INTAKE:

FOOD/BEVERAGES	CALORIES	FAT	CARBS
DAILY TOTALS:			

NOTES/REMINDERS:

DATE: ___ / ___ / ___

SUNDAY

WEEK
18

························· **Daily Tip** ·························

Prepare your own meals as often as you can.
You can control exactly what goes into each
meal if you make it yourself.

DAILY NUTRITIONAL INTAKE:

FOOD/BEVERAGES	CALORIES	FAT	CARBS
DAILY TOTALS:			

WEIGHT:

WATER INTAKE:
# of 8oz. glasses
☐ ☐ ☐ ☐
☐ ☐ ☐ ☐

**VITAMINS &
SUPPLEMENTS:**

ENERGY LEVEL:
☐ low
☐ medium
☐ high

CALORIES BURNED:

NOTES/REMINDERS:

End-of-the-Week
WRAP-UP

START WEIGHT: **END WEIGHT:**   **WEEKLY ENERGY LEVEL:**   **WEEKLY CALORIES BURNED:**

☐ low ☐ med ☐ high

DAYS I TRACKED MY DIET:
☐ Monday ☐ Tuesday ☐ Wednesday ☐ Thursday ☐ Friday ☐ Saturday ☐ Sunday

HOW I FELT THIS WEEK:

_____

_____

_____

_____

_____

_____

_____

_____

GOALS FOR NEXT WEEK:

_____

_____

_____

_____

_____

_____

_____

_____

NOTES/REMINDERS:

MONDAY

DATE:

____ / ____ / ____

Don't think of how much more weight you have to lose,
but rather think about how much you've already lost!

DAILY NUTRITIONAL INTAKE:

FOOD/BEVERAGES	CALORIES	FAT	CARBS
DAILY TOTALS:			

WEIGHT:

WATER INTAKE:
# of 8oz. glasses

☐ ☐ ☐ ☐
☐ ☐ ☐ ☐

VITAMINS & SUPPLEMENTS:

ENERGY LEVEL:
☐ low
☐ medium
☐ high

CALORIES BURNED:

NOTES/REMINDERS:

TUESDAY

DATE: ___ / ___ / ___

·· **Daily Tip** ··

Congratulate yourself every time you get a
step closer to your weight-loss goal.

WEIGHT:

WATER INTAKE:
# of 8oz. glasses

☐ ☐ ☐ ☐
☐ ☐ ☐ ☐

**VITAMINS &
SUPPLEMENTS:**

ENERGY LEVEL:
☐ low
☐ medium
☐ high

CALORIES BURNED:

DAILY NUTRITIONAL INTAKE:

FOOD/BEVERAGES	CALORIES	FAT	CARBS
DAILY TOTALS:			

NOTES/REMINDERS:

················· **Daily Tip** ·················

Don't rule out foods because of the time of day.

···

DAILY NUTRITIONAL INTAKE:

FOOD/BEVERAGES	CALORIES	FAT	CARBS
DAILY TOTALS:			

WEIGHT:

WATER INTAKE:
# of 8oz. glasses
☐ ☐ ☐ ☐
☐ ☐ ☐ ☐

VITAMINS & SUPPLEMENTS:

ENERGY LEVEL:
☐ low
☐ medium
☐ high

CALORIES BURNED:

NOTES/REMINDERS:

THURSDAY

DATE: ___ / ___ / ___

······························· **Daily Tip** ·······························

Avoid going to a candy store or an ice cream shop,
where you will be tempted to stray from your diet.

WEIGHT:

WATER INTAKE:
# of 8oz. glasses

☐ ☐ ☐ ☐
☐ ☐ ☐ ☐

**VITAMINS &
SUPPLEMENTS:**

ENERGY LEVEL:
☐ low
☐ medium
☐ high

CALORIES BURNED:

DAILY NUTRITIONAL INTAKE:

FOOD/BEVERAGES	CALORIES	FAT	CARBS
DAILY TOTALS:			

NOTES/REMINDERS:

FRIDAY

· **Daily Tip** ·

Instead of simply swearing off chips, cookies, cake, or candy, find healthy alternatives and have them available when you feel like snacking.

· ·

DAILY NUTRITIONAL INTAKE:

FOOD/BEVERAGES	CALORIES	FAT	CARBS
DAILY TOTALS:			

WEIGHT:

WATER INTAKE:
# of 8oz. glasses

☐ ☐ ☐ ☐
☐ ☐ ☐ ☐

VITAMINS & SUPPLEMENTS:

_____
_____
_____
_____
_____
_____
_____
_____
_____

ENERGY LEVEL:
☐ low
☐ medium
☐ high

CALORIES BURNED:

NOTES/REMINDERS:

WEEK 19

SATURDAY

DATE: ___ / ___ / ___

········· **Daily Tip** ·········

Walking at least 3 miles a day can contribute
significantly to your weight-loss program.

WEIGHT:

WATER INTAKE:
# of 8oz. glasses
☐ ☐ ☐ ☐
☐ ☐ ☐ ☐

**VITAMINS &
SUPPLEMENTS:**

ENERGY LEVEL:
☐ low
☐ medium
☐ high

CALORIES BURNED:

DAILY NUTRITIONAL INTAKE:

FOOD/BEVERAGES	CALORIES	FAT	CARBS

DAILY TOTALS:

NOTES/REMINDERS:

DATE:
_____ / _____ / _____

SUNDAY

Daily Tip

Stock your freezer with healthy frozen entrees.

DAILY NUTRITIONAL INTAKE:

FOOD/BEVERAGES	CALORIES	FAT	CARBS
DAILY TOTALS:			

WEIGHT:

WATER INTAKE:
# of 8oz. glasses
☐ ☐ ☐ ☐
☐ ☐ ☐ ☐

VITAMINS & SUPPLEMENTS:

ENERGY LEVEL:
☐ low
☐ medium
☐ high

CALORIES BURNED:

NOTES/REMINDERS:

End-of-the-Week

WRAP-UP

START WEIGHT: **END WEIGHT:**   **WEEKLY ENERGY LEVEL:**   **WEEKLY CALORIES BURNED:**

☐ low ☐ med ☐ high

DAYS I TRACKED MY DIET:
☐ Monday ☐ Tuesday ☐ Wednesday ☐ Thursday ☐ Friday ☐ Saturday ☐ Sunday

HOW I FELT THIS WEEK:

GOALS FOR NEXT WEEK:

NOTES/REMINDERS:

DATE:

_____ / _____ / _____

MONDAY

WEEK
20

······························· **Daily Tip** ·······························

Add strength training to your aerobic workout.
You will burn fat faster in the areas you build muscle.

···

DAILY NUTRITIONAL INTAKE:

FOOD/BEVERAGES	CALORIES	FAT	CARBS
DAILY TOTALS:			

WEIGHT:

WATER INTAKE:
# of 8oz. glasses
☐ ☐ ☐ ☐
☐ ☐ ☐ ☐

VITAMINS & SUPPLEMENTS:

_____

_____

_____

_____

_____

_____

_____

ENERGY LEVEL:
☐ low
☐ medium
☐ high

CALORIES BURNED:

NOTES/REMINDERS:

TUESDAY

DATE: _____ / _____ / _____

······························ Daily Tip ······························

Before strength training, consult a trainer who can guide you in the
safety procedures and correct way to use exercise machines.

··

WEIGHT:

WATER INTAKE:
# of 8oz. glasses

☐ ☐ ☐ ☐
☐ ☐ ☐ ☐

VITAMINS & SUPPLEMENTS:

ENERGY LEVEL:
☐ low
☐ medium
☐ high

CALORIES BURNED:

DAILY NUTRITIONAL INTAKE:

FOOD/BEVERAGES	CALORIES	FAT	CARBS
DAILY TOTALS:			

NOTES/REMINDERS:

DATE:

_____ / _____ / _____

WEDNESDAY

· **Daily Tip** ·

You won't need to rely on take-out, fast food, or delivery if your kitchen is stocked with nutritious foods that are easy to prepare.

· ·

DAILY NUTRITIONAL INTAKE:

FOOD/BEVERAGES	CALORIES	FAT	CARBS
DAILY TOTALS:			

WEIGHT:

WATER INTAKE:
# of 8oz. glasses

☐ ☐ ☐ ☐
☐ ☐ ☐ ☐

VITAMINS & SUPPLEMENTS:

_____
_____
_____
_____
_____
_____
_____
_____

ENERGY LEVEL:
☐ low
☐ medium
☐ high

CALORIES BURNED:

NOTES/REMINDERS:

THURSDAY

DATE: ___/___/___

········· **Daily Tip** ·········

Don't cut too many calories out of your diet. If you feel
deprived or unsatisfied, you are more likely to cheat.

WEIGHT:

WATER INTAKE:
# of 8oz. glasses

☐ ☐ ☐ ☐
☐ ☐ ☐ ☐

**VITAMINS &
SUPPLEMENTS:**

ENERGY LEVEL:
☐ low
☐ medium
☐ high

CALORIES BURNED:

DAILY NUTRITIONAL INTAKE:

FOOD/BEVERAGES	CALORIES	FAT	CARBS
DAILY TOTALS:			

NOTES/REMINDERS:

FRIDAY

WEEK
20

Include a healthy treat into your weight-loss plan
so you don't feel deprived. Try to keep these
foods between 200 and 250 calories.

DAILY NUTRITIONAL INTAKE:

FOOD/BEVERAGES	CALORIES	FAT	CARBS
DAILY TOTALS:			

WEIGHT:

WATER INTAKE:
# of 8oz. glasses

☐ ☐ ☐ ☐
☐ ☐ ☐ ☐

VITAMINS & SUPPLEMENTS:

ENERGY LEVEL:
☐ low
☐ medium
☐ high

CALORIES BURNED:

NOTES/REMINDERS:

SATURDAY

DATE: ___ / ___ / ___

························· **Daily Tip** ·························

Varying your physical activity keeps your workout
routine interesting and fun and keeps your
body working at its peak potential.

WEIGHT:

WATER INTAKE:
# of 8oz. glasses

☐ ☐ ☐ ☐
☐ ☐ ☐ ☐

**VITAMINS &
SUPPLEMENTS:**

_____
_____
_____
_____
_____
_____
_____
_____

ENERGY LEVEL:
☐ low
☐ medium
☐ high

CALORIES BURNED:

DAILY NUTRITIONAL INTAKE:

FOOD/BEVERAGES	CALORIES	FAT	CARBS
DAILY TOTALS:			

NOTES/REMINDERS:

DATE:
____ / ____ / ____

SUNDAY

········· **Daily Tip** ·········

Make a list of all the foods you like that fit within your
diet program so you can easily plan meals.

DAILY NUTRITIONAL INTAKE:

FOOD/BEVERAGES	CALORIES	FAT	CARBS
DAILY TOTALS:			

WEIGHT:

WATER INTAKE:
# of 8oz. glasses

☐ ☐ ☐ ☐
☐ ☐ ☐ ☐

**VITAMINS &
SUPPLEMENTS:**

ENERGY LEVEL:
☐ low
☐ medium
☐ high

CALORIES BURNED:

NOTES/REMINDERS:

End-of-the-Week

WRAP-UP

START WEIGHT:

END WEIGHT:

WEEKLY ENERGY LEVEL:
☐ low ☐ med ☐ high

WEEKLY CALORIES BURNED:

DAYS I TRACKED MY DIET:
☐ Monday ☐ Tuesday ☐ Wednesday ☐ Thursday ☐ Friday ☐ Saturday ☐ Sunday

HOW I FELT THIS WEEK:

_____
_____
_____
_____
_____
_____
_____
_____
_____

GOALS FOR NEXT WEEK:

_____
_____
_____
_____
_____
_____
_____
_____

NOTES/REMINDERS:

OTHER HEALTH & FITNESS BOOKS
BY ALEX A. LLUCH

THE COMPLETE CALORIE, FAT & CARB COUNTER

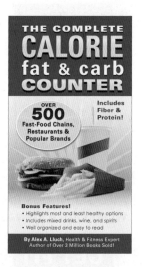

LOSE WEIGHT NOW! DIET JOURNAL & ORGANIZER

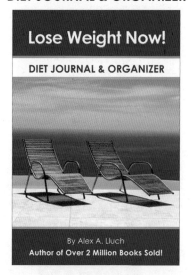

DAILY PLANNER DIET JOURNAL

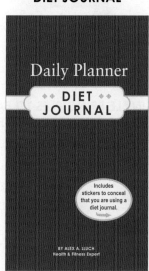

DAILY PLANNER WORKOUT JOURNAL

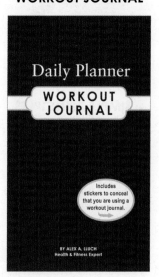

Visit www.WSPublishingGroup.com for more information.

OTHER HEALTH & FITNESS BOOKS
BY ALEX A. LLUCH

I WILL LOSE WEIGHT THIS TIME! DIET JOURNAL

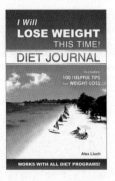

THE ULTIMATE POCKET DIET JOURNAL

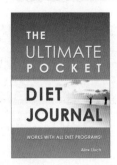

THE ULTIMATE POCKET WORKOUT JOURNAL

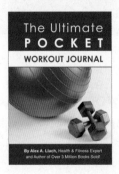

I WILL GET FIT THIS TIME! WORKOUT JOURNAL

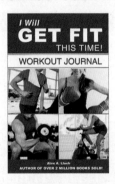

SIMPLE PRINCIPLES TO GET FIT

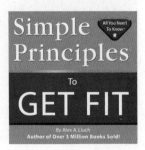

SIMPLE PRINCIPLES TO EAT SMART AND LOSE WEIGHT

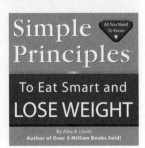